Pharmacological Foundations of Parkinson's Disease

Pharmacological Foundations of Parkinson's Disease

From Mechanisms to Clinical Practice

Edited by

Wael Mohamed

Clinical Pharmacology Department, Menoufia Medical School, Menoufia University, Egypt

Basic Medical science department, Kulliyyah of Medicine, International Islamic University Malaysia (IIUM), Malaysia

ELSEVIER

ACADEMIC PRESS

An imprint of Elsevier

Academic Press is an imprint of Elsevier
125 London Wall, London EC2Y 5AS, United Kingdom
50 Hampshire Street, 5th Floor, Cambridge, MA 02139, United States

ISBN: 978-0-443-27702-3

For information on all Academic Press publications visit our website at https://www.elsevier.com/books-and-journals

Publisher: Megan R. Ball
Acquisitions Editor: Simonetta Harrison,
Editorial Project Manager: Himanshi Yadav
Production Project Manager: Kaviya Karthik
Cover Designer: Gopalakrishnan Venkatraman

Typeset by TNQ Tech

Dedication

*To my beloved parents, **Mohamed** and **Nawal**.*
Your unwavering love, sacrifices, and endless encouragement
have been the foundation of every step I have taken.
Thank you for your tireless efforts, your patience, and your faith
in me—even when the path was uncertain.
This work is as much yours as it is mine, a reflection of the values
and strength you instilled in me.
*May **Allah SWT** forgive all your sins and shower you with*
His infinite blessings, mercy, and everlasting peace.

With deepest gratitude and love,

Wael Mohamed
Pahang
Malaysia

Contents

Contributors

Eman K. Abdelhadi
Faculty of Pharmacy, Clinical Pharmacy Department, Suez Canal University, Ismaïlia, Egypt

Ahmed Abdelkader
Faculty of Medicine, New Vision University, Tbilisi, Georgia

Sulhi Abidin
Department of Prosthodontics, Kulliyyah of Dentistry, International Islamic University of Malaysia, Kuantan, Pahang, Malaysia

Dina Essam Abo-elnour
Faculty of Medicine, Zagazig University, Zagazig, Egypt

Moaz Elsayed Abouelmagd
Kasr-Alainy Faculty of Medicine, Cairo University, Cairo, Egypt

Esther Abosede Adewumi
School of Science, Environment and Engineering, University of Salford, Manchester, United Kingdom

Basant Atef Ahmed
Faculty of Medicine, Tanta University, Tanta, Egypt

Yusuf Olalekan Ahmed
Department of Clinical Pharmacology and Therapeutics, Faculty of Basic Clinical Sciences, Federal University of Health Sciences Azare, Azare, Bauchi, Nigeria

Edre Mohamad Aidid
Department of Community Medicine, Kulliyyah of Medicine, International Islamic University of Malaysia, Kuantan, Pahang, Malaysia

Abayomi Oyeyemi Ajagbe
Department of Anatomy, Nile University of Nigeria, Abuja, Nigeria

Ebele Joan Ajagun
Bioresources Development Centre, National Biotechnology Research and Development Agency, Ogbomoso, Oyo, Nigeria

Nada Mostafa Al-dardery
Faculty of Medicine, Fayoum University, Fayoum, Egypt

Ahmed Tharwat Al-Namrouti
Faculty of Medicine, Galala University, New Galala City, Suez, Egypt

Gideon S. Alex
University of Port Harcourt, Rivers State, Nigeria

Hamza K. Alsalhi
The Hashemite University, Zarqa, Jordan

Sakhr Alshwayyat
Kern Medical (UCLA David Geffen School of Medicine Affiliate), Bakersfield, CA, United States; Applied Science Research Center, Applied Science Private University, Amman, Jordan; King Hussein Cancer Center, Amman, Jordan

Ganna Ameen
Biophysics Department, Faculty of Science, Cairo University, Cairo, Egypt

Muhammad Aminu
School of Public Health, Fujian Medical University, Fuzhou, Fujian, China

Abraham Olufemi Asuku
Bioresources Development Centre, National Biotechnology Research and Development Agency, Ogbomoso, Oyo, Nigeria

Darin W. Aswa
Faculty of Medicine, Galala University, New Galala City, Suez, Egypt

Hadeer N. Atalah
Institute of Global Health and Human Ecology, School of Science and Engineering, The American University in Cairo, Cairo, Egypt

Maha Awan
Sulaiman Al Rajhi University, Al Bukayriyah, Saudi Arabia

Mai Barakat
Institute of Global Health and Human Ecology, School of Science and Engineering, The American University in Cairo, Cairo, Egypt

Muhammad Danial Bin Che Ramli
Management and Science University, Department of Diagnostic and Allied Health Science, Faculty of Health and Life Sciences, Shah Alam, Malaysia

Ziad E. Farouk
Faculty of Medicine, Galala University, New Galala City, Suez, Egypt

Shaimaa El-Jaafary
Cairo University, Cairo, Egypt

Manar T. El-Morsy
Biotechnology Department, Faculty of Postgraduate Studies for Nanotechnology, Cairo University, Giza, Egypt

Esraa A. Elgayar
Faculty of Biotechnology, Nile University, Sheikh Zayed, Cairo, Egypt

Ahmed T. Elhendawy
Physics Department, Faculty of Science, Galala University, New Galala City, Suez, Egypt

Nada Fath
School of Basic Medical Sciences, Fujian Medical University, Fuzhou, China

Hairul Aini Hamzah
Department of Basic Medical Sciences, Kulliyyah of Medicine, International Islamic University of Malaysia, Kuantan, Pahang, Malaysia

Mahmoud Tarek Hefnawy
Faculty of Medicine, Zagazig University, Zagazig, Egypt

Mohamed Mohsen Helal
Faculty of Medicine, Zagazig University, Zagazig, Egypt

Ibilola Funsho Itiolu
Pharmacology and Therapeutics Department, Faculty of Basic Clinical Sciences University of Ilorin, Ilorin, Kwara State, Nigeria

Doaa S.R. Khafaga
Department of Basic Medical Sciences, Health Sector, Galala University, New Galala City, Suez, Egypt

Ismail Louragli
Higher Institute of Nursing and Health Techniques, Ministry of Health and Social Protection, Dakhla, Morocco

Amera M. Ghazi
Faculty of Science, Microbiology and Chemistry Department, Al-Azhar University, Cairo, Egypt

Tumelo Elina Mauta
Management and Science University, Department of Diagnostic and Allied Health Science, Faculty of Health and Life Sciences, Shah Alam, Malaysia

Yasser Mecheri
Department of Neurology, Dr Benbadis University Hospital, Constantine, Algeria; Department of Medicine, Salah Boubnider Constantine 3 University, Constantine, Algeria

Adejoke Elizabeth Memudu
Anatomy Department, Faculty of Basic Medical Sciences Edo State University, Iyamho, Edo State, Nigeria

Salma K. Mohamed
Faculty of Medicine, Galala University, New Galala City, Suez, Egypt

Wael Mohamed
Basic Medical Science Department, Kulliyyah of Medicine, International Islamic University Malaysia (IIUM), Kuantan, Pahang, Malaysia; Clinical Pharmacology Department, Menoufia Medical School, Menoufia University, Menoufia, Egypt

Kholoud Mohamed Ibrahim
Biophysics Department, Faculty of Science, Cairo University, Cairo, Egypt

Nur Sabrina Ameerah Mohd Nazri
Kulliyyah of Medicine, International Islamic Univeristy of Malaysia, Kuantan, Pahang, Malaysia

Yomna Mostafa
Biophysics Department, Faculty of Science, Cairo University, Cairo, Egypt

Ramli Musa
Department of Psychiatry, Kulliyyah of Medicine, International Islamic University of Malaysia, Kuantan, Pahang, Malaysia

Kenechukwu Emmanuel Nwanama
Sancta Maria Catholic College of Nursing Sciences, Uzairue, Edo State, Nigeria

Blaire Okunsai
School of Graduate Studies, Management and Science University, Shah Alam, Malaysia

Peace Ayo Olaoluwa
Department of Physiology, Faculty of Basic Medical Sciences, University of Ilorin, Ilorin, Kwara, Nigeria

Baliqis Adejoke Olukade
Department of Molecular Medicine, Morsani College of Medicine, University of South Florida, Tampa, FL, United States

Sara Omar
John D. Dingell VA Medical Center, Detroit, MI, United States; Wayne State University, Neurology Department, Detroit, MI, United States

Kenneth Chiedozie Oparaji
Department of Physiology, Faculty of Basic Medical Sciences, Alex Ekwueme Federal University Ndufu-Alike (AE-FUNAI), Abakaliki, Ebonyi State, Nigeria

Basant Osama
Biophysics Department, Faculty of Science, Cairo University, Cairo, Egypt

Tiago Fleming Outeiro
University Medical Center Göttingen, Department of Experimental Neurodegeneration, Göttingen, Germany; Faculdade de Medicina e Ciências Biomédicas, Algarve Biomedical Center Research Institute, Universidade do Algarve, Faro, Portugal

Mohammad Ammar Qaed
School of Health Management, Fujian Medical University, Fuzhou, Fujian, China

Esraa M. Qansuwa
Institute of Global Health and Human Ecology, School of Science and Engineering, The American University in Cairo, Cairo, Egypt; Universal Health Insurance Authority (UHIA), Presidency of the Council of Ministers, Cairo, Egypt

Esraa M. Sakr
Biophysics Department, Faculty of Science, Cairo University, Cairo, Egypt

Radwa N. Selim
Biotechnology Department, Faculty of Postgraduate Studies for Nanotechnology, Cairo University, Giza, Egypt

Mohd Shaiful Ehsan Shalihin
Department of Family Medicine, Kulliyyah of Medicine, International Islamic University of Malaysia, Kuantan, Pahang, Malaysia

Genevieve Simboh Anak Umbar
Management and Science University, Department of Diagnostic and Allied Health Science, Faculty of Health and Life Sciences, Shah Alam, Malaysia

Zakirah Zainal Abidin
School of Graduate Studies, Management and Science University, Shah Alam, Malaysia

Preface

> Acceptance doesn't mean resignation; it means understanding that something is what it is and that there's got to be a way through it.
>
> — **Michael J. Fox**

The quest to understand and alleviate movement disorders is as ancient as medicine itself. Long before James Parkinson formally described the "shaking palsy" in 1817, royal physicians in the court of Egyptian Pharaohs documented motor dysfunctions and "trembling disease" in medical scrolls like the *Ebers Papyrus* (c. 1550 BCE). In their pursuit to restore control over rigid limbs, these early healers administered plant remedies rich in tropane alkaloids—unknowingly delivering the earliest anticholinergic therapies millennia before the birth of modern neurochemistry.

As science advanced from botanical remedies to cellular networks, pioneers like Santiago Ramón y Cajal revolutionized neuroscience by demonstrating that signals flow **unidirectionally** across neuronal synapses. This understanding of directional signaling unlocked the secrets of the basal ganglia, revealing how the selective degeneration of dopaminergic neurons in the substantia nigra leads to the complex motor and cognitive hallmarks of Parkinson's disease. Today, managing this condition demands a far more sophisticated, multi-targeted pharmacological strategy.

Pharmacological Foundations of Parkinson's Disease: From Mechanisms to Clinical Practice bridges the gap between laboratory benchwork and real-world clinical care. **Section I: Foundations and Pharmacological Principles** establishes the biological core, featuring novel zebrafish disease models, molecular pathogenesis, environmental neurotoxins, circadian rhythm disruptions, and the emerging influence of the oral bacteriome on cognitive decline. It integrates these mechanisms with pharmacokinetics, pharmacodynamics, and cross-cultural considerations for a holistic understanding of drug behavior.

Section II: Established Pharmacotherapies and Future Horizons translates foundational science into clinical action. It examines core dopaminergic strategies, COMT inhibitors, non-dopaminergic pathways, motor and non-motor management, and practical clinical case studies. Looking ahead, it highlights emergent therapeutic agents and next-generation biological interventions.

We stand on the threshold of a revolution in neurotherapeutics. As precision neuropharmacology, targeted gene therapies, and regenerative medicine converge, our horizon shifts from merely slowing neurodegeneration to halting and actively repairing it. This volume is dedicated to empowering the clinicians, pharmacologists, and researchers shaping that future—paving the path toward a world where Parkinson's disease is no longer a lifelong sentence of management, but a fully curable chapter in medical history.

Editor:
Wael Mohamed
Pahang
Malaysia

Acknowledgments

The editor extends sincere gratitude to all contributors whose dedication, expertise, and scholarly commitment have made this volume possible. Each chapter represents a collective effort to advance our understanding of Parkinson's disease and to bridge the gap between molecular science and clinical practice.

Special appreciation is given to the institutions, research groups, and collaborators whose continuous support and encouragement fostered this academic endeavor. In particular, heartfelt thanks are due to members of the **AfrAbia Parkinson's Disease Genomic Consortium (AA-PD-GC)**, whose shared vision and collaborative spirit continue to promote scientific excellence and inclusivity across regions.

The editor also acknowledges the invaluable contributions of patients and their families, whose resilience, hope, and courage in the face of Parkinson's disease remain the truest sources of inspiration behind this work.

With profound personal gratitude, the editor dedicates this achievement to his parents, **Mohamed** and **Nawal**, for their lifelong sacrifices, wisdom, and unwavering prayers. May **Allah SWT** forgive all their sins and shower them with His blessings, mercy, and eternal peace.

Wael Mohamed
Pahang
Malaysia

SECTION

I

Foundations and pharmacological principles

CHAPTER

Zebrafish models provide insight into the biological classification of Parkinson's disease

1

Wael Mohamed[1, 2] and Tiago Fleming Outeiro[3, 4]

[1]*Basic Medical Science Department, Kulliyyah of Medicine, International Islamic University Malaysia (IIUM), Kuantan, Pahang, Malaysia;* [2]*Clinical Pharmacology Department, Menoufia Medical School, Menoufia University, Menoufia, Egypt;* [3]*University Medical Center Göttingen, Department of Experimental Neurodegeneration, Göttingen, Germany;* [4]*Faculdade de Medicina e Ciências Biomédicas, Algarve Biomedical Center Research Institute, Universidade do Algarve, Faro, Portugal*

1.1 Introduction

Our understanding of Parkinson's disease (PD) has significantly increased since James Parkinson first described as a 'Shaking palsy', over 200 years ago, simply based on his clinical observations (Parkinson, 2002). Although PD was initially classified as a movement/motor disorder, it is now widely recognised that the clinical presentations extend far beyond the characteristic motor symptoms, which remain the primary prerequisite for the clinical diagnosis (Postuma et al., 2015).

Advances in neuropathology and the identification of genetic factors have greatly influenced our understanding of the biological mechanisms involved and enabled us to explore the molecular underpinnings of the illness. However, despite tremendous advancements in the field, many concepts are still overlooked and propagated, leading to misconceptions and the use of terminology that does not distinguish between different types of PD. Importantly, we now have access to a wealth of information that can be used to better define PD. Therefore, we should ask difficult but important questions, such as: ***Should motor symptoms continue to be the basis for diagnosis? What distinguishes various forms of parkinsonism from PD? Should we continue to use the term "idiopathic" to describe PD forms that have recognised genetic roots? How can we reinterpret and classify PD by combining clinical features with biological concepts?***

The current description of PD states that nigral degeneration and axonal retraction of dopamine-producing neurones are the ultimate result of the convergence of several biological processes (Halliday et al., 1990; Jellinger, 1987; Mann & Yates, 1983) (Fig. 1.1). Although nigral degeneration is not the sole feature that sets PD apart, it provides the basis for the efficacy of dopamine replacement therapy in these patients (Tolosa et al., 2006). This has greatly influenced the "nigrocentric" concept of PD, since it is so amazing and rare for a neurodegenerative illness that dopaminergic medications may reduce symptoms (even if temporarily) for many of the disease's motor components.

Pharmacological Foundations of Parkinson's Disease. https://doi.org/10.1016/B978-0-443-27702-3.00032-7

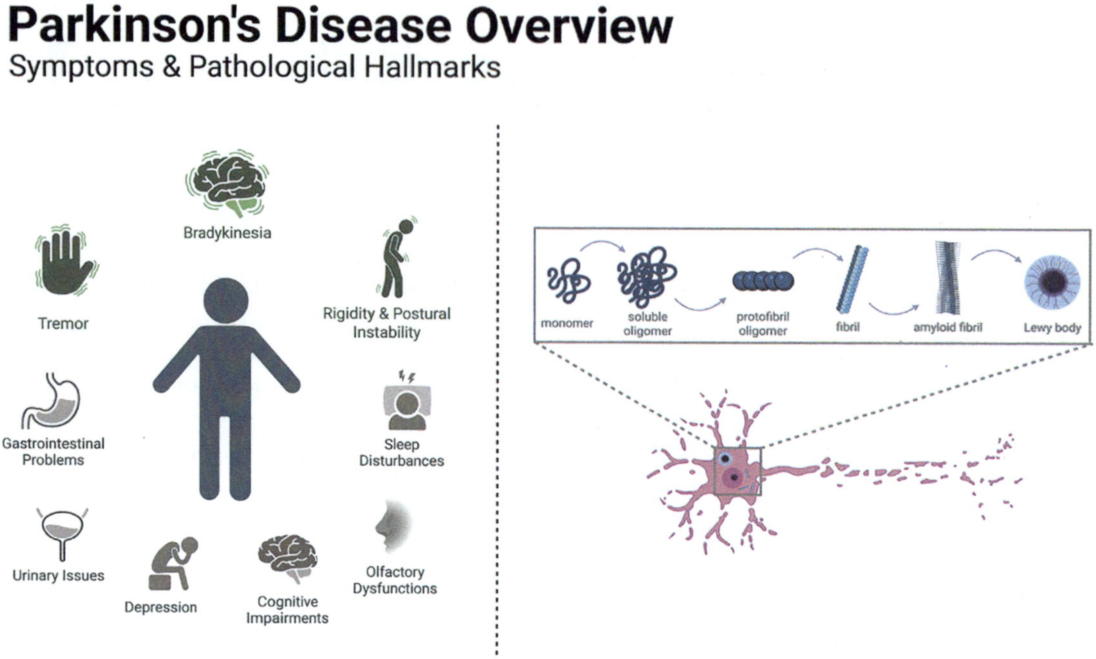

FIGURE 1.1 Clinical Definition of PD.

A. Clinical characterization of PD as a progressive neurodegenerative disorder primarily affecting the dopaminergic neurons in the substantia nigra. The diagnosis is based on core motor features—particularly bradykinesia, in combination with either resting tremor or rigidity—and a positive response to dopaminergic therapy. PD is also recognized by its progressive nature and the eventual emergence of non-motor symptoms.

According to clinical criteria (e.g., the UK Brain Bank Criteria) (Hughes et al., 1992), the majority of patients' brains will have Lewy body (LB) pathology even in rare, Mendelian forms of the disease. They may also exhibit more varied disease phenotypes (von Coelln & Shulman, 2016). Although symptoms may be more variable, most patients' brains will contain LBs, even in situations of uncommon, Mendelian variations of the condition (von Coelln & Shulman, 2016). Here, we provide a range of operational definitions of PD based on many perspectives in order to draw attention to the complexity of the issue and promote a scientific discussion that ought to produce a single, comprehensive explanation of the condition.

1.2 Redefining PD: A biological perspective

The current definition of PD has enabled it to be a diverse neurologic condition with a broad range of clinical symptoms and progressions in both clinical practice and research. Other often used terms for the clinical entity PD include juvenile-onset PD, which refers to patients whose start happens before the age of 21, and young-onset PD/early-onset PD (EOPD), which refers to patients whose onset occurs between the ages of 21 and 50 (Mehanna et al., 2022; Schrag et al., 1998). When we look at the pathophysiological basis for this classification, we find that the suggested cut off age to differentiate between juvenile- and early-onset parkinsonism is based on a higher risk of familial parkinsonism in patients with onset before 21 years of age and the lack of known hereditary factors identified over 21 years of age (Schrag et al., 1998). Although these terms were originally used in 1987, the first gene mutation associated with PD was not identified until 1997 (Polymeropoulos et al., 1997). Some have called the sickness "EOPD," and the cut-off ages are between 40 and 60 (Mehanna et al., 2022; Muthane et al., 1994). Since EOPD is a topic that requires more research, the MDS actually established a work force to address this problem and define it appropriately (Mehanna et al., 2022; Vollstedt et al., 2023).

Even though "parkinsonism" is a commonly used word, no accepted definition exists. It often refers to a clinical condition that includes bradykinesia along with two or three characteristics: postural instability, muscle stiffness, and/or resting tremor that occurs between four and 6 Hz (Hughes et al., 1992). The most prevalent neurological cause of parkinsonism is PD. "Atypical parkinsonism" is a colloquial word for several neurodegenerative diseases linked to parkinsonism, such as multiple system atrophy [type P], progressive supranuclear palsy [PSP], and corticobasal degeneration. Compared to the majority of individuals with typical PD, they usually have a poorer prognosis (i.e., a shorter life span), react less effectively to dopaminergic therapies, and have less dyskinesia after chronic levodopa medication (Lees, 2009). A variety of vascular, drug-related, viral, toxic, structural, or other factors that result in "secondary parkinsonism" may also produce the motor syndrome.

The term prodromal refers to a phase when early signs or symptoms of neurodegeneration are present but do not yet permit a clinical diagnosis based on motor parkinsonism. Anticipating that a more precise diagnosis and categorization of the "premotor" and early stages of PD would be necessary for the clinical development of disease-modifying medicines, the MDS formed a task force to produce research criteria for prodromal PD. These criteria provided a new way to assess an individual's risk of prodromal PD based on the likelihood that prodromal sickness would appear. These include motor and non-motor clinical complaints, auxiliary diagnostic tests, and clinical markers (Berg et al., 2015; Heinzel et al., 2019). According to these criteria, the following conditions are considered high-risk indicators for prodromal PD: hyper-echogenicity of the substantia nigra; probable rapid eye movement sleep behavior disorder (RBD) as indicated by a polysomnogram; abnormal dopaminergic positron emission tomography/single-photon emission computed tomography (PET/SPECT) (i.e., the presence of one clinical sign, such as bradykinesia); olfactory loss (Berg et al., 2015; Heinzel et al., 2019). The formal inclusion of substantia nigra hyperechogenicity and dopamine transporter (DAT) scan as risk indicators for PD created the first association between clinical criteria and a potential physiopathological marker. The proposed criteria have a good specificity in detecting prodromal PD, according to recent data, mainly because RBD is a nonmotor symptom with a high specificity. But only at later, unknown times would the discovered individuals fulfill the clinical criteria for PD (Mirelman et al., 2018; Pilotto et al., 2017). Nevertheless, we think that by adding nonmotor problems to the list of "cardinal signs," the concept of prodromal PD will evolve in the future and enable the identification of PD prior to the onset of the distinctive motor symptoms.

The most prevalent clinical features and data-driven research have prompted the creation of many PD subtype classifications. There is ongoing discussion on the most appropriate classification for PD subtypes in clinical practice and research, as well as the one that best reflects the many paths taken by the physiopathological processes of the illness. Based on the most prevalent motor symptoms at an early stage, the original hypothesis distinguished between the tremor-dominant and akinetic-rigid dominant clinical categories (Jankovic et al., 1990). A distinct subgroup was then proposed, called postural instability gait disorders [PIGD], which showed relevant axial symptoms such postural instability and abnormalities in gait. Other features of the PIGD subtype include higher cognitive progress, more frequent hallucinations, psychosis, and more severe sickness symptoms upon diagnosis (Van Der Heeden et al., 2016). A Montreal prospective cohort study distinguished three subtypes: motor/slow progression, diffuse/malignant, and intermediate. At baseline, individuals with the diffuse/malignant phenotype were more likely to have RBD, orthostatic hypotension, and mild cognitive impairment. According to(Fereshtehnejad et al., 2015), they had more severe motor symptoms and signs, more nonmotor symptoms, worse global composite outcomes, and a quicker pace of cognitive decline at follow-up. Using data from the Parkinson's Progression Markers Initiative (PPMI), another study (Fereshtehnejad et al., 2017). classified people as having a "mild motor-predominant," "diffuse malignant," or "intermediate" kind. The main classifiers in a hierarchical cluster analysis were a motor summary score and three nonmotor traits: dysautonomia, RBD, and cognitive impairment. Patients with the diffuse malignant subtype have a faster overall prognosis and a greater decline in cognition and dopamine functional neuroimaging after an average of 2.7 years. Individuals with diffuse malignant PD also had the highest brain network atrophy and the lowest levels of amyloid-β and amyloid-β/total tau ratio (AD-like CSF profile). In another study that employed PPMI data, the motor assessment items identified five distinct motor subtypes: tremor dominant, axial dominant, appendicular dominant, stiffness dominant, and postural and instability gait disorder dominant (Eisinger et al., 2017). Notably, a study that looked at all published research on data-driven PD subtype classification failed to demonstrate consistency in the Longitudinal and Biomarker Study in PD systems, a cohort intended for clinical studies. These results raise questions about the validity and generalizability of these data-driven approaches for classifying PD subtypes (Mestre et al., 2018). Using a semi-mechanistic model of PD that is focused on the development of functional impairment rather than particular clinical scales would be an alternative strategy. In addition to identifying different techniques to treat the underlying disease, this would reveal each cohort's unique pathogenetic and genetic fingerprints.

The principal morphological correlate of clinical Parkinson's syndrome is the substantial dysfunction or depletion of nigral dopaminergic neurones projecting to the basal ganglia, as shown in normal-pressure hydrocephalus or neuroleptic exposure. The dorsal and medial neurones exhibit more resilience, while the ventrolateral neurones have increased susceptibility (Dickson et al., 2009). While LB pathology (LBP) is associated with neuronal loss in PD, loss of nigral neurones with parkinsonism may manifest in several other conditions (Dickson, 2018). The spectrum of Lewy Body disease (LBD), which includes dementia with Lewy Bodies (DLB) and PD dementia (PDD), covers PD. All of these illnesses exhibit a neuropathological feature termed LBP, characterized by the presence of α-synuclein (αSyn) aggregates in neuronal cell bodies and processes, referred to as Lewy neurites and LBs, respectively. The Braak stages for the evolution of LBP in PD are delineated by(Braak et al., 2003). LBP first presents in the anterior olfactory nucleus (olfactory bulb) and the dorsal motor nucleus of the vagus nerve (medulla oblongata). It then disseminates to the locus coeruleus (pons) and substantia nigra, resulting in considerable cellular degeneration and parkinsonism. LBP may progress to clinical dementia in advanced stages and include limbic and neocortical areas. Recent research indicates that aSyn aggregates may be present in several peripheral organs at the time of diagnosis, challenging the spreading hypothesis first presented by Braak for PD (Vacchi et al., 2021; Zheng et al., 2022). The distinction between DLB and PDD is predicated on clinical observations: in DLB, cognitive decline manifests prior to, concurrently with, or within 1 year of the onset of parkinsonism, suggesting that the Braak stages for the advancement of LBP are inapplicable to DLB, where significant LBP may initially emerge in limbic and neocortical regions. In PDD, parkinsonism must begin at least 1 year prior to the onset of dementia (Attems et al., 2021). The investigation of individuals with PD and PD dementia (PDD), excluding those with dementia with Lewy bodies (DLB), fundamentally informed the idea of the Braak phases. The predominant etiologies of parkinsonism, accounting for almost 50%, are Dementia with Lewy Bodies and PD (Dickson, 2018). Syn aggregates mostly appear as glial inclusions (Papp Lantos bodies) in many parkinsonian illnesses, including multiple system atrophy (MSA). TAR DNA-binding protein (TDP)-43 proteinopathies, such as frontotemporal lobar degeneration TDP and Perry syndrome, along with tauopathies, including progressive supranuclear palsy, corticobasal degeneration, Guam Parkinson's dementia complex, and chronic traumatic encephalopathy, often exhibit synaptic inclusions. Additionally, many genetic illnesses associated with mutations in *PINK1*, *PRKN*, *POLG*, and specific variants of *LRRK2* manifest parkinsonism and degeneration of nigral neuronal cells in the absence of certain protein accumulations. As previously stated, nondegenerative causes such as vascular (vascular parkinsonism), toxic (manganese poisoning), drug-induced (antipsychotic medications), and viral (post-encephalitic parkinsonism or SARS-CoV-2) may also result in parkinsonism (Lippi et al., 2020; Jellinger, 2019). Although LBP is the principal pathology of LBD, other age-related neuropathological changes may also manifest, with their prevalence in LBD increasing as individuals age, aligning with findings in the broader population (Spires-Jones et al., 2017; Attems, 2017; Walker et al., 2019). Consistent with expectations, the characteristic pathologies of Alzheimer's disease (AD), namely hyperphosphorylated tau (e.g., neurofibrillary tangles) and amyloid-β (e.g., amyloid plaques), are prevalent in LBD, with over 20% displaying limbic-predominant age-related TDP-43 encephalopathy and up to 50% demonstrating significant additional AD pathology (Irwin et al., 2017; McAleese et al., 2021; Nelson et al., 2019). Although more prevalent and severe in DLB than in PD/PDD, these diseases influence clinical symptoms and biomarker profiles, alongside cerebrovascular illness, providing a neuropathological rationale for the heterogeneity of the PD phenotype (Walker et al., 2019). The term PD may sometimes be used to denote parkinsonism broadly, irrespective of the underlying pathology (e.g., "genetic PD"). While parkinsonism may stem from several sources and associated disorders, the present neuropathological diagnosis of PD is characterized by nigral neuronal loss and Lewy body pathology (LBP).

The Biological Definition of PD refers to the work group created by the International Parkinson and Movement Disorder Society (MDS). The primary objectives of this task force were to: (1) delineate typical PD clinically through a more precise definition of motor and nonmotor symptoms; (2) differentiate between complex and monogenic forms of PD utilizing genomic sequence-based elements; (3) revise the neuropathological hallmark criteria for various variants that fulfill the clinical diagnosis of PD; and (4) aggregate the essential characteristics of PD variants to inform the development of practical laboratory models.

Genome-wide association studies (GWAS) have found around 100 genetic loci associated with the susceptibility to PD (Nalls et al., 2019). Despite the presence of these differences in the population, their impact is negligible (odds ratios typically range from 1.05 to 1.3). Algorithms that include several risk variants in a calculated polygenic risk score (PRS) may be very informative, even if each variable individually contributes only little to the risk of PD. PRS has so far been associated with the age of onset, rate of progression (in motor function and cognition), and the risk of PD (Ibanez et al., 2017;

Paul et al., 2018). Furthermore, PRS is associated with disease status, or penetrance, in *LRRK2*(Lai, Alipanahi, et al., 2021; Lai, Kim, et al., 2021) and the expressivity of Gaucher disease, which is caused by biallelic variations at the *GBA1* locus, even in the presence of high-effect-size variants (also referred to as Mendelian forms of PD) (Blauwendraat et al., 2023). In contrast, objective genome-wide studies of rare, large families with several clinically confirmed PD patients have revealed multiple genes whose alterations may lead to monogenic (Mendelian) variations of the disorder (see to Puschmann, 2017). Although these forms are often rare, their discovery has resulted in new and substantial insights into the molecular processes and mechanisms associated with the neurodegenerative process. Moreover, they have impacted and invigorated contemporary biological research, perhaps leading to novel targets for disease modification (Sardi & Simuni, 2019). This variance produces clinical presentations distinct from those seen in "classical PD," such as atypical parkinsonism resembling PSP, frontotemporal dementia (FTD), or a dementing illness akin to LBD (Bougea et al., 2017; Wider et al., 2010). Mutations in the *SNCA* gene, which encodes αSyn, are characteristic of hereditary PD. Point mutations (including A30P, E46K, G51D, and A53 T/E) and gene multiplexations (duplications or triplications) exemplify these autosomal dominant variants. Due to the infrequency of other point mutations, obtaining a comprehensive understanding of their phenotypic spectrum is challenging, save for the *p.A53T* mutation, which is prevalent among individuals of Greek descent. Despite reports of cases exhibiting DLB-like or FTD-like presentations, individuals with the *p.A53T* mutation often have a distinctive motor beginning of PD (Papadimitriou et al., 2016; Morfis & Cordato, 2006). This kind often presents more severely than idiopathic PD (iPD) due to an earlier onset, accelerated progression, and pronounced nonmotor features associated with neuropsychiatric illnesses, dysautonomia, and dementia (Koros et al., 2018). Although instances of duplication have a more diverse presentation and development, cases of *SNCA* triplication are likewise rather severe, maybe even more so than *p.A53T* patients (Gwinn et al., 2011). From a neuropathological perspective, hereditary *SNCA* patients exhibit similarities to prevalent synucleinopathies, although they may also present with oligodendroglial αSyn deposition, heightened tau pathology, and significant neuronal involvement. With a few significant exceptions, these instances do not provide a conceptual problem when seen in the largest context. They are regarded as quintessential synucleinopathies from both clinical and neuropathological perspectives, offering a substantial area of research to understand how PD arises from a hereditary mutation in the *SNCA* gene. The predominant cause of a monogenic type of clinically typical PD is mutations in *LRRK2*. It is conceivable that a smaller proportion of asymptomatic carriers exhibit symptoms than previously assumed (Simuni et al., 2022). Notably, LBs are absent in a substantial number of postmortem patients with *LRRK2* mutations, a finding corroborated in people with several pathogenic variants in this gene (Hasegawa et al., 2009). A subset of these *LRRK2* patients exhibits tau-positive disease (Henderson et al., 2019). Some have no distinctive protein aggregation and only demonstrate neuronal death in the substantia nigra (Takanashi et al., 2018; Vilas et al., 2019). This extensive pleomorphism unequivocally undermines the current pathogenic diagnosis of PD. Utilizing *LRRK2* as a model for idiopathic PD suggests that Lewy bodies are not an essential pathogenic characteristic nor a consistent feature associated with cellular demise, and it also indicates that some people with late-onset PD may lack Lewy body pathology. Third, LBs are increasingly identified in several monogenic neurodegenerative disorders that are clinically differentiated from the established criteria of PD. These include juvenile-onset, quickly progressing parkinsonism, dystonic parkinsonism, or parkinsonism-related dementia. Significant brain iron accumulation is sometimes associated with these conditions, as observed in individuals with PLA2G6-associated neurodegeneration

(Paisan-Ruiz et al., 2012), mitochondrial membrane protein-associated neurodegeneration (attributable to *c9orf12* mutations), *RAB39B* mutations (Gao et al., 2020), and *VPS13C* mutations (Lesage et al., 2016). Several variations in the glucocerebrosidase (*GBA1*) gene (Do et al., 2019) and one in *LRRK2* (*G2019S*) (Kluss et al., 2019) appear to be conceptually distinct, serving as significant genetic determinants of disease that demonstrate intermediate frequency and effect size, situated between common small-effect risk variants identified in GWAS and classical rare, highly penetrant Mendelian variants. Approximately 30%–40% of typical iPD patients from certain ethnic groups, including Ashkenazi Jews and North African Berbers, possess the *LRRK2-G2019S* mutation, which may present in both familial and sporadic forms (Correia et al., 2010, 2017). Diverse motor features and lower back pain are also seen in other monogenic forms of PD, indicating a complex underlying biology. We should consider the potential that PD and some cases presenting as separate neurodegenerative disorders, such as dementia with Lewy bodies or progressive supranuclear palsy, may really have a common biological basis if the extensive clinical variability associated with monogenic forms applies to the disease in its entirety. Understanding this might enhance the precision of our treatment for the PD.

1.3 The contribution of model organisms toward PD conceptualization

The four phases of PD progression are: (1) the prodromal phase; (2) the newly introduced risk phase; (3) the pre-clinical phase; and (4) the clinical (post-diagnosis) phase (Dommershuijsen et al., 2021; Mantri et al., 2019). The stage preceding the prodromal phase of PD, known as the "newly introduced risk phase," is when people are asymptomatic but have observable biological, environmental, or genetic risk factors—like *GBA1* or *LRRK2* mutations, family history, or particular exposures—that raise their chance of getting the disease. This stage differs from the prodromal stage, which comes before the clinical stage characterized by motor manifestations and is when early non-motor symptoms (such as constipation, hyposmia, and REM sleep behavior disorder) start to appear. Understanding the risk phase highlights chances for early intervention and prevention before serious neurodegeneration takes place. The clinical phase has garnered the greatest focus among these phases, both in laboratory models and in human subjects. A significant limitation of focusing on the clinical stage is that the detected molecular abnormalities likely reflect the disease's consequences rather than its initial pathogenic origins. Therefore, these findings may not comprehensively reflect the first biological pathways associated with the start of disease. The last three stages include the pre-diagnostic phases of PD, which are crucial for understanding disease progression and for identifying potential preventive or disease-modifying interventions. The limited availability of brain tissue from presymptomatic periods and the non-specificity of prodromal symptoms hinder the acquisition of human-based evidence about the molecular mechanisms involved in the early stages of PD progression. Consequently, the resolution to this problem resides in research models that emulate this historical epoch. Cell lines and non-human primates (NHPs) exemplify the many complexities of research models used to study PD. These models include the administration of proteins or toxins that elicit various PD-like symptoms. Numerous reviews delineate the methodologies employed to simulate the disease, encompassing the following subjects: the animal model (Pingale & Gupta, 2020), the route of administration (Innos & Hickey, 2021; Zeng et al., 2018; Johnson & Bobrovskaya, 2015), the dosages of the inducing agent, the timing of motor sign development and dopamine loss (Meredith et al., 2008), non-motor characteristics, and the influence of the animal's age on the resultant phenotype (Klaestrup et al., 2022). The accessibility of pre-clinical phases, when research is already available, will be of special significance. The objective is to critically assess if the actual modeling of PD endeavors to explore the sequence of events that lead to the progression of the illness. Developing preventive and disease-modifying strategies requires this. An effective animal model of PD must include αSyn, motor deficits, the formation of LBs, and/or the loss of dopamine/dihydroxyphenylalanine, in accordance with clinical and pathological features. In vitro and in vivo investigations of PD models often concentrate on three primary pathogenic mechanisms: protein misfolding, inflammation, and redox dysfunction. The primary aim of this chapter is to establish a novel framework for identifying (1) the pathogenetic cause, (2) biomarkers of disease state, (3) markers of disease progression, (4) therapeutic intervention targets tailored to each patient's distinct disease mechanisms, and (5) strategies for redefining PD based on molecular insights obtained using the zebrafish (ZF) model.

1.3.1 Limitations of traditional models in PD research

Animal and cellular models are very useful for deciphering the molecular mechanisms associated with many different diseases. In fact, preclinical research using animals and cells is often required prior to the initiation of clinical trials, since models are crucial for identifying and assessing pathophysiological pathways that cannot be studied in humans (Fig. 1.2) (Bras et al., 2020; Marvian et al., 2019). However, modeling a condition like PD has proven hard due to the aforementioned considerations, since it is not always clear which characteristics of the illness should be represented (Marvian et al., 2019). Since the 1960s, conventional animal models of PD have relied on the localized or systemic application of toxins that obliterate nigrostriatal dopaminergic neurones. 6-hydroxydopamine, 1-methyl-4-phenyl-1,2,3,6-tetrahydropyridine, and, to a lesser extent, rotenone and paraquat are the most often used toxins. The advancement and assessment of treatments for the main motor deficits of PD have been enhanced by the use of these toxin-based models. Consequently, these models have facilitated the development of deep brain stimulation and dopamine agonists. They also provide valuable information for developing therapeutics for levodopa-induced dyskinesia. Nevertheless, since these models are improbable to emulate the pathophysiological foundations of the disease, they have failed to forecast the clinical efficacy of neuroprotective treatments.

The difficulties in characterizing PD clearly indicate that there is no "ideal" framework for this complex disease. An effective model must, at a minimum, be based on a mechanism shown in human studies to be relevant to specific illness symptoms. Uncommon genetic variants have elucidated processes that enhance our understanding of sporadic PD. Consequently, genetic models are crucial for assessing hypotheses and neuroprotective treatments. Identifying the elements or characteristics of PD necessary for a model to qualify as an accurate picture of the condition remains difficult. A diverse array of animal models is essential for investigating specific aspects of the condition. Mammalian models, including mice, rats, and rarely nonhuman primates, are crucial for replicating circuit-level alterations, although versatile model species like as the invertebrates *Caenorhabditis elegans* and Drosophila are valuable for elucidating genetic relationships and processes. In conclusion, instead than seeking an elusive animal model that replicates every phenotypic characteristic of PD, the optimal model is the one that most effectively addresses the specific research question. An effective model should reproduce disease-relevant processes and align with the intended treatment goal, but these features may not be universally present across all persons or disease types. Consequently, the current issue is to provide a direct and disease-specific drug that aligns with the intended pharmacological

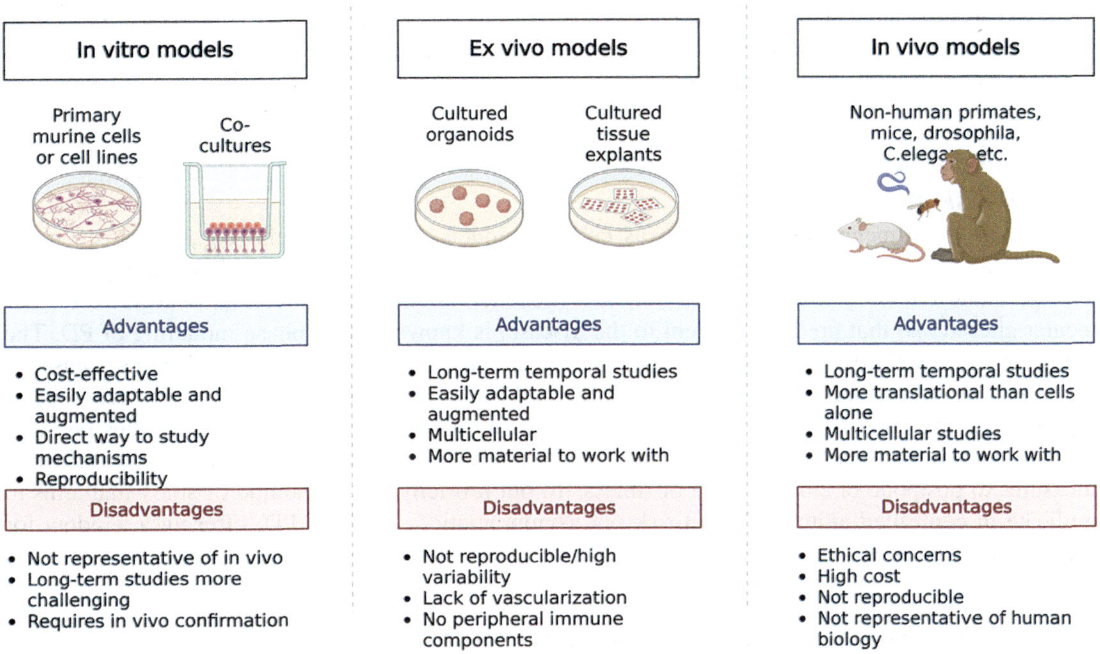

FIGURE 1.2 Preclinical models of neurodegenerative diseases.

This figure provides an overview of the main experimental models used to study neurodegenerative diseases, including PD and Alzheimer's disease. In vivo models involve the use of whole organisms—commonly rodents, ZF, and Drosophila—to replicate disease pathology and assess behavioral, molecular, and pharmacological responses in a physiologically relevant environment. Ex vivo models utilize isolated tissues (e.g., brain slices or organotypic cultures) that preserve native cellular architecture, allowing for real-time studies of synaptic activity, neurodegeneration, and drug effects. In vitro models involve cultured neuronal or glial cells (primary cells, immortalized lines, or stem cell-derived neurons), enabling high-throughput analysis of cellular mechanisms, genetic manipulation, and compound screening under controlled conditions. Together, these complementary models offer valuable platforms for understanding disease mechanisms and evaluating potential therapeutic strategies.

target. Thus, the current problem of delineating PD in a clear and universal manner underscores the need for several models and the rigorous evaluation of the primary pathologies and phenotypes within each model. What specific characteristics or parts of the PD does it replicate? What is the reliability and significance of the endpoints? To what extent are the findings from this particular model relevant to other forms of PD? Basic and translational scientists must discern the suitability of a certain model for investigating particular aspects of this complex ailment, analogous to a physician's ability to recognize PD amongst many clinical manifestations and putative etiologies. Subsequently, any genetically relevant models for PD must be regarded as beneficial for elucidating the processes underlying both central and peripheral symptoms and pathologies. Cell models of autosomal dominant variations of genetic PD, which rely on the synthesis of wild-type or mutant protein forms, are invaluable for assessing specific biochemical alterations (Agin-Liebes et al., 2020). Cell-based models are essential for continuous and comprehensive study into the molecular pathways that underlie the pathophysiology of PD.

1.3.2 Modeling of various PD phases

1.3.2.1 Risk phase modeling

The use of experimental systems, such as cellular models, animal models (e.g., zebrafish, mice, Drosophila), or computer simulations, to replicate and study the earliest stage of PD, when people are asymptomatic but carry identifiable risk factors (genetic variants, environmental exposures, or molecular alterations) that predispose them to the disease, is known as risk phase modeling of PD. The objectives of modeling the risk phase are to: 1)Simulate preclinical susceptibility prior to the onset of prodromal or motor signs., 2) Recognize early cellular and molecular abnormalities (e.g., αSyn biology, synaptic modifications, mitochondrial malfunction)., 3) Examine the relationships between genes and the environment that lead to heightened sensitivity, and 4)Create and evaluate preventative measures to postpone or stop the start of illness. To put it briefly, it is a method of study that aims to replicate in controlled animals the "at-risk but asymptomatic" period of PD, offering a window for early identification and treatment prior to irreversible neurodegeneration (Table 1.1).

Table 1.1 Comparative overview: Modeling of various PD phases.

PD phase	Key features	Modeling approaches	Applications/Insights
1. **Risk phase modeling**	Genetic susceptibility, environmental exposures, pre-pathological state	- Transgenic zebrafish/ Drosophila with PD-risk genes (e.g., *LRRK2*, *SNCA*, *PINK1*, *GBA*) - CRISPR-based editing - exposure to pesticides (e.g., rotenone)	Understanding gene-environment interactions; screening early biomarkers
2. **Prodromal phase modeling**	Non-motor symptoms (e.g., sleep disturbance, GI issues, hyposmia)	- αSyn aggregation in enteric nervous system or olfactory bulb - ZF gut-brain axis models - behavioral analysis for sleep/cognition	Exploring early pathogenesis; targeting early intervention and diagnosis
3. **Initial clinical PD**	Onset of motor symptoms; partial nigrostriatal degeneration	- MPTP/6-OHDA-induced dopaminergic cell loss - genetic + toxin hybrid models in ZF and Drosophila - Quantitative locomotion assays	Testing neuroprotective strategies; validation of clinical diagnostic criteria
4. **Advanced PD**	Widespread neurodegeneration, motor and non-motor complications	- Chronic MPTP exposure - high-dose αSyn overexpression - models with cumulative oxidative stress/ inflammation	Assessing long-term disease progression; studying complications; evaluating disease-modifying therapies

Tests using intragastric rotenone have demonstrated encouraging results for the Braak hypothesis, which states that PD synucleinopathy starts in the gastrointestinal tract and moves to the brain via the vagus nerve, where it spreads like a prion (Braak & Braak, 2000; Rietdijk et al., 2017; Visanji et al., 2013). Olfactory impairment is a well-known PD symptom that affects 90%–96% of people with the illness (Doty, 2012). Because there are no suitable models, post mortem samples from PD patients are the only ones accessible for the study of olfactory pathology. However, during the prediagnostic and prodromal phases of PD, organotypic olfactory bulb cultures experience monoamine-induced DA depletion. The main reasons of this include oxidative stress, mitochondrial dysfunction, and transcriptional alterations (Bagnoli et al., 2023). The alterations include the overexpression of the amyloid-beta precursor protein (APP), the hyperexpression of BDNF, and the dysregulation of PARK genes, such as PINK1 and DJ-1/PARK7, which are crucial for mitochondrial function and the regulation of oxidative stress (Bango(Li et al., 2023). PD has a number of genetic models, many of which cannot reproduce all of the classic clinical symptoms (Breger & Fuzzati Armentero, 2019; Dawson et al., 2010). This supports the idea that only a tiny portion of PD cases are purely genetic in origin. In short, mutations in DJ1/PARK7, a part of the antioxidant defense system, cause a moderate PD phenotype without DA loss (Meredith et al., 2008). One of the main molecular markers of PD, mitochondrial dysfunction, is solely responsible for the behavioral deficits in the DJ1 genetic model in ZF (Razali et al., 2021; Sallinen et al., 2010). In line with DJ1's function in redox-mediated disease processes, rodents with DJ1 KO challenged with 6-OHDA had lower performance in behavioral tests, higher DA depletion, and loss of TH + neurones compared to WT mice treated with 6-OHDA (Lev et al., 2013). These findings support the hypothesis that this mutation is a risk factor for redox stress (Xia et al., 2022), which occurs often in a variety of neurodegenerative diseases due to interactions between genes and environment. Since they are a component of the PINK1–PARKIN protein complex, which is required for the removal of damaged mitochondria, their failure leads to a secondary lack of autophagy and accumulation of αSyn (Xia et al., 2022). According to Mata et al. (2004), PARKIN, an E3 ubiquitin ligase, particularly brings about proteasomal dysfunctions and the accumulation of parkin substrates, such as cyclin E, synphilin-1, O-glycosylated αSyn, Pael-R, CHIP, cdc-Rel1A, and synaptotagmin X1. The genetic models, however, cannot reproduce LB development and neurodegeneration (Dawson et al., 2010; Pingale & Gupta, 2020). Once again, only the PARKINQ311X-DAT-BAC mice show growing motor deficits and loss of nigrostriatal DA neurones. According to (Van Rompuy et al., 2014), rats with this mutation also suffer from dose-dependent neurodegeneration. Only behavioral impairments and mitochondrial dysfunction are seen in ZF with PINK1 mutations (Razali et al., 2021). These mice have no DOPAn loss in SN, modest anxiety behaviors (Decourt et al., 2021; Neha et al., 2023), and slight locomotor deficits (Dawson et al., 2010; Pingale & Gupta, 2020). Furthermore, SN neurones may become more prone to inflammation as a result of PARKIN depletion. This was supported by a study that showed that injecting LPS into PARKIN ± improved TH + rescue, reduced inflammation, and damaged neurones compared to WT mice who received the same therapy. This illustrates the regulation of the inflammasome by PARKIN (Wang et al., 2024). Most studies focus on microglia activation and inflammatory markers instead of behavioral testing, and DA depletion is not always present in *SNCA* models (Blesa & Przedborski, 2014; Meredith et al., 2008; Neha et al., 2023; Pingale & Gupta, 2020). The ZF *SNCA* model exhibits reduced DA, mitochondrial activity, and motor deficits (O'Donnell et al., 2014; Razali et al., 2021; Robea et al., 2020; Milanese et al., 2012). As discussed in the clinical section, it is now believed that the most likely cause of PD development is the combination of hereditary, environmental, and behavioral factors. Therefore, in a mouse αSyn transgenic model, LPS led to a slow deterioration of the nigrostriatal dopamine pathway, αSyn aggregation, and LBs formation that was not present in the pure genetic model (Gao et al., 2011). Interestingly, rotenone therapy mimics the symptoms of clinical PD in αSyn genetic models. It is possible that αSyn overexpression makes DA more susceptible to oxidative stress and mitochondrial malfunction since a single inducer cannot do this (Johnson & Bobrovskaya, 2015). However, similar to the other PD-linked mutations, iPSCs derived from patients with *SNCA* variants are useful tools for developing individualized treatment plans (Chia et al., 2020; Devine et al., 2011). In animal models, mutations in LRRK2 do not cause neurodegeneration, LB and αSyn development, or evident motor impairments, but they frequently cause oxidative stress, inflammation, autophagy, mitochondrial dysfunction, and proteasomal dysfunction (Lama et al., 2021). DOPAn loss in SN only occurs in mice with the *G2019S LRRK2* mutation (Volpicelli-Daley et al., 2016). This mutation in iPSCs promotes cell death and reduces branching complexity in DOPAn (Bose et al., 2022). The ZF with an LRRK2 mutation exhibit a more complete typical PD phenotype, which is identical to αSyn and includes motor deficits, αSyn aggregation, and neuronal death. According to(Nguyen et al., 2011), the iPSC cells of a patient with early-onset PD and LRRK2 mutations displayed increased expression of the αSyn protein and other oxidative stress-related genes. More people are beginning to see inflammation as a potential cause of clinical PD, and new studies are beginning to look at this notion(Choi et al., 2009). reported that rats given LPS injections gradually reduced the number of TH + cells in SN (21%, 38%, and 41% after 1, 2, and 4 weeks, respectively) compared to the non-injected side. Both mice (Hunter et al., 2009) and rats (Choi et al., 2009; Hunter et al., 2007, 2017)have reported similar results, indicating that the model is repeatable. Importantly, our results are one of the few experimental studies that monitor PD readouts over time, providing valuable information on temporal mechanisms that might account for how PD develops. More relevant to the danger phase, intrauterine injection of LPS in pregnant rats results in a decrease in dopamine (DA) in the brains of the offspring and enhanced damage from pro-inflammatory stimuli administered in the postnatal period (Ling et al., 2006). This is in line with the discovery that in OBCs treated with modest doses of rotenone to mimic a progressive degenerative form of PD, inflammation—more specifically, TNFα—is the determinant of DOPAn demise (Jayanti et al., 2022). Remarkably, TNFα overexpression in SN results in microgliosis, motor complaints, and progressive neurodegeneration, suggesting that this cytokine is essential for the loss of DA. Insulin growth factor binding protein 5 (IGFBP5) silencing almost completely cures cell death in PC12 cells exposed to 6-OHDA, and diabetes has low systemic inflammation in addition to risk factors (Guo et al., 2024). These results have been confirmed in vivo, where wild-type (WT) rats exposed to 6-OHDA showed motor deficits and a decrease in TH+, but not IGFBP5−/− animals (Guo et al., 2024). Accordingly, studies on aging have connected IGFBP5 to cognitive decline, which is also seen in PD (Capuano et al., 2019). The following are debatable risk factors for PD in humans, as others have pointed out: age, obesity, pre-diabetes, type 2 diabetes, and insulin resistance (Calabrese et al., 2018; Lewitt & Boyd, 2024; Li et al., 2023; Russo & Riessland, 2022; Yu et al., 2022). However, low-dose LPS preconditioning to midbrain OBCs protected DOPAn against inflammatory damage by decreasing microglial activation and generating pro-inflammatory chemicals (Yang et al., 2020). As part of a complementary in vitro approach, co-culturing SH-SY5Y cells, BV2 cells, and primary microglia demonstrated that the adaptive anti-inflammatory behavior results from the suppression of the MAPK p38 and TLR4-mediated NF-κB signaling pathways (Yang et al., 2020). This suggests that the level of inflammation (and perhaps TNFα) may determine whether PD has a protective or harmful sequence.

1.3.2.2 Prodromal phase modeling

The collection of non-motor symptoms that manifest during the prodromal phase of PD presents opportunities to establish an early therapy window (Table 1.1). In regions of the brain other than the nigrostriatal pathway, pathology in DA and non-DA pathways results in these symptoms (Decourt et al., 2021; Miyazaki & Asanuma, 2020; Tieu, 2011).

In vivo models (6-OHDA; MPTP; paraquat; rotenone; reserpine; and *VMAT2*, *LRRK2*, and *hA53T* αSyn models) have reproduced the pre-diagnosis symptoms as well as NA, SE, and Chol dysfunction in extra nigrostriatal regions. For example, hyposmia occurs when rats receive a small dose of MPTP via intranasal infusion. Following TH + decreases in the olfactory bulb, SN, striatum, and prefrontal cortex that accompanied hyposmia, there were cognitive and motor deficits. This concept is noteworthy since these effects, which result from an environmental poison entering the brain via the olfactory tract, repeat the prodromal stage, the symptomatic PD stage, and the risk phase. Rats stereotaxically-injected with rotenone in the nigra have shown similar results. The theory relates hyposmia and reduced DA in the SN to anomalies in rapid eye movement (REM) sleep (Rodrigues et al., 2014). Furthermore, 6-OHDA disrupts the sleep of NHP (Barraud et al., 2009; Verhave et al., 2011)and rats (Vo et al., 2014). In the prefrontal cortex, hippocampus, and VTA—significant cognitive and affective nuclei linked to prodromal and late PD symptoms—reserpine blockage of ex vivo (OBCs) VMAT2 inhibits glutamatergic and dopaminergic synaptic activity. Applying DA restored synaptic activity early in the reserpine challenge but not later, which is consistent with L-DOPA therapy in the clinical setting (Kroener et al., 2009). According to thorough clinical results in prodromal PD, OBCs have shown decreased neurite length and quantity when treated with rotenone (Dal Ben et al., 2019) and decreased synaptic spine number when treated with MPTP. According to the 18-F Dopa scan/PET scan, these ex vivo slow degenerating mice are beneficial for studying the prodromal processes of PD because they mimic the decreased synaptic DA that occurs before DOPAn loss in the clinic. According to(Drukarch et al., 1996), GSH has a protective antioxidant effect on DA both intracellularly and in the extracellular matrix. In PC12 cells exposed to reserpine, intracellular DA depletion results in increased intracellular GSH levels, whereas GSH depletion induces DA death. Despite very limited studies, the blood–brain barrier (BBB) may have a role in PD. The discovery that damage may be repaired by exposing the cells to a pericyte-conditioned medium in the Lund Human Mesencephalic (LUHMES) cell model with a modest lesion caused by 6-OHDA and MPTP highlights the importance of cells surrounding the BBB in the early stages of the illness (Gaceb et al., 2020). Constipation and decreased intestinal motility are among the gastrointestinal abnormalities reported in mice and primates exposed to continuous doses of MPTP and rotenone. These abnormalities are thought to occur before the typical symptoms of PD in humans (Chaumette et al., 2009; Drolet et al., 2009; Greene et al., 2009). It's interesting to note that these models alter the intestinal DA level as well. Enteric DA has an immunomodulatory role (Jayanti et al., 2023), hence PD-induced DA modulation supports another link between PD and inflammation. Given the possible role of the gastroenteric system in the risk phase of the illness, more attention should be paid to the causative association between gastrointestinal problems, inflammation, DA depletion, and PD symptoms.

1.3.2.3 Modeling of the early phases of clinical PD

Rodents and ZF exposed to 6-OHDA may exhibit motor symptoms (rigidity and akinesia) in addition to a DOPAn loss of up to 75% in SN (Feng et al., 2014; Hughes et al., 2020; Lam et al., 2005; Makhija & Jagtap, 2014; Meredith et al., 2008; Razali et al., 2021; Vaz et al., 2018; Wasel & Freeman, 2020;

Zeng et al., 2018). Rotenone is rarely, if ever, used in NHP, but it mimics key features of both early and late clinical PD in rats and zebrafish, such as DA depletion, αSyn inclusions in nigral neurones, and motor abnormalities in LBs (Blesa & Przedborski, 2014; Cannon et al., 2009; Innos & Hickey, 2021; Johnson & Bobrovskaya, 2015; Lv et al., 2019; Miyazaki & Asanuma, 2020; Neha et al., 2023; Pingale & Gupta, 2020; Rocha et al., 2022; Thomas Broome & Castorina, 2022; Van Laar et al., 2023; Wang et al., 2015). Acute (high dosage, short duration) MPTP treatment causes bradykinesia, stiffness, stooped posture, and mild postural instability in mice and NHP. Additionally, the DOPAn degrades quickly (Konnova & Swanberg, 2018, pp. 83–106; Li et al., 2023; Blessa and Przedborski, 2014; Sanf). A sustained challenge with lower doses of MPTP results in a decrease in DOPAn levels and clinical motor symptoms in middle-aged NHP. Remarkably, in acute 6-OHDA and MPTP, as well as in reserpine models, the initial decrease in tyrosine hydroxylase (TH+, DA precursor) may reversed, suggesting a decrease in DA generation rather than neurone death (De Freitas et al., 2016; Meredith et al., 2008; Neha et al., 2023; Pingale & Gupta, 2020). Moreover, acute dosing regimens are seldom linked to toxicity that might be fatal. This makes it abundantly evident that acute dose schedules do not fairly represent the etiopathogenesis of PD in people. This might limit both the translational usefulness of understanding PD processes and the capacity to develop and assess therapeutic choices. In addition to their well-known pro-oxidant effect, which causes endoplasmic reticulum stress and the upregulation of chaperones linked to cell death (Xie et al., 2016), MPTP and 6-OHDA mechanistically give proteasome inhibition (Jang & Chung, 2022). Since proteasome inhibitors in vivo result in αSyn accumulation, DOPAn loss, and motor deficits, the notion of protein misfolding in PD is intimately linked to proteasome suppression (Cenci & Bjorklund, 2020). It is unknown if αSyn is harmful in these species, although tiny inclusion bodies were also seen in c. elegans, rats, minipigs, and NHPs exposed to 6-OHDA and proteosome inhibitors, for instance. In vitro protease suppression results in intracellular accumulation of p52, a mediator that facilitates apoptosis (Lopes et al., 1997; Nair et al., 2006). Protease inhibitors can therefore initiate the mitochondrial apoptotic signaling cascade, which activates caspase three and caspase nine and increases the synthesis of cytochrome C, ROS, and Bcl-2-associated X (BAX) (Lee et al., 2005; Perez-Alvarez et al., 2009). Interestingly, rotenone and 6-OHDA induce apoptosis in the MN9D cell line and primary cultures, whereas MPTP does not (Lopes et al., 1997; Nair et al., 2006), showing how the chemical used to induce PD may affect the results and their clinical application. Protease inhibitors, especially actacystin, and rotenone both reduce intracellular ATP and hinder mitochondrial function (Bir et al., 2014; Kang et al., 2012). This might impede vesicular trafficking and the elimination of misfolded proteins, potentially leading to an accumulation of αSyn (Yamamoto et al., 2007). In a cellular model of PD caused by rotenone, transcriptome sequencing revealed that PTEN-induced putative kinase 1 (*PINK1*) was one of the most altered mitophagy pathways, suggesting a potential involvement in this specific disease mechanism (Zhang et al., 2024). Notably, in animal models of the early PD phase that replicate the presence of αSyn, 6-OHDA (regardless of injection site and dosage) and MPTP (at least in acute schemes) do not cause LBs, even in the presence of motor abnormalities (Doppler et al., 2021; Pingale & Gupta, 2020; Neha et al., 2023; De Freitas et al., 2016; Blesa & Przedborski, 2014; Li et al., 2023; Meredith et al., 2008; Konnove and Swanberg, 2018; Khan et al., 2023; Sanf). Rats that get several injections of paraquat 8 weeks apart show no LBs but a 50% reduction in TH + cells and αSyn present (Blesa et al., 2012; Dauer & Przedborski, 2003; Tieu, 2011). Even genetic models often fail to meet this objective, save for the SNCA gene, which codes for αSyn. Either a model failure or evidence that αSyn is not the cause of PD symptoms are the two possible interpretations of these results. Critiques of a mechanistic role of αSyn and LBs in clinical PD are supported by the findings that injecting αSyn preformed fibrils into the mouse striatum unilaterally causes neuroinflammation prior to the accumulation of the pathologic form of αSyn, followed by neurodegeneration and motor deficits (Lai, Alipanahi, et al., 2021; Lai, Kim, et al., 2021) and that moderate/chronic doses of MPTP cause αSyn aggregation in mice but not DOPAn loss or motor symptoms (Konnove and Swanberg, 2018). According to Blesa et al. (2012), this highlights the importance of experimental setup and analysis (e.g., physiologic protein, fibrils, and αSyn gene expression) in elucidating translational pathologic pathways. Interestingly, the pathophysiological effects of the side injected with αSyn produced fibrils are similar to those of the non-injected contralateral striatum (Lai, Alipanahi, et al., 2021; Lai, Kim, et al., 2021). This suggests that inflammatory mediators are important in the development of the disease, according to certain interpretations (Dauer & Przedborski, 2003; Pingale & Gupta, 2020; Lai, Alipanahi, et al., 2021; Lai, Kim, et al., 2021; Meredith et al., 2008; Sacino et al., 2014a, 2014b).

1.3.2.4 Modeling of advanced stages of PD

Advanced stages of PD include both motor and non-motor symptoms. In addition to aphagia, adipsia, and death, the therapy of 6-OHDA and MPTP may result in behaviors that resemble anxiety, despair, and apathy. Neural loss occurs continuously in mice injected intracisternally (NE loss up to 75%; DA 83%–98%) (Decourt et al., 2021; Meredith et al., 2008; Pingale & Gupta, 2020; Razali et al., 2021; Tieu, 2011). According to (Carvalho et al., 2013; Razali et al., 2021; Vaz et al., 2020; Wang et al., 2015; Zeng et al., 2018), ZF have parallel effects. NE depletion, NMDA-linked parkinsonian symptoms (Bonnet, 2000; Graham et al., 1990), and non-motor PD markers (Masilamoni & Smith, 2018) are all consequences of chronic MPTP therapy in NHPs. Nigrostriatal DOPAn degradation results in increased GABAergic activity in the striatum (Levy et al., 1995). In OBCs from the dorsal striatum, cortex, ventral mesencephalon, and nucleus of Meyert, rotenone treatment results in cholinergic cell death (Ullrich & Humpel, 2009). PD has been linked to non-motor symptoms like gastrointestinal dysfunctions (Dauer & Przedborski, 2003; Innos & Hickey, 2021; Johnson & Bobrovskaya, 2015; Konnova & Swanberg, 2018; Miyazaki & Asanuma, 2020; Müller & Bohnen, 2013; Rocha et al., 2022; Xu et al., 2023; Thomas Broome & Castorina, 2022). These symptoms have been linked to the loss of SE, Chol, and NE neurones (Blesa et al., 2012; Tang et al., 2023). Recent studies suggest that systems associated to cholinergic control mediate the effects of MPP + on DA release (Zhao et al., 2024). The use of rotenone in rats has been challenging due to the long period required for chronic administration, the high mortality rate with acute treatment, and differences in the percentage of animals affected (Innos & Hickey, 2021). Using middle-aged rats and the medium-chain triglyceride Miglyol 812 N as an adjuvant has eliminated these limitations. With this treatment, all animals show signs of PD after 3 weeks, and the severity of the sickness varies little from person to person (Cannon et al., 2009; Klaestrup et al., 2022). Given the completeness of phenotypic markers and the consistency in their development, this is likely one of the finest models currently available for doing time course evaluations of biomolecular processes occurring in the connected CNS circuits. Additionally, it provides valuable insights on the onset and progression of sickness without requiring any ethical or financial investment.

1.4 Redefining PD: insights from ZF models into risk, prodromal, and clinical phases

In comparison to their invertebrate counterparts, *C. elegans and D. melanogaster*, ZF demonstrate a significantly closer physical relationship to humans. The measurable characteristics and pathologies of ZF and humans are very similar. The mapping of the dopaminergic nervous system in ZF has been the result of extensive research since its initial designation as a model organism in 1998 (Tay et al., 2011). At 19 h post-fertilization (hpf), dopaminergic neurones were initially characterized in the posterior tuberculum of the ventral diencephalon of ZF embryos (Fig. 1.3). This region is analogous to the human substantia nigra (SN). The ventral telencephalon, which corresponds to the human striatum,

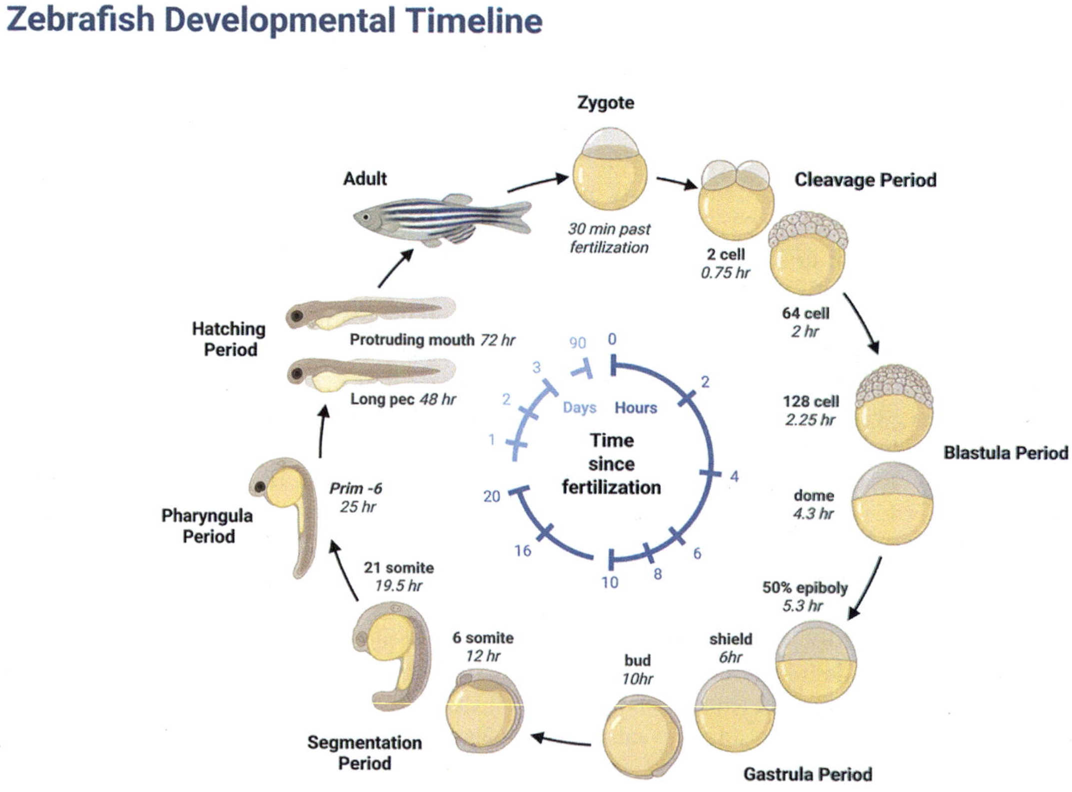

FIGURE 1.3 ZF developmental timeline.

A schematic overview of key stages in ZF embryonic and larval development, from fertilization through early organogenesis and neurodevelopment. The timeline highlights critical windows for central nervous system formation, including dopaminergic neuron differentiation in the diencephalon. ZF serve as a powerful in vivo model for PD due to their conserved dopaminergic pathways, rapid development, and genetic tractability. Early developmental stages enable high-throughput screening of PD-related genetic mutations, neurotoxicity assays, and evaluation of potential neuroprotective compounds.

was demonstrated to be the destination of this group of neurones. This process is a prime example of the nigrostriatal dopaminergic neural system, which is of paramount importance in the pathogenesis of PD (Flinn et al., 2008). The ZF brain's exhaustive data on dopaminergic neural projections, in conjunction with its susceptibility to experimental manipulations, renders this species an advantageous specimen for the investigation of molecular pathways associated with PD.

ZF are a critical model for the investigation of a variety of neurological disorders due to their rapid maturation, substantial brood sizes, and economical husbandry. The human brain and ZF brain exhibit numerous homologous and highly conserved structures, despite their differences in configuration (Diotel et al., 2020). Experiments that utilize ZF to generate PD models frequently involve the regions associated with the disease in humans. The olfactory bulb and telencephalon are among the regions. The olfactory bulb is a brain region that is abundant in dopaminergic neurones and is closely associated with memory and learning. It plays a crucial role in the sense of smell (Diotel et al., 2020; Kozol et al., 2016). In humans, the telencephalon, or cerebrum, is a significant component of the brain that is responsible for the preponderance of sensory processing and all voluntary motor control. Comparable to the substantia nigra in humans, the diencephalon is a neuron-rich region of the brain that is responsible for the regulation of virtually all coordinated movements in fish. *Danio rerio* are vertebrate teleosts that contain orthologs for over 78% of human genes, in contrast to commonly used invertebrate models such as *Drosophila melanogaster* and *C. elegans*(Ellis & Soanes, 2012).

The process in this model is nearly identical to that in humans due to the highly conserved catecholamine production cascade and the observed high genetic homology. Vesicular monoamine transporter 2 (VMAT2) facilitates the transmission of dopamine as a signal between neurones. The synaptic cleft of signaling neurones is where the dopamine transporter (DAT) is located, which facilitates the release of dopamine into the synapse. Dopamine is bound to the dopamine receptor (D1 Receptor) on the dendritic end of a receiving neurone, which results in the activation of cyclic adenosine monophosphate (cAMP). cAMP functions as a secondary mediator that enables signal transduction between neurones in the central nervous system (Lebowitz & Khoshbouei, 2020). The neurotransmitter pathways for noradrenergic, serotonergic, histaminergic, and dopaminergic systems in ZF exhibit substantial conservation and are pertinent to discussions regarding PD (Anichtchik et al., 2003; Tay et al., 2011). The meticulous investigation of dopamine's synthesis is necessary for the study of PD. Tyrosine, an indispensable amino acid, serves as the precursor to dopamine. The enzyme tyrosine hydroxylase (TH) catalyzes the hydroxylation of L-tyrosine, a rate-limiting step that results in the production of the dopamine precursor, L-DOPA (Albarran et al., 2014). In microglia and TH-positive neurones, aromatic amino acid decarboxylase converts L-DOPA to dopamine.

Research utilizing adult ZF as a model for human neurological diseases has proven advantageous for drug development and the study of genetic disorders. ZF serve as an effective model for assessing medicinal efficacy in a high-throughput, in vivo context, attributed to their notable genetic similarity to humans, economical care requirements, relatively swift breeding cycles, and considerable embryo production. Currently, most research utilizing ZF models for PD induces the condition in larval or embryonic specimens due to the ease of administration, with developmental progression occurring within a few days. The utilisation of early-stage organisms limits the applicability of ZF as models for adult diseases, especially those related to age-associated neurodegeneration. Researchers have recently sought to improve the use of ZF as models for PD. 1-Methyl-4-phenyl-1,2,3,6-tetrahydropyridine (MPTP) is recognised as a prodrug that, upon administration, encapsulates the biochemical processes and symptoms associated with PD. The use of MPTP in an adult ZF model may advance research in PD. This article highlights recent research on this model, comparing it with the human variant of PD.

The lack of experimentation on adult ZF suggests inconsistencies in procedural setups and fish characteristics, which may result in variability in behavioral and neurochemical observations. The application of MPTP in ZF is increasingly recognised as a valuable research avenue for animal models of PD. Various research groups, including ours (Razali et al., 2021, 2022, 2023, 2024), are contributing essential insights that may facilitate the development of a more standardised model. The age, gender, and strain of ZF used in experiments demonstrate considerable variability. In zebrafish, "adult" typically denotes the achievement of sexual maturity, which occurs around 3 months of age (Singleman & Holtzman, 2014). The aging process in ZF is being studied and is linked to functional changes (Kishi, 2004), which may impact study outcomes and make comparisons of findings unsuitable.

ZF models exhibit specific characteristics of parkinsonism due to anatomical, biochemical, and cellular pathological similarities with human systems. Nonetheless, they may not fully capture the diversity present in the etiology of human PD (Gialluisi et al., 2021). The mechanisms of disease induction in these fish fail to sufficiently account for the gradual and progressive features of human PD. PD in humans is characterized by the progressive degeneration of dopaminergic neurones and the accumulation of αSyn over time (DeMaagd & Philip, 2015). ZF models demonstrate accelerated symptom onset after toxin exposure, thereby complicating the exploration of long-term, age-related factors in PD (Cassar et al., 2020). There are notable differences in the pharmacokinetics of drug metabolism, the characteristics of the blood–brain barrier, and drug responses when comparing ZF and humans. As a result, findings from drug testing may not directly translate and necessitate validation in mammalian models before proceeding with further development (Cassar et al., 2020; Knap et al., 2023). ZF models offer significant benefits, including accelerated development, optical transparency, and the ability for genetic modification. These models are particularly useful for investigating the basic mechanisms of neurodegeneration and for performing drug screening (Kim & Jin, 2012). Integrating insights from ZF with other animal models and human studies is crucial for a comprehensive understanding of PD. The homology of the catecholamine cascade indicates that neurotoxin models in ZF are advantageous for the development of effective therapeutics for PD. This discussion focusses on the use of the neurotoxin 1-Methyl-4-phenyl-1,2,3,6-tetrahydropyridine (MPTP) as a model for PD, highlighting its straightforward administration in zebrafish. While MPTP neurotoxin clearly contributes to the manifestation of PD symptoms in zebrafish, several challenges related to its application warrant attention. Previous studies utilizing the MPTP-induced paradigm have demonstrated that the effects of this neurotoxin are transient (Godoy et al., 2020; Sarath Babu et al., 2016; Wasel & Freeman, 2020). In summary, the neurochemical changes resulting from MPTP injection caused a temporary dysfunction of dopaminergic neurones. Continuous exposure to MPTP is required in the ZF model to sustain the effects of MPTP. The different methods of administering MPTP to ZF models may lead to inconsistencies in dosage and exposure duration. For example, despite equivalent dosages, a lesser amount of MPTP will arrive at the target area when delivered intraperitoneally compared to intracerebellar injection, due to the increased travel distance. A similar example is observed in ZF embryos or larvae. The immersion induced MPTP may lead to varying levels of compound absorption in individual embryos or larvae. Careful precautions are essential, as this issue may influence the interpretation of results and the overall success of the research. Despite the challenges, MPTP has provided significant insights into the development of ZF as a model for PD. The combination of gene knockdown and MPTP exposure has enabled the investigation of the relationships between genetic and environmental factors in the onset of PD. This neurotoxin has enabled substantial discoveries, allowing researchers to enhance their understanding of the mechanisms and pathology of PD.

The toxic mechanism of MPTP and its conversion to MPP + offers a valuable framework for the development of animal models of PD in research, as it replicates several key pathological characteristics of the disorder (Mustapha & Taib, 2021). The progression of MPTP-induced parkinsonism generally occurs more rapidly and severely than that of idiopathic PD in humans. MPTP is not considered a causative factor in idiopathic PD among human patients. MPTP, despite its limitations, has demonstrated significant value in PD research due to its pharmacodynamic properties in neural tissues (Vaz et al., 2018). MPTP is beneficial as it accurately mimics the effects on catecholaminergic production, as well as behavioral and motor deficits. Most MPTP ZF models predominantly employ fish in early developmental stages. The ZF embryonic model of PD is preferred mainly because of the straightforward nature of MPTP induction, which can be readily dissolved in tank water at appropriate dilutions. Embryonic ZF can absorb the neurotoxin MPTP through their gill capillaries, leading to irreversible neurological deficits within a few hours. Numerous studies have utilized this method, allowing fish to reach sexual maturity after incubation in MPTP during the larval developmental phase (Razali et al., 2021; Vaz et al., 2018).

Many questions remain and articulating them could encourage experiments to seek answers. Is sporadic PD caused by toxicants that penetrate the brain, or does it have its origins in the gut, as proposed by certain researchers? The narrative suggests that unidentified toxicants may penetrate the blood-brain barrier and interfere with the interconnected pathways of glutathione and metal disposition. What explains the variations in mechanistic evaluations of rotenone, MPP+, and 6HD, given their shared inhibition of Complex I in mitochondria? Do sporadic PD and non-Lewy body parkinsonism share common etiological factors, and what is the relevance of Lewy bodies in this context? What is the role of neuromelanin? Does it serve a protective function, or does it act as a repository for readily oxidized catecholamines that were utilized as neurotransmitters before the evolution of long-lived animals? What explains the relative deficiency of metallothionein and glutathione in healthy neurones? Do they interfere with neurotransmission, which relies on zinc mobilization, or is this simply another instance of neurones depending on astrocytes, which contain substantial amounts of metallothionein and glutathione, for protection? Is there a specific reductase enzyme that reduces oxidized sulfhydryl groups in metallothionein to restore functionality? Does this reaction also utilize GSH? What roles do MTF1 and MTF2 play in transcriptional regulation and resilience to threats? In conclusion, a notable question emerges: Is there a therapeutic strategy to prevent neurodegeneration after a substantial loss of neurones has occurred and symptoms have presented? Should resources be directed toward the identification of causes and the prevention of neurodegenerative diseases instead? Neurodegenerative diseases display variability; nonetheless, they consistently lead to the degeneration of particular neuronal groups. PD and parkinsonism are environmental disorders marked by the selective degeneration of dopaminergic neurones in the substantia nigra, noted in individuals exposed to agents like rotenone or MPTP, as well as in animals administered these substances or 6-hydroxydopamine (6HD). This disease allows for the identification of environmental causes through chemical methods to reveal neuronal vulnerabilities. The observation that metallothionein genes were markedly induced by seven neurotoxicants, including rotenone, 6HD, MPP+, and methylmercury, indicates a potential connection between the metal disposition pathway and the glutathione pathway. Metallothionein detects reactive oxygen species (ROS), oxidized glutathione (GSSG), and free metals, including iron, and subsequently responds by releasing zinc ions. MTF1 binds to free zinc and activates the transcription of genes that adapt to stress, such as metallothionein and reductases. Neurones have restricted levels of GSH and low amounts of metallothionein, limiting their ability to tolerate free iron and reactive oxygen species (ROS). Neurones, especially large striatal dopaminergic neurones, necessitate considerable aerobic metabolism, resulting in significant production of reactive oxygen species (ROS). Low levels of glutathione (GSH) and metallothionein seem to make neurones vulnerable to disruptions in these metabolic pathways, increasing their dependence on astrocytes for protective assistance. Neurones typically exhibit a deficiency in metallothionein and glutathione.

The question now is: How can ZF help us rethink PD?

By transforming PD from a precisely defined motor problem to a complicated, whole-body ailment, the ZF model is transforming our understanding of the illness. According to conventional wisdom, PD is a neurodegenerative illness that strikes adults and is characterized by the death of dopaminergic neurones. But new knowledge from studies on ZF is reframing PD as a multifaceted, multi-pathway illness with potential neurodevelopmental causes. ZF research is redefining the long-standing genetic versus environmental argument as a model of gene–environment interaction. Importantly, by shifting diagnosis from post-symptom to pre-symptomatic phases, the paradigm also provides opportunities for early identification using biomarkers. Finally, PD is now seen as a diverse, spectrum-based, whole-body illness rather than a uniform one—a revolutionary viewpoint made possible by this little but powerful aquatic creature (Fig. 1.4).

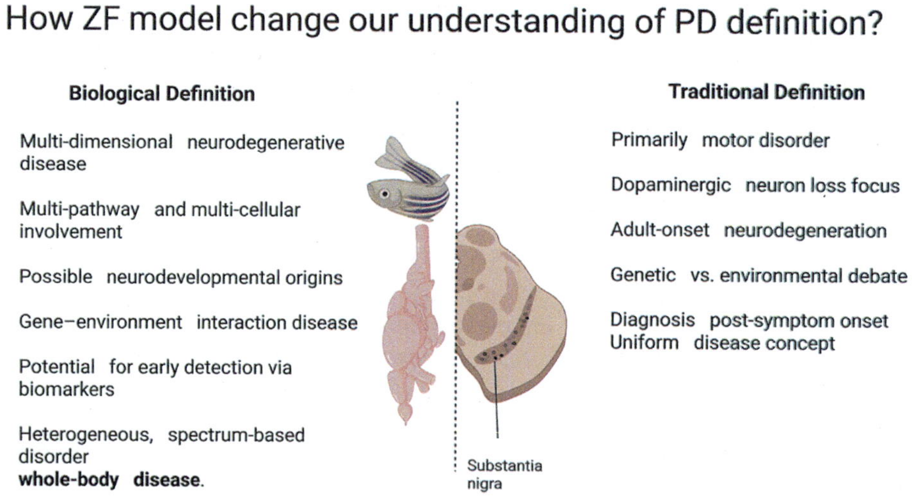

FIGURE 1.4

How can the ZF model change our understanding of PD definition? Comparison of definitions of PD. The conventional definition highlights motor symptoms including tremor, stiffness, and bradykinesia. The traditional definition emphasizes neuropathological characteristics, such as the degeneration of dopaminergic neurones and the production of Lewy bodies. The biological definition, based on the ZF model, incorporates molecular, genetic, and environmental causes, emphasizing PD as a complex condition that transcends clinical and pathological limits.

ZF provides numerous advantages that have led to important observations and new discoveries. However, several limitations must be recognised when utilizing this species as a research model. The external development of ZF embryos enables real-time observation; however, the uptake of chemicals by individual embryos may vary, especially with oral administration. Additionally, the metabolic pathways and absorption rates of specific substances or chemicals in embryos grown externally may differ from those in human embryos. A comprehensive assessment is essential to determine the effective dosage and avoid misinterpretation of results. ZF possess an intrinsic ability for regeneration and neurogenesis, enabling the replacement of cellular damage or loss. Dopaminergic neurodegeneration caused by 6-OHDA was repopulated 30 days post neurotoxin administration. This phenomenon presents challenges to investigations of degenerative diseases, as it directly contradicts the concept of degeneration (Vaz et al., 2018). This understanding provides a new and promising basis for research in neural regeneration.

The diseases and quantifiable traits of humans and ZF are quite similar. Since ZF were first identified as a model organism in 1998, a great deal of research has been conducted to map their dopaminergic nervous system (Tay et al., 2011). The posterior tuberculum of the ventral diencephalon of ZF embryos revealed dopaminergic neurones at 19 h post-fertilization (hpf). This area is comparable to the substantia nigra (SN) in humans. They showed that this set of neurones travels to the ventral telencephalon, which is equivalent to the human striatum. The pathophysiology of PD heavily relies on the nigrostriatal dopaminergic brain system, of which this process is an excellent illustration (Flinn et al., 2008). Because of its extensive information on dopaminergic neuronal projections and its vulnerability to experimental manipulation, the ZF brain is a useful model organism for studying the molecular mechanisms linked to PD (Fig. 1.5).

Zebrafish's quick maturity, large brood numbers, and cost-effective care make them an essential model for studying a range of neurological conditions. Despite their different configurations, the human and ZF brains share many homologous and highly conserved components (Diotel et al., 2020). Studies that use ZF to create models of PD often focus on the areas linked to the condition in humans. Among the areas are the telencephalon and olfactory bulb. A part of the brain that is rich in dopaminergic neurones and intimately related to memory and learning is the olfactory bulb. The sense of smell depends on it (Diotel et al., 2020; Kozol et al., 2016). A major part of the human brain, the telencephalon, also known as the cerebrum, is in charge of all voluntary motor control and the majority of sensory processing. The diencephalon, a neuron-rich area of the brain that controls almost all coordinated movements in fish, is comparable to the substantia nigra in humans. Unlike widely used invertebrate models like Drosophila melanogaster and Caenorhabditis elegans (Ellis & Soanes, 2012), Danio rerio are vertebrate teleosts that have orthologs for more than 78% of human genes.

Because of the found high genetic homology and the highly conserved catecholamine synthesis cascade, the procedure in this model is almost the same as that in humans. Vesicular monoamine transporter 2 (VMAT2) helps dopamine go from neurone to neurone as a signal. Located in the synaptic cleft of signaling neurones, the dopamine transporter (DAT) promotes dopamine release into the synapse. Dopamine activates cyclic adenosine monophosphate (cAMP) when it binds to the dopamine receptor (D1 Receptor) on the dendritic end of a receiving neurone. In the central nervous system, cAMP serves as a secondary mediator that permits signal transmission between neurones (Lebowitz & Khoshbouei, 2020). The ZF noradrenergic, serotonergic, histaminergic, and dopaminergic neurotransmitter pathways are highly conserved and relevant to PD debates (Anichtchik et al., 2003; Tay et al., 2011). The study of PD requires a careful examination of dopamine production. The

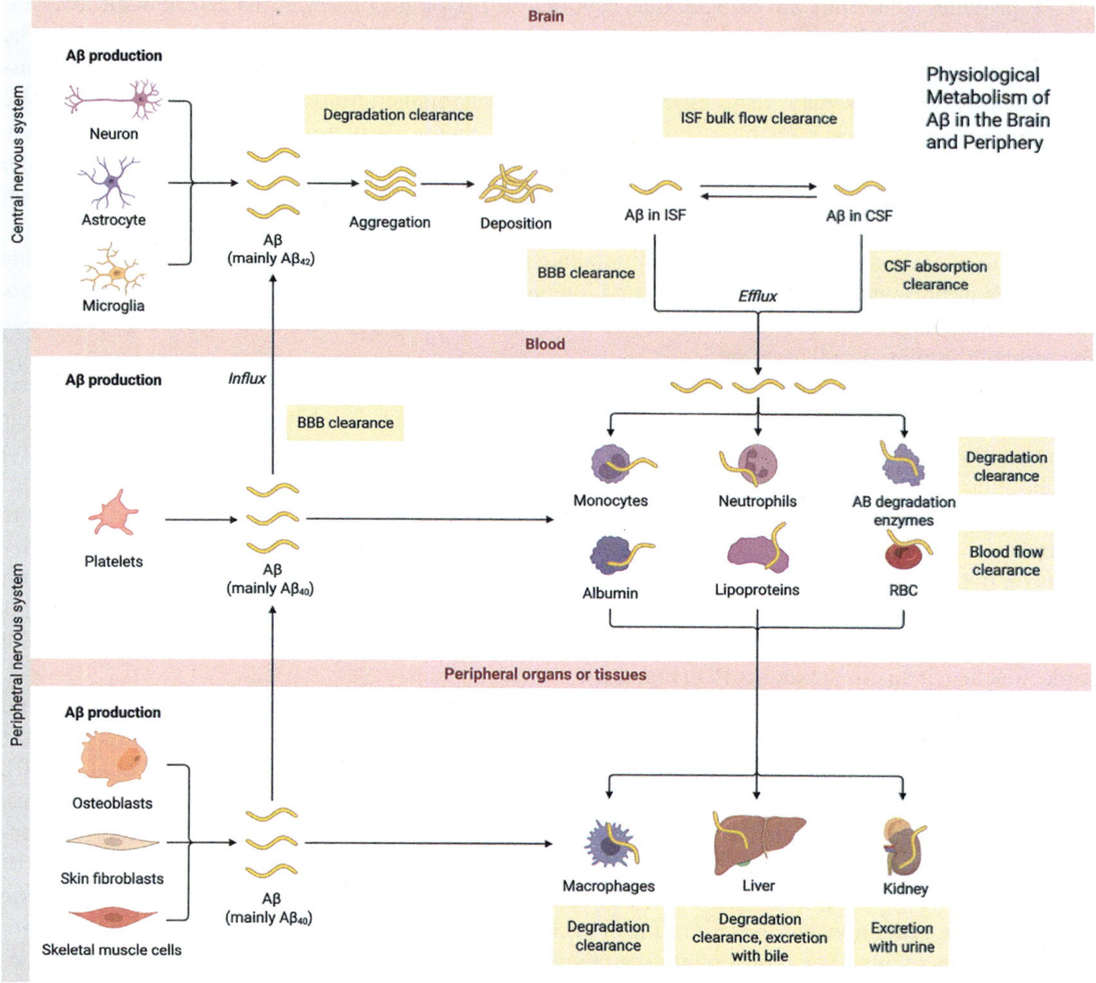

FIGURE 1.5 Physiological Metabolism of Amyloid-β (Aβ) in the Brain and Periphery and Its Relevance to PD Biomarkers.

This figure illustrates the normal production, clearance, and transport pathways of amyloid-β (Aβ) peptides within the central nervous system and peripheral circulation. In the brain, Aβ is generated through enzymatic cleavage of amyloid precursor protein (APP) and is cleared via enzymatic degradation, glymphatic drainage, and transport across the blood–brain barrier (BBB) into the periphery. Peripheral organs, such as the liver and kidneys, also contribute to Aβ clearance. Dysregulation in any of these pathways can lead to Aβ accumulation and altered systemic levels, which have been implicated not only in Alzheimer's disease but also in the pathology and progression of PD, particularly in PD patients with cognitive decline. Monitoring Aβ dynamics in cerebrospinal fluid (CSF) and blood may offer valuable non-invasive biomarkers for early detection, disease progression, and subtype differentiation in PD.

precursor of dopamine is tyrosine, an essential amino acid. Tyrosine hydroxylase (TH) is an enzyme that catalyzes the hydroxylation of L-tyrosine, a rate-limiting step that produces L-DOPA, the precursor to dopamine (Albarran et al., 2014). Aromatic amino acid decarboxylase transforms L-DOPA into dopamine in TH-positive neurones and microglia.

The creation of symptomatic treatments for PD patients has advanced significantly during the last several decades (Bloem et al., 2021). Nevertheless, there is currently no single treatment option available, and efforts to create disease-modifying treatments (DMTs) to slow or halt the disease's course have resulted in a string of unfortunate failures (Bloem et al., 2021). While neurotransmitter restoration is the primary stay of symptomatic therapy techniques, DMTs seek to disrupt the physiological and molecular processes that cause neuronal dysfunction and degeneration. Scientific developments in recent years have provided a multitude of insights into the molecular pathways underlying illness, consequently revealing promising targets for therapeutic approaches (Bloem et al., 2021; Poewe et al., 2017). The general idea that PD is a complex condition that can arise from a variety of genetic predispositions and environmental triggers, may or may not be linked to pathological αSyn aggregation, may affect different parts of the central and peripheral nervous systems in different sequential orders, and may evoke a wide range of symptoms in the motor, sensory, autonomic, sleep, and cognitive domains has emerged based on this knowledge (Poewe et al., 2017; Postuma & Berg, 2016). In particular, it has been shown that the molecular processes underlying PD remain active, disrupting neuronal function and causing neurodegeneration years or even decades before the symptoms and clinical indicators show up (Poewe et al., 2017; Postuma & Berg, 2016). As a result, the idea that the illness should be defined biologically rather than clinically has surfaced for many reasons.

1. Objectivity: Compared to criteria based on clinical characteristics, the biological criteria are probably more objective and, thus, less likely to be misclassified.
2. Homogeneity: Due to varying pathologies, patients who meet the criteria for biological illness classifications are unlikely to exhibit clinical phenocopies, which homogenizes populations for observational and therapeutic research.
3. Early diagnosis: Patients who satisfy biological criteria may get a diagnosis well in advance of the development of severe neurodegeneration and symptoms, increasing their likelihood of benefiting from a disease-modifying treatment.
4. Mechanistic stratification: Precision medicine requires that patients who meet certain biological disease criteria have an abnormal activation of a particular disease mechanism. As a result, they may be more responsive to interventions that target the precise pathway.

Any notion of biological illness characterization in this context may accomplish one or more of the following goals.

1. The biological definition is a set of objective conceptual biological standards used to identify the traits that characterize a disease entity.
2. Biological diagnosis: Operationalized biological test criteria for determining whether a patient is ill or not are known as biological diagnosis.
3. Biological categorization, which uses objective biological standards to divide individuals into smaller groups within a disease entity based on the processes underlying the illness.
4. Biological staging: Using objective biological standards to group individuals into disease entities based on a series of illness occurrences.

Biological PD criteria may therefore be useful to define the disease entity, for objective and early diagnosis, ideally prior to symptom onset, for harmonization and stratification of patient groups by active disease mechanisms, for demonstrating the presence of targets for specific therapeutic interventions, and possibly for disease staging with the implicit possibility of measuring disease progression, in contrast to the currently prevalent clinically defined disease concepts of PD (Berg et al., 2015; Gibb & Lees, 1988; Postuma et al., 2015).The SynNeurGe criteria and NDS are two newly suggested biology-based research criteria for PD. Each has advantages and disadvantages (see Höglinger & Lang, 2024 for further information).

1.5 Outlook

There is now a great deal of scientific disagreement on the creation of a biological staging and classification system for PD. A recent task force from the International Parkinson and Movement Disorder Society (MDS) emphasized the need for a biological definition of PD by highlighting the illness's clinical, genetic, molecular, and neuropathological variability (Outeiro et al., 2023). This chapter hopes to assess the suggested concepts, investigates the possibility of unified classification criteria, and emphasizes the need for data to fill in current knowledge gaps, which highlights our proposal for a biological classification of PD using ZF model of PD and contrasts it with another proposal for a biological definition and staging system (Höglinger et al., 2024; Simuni et al., 2024). In order to improve communication between clinicians and fundamental scientists and update terminologies in the area of PD based on our most recent understanding, we identify a number of open questions in the field below.

The intricate nature of PD restricts current therapeutic therapy mostly to symptom alleviation. There is a notable deficiency of preventive programs and disease-modifying methods. To rectify these deficiencies, current PD models must be used more comprehensively and strategically. Clinical knowledge need to function as a validation instrument for evaluating the repeatability of newly generated models, rather than being the ultimate objective. There is an urgent need to precisely replicate the chronic course of PD, particularly to examine the pre-diagnostic stages for the identification of biomolecular alterations in the first phases. Our research underscores a notable deficiency of studies spanning from risk assessment to preclinical phases.

Essential observations about the primary shortcomings and limitations of the existing models include.

1. The acute schemes technique fails to reliably replicate the etiopathogenesis of human PD. This constrains the translational significance in comprehending the illness and screening therapeutics.
2. Concentrate on synucleopathy. The significance of synucleopathy is contentious, perhaps applicable just to a subtype of PD. Potentially a delayed occurrence.
3. So far, much focus has been directed into the molecular processes occurring post-diagnosis. Requirement for exploratory methodologies, essential in investigating the first phases.
4. Complexity of diseases. Various processes and neurotransmitters are implicated, operating on distinct temporal scales. Requirement for experimental designs investigating many stages within a singular investigation.
5. Requirement for intricate models. The temporal duration of human PD is too prolonged for experimental investigations. Models are essential and foundational.

6. Requirement for robust, repeatable, and collaborative models. Previous research provide the foundation for understanding how to accurately replicate real PD. Utilizing this foundation to pursue the aims outlined in the preceding sections by developing gradual degenerative models, employing standardised techniques, and ensuring data comparability and possible complementarity may be advantageous.

Researchers often have difficulties in identifying the best suitable model, since the primary emphasis continues to be on the clinical (symptomatic) stage of PD. Research often examines specific pathways in isolation, neglecting their integration into the wider, interrelated context of PD. Contemporary understanding reveals the profound intricacy of PD. Numerous and interrelated neurotransmitter systems are engaged. Numerous non-motor symptoms identified are evident in both the prodromal and advanced stages. The additional origin from the central nervous system is increasingly accepted, not just the Braak ideas, but also the interaction of genes with inflammation, for instance. The most promising strategy to address the gap seems to be the use of several PD models with milder disease triggers that replicate the early phases, both in vitro and in vivo. The examination of various trial durations in gradual degenerative models using a discovery methodology would be optimal. In vitro models are essential for studying intrinsic cellular signaling mechanisms. Genetic models, although not entirely typical of all PD symptoms or outcomes, are essential for investigating the pathogenic effects of individual mutations and the interplay between genetic variations, environmental factors, and lifestyle choices. The ongoing development and utilisation of intricate in vivo models, notwithstanding the ethical dilemmas they provide, is essential to surpass the constraints of specimens, protracted durations, and the ethical issues associated with clinical trials involving PD sufferers. A holistic perspective that harmonizes complexity with clinical relevance and repeatability is crucial. Notwithstanding its prominent public visibility, PD remains mostly perplexing from a biological perspective. Clinical and fundamental research must persist in exploring its processes, using novel omics tools for disease discovery.

References

Agin-Liebes, J., Cortes, E., Vonsattel, J. P., Marder, K., & Alcalay, R. N. (2020). Movement disorders rounds: A case of missing pathology in a patient with LRRK2 parkinson's disease. *Parkinsonism & Related Disorders, 74*, 76–77. https://doi.org/10.1016/j.parkreldis.2019.11.006

Albarran, S., Rangel-Barajas, C., & Garduo, B. F. (2014). Pathophysiology of L-Dopa induced dyskinesia — Changes in D1/D3 receptors and their signaling pathway. In A. Q. Rana (Ed.), *A synopsis of Parkinson's disease*. London: IntechOpen Limited.

Anichtchik, O. V., Kaslin, J., Peitsaro, N., Scheinin, M., & Panula, P. (2003). Neurochemical and behavioural changes in zebrafish *Danio rerio* after systemic administration of 6-hydroxydopamine and 1-methyl-4-phenyl-1,2,3,6-tetrahydropyridine. *Journal of Neurochemistry, 88*, 443–453.

Attems, J. (2017). The multi-morbid old brain. *Acta Neuropathologica, 134*(2), 169–170.

Attems, J., Toledo, J. B., Walker, L., Gelpi, E., Gentleman, S., Halliday, G., Hortobagyi, T., Jellinger, K., Kovacs, G. G., Lee, E. B., Love, S., McAleese, K. E., Nelson, P. T., Neumann, M., Parkkinen, L., Polvikoski, T., Sikorska, B., Smith, C., Grinberg, L. T., … McKeith, I. G. (2021). Neuropathological consensus criteria for the evaluation of lewy pathology in post-mortem brains: A multi-centre study. *Acta Neuropathologica, 141*(2), 159–172. https://doi.org/10.1007/s00401-020-02255-2

Bagnoli, E., Trotier, A., McMahon, J., Quinlan, L. R., Biggs, M., Pandit, A., & FitzGerald, U. (2023). Prodromal parkinson's disease and the catecholaldehyde hypothesis: Insight from olfactory bulb organotypic cultures. *FASEB Journal, 37*(12). https://doi.org/10.1096/fj.202301253R

Barraud, Q., Lambrecq, V., Forni, C., McGuire, S., Hill, M., Bioulac, B., Balzamo, E., Bezard, E., Tison, F., & Ghorayeb, I. (2009). Sleep disorders in parkinson's disease: The contribution of the MPTP non-human primate model. *Experimental Neurology, 219*(2), 574–582. https://doi.org/10.1016/j.expneurol.2009.07.019

Berg, D., Postuma, R. B., Adler, C. H., Bloem, B. R., Chan, P., Dubois, B., Gasser, T., Goetz, C. G., Halliday, G., Joseph, L., Lang, A. E., Liepelt-Scarfone, I., Litvan, I., Marek, K., Obeso, J., Oertel, W., Olanow, C. W., Poewe, W., Stern, M., & Deuschl, G. (2015). MDS research criteria for prodromal parkinson's disease. *Movement Disorders, 30*(12), 1600–1611. https://doi.org/10.1002/mds.26431

Bir, A., Sen, O., Anand, S., Khemka, V. K., Banerjee, P., Cappai, R., Sahoo, A., & Chakrabarti, S. (2014). α-synuclein-induced mitochondrial dysfunction in isolated preparation and intact cells: Implications in the pathogenesis of parkinson's disease. *Journal of Neurochemistry, 131*(6), 868–877. https://doi.org/10.1111/jnc.12966

Blauwendraat, C., Tayebi, N., Woo, E. G., Lopez, G., Fierro, L., Toffoli, M., Limbachiya, N., Hughes, D., Pitz, V., Patel, D., Vitale, D., Koretsky, M. J., Hernandez, D., Real, R., Alcalay, R. N., Nalls, M. A., Morris, H. R., Schapira, A. H. V., Balwani, M., & Sidransky, E. (2023). Polygenic parkinson's disease genetic risk score as risk modifier of parkinsonism in gaucher disease. *Movement Disorders, 38*(5), 899–903. https://doi.org/10.1002/mds.29342

Blesa, J., Phani, S., Jackson-Lewis, V., & Przedborski, S. (2012). Classic and new animal models of parkinson's disease. *Journal of Biomedicine and Biotechnology, 2012*, 1–10. https://doi.org/10.1155/2012/845618

Blesa, J., & Przedborski, S. (2014). .Parkinson's disease: Animal models and dopaminergic cell vulnerability. *Frontiers in Neuroanatomy, 8*, 155.

Bloem, B. R., Okun, M. S., & Klein, C. (2021). Parkinson's disease. *Lancet, 397*, 2284–2303.

Bonnet, A.-M. (2000). Involvement of non-dopaminergic pathways in parkinson???s disease. *CNS Drugs, 13*(5), 351–364. https://doi.org/10.2165/00023210-200013050-00005

Bose, A., Petsko, G. A., & Studer, L. (2022). Induced pluripotent stem cells: A tool for modeling parkinson's disease. *Trends in Neurosciences, 45*, 608–620.

Bougea, A., Koros, C., Stamelou, M., Simitsi, A., Papagiannakis, N., Antonelou, R., Papadimitriou, D., Breza, M., Tasios, K., Fragkiadaki, S., Geronicola Trapali, X., Bourbouli, M., Koutsis, G., Papageorgiou, S. G., Kapaki, E., Paraskevas, G. P., & Stefanis, L. (2017). Frontotemporal dementia as the presenting phenotype of p.A53T mutation carriers in the alpha-synuclein gene. *Parkinsonism & Related Disorders, 35*, 82–87. https://doi.org/10.1016/j.parkreldis.2016.12.002

Braak, H., & Braak, E. (2000). Pathoanatomy of Parkinson's disease. *Journal of Neurology, 247*(S2), II3. https://doi.org/10.1007/pl00007758

Braak, H., Del Tredici, K., Rüb, U., De Vos, R. A. I., Jansen Steur, E. N. H., & Braak, E. (2003). Staging of brain pathology related to sporadic parkinson's disease. *Neurobiology of Aging, 24*(2), 197–211. https://doi.org/10.1016/S0197-4580(02)00065-9

Bras, I. C., Dominguez-Meijide, A., Gerhardt, E., et al. (2020). Synucleinopathies: Where we are and where we need to go. *Journal of Neurochemistry, 153*(4), 433–454.

Breger, L. S., & Fuzzati Armentero, M. T. (2019). Genetically engineered animal models of parkinson's disease: From worm to rodent. *European Journal of Neuroscience, 49*, 533–560.

Calabrese, V., Santoro, A., Monti, D., Crupi, R., Di Paola, R., Latteri, S., Cuzzocrea, S., Zappia, M., Giordano, J., Calabrese, E. J., & Franceschi, C. (2018). Aging and parkinson's disease: Inflammaging, neuroinflammation and biological remodeling as key factors in pathogenesis. *Free Radical Biology and Medicine, 115*, 80–91. https://doi.org/10.1016/j.freeradbiomed.2017.10.379

Cannon, J. R., Tapias, V., Na, H. M., Honick, A. S., Drolet, R. E., & Greenamyre, J. T. (2009). A highly reproducible rotenone model of parkinson's disease. *Neurobiology of Disease, 34*(2), 279–290. https://doi.org/10.1016/j.nbd.2009.01.016

Capuano, A. W., Wilson, R. S., Honer, W. G., Petyuk, V. A., Leurgans, S. E., Yu, L., Gatchel, J. R., Arnold, S., Bennett, D. A., & Arvanitakis, Z. (2019). Brain IGFBP-5 modifies the relation of depressive symptoms to decline in cognition in older persons. *Journal of Affective Disorders, 250*, 313–318. https://doi.org/10.1016/j.jad.2019.03.051

Carvalho, M. M., Campos, F. L., Coimbra, B., Pêgo, J. M., Rodrigues, C., Lima, R., Rodrigues, A. J., Sousa, N., & Salgado, A. J. (2013). Behavioral characterization of the 6-hydroxidopamine model of parkinson's disease and pharmacological rescuing of non-motor deficits. *Molecular Neurodegeneration, 8*(1). https://doi.org/10.1186/1750-1326-8-14

Cassar, S., Adatto, I., Freeman, J. L., Gamse, J. T., Iturria, I., Lawrence, C., Muriana, A., Peterson, R. T., Van Cruchten, S., & Zon, L. I. (2020). Use of zebrafish in drug discovery toxicology. *Chemical Research in Toxicology, 33*(1), 95–118. https://doi.org/10.1021/acs.chemrestox.9b00335

Cenci, M. A., & Bjorklund, A. (2020). Animal models for preclinical Parkinson's research: An update and critical appraisal. *Progress in Brain Research, 252*, 27–59.

Chaumette, T., Lebouvier, T., Aubert, P., Lardeux, B., Qin, C., Li, Q., Accary, D., Bézard, E., Bruley Des Varannes, S., Derkinderen, P., & Neunlist, M. (2009). Neurochemical plasticity in the enteric nervous system of a primate animal model of experimental parkinsonism. *Neuro-Gastroenterology and Motility, 21*(2), 215–222. https://doi.org/10.1111/j.1365-2982.2008.01226.x

Chia, S. J., Tan, E.-K., & Chao, Y.-X. (2020). Historical perspective: Models of parkinson's disease. *International Journal of Molecular Sciences, 21*, 2464.

Choi, D. Y., Liu, M., Hunter, R. L., Cass, W. A., Pandya, J. D., Sullivan, P. G., Shin, E. J., Kim, H. C., Gash, D. M., & Bing, G. (2009). Striatal neuroinflammation promotes parkinsonism in rats. *PLoS One, 4*(5). https://doi.org/10.1371/journal.pone.0005482

Correia, G. L., Ferreira, J. J., Rosa, M. M., Coelho, M., Bonifati, V., & Sampaio, C. (2010). Worldwide frequency of G2019S LRRK2 mutation in parkinson's disease: A systematic review. *Parkinsonism Relat Disord, 16*(4), 237–242.

Correia, G. L., Reimão, S., Paulino, P., et al. (2017). Neuromelanin magnetic resonance imaging of the substantia nigra in LRRK2-related parkinson's disease. *Movement Disorders, 32*(9), 1331–1333.

Dal Ben, M., Bongiovanni, R., Tuniz, S., Fioriti, E., Tiribelli, C., Moretti, R., & Gazzin, S. (2019). Earliest mechanisms of dopaminergic neurons sufferance in a novel slow progressing Ex vivo model of parkinson disease in rat organotypic cultures of substantia nigra. *International Journal of Molecular Sciences, 20*(9), 2224. https://doi.org/10.3390/ijms20092224

Dauer, W., & Przedborski, S. (2003). Parkinson's disease: Mechanisms and models. *Neuron, 39*(6), 889–909. https://doi.org/10.1016/S0896-6273(03)00568-3

Dawson, T. M., Ko, H. S., & Dawson, V. L. (2010). Genetic animal models of parkinson's disease. *Neuron, 66*, 646–661.

De Freitas, C. M., Busanello, A., Schaffer, L. F., Peroza, L. R., Krum, B. N., Leal, C. Q., Ceretta, A. P. C., Da Rocha, J. B. T., & Fachinetto, R. (2016). Behavioral and neurochemical effects induced by reserpine in mice. *Psychopharmacology, 233*(3), 457–467. https://doi.org/10.1007/s00213-015-4118-4

Decourt, M., Jiménez-Urbieta, H., Benoit-Marand, M., & Fernagut, P. O. (2021). Neuropsychiatric and cognitive deficits in parkinson's disease and their modeling in rodents. *Biomedicines, 9*(6). https://doi.org/10.3390/biomedicines9060684

DeMaagd, G., & Philip, A. (2015). Parkinson's disease and its management part 1: Disease entity, risk factors, pathophysiology, clinical presentation, and diagnosis. *P and T, 40*(8), 504–532.

Devine, M. J., Ryten, M., Vodicka, P., Thomson, A. J., Burdon, T., Houlden, H., Cavaleri, F., Nagano, M., Drummond, N. J., Taanman, J. W., Schapira, A. H., Gwinn, K., Hardy, J., Lewis, P. A., & Kunath, T. (2011).

Parkinson's disease induced pluripotent stem cells with triplication of the α-synuclein locus. *Nature Communications, 2*(1). https://doi.org/10.1038/ncomms1453

Dickson, D. W. (2018). Neuropathology of parkinson disease. *Parkinsonism Relat Disord, 46*(Suppl. 1), S30–S33.

Dickson, D. W., Braak, H., Duda, J. E., Duyckaerts, C., Gasser, T., Halliday, G. M., Hardy, J., Leverenz, J. B., Del Tredici, K., Wszolek, Z. K., & Litvan, I. (2009). Neuropathological assessment of parkinson's disease: Refining the diagnostic criteria. *The Lancet Neurology, 8*(12), 1150–1157. https://doi.org/10.1016/S1474-4422(09)70238-8

Diotel, N., Lübke, L., Strähle, U., & Rastegar, S. (2020). Common and distinct features of adult neurogenesis and regeneration in the telencephalon of zebrafish and mammals. *Frontiers in Neuroscience, 14*. https://doi.org/10.3389/fnins.2020.568930

Do, J., McKinney, C., Sharma, P., & Sidransky, E. (2019). Glucocerebrosidase and its relevance to parkinson disease. *Molecular Neurodegeneration, 14*(1). https://doi.org/10.1186/s13024-019-0336-2

Dommershuijsen, L. J., Boon, A. J. W., & Ikram, M. K. (2021). Probing the pre-diagnostic phase of parkinson's disease in population-based studies. *Frontiers in Neurology, 12*, Article 702502.

Doppler, C. E. J., Smit, J. A. M., Hommelsen, M., Seger, A., Horsager, J., Kinnerup, M. B., Hansen, A. K., Fedorova, T. D., Knudsen, K., Otto, M., Nahimi, A., Borghammer, P., & Sommerauer, M. (2021). Microsleep disturbances are associated with noradrenergic dysfunction in parkinson's disease. *Sleep, 44*(8). https://doi.org/10.1093/sleep/zsab040

Doty, R. L. (2012). Olfaction in parkinson's disease and related disorders. *Neurobiology of Disease, 46*(3), 527–552. https://doi.org/10.1016/j.nbd.2011.10.026

Drolet, R. E., Cannon, J. R., Montero, L., & Greenamyre, J. T. (2009). Chronic rotenone exposure reproduces parkinson's disease gastrointestinal neuropathology. *Neurobiology of Disease, 36*(1), 96–102. https://doi.org/10.1016/j.nbd.2009.06.017

Drukarch, B., Jongenelen, C. A. M., Schepens, E., Langeveld, C. H., & Stoof, J. C. (1996). Glutathione is involved in the granular storage of dopamine in rat PC12 pheochromocytoma cells: Implications for the pathogenesis of parkinson's disease. *Journal of Neuroscience, 16*(19), 6038–6045. https://doi.org/10.1523/jneurosci.16-19-06038.1996

Eisinger, R., Martinez-Ramirez, D., Hess, C., Okun, M., & Gunduz, A. (2017). Changes in motor subtype designation of early parkinson's disease patients. *Movement Disorders, 32*, S1.

Ellis, L. D., & Soanes, K. H. (2012). A larval zebrafish model of bipolar disorder as a screening platform for neurotherapeutics. *Behavioural Brain Research, 233*(2), 450–457. https://doi.org/10.1016/j.bbr.2012.05.043

Feng, C. W., Wen, Z. H., Huang, S. Y., Hung, H. C., Chen, C. H., Yang, S. N., Chen, N. F., Wang, H. M., Hsiao, C. D., & Chen, W. F. (2014). Effects of 6-hydroxydopamine exposure on motor activity and biochemical expression in zebrafish (Danio rerio) larvae. *Zebrafish, 11*(3), 227–239. https://doi.org/10.1089/zeb.2013.0950

Fereshtehnejad, S. M., Romenets, S. R., Anang, J. B. M., Latreille, V., Gagnon, J. F., & Postuma, R. B. (2015). New clinical subtypes of parkinson disease and their longitudinal progression a prospective cohort comparison with other phenotypes. *JAMA Neurology, 72*(8), 863–873. https://doi.org/10.1001/jamaneurol.2015.0703

Fereshtehnejad, S. M., Zeighami, Y., Dagher, A., & Postuma, R. B. (2017). Clinical criteria for subtyping parkinson's disease: Biomarkers and longitudinal progression. *Brain, 140*(7), 1959–1976. https://doi.org/10.1093/brain/awx118

Flinn, L., Bretaud, S., Lo, C., Ingham, P. W., & Bandmann, O. (2008). Zebrafish as a new animal model for movement disorders. *Journal of Neurochemistry, 106*(5), 1991–1997. https://doi.org/10.1111/j.1471-4159.2008.05463.x

Gaceb, A., Barbariga, M., & Paul, G. (2020). An in vitro partial lesion model of differentiated human mesencephalic neurons: Effect of pericyte secretome on phenotypic markers. *J. Mol. Neurosci. MN, 70*, 1914–1925.

Gao, Y., Wilson, G. R., Stephenson, S. E. M., Oulad-Abdelghani, M., Charlet-Berguerand, N., Bozaoglu, K., McLean, C. A., Thomas, P. Q., Finkelstein, D. I., & Lockhart, P. J. (2020). Distribution of parkinson's disease associated RAB39B in mouse brain tissue. *Molecular Brain, 13*(1). https://doi.org/10.1186/s13041-020-00584-7

Gao, H. M., Zhang, F., Zhou, H., Kam, W., Wilson, B., & Hong, J. S. (2011). Neuroinflammation and α-synuclein dysfunction potentiate each other, driving chronic progression of neurodegeneration in a mouse model of parkinson's disease. *Environmental Health Perspectives, 119*(6), 807–814. https://doi.org/10.1289/ehp.1003013

Gialluisi, A., Reccia, M. G., Modugno, N., Nutile, T., Lombardi, A., Di Giovannantonio, L. G., Pietracupa, S., Ruggiero, D., Scala, S., Gambardella, S., Noyce, A. J., Kaiyrzhanov, R., Middlehurst, B., Kia, D. A., Tan, M., Houlden, H., Morris, H. R., Plun-Favreau, H., Holmans, P., ... Esposito, T. (2021). Identification of sixteen novel candidate genes for late onset Parkinson's disease. *Molecular Neurodegeneration, 16*(1). https://doi.org/10.1186/s13024-021-00455-2

Gibb, W. R., & Lees, A. J. (1988). The relevance of the lewy body to the pathogenesis of idiopathic Parkinson's disease. *Journal of Neurology Neurosurgery and Psychiatry, 51*, 745–752.

Godoy, R., Hua, K., Kalyn, M., Cusson, V. M., Anisman, H., & Ekker, M. (2020). Dopaminergic neurons regenerate following chemogenetic ablation in the olfactory bulb of adult zebrafish (Danio rerio). *Scientific Reports, 10*(1). https://doi.org/10.1038/s41598-020-69734-0

Graham, W. C., Robertson, R. G., Sambrook, M. A., & Crossman, A. R. (1990). Injection of excitatory amino acid antagonists into the medial pallidal segment of a 1-methyl-4-phenyl-1,2,3,6-tetrahydropyridine (MPTP) treated primate reverses motor symptoms of parkinsonism. *Life Sciences, 47*(18), PL91. https://doi.org/10.1016/0024-3205(90)90376-3

Greene, J. G., Noorian, A. R., & Srinivasan, S. (2009). Delayed gastric emptying and enteric nervous system dysfunction in the rotenone model of parkinson's disease. *Experimental Neurology, 218*, 154–161.

Guo, S., Qi, L., Yang, Q., & Chen, R. (2024). IGFBP5 promotes neuronal apoptosis in a 6-OHDA-Toxicant model of parkinson's disease by inhibiting the sonic hedgehog signaling pathway. *Medical Principles and Practice, 33*(3), 269–280. https://doi.org/10.1159/000538467

Gwinn, K., Devine, M. J., Jin, L. W., Johnson, J., Bird, T., Muenter, M., Waters, C., Adler, C. H., Caselli, R., Houlden, H., Lopez, G., Singleton, A., Hardy, J., & Singleton, A. (2011). Clinical features, with video documentation, of the original familial lewy body parkinsonism caused by α-synuclein triplication (Iowa kindred). *Movement Disorders, 26*(11), 2134–2136. https://doi.org/10.1002/mds.23776

Halliday, G. M., Li, Y. W., Blumbergs, P. C., Joh, T. H., Cotton, R. G. H., Howe, P. R. C., Blessing, W. W., & Geffen, L. B. (1990). Neuropathology of immunohistochemically identified brainstem neurons in parkinson's disease. *Annals of Neurology, 27*(4), 373–385. https://doi.org/10.1002/ana.410270405

Hasegawa, K., Stoessl, A. J., Yokoyama, T., Kowa, H., Wszolek, Z. K., & Yagishita, S. (2009). Familial parkinsonism: Study of original sagamihara PARK8 (I2020T) kindred with variable clinicopathologic outcomes. *Parkinsonism & Related Disorders, 15*(4), 300–306. https://doi.org/10.1016/j.parkreldis.2008.07.010

Heinzel, S., Berg, D., Gasser, T., Chen, H., Yao, C., & Postuma, R. B. (2019). Update of the MDS research criteria for prodromal parkinson's disease. *Movement Disorders, 34*(10), 1464–1470.

Henderson, M. X., Sengupta, M., Trojanowski, J. Q., & Lee, V. M. Y. (2019). Alzheimer's disease tau is a prominent pathology in LRRK2 parkinson's disease. *Acta Neuropathologica Communications, 7*(1). https://doi.org/10.1186/s40478-019-0836-x

Höglinger, G. U., Adler, C. H., Berg, D., et al. (2024). A biological classification of parkinson's disease: The SynNeurGe research diagnostic criteria. *Lancet Neurology, 23*, 191–204.

Höglinger, G. U., & Lang, A. E. (2024). SynNeurGe: The road ahead for a biological definition of Parkinson's disease. *Journal of Parkinson's Disease, 0*(0).

Hughes, A. J., Daniel, S. E., Kilford, L., & Lees, A. J. (1992). Accuracy of clinical diagnosis of idiopathic parkinson's disease: A clinico-pathological study of 100 cases. *Journal of Neurology, Neurosurgery & Psychiatry, 55*(3), 181–184. https://doi.org/10.1136/jnnp.55.3.181

Hughes, G. L., Lones, M. A., Bedder, M., Currie, P. D., Smith, S. L., & Pownall, M. E. (2020). Machine learning discriminates a movement disorder in a zebrafish model of Parkinson's disease. *DMM Disease Models and Mechanisms, 13*(10). https://doi.org/10.1242/dmm.045815

Hunter, R. L., Cheng, B., Choi, D. Y., Liu, M., Liu, S., Cass, W. A., & Bing, G. (2009). Intrastriatal lipopolysaccharide injection induces parkinsonism in C57/B6 mice. *Journal of Neuroscience Research, 87*(8), 1913–1921. https://doi.org/10.1002/jnr.22012

Hunter, R. L., Dragicevic, N., Seifert, K., Choi, D. Y., Liu, M., Kim, H. C., Cass, W. A., Sullivan, P. G., & Bing, G. (2007). Inflammation induces mitochondrial dysfunction and dopaminergic neurodegeneration in the nigrostriatal system. *Journal of Neurochemistry, 100*(5), 1375–1386. https://doi.org/10.1111/j.1471-4159.2006.04327.x

Hunter, R., Ojha, U., Bhurtel, S., Bing, G., & Choi, D. Y. (2017). Lipopolysaccharide-induced functional and structural injury of the mitochondria in the nigrostriatal pathway. *Neuroscience Research, 114*, 62–69. https://doi.org/10.1016/j.neures.2016.09.007

Ibanez, L., Dube, U., Saef, B., Budde, J., Black, K., Medvedeva, A., Del-Aguila, J. L., Davis, A. A., Perlmutter, J. S., Harari, O., Benitez, B. A., & Cruchaga, C. (2017). Parkinson disease polygenic risk score is associated with parkinson disease status and age at onset but not with alpha-synuclein cerebrospinal fluid levels. *BMC Neurology, 17*(1). https://doi.org/10.1186/s12883-017-0978-z

Innos, J., & Hickey, M. A. (2021). Using rotenone to model parkinson's disease in mice: A review of the role of pharmacokinetics. *Chemical Research in Toxicology, 34*(5), 1223–1239. https://doi.org/10.1021/acs.chemrestox.0c00522

Irwin, D. J., Grossman, M., Weintraub, D., Hurtig, H. I., Duda, J. E., Xie, S. X., Lee, E. B., Deerlin, V. M Van, Lopez, O. L., Kofler, J. K., Nelson, P. T., Jicha, G. A., Woltjer, R., Quinn, J. F., Kaye, J., Leverenz, J. B., Tsuang, D., Longfellow, K., Yearout, D., … Trojanowski, J. Q. (2017). Neuropathological and genetic correlates of survival and dementia onset in synucleinopathies: A retrospective analysis. *The Lancet Neurology, 16*(1), 55–65. https://doi.org/10.1016/s1474-4422(16)30291-5

Jang, H. J., & Chung, K. C. (2022). The ubiquitin–proteasome system and autophagy mutually interact in neurotoxin-induced dopaminergic cell death models of parkinson's disease. *FEBS Letters, 596*(22), 2898–2913. https://doi.org/10.1002/1873-3468.14479

Jankovic, J., McDermott, M., Carter, J., Gauthier, S., Goetz, C., Golbe, L., Huber, S., Koller, W., Olanow, C., Shoulson, I., Stern, M., Tanner, C., & Weiner, W. (1990). Variable expression of parkinson's disease: A baseline analysis of the DAT ATOP cohort. *Neurology, 40*(10). https://doi.org/10.1212/WNL.40.10.1529, 1529–1529.

Jayanti, S., Dalla Verde, C., Tiribelli, C., Gazzin, S., & Inflammation. (2023). Dopaminergic brain and bilirubin. *International Journal of Molecular Sciences, 24*(14), Article 11478. https://doi.org/10.3390/ijms241411478

Jayanti, S., Moretti, R., Tiribelli, C., & Gazzin, S. (2022). Bilirubin prevents the TH+ dopaminergic neuron loss in a parkinson's disease model by acting on TNF-α. *International Journal of Molecular Sciences, 23*(22), Article 14276. https://doi.org/10.3390/ijms232214276

Jellinger, K. (1987). Overview of morphological changes in parkinson's disease. *Advances in Neurology, 45*, 1–18.

Jellinger, K. A. (2019). Neuropathology and pathogenesis of extrapyramidal movement disorders: A critical update. II. Hyperkinetic disorders. *Journal of Neural Transmission, 126*(8), 997–1027.

Johnson, M. E., & Bobrovskaya, L. (2015). An update on the rotenone models of parkinson's disease: Their ability to reproduce the features of clinical disease and model gene-environment interactions. *NeuroToxicology, 46*, 101–116. https://doi.org/10.1016/j.neuro.2014.12.002

Kang, H. W., Han, B. S., Kim, S. J., & Oh, Y. J. (2012). Mechanisms to prevent caspase activation in rotenone-induced dopaminergic neurodegeneration: Role of ATP depletion and procaspase-9 degradation. *Apoptosis, 17*(5), 449–462. https://doi.org/10.1007/s10495-012-0699-0

Khan, E., Hasan, I., & Haque, M. E. (2023). Parkinson's disease: Exploring different animal model systems. *International Journal of Molecular Sciences, 24*, 9088.

Kim, H. J., & Jin, C. Y. (2012). Stem cells in drug screening for neurodegenerative disease. *Korean Journal of Physiology and Pharmacology, 16*(1), 1–9. https://doi.org/10.4196/kjpp.2012.16.1.1

Kishi, S. (2004). Functional aging and gradual senescence in zebrafish. *Annals of the New York Academy of Sciences, 1019*, 521–526. https://doi.org/10.1196/annals.1297.097

Klaestrup, I. H., Just, M. K., Holm, K. L., Alstrup, A. K. O., Romero-Ramos, M., Borghammer, P., & Van Den Berge, N. (2022). Impact of aging on animal models of parkinson's disease. *Frontiers in Aging Neuroscience, 14*, Article 909273.

Kluss, J. H., Mamais, A., & Cookson, M. R. (2019). LRRK2 links genetic and sporadic parkinson's disease. *Biochemical Society Transactions, 47*(2), 651–661.

Knap, B., Nieoczym, D., Kundap, U., Kusio-Targonska, K., Kukula-Koch, W., Turski, W. A., & Gawel, K. (2023). Zebrafish as a robust preclinical platform for screening plant-derived drugs with anticonvulsant properties—a review. *Frontiers in Molecular Neuroscience, 16*. https://doi.org/10.3389/fnmol.2023.1221665

Konnova, E. A., & Swanberg, M. (2018). *Animal models of parkinson's disease parkinson's disease: Pathogenesis and clinical aspects*. Sweden: Exon Publications. https://doi.org/10.15586/codonpublications.parkinsonsdisease.2018.ch5

Koros, C., Stamelou, M., Simitsi, A., Beratis, I., Papadimitriou, D., Papagiannakis, N., Fragkiadaki, S., Kontaxopoulou, D., Papageorgiou, S. G., & Stefanis, L. (2018). Selective cognitive impairment and hyposmia in p.A53T SNCA PD vs typical PD. *Neurology, 90*(10). https://doi.org/10.1212/wnl.0000000000005063

Kozol, R. A., Abrams, A. J., James, D. M., Buglo, E., Yan, Q., & Dallman, J. E. (2016). Function over form: Modeling groups of inherited neurological conditions in zebrafish. *Frontiers in Molecular Neuroscience, 9*. https://doi.org/10.3389/fnmol.2016.00055

Kroener, S., Chandler, J. L., Phillips, P. E. M., & Seamans, J. K. (2009). Dopamine modulates persistent synaptic activity and enhances the signal-to-noise ratio in the prefrontal cortex. *PLoS One, 4*(8). https://doi.org/10.1371/journal.pone.0006507

Lai, D., Alipanahi, B., Fontanillas, P., et al. (2021a). Genomewide association studies of LRRK2 modifiers of parkinson's disease. *Annals of Neurology, 90*(1), 76–88.

Lai, T. T., Kim, Y. J., Nguyen, P. T., Koh, Y. H., Nguyen, T. T., Ma, H. I., & Kim, Y. E. (2021b). Temporal evolution of inflammation and neurodegeneration with alpha-synuclein propagation in parkinson's disease mouse model. *Frontiers in Integrative Neuroscience*, 15. https://doi.org/10.3389/fnint.2021.715190

Lam, C. S., Korzh, V., & Strahle, U. (2005). Zebrafish embryos are susceptible to the dopaminergic neurotoxin MPTP. *European Journal of Neuroscience, 21*, 1758–1762.

Lama, Buhidma, Fletcher, & Duty. (2021). Animal models of parkinson's disease: A guide to selecting the optimal model for your research. *Neuronal Signaling, 5*.

Lebowitz, J. J., & Khoshbouei, H. (2020). Heterogeneity of dopamine release sites in health and degeneration. *Neurobiology of Disease, 134*, Article 104633. https://doi.org/10.1016/j.nbd.2019.104633

Lee, H. J., Patel, S., & Lee, S. J. (2005). Intravesicular localization and exocytosis of α-synuclein and its aggregates. *Journal of Neuroscience, 25*(25), 6016–6024.

Lees, A. J. (2009). The parkinson chimera. *Neurology, 72*(Issue 7, Suppl. 2), S2. https://doi.org/10.1212/WNL.0b013e318198daec

Lesage, S., Drouet, V., Majounie, E., Vincent, D., Jacoupy, M., Nicolas, A., Cormier-Dequaire, F., Hassoun, S. M., Pujol, C., Ciura, S., Erpapazoglou, Z., Usenko, T., Maurage, C.-A., Sahbatou, M., Liebau, S., Ding, J., Bilgic, B., Emre, M., Erginel-Unaltuna, N., … Brice, A. (2016). Loss of VPS13C function in autosomal-recessive parkinsonism causes mitochondrial dysfunction and increases PINK1/Parkin-Dependent mitophagy. *The American Journal of Human Genetics, 98*(3), 500–513. https://doi.org/10.1016/j.ajhg.2016.01.014

Lev, N., Barhum, Y., Ben-Zur, T., Melamed, E., Steiner, I., & Offen, D. (2013). Knocking out DJ-1 attenuates astrocytes neuroprotection against 6-Hydroxydopamine toxicity. *Journal of Molecular Neuroscience, 50*(3), 542–550. https://doi.org/10.1007/s12031-013-9984-9

Levy, R., Herrero, M. T., Ruberg, M., Villares, J., Faucheux, B., Guridi, J., Guillen, J., Luquin, M. R., Javoy-Agid, F., Obeso, J. A., Agid, Y., & Hirsch, E. C. (1995). Effects of nigrostriatal denervation and l-dopa therapy on the GABAergic neurons of the striatum in MPTP-treated monkeys and parkinson's disease: An in situ hybridization study of GAD 67 mRNA. *European Journal of Neuroscience, 7*(6), 1199–1209. https://doi.org/10.1111/j.1460-9568.1995.tb01110.x

Lewitt, M. S., & Boyd, G. W. (2024). Role of the insulin-like growth factor system in neurodegenerative disease. *International Journal of Molecular Sciences, 25*(8). https://doi.org/10.3390/ijms25084512

Li, X., Li, C., Zhang, W., Wang, Y., Qian, P., & Huang, H. (2023). Inflammation and aging: Signaling pathways and intervention therapies. *Signal Transduction and Targeted Therapy, 8*(1). https://doi.org/10.1038/s41392-023-01502-8

Ling, Z., Zhu, Y., Tong, C.w., Snyder, J. A., Lipton, J. W., & Carvey, P. M. (2006). Progressive dopamine neuron loss following supra-nigral lipopolysaccharide (LPS) infusion into rats exposed to LPS prenatally. *Experimental Neurology, 199*(2), 499–512. https://doi.org/10.1016/j.expneurol.2006.01.010

Lippi, A., Domingues, R., Setz, C., Outeiro, T. F., & Krisko, A. (2020). SARS-CoV-2: At the crossroad between aging and neurodegeneration. *Movement Disorders, 35*(5), 716–720. https://doi.org/10.1002/mds.28084

Lopes, U. G., Erhardt, P., Yao, R., & Cooper, G. M. (1997). p53-dependent induction of apoptosis by proteasome inhibitors. *Journal of Biological Chemistry, 272*(20), 12893–12896. https://doi.org/10.1074/jbc.272.20.12893

Lv, D.j., Li, L.x., Chen, J., Wei, S. Z., Wang, F., Hu, H., Xie, A. M., & Liu, C. F. (2019). Sleep deprivation caused a memory defects and emotional changes in a rotenone-based zebrafish model of parkinson's disease. *Behavioural Brain Research*, 372. https://doi.org/10.1016/j.bbr.2019.112031

Makhija, D. T., & Jagtap, A. G. (2014). Studies on sensitivity of zebrafish as a model organism for Parkinson's disease: Comparison with rat model. *Journal of Pharmacology and Pharmacotherapeutics, 5*(1), 39–46. https://doi.org/10.4103/0976-500X.124422

Mann, D. M. A., & Yates, P. O. (1983). Pathological basis for neurotransmitter changes in Parkinson's disease. *Neuropathology and Applied Neurobiology, 9*(1), 3–19. https://doi.org/10.1111/j.1365-2990.1983.tb00320.x

Mantri, S., Morley, J. F., & Siderowf, A. D. (2019). The importance of preclinical diagnostics in parkinson disease. *Parkinsonism Relat. Disord., 64*, 20–28.

Marvian, A. T., Koss, D. J., Aliakbari, F., Morshedi, D., & Outeiro, T. F. (2019). Vitro models of synucleinopathies: Informing on molecular mechanisms and protective strategies. *Journal of Neurochemistry, 150*(5), 535–565. https://doi.org/10.1111/jnc.14707

Masilamoni, G. J., & Smith, Y. (2018). Chronic MPTP administration regimen in monkeys: A model of dopaminergic and non-dopaminergic cell loss in Parkinson's disease. *Journal of Neural Transmission, 125*(3), 337–363. https://doi.org/10.1007/s00702-017-1774-z

Mata, I. F., Lockhart, P. J., & Farrer, M. J. (2004). Parkin genetics: One model for parkinson's disease. *Human Molecular Genetics, 13*, R127–R133.

McAleese, K. E., Colloby, S. J., Thomas, A. J., Al-Sarraj, S., Ansorge, O., Neal, J., Roncaroli, F., Love, S., Francis, P. T., & Attems, J. (2021). Concomitant neurodegenerative pathologies contribute to the transition from mild cognitive impairment to dementia. *Alzheimer's & Dementia, 17*(7), 1121–1133. https://doi.org/10.1002/alz.12291

Mehanna, R., Smilowska, K., Fleisher, J., Post, B., Hatano, T., Piemonte, M. E. P., Raj Kumar, K., McConvey, V., Zhang, B., Tan, E.-K., & Savica, R. (2022). Age cutoff for early-onset parkinson's disease: Recommendations from the international parkinson and movement disorder society task force on early onset parkinson's disease. *Movement Disorders Clinical Practice, 9*(7), 869–878. https://doi.org/10.1002/mdc3.13523

Meredith, G. E., Sonsalla, P. K., & Chesselet, M.-F. (2008). Animal models of parkinson's disease progression. *Acta Neuropathologica, 115*, 385–398.

Mestre, T. A., Eberly, S., Tanner, C., Grimes, D., Lang, A. E., Oakes, D., & Marras, C. (2018). Reproducibility of data-driven parkinson's disease subtypes for clinical research. *Parkinsonism & Related Disorders, 56*, 102–106. https://doi.org/10.1016/j.parkreldis.2018.07.009

Milanese, C., Sager, J. J., Bai, Q., Farrell, T. C., Cannon, J. R., Greenamyre, J. T., & Burton, E. A. (2012). Hypokinesia and reduced dopamine levels in zebrafish lacking β- and γ1-Synucleins. *Journal of Biological Chemistry, 287*, 2971–2983.

Mirelman, A., Saunders-Pullman, R., Alcalay, R. N., Shustak, S., Thaler, A., Gurevich, T., Raymond, D., Mejia-Santana, H., Orbe Reilly, M., Ozelius, L., Clark, L., Gana-Weisz, M., Bar-Shira, A., Orr-Utreger, A., Bressman, S. B., Marder, K., & Giladi, N. (2018). Application of the movement disorder society prodromal criteria in healthy G2019S-LRRK2 carriers. *Movement Disorders, 33*(6), 966–973. https://doi.org/10.1002/mds.27342

Miyazaki, I., & Asanuma, M. (2020). The rotenone models reproducing central and peripheral features of parkinson's disease. *NeuroSci, 1*(1), 1–14. https://doi.org/10.3390/neurosci1010001

Morfis, L., & Cordato, D. J. (2006). Dementia with lewy bodies in an elderly Greek male due to α-synuclein gene mutation. *Journal of Clinical Neuroscience, 13*(9), 942–944.

Mustapha, M., & Taib, C. N. M. (2021). MPTP-induced mouse model of Parkinson's disease: A promising direction for therapeutic strategies. *Bosnian Journal of Basic Medical Sciences, 21*(4), 422–433. https://doi.org/10.17305/bjbms.2020.5181

Muthane, U. B., Swamy, H. S., Satishchandra, P., Subhash, M. N., Rao, S., & Subbakrishna, D. (1994). Early onset parkinson's disease: Are juvenile- and young-onset different? *Movement Disorders, 9*(5), 539–544. https://doi.org/10.1002/mds.870090506

Müller, M. L. T. M., & Bohnen, N. I. (2013). Cholinergic dysfunction in parkinson's disease. *Current Neurology and Neuroscience Reports, 13*, 377.

Nair, V. D., McNaught, K. S. P., González-Maeso, J., Sealfon, S. C., & Olanow, C. W. (2006). p53 mediates nontranscriptional cell death in dopaminergic cells in response to proteasome inhibition. *Journal of Biological Chemistry, 281*(51), 39550–39560. https://doi.org/10.1074/jbc.M603950200

Nalls, M. A., Blauwendraat, C., Vallerga, C. L., Heilbron, K., Bandres-Ciga, S., Chang, D., Tan, M., Kia, D. A., Noyce, A. J., Xue, A., Bras, J., Young, E., von Coelln, R., Simón-Sánchez, J., Schulte, C., Sharma, M., Krohn, L., Pihlstrøm, L., Siitonen, A., … Zhang, F. (2019). Identification of novel risk loci, causal insights, and heritable risk for parkinson's disease: A meta-analysis of genome-wide association studies. *The Lancet Neurology, 18*(12), 1091–1102. https://doi.org/10.1016/S1474-4422(19)30320-5

Neha, S., Ahmad, M., Kumari, B., Ali, M. Z., & Dholaniya, P. S. (2023). Early diagnosis of Parkinson's disease: Utility of animal models. In S. C. Yenisetti, Z. Koza, D. Kumar, S. K. Singh, & A. Ganeshpurkar (Eds.), *Parkinson's disease - animal models, current therapies and clinical trials*. IntechOpen. https://doi.org/10.5772/intechopen.107887

Nelson, P. T., Dickson, D. W., Trojanowski, J. Q., Jack, C. R., Boyle, P. A., Arfanakis, K., Rademakers, R., Alafuzoff, I., Attems, J., Brayne, C., Coyle-Gilchrist, I. T. S., Chui, H. C., Fardo, D. W., Flanagan, M. E., Halliday, G., Hokkanen, S. R. K., Hunter, S., Jicha, G. A., Katsumata, Y., … Schneider, J. A. (2019). Limbic-predominant age-related TDP-43 encephalopathy (LATE): Consensus working group report. *Brain, 142*(6), 1503–1527. https://doi.org/10.1093/brain/awz099

Nguyen, H. N., Byers, B., Cord, B., Shcheglovitov, A., Byrne, J., Gujar, P., Kee, K., Schüle, B., Dolmetsch, R. E., Langston, W., Palmer, T. D., & Pera, R. R. (2011). LRRK2 mutant iPSC-derived da neurons demonstrate increased susceptibility to oxidative stress. *Cell Stem Cell, 8*(3), 267–280. https://doi.org/10.1016/j.stem.2011.01.013

O'Donnell, K. C., Lulla, A., Stahl, M. C., Wheat, N. D., Bronstein, J. M., & Sagasti, A. (2014). Axon degeneration and PGC-1α-mediated protection in a zebrafish model of α-synuclein toxicity. *DMM Disease Models and Mechanisms, 7*(5), 571–582. https://doi.org/10.1242/dmm.013185

Outeiro, T. F., Alcalay, R. N., Antonini, A., Attems, J., Bonifati, V., Cardoso, F., Chesselet, M. F., Hardy, J., Madeo, G., McKeith, I., Mollenhauer, B., Moore, D. J., Rascol, O., Schlossmacher, M. G., Soreq, H., Stefanis, L., & Ferreira, J. J. (2023). Defining the riddle in order to solve it: There is more than one "Parkinson's Disease". *Movement Disorders, 38*(7), 1127–1142. https://doi.org/10.1002/mds.29419

Paisan-Ruiz, C., Li, A., Schneider, S. A., et al. (2012). Widespread lewy body and tau accumulation in childhood and adult onset dystonia-parkinsonism cases with PLA2G6 mutations. *Neurobiology of Aging, 33*(4), 814–823.

Papadimitriou, D., Antonelou, R., Miligkos, M., Maniati, M., Papagiannakis, N., Bostantjopoulou, S., Leonardos, A., Koros, C., Simitsi, A., Papageorgiou, S. G., Kapaki, E., Alcalay, R. N., Papadimitriou, A., Athanassiadou, A., Stamelou, M., & Stefanis, L. (2016). Motor and nonmotor features of carriers of the p. A53T alpha-synuclein mutation: A longitudinal study. *Movement Disorders, 31*(8), 1226–1230. https://doi.org/10.1002/mds.26615

Parkinson, J. (2002). An essay on the shaking palsy. *Journal of Neuropsychiatry, 14*(2), 223–236. https://doi.org/10.1176/appi.neuropsych.14.2.223

Paul, K. C., Schulz, J., Bronstein, J. M., Lill, C. M., & Ritz, B. R. (2018). Association of polygenic risk score with cognitive decline and motor progression in parkinson disease. *JAMA Neurology, 75*(3), 360–366. https://doi.org/10.1001/jamaneurol.2017.4206

Perez-Alvarez, S., Solesio, M. E., Manzanares, J., Jordán, J., & Galindo, M. F. (2009). Lactacystin requires reactive oxygen species and bax redistribution to induce mitochondria-mediated cell death. *British Journal of Pharmacology, 158*(4), 1121–1130. https://doi.org/10.1111/j.1476-5381.2009.00388.x

Pilotto, A., Heinzel, S., Suenkel, U., Lerche, S., Brockmann, K., Roeben, B., Schaeffer, E., Wurster, I., Yilmaz, R., Scarfone, I. L., von Thaler, A.-K., Metzger, F. G., Eschweiler, G. W., Postuma, R. B., Maetzler, W., & Berg, D. (2017). Application of the movement disorder society prodromal parkinson's disease research criteria in 2 independent prospective cohorts. *Movement Disorders, 32*(7), 1025–1034. https://doi.org/10.1002/mds.27035

Pingale, T., & Gupta, G. L. (2020). Classic and evolving animal models in parkinson's disease. *Pharmacology Biochemistry and Behavior, 199*, Article 173060. https://doi.org/10.1016/j.pbb.2020.173060

Poewe, W., Seppi, K., Tanner, C. M., Halliday, G. M., Brundin, P., Volkmann, J., Schrag, A. E., & Lang, A. E. (2017). Parkinson disease. *Nature Reviews Disease Primers*, (3), 1–21. https://doi.org/10.1038/nrdp.2017.13

Polymeropoulos, M. H., Lavedan, C., Leroy, E., Ide, S. E., Dehejia, A., Dutra, A., Pike, B., Root, H., Rubenstein, J., Boyer, R., Stenroos, E. S., Chandrasekharappa, S., Athanassiadou, A., Papapetropoulos, T., Johnson, W. G., Lazzarini, A. M., Duvoisin, R. C., Di Iorio, G., Golbe, L. I., & Nussbaum, R. L. (1997). Mutation in the α-synuclein gene identified in families with parkinson's disease. *Science, 276*(5321), 2045–2047. https://doi.org/10.1126/science.276.5321.2045

Postuma, R. B., & Berg, D. (2016). Advances in markers of prodromal parkinson disease. *Nature Reviews Neurology, 12*(11), 622–634. https://doi.org/10.1038/nrneurol.2016.152

Postuma, R. B., Berg, D., Stern, M., Poewe, W., Olanow, C. W., Oertel, W., Obeso, J., Marek, K., Litvan, I., Lang, A. E., Halliday, G., Goetz, C. G., Gasser, T., Dubois, B., Chan, P., Bloem, B. R., Adler, C. H., & Deuschl, G. (2015). MDS clinical diagnostic criteria for parkinson's disease. *Movement Disorders, 30*(12), 1591–1601. https://doi.org/10.1002/mds.26424

Puschmann, A. (2017). New genes causing hereditary parkinson's disease or parkinsonism. *Current Neurology and Neuroscience Reports, 17*(6), 1–11.

Razali, K., Kumar, J., & Mohamed, W. M. Y. (2024). Characterizing the adult zebrafish model of parkinson's disease: A systematic review of dynamic changes in behavior and physiology post-MPTP administration. *Frontiers in Neuroscience, 18*, Article 1432102. https://doi.org/10.3389/fnins.2024.1432102

Razali, K., Mohd Nasir, M. H., Kumar, J., & Mohamed, W. M. Y. (2023). Mitophagy: A bridge linking HMGB1 and Parkinson's disease using adult zebrafish as a model organism. *Brain Sciences, 13*(7), 1076. https://doi.org/10.3390/brainsci13071076

Razali, K., Mohd Nasir, M. H., Othman, N., Doolaanea, A. A., Kumar, J., Ibrahim, W. N., & Mohamed, W. M. Y. (2022). Characterization of neurobehavioral pattern in a zebrafish 1-methyl-4-phenyl-1,2,3,6-tetrahydropyridine (MPTP)-induced model: A 96-hour behavioral study. *PLoS One, 17*(10), Article e0274844. https://doi.org/10.1371/journal.pone.0274844

Razali, K., Othman, N., Mohd Nasir, M. H., Doolaanea, A. A., Kumar, J., Ibrahim, W. N., Mohamed Ibrahim, N., & Mohamed, W. M. Y. (2021). The promise of the zebrafish model for parkinson's disease: Today's science and tomorrow's treatment. *Frontiers in Genetics, 12*. https://doi.org/10.3389/fgene.2021.655550

Rietdijk, C. D., Perez-Pardo, P., Garssen, J., van Wezel, R. J. A., & Kraneveld, A. D. (2017). Exploring braak's hypothesis of Parkinson'S disease. *Frontiers in Neurology, 8*. https://doi.org/10.3389/fneur.2017.00037

Robea, M. A., Balmus, I. M., Ciobica, A., Strungaru, S., Plavan, G., Gorgan, L. D., Savuca, A., & Nicoara, M. (2020). Parkinson's disease-induced zebrafish models: Focussing on oxidative stress implications and sleep processes. *Oxidative Medicine and Cellular Longevity, 2020*. https://doi.org/10.1155/2020/1370837

Rocha, S. M., Bantle, C. M., Aboellail, T., Chatterjee, D., Smeyne, R. J., & Tjalkens, R. B. (2022). Rotenone induces regionally distinct α-synuclein protein aggregation and activation of glia prior to loss of dopaminergic neurons in C57Bl/6 mice. *Neurobiology of Disease, 167*. https://doi.org/10.1016/j.nbd.2022.105685

Rodrigues, L. S., Targa, A. D. S., Noseda, A. C. D., Aurich, M. F., Da Cunha, C., & Lima, M. M. S. (2014). Olfactory impairment in the rotenone model of parkinson's disease is associated with bulbar dopaminergic D2 activity after REM sleep deprivation. *Frontiers in Cellular Neuroscience, 8*. https://doi.org/10.3389/fncel.2014.00383

Russo, T., & Riessland, M. (2022). Age-Related midbrain inflammation and senescence in parkinson's disease. *Frontiers in Aging Neuroscience, 14*, Article 917797.

Sacino, A. N., Brooks, M., McKinney, A. B., Thomas, M. A., Shaw, G., Golde, T. E., & Giasson, B. I. (2014). Brain injection of α-synuclein induces multiple proteinopathies, gliosis, and a neuronal injury marker. *J. Neurosci. Off. J. Soc. Neurosci., 34*, 12368–12378.

Sacino, A. N., Brooks, M., Thomas, M. A., McKinney, A. B., Lee, S., Regenhardt, R. W., McGarvey, N. H., Ayers, J. I., Notterpek, L., Borchelt, D. R., et al. (2014). Intramuscular injection of α-synuclein induces CNS α-synuclein pathology and a rapid-onset motor phenotype in transgenic mice. *Proceedings of the National Academy of Sciences, 111*, 10732–10737.

Sallinen, V., Kolehmainen, J., Priyadarshini, M., Toleikyte, G., Chen, Y. C., & Panula, P. (2010). Dopaminergic cell damage and vulnerability to MPTP in Pink1 knockdown zebrafish. *Neurobiology of Disease, 40*(1), 93–101. https://doi.org/10.1016/j.nbd.2010.06.001

Sarath Babu, N., Murthy, C. L. N., Kakara, S., Sharma, R., Brahmendra Swamy, C. V., & Idris, M. M. (2016). 1-Methyl-4-phenyl-1,2,3,6-tetrahydropyridine induced parkinson's disease in zebrafish. *Proteomics, 16*(9), 1407–1420. https://doi.org/10.1002/pmic.201500291

Sardi, S. P., & Simuni, T. (2019). New era in disease modification in parkinson's disease: Review of genetically targeted therapeutics. *Parkinsonism Relat Disord, 59*, 32–38.

Schrag, A., Ben-Shlomo, Y., Brown, R., Marsden, C. D., & Quinn, N. (1998). Young-onset parkinson's disease revisited - Clinical features, natural history, and mortality. *Movement Disorders, 13*(6), 885–894. https://doi.org/10.1002/mds.870130605

Simuni, T., Chahine, L. M., Poston, K., Brumm, M., Buracchio, T., Campbell, M., Chowdhury, S., Coffey, C., Concha-Marambio, L., Dam, T., DiBiaso, P., Foroud, T., Frasier, M., Gochanour, C., Jennings, D., Kieburtz, K., Kopil, C. M., Merchant, K., Mollenhauer, B., … Marek, K. (2024). A biological definition of neuronal α-synuclein disease: Towards an integrated staging system for research. *The Lancet Neurology, 23* (2), 178–190. https://doi.org/10.1016/S1474-4422(23)00405-2

Simuni, T., Merchant, K., Brumm, M. C., Cho, H., Caspell-Garcia, C., Coffey, C. S., Chahine, L. M., Alcalay, R. N., Nudelman, K., Foroud, T., Mollenhauer, B., Siderowf, A., Tanner, C., Iwaki, H., Sherer, T., Marek, K., Siderowf, A., Seibyl, J., Coffey, C., … Tauscher, J. (2022). Longitudinal clinical and biomarker characteristics of non-manifesting LRRK2 G2019S carriers in the PPMI cohort. *Npj Parkinson's Disease, 8* (1). https://doi.org/10.1038/s41531-022-00404-w

Singleman, C., & Holtzman, N. G. (2014). Growth and maturation in the zebrafish, danio rerio: A staging tool for teaching and research. *Zebrafish, 11*(4), 396–406. https://doi.org/10.1089/zeb.2014.0976

Spires-Jones, T. L., Attems, J., & Thal, D. R. (2017). Interactions of pathological proteins in neurodegenerative diseases. *Acta Neuropathologica, 134*(2), 187–205.

Takanashi, M., Funayama, M., Matsuura, E., Yoshino, H., Li, Y., Tsuyama, S., Takashima, H., Nishioka, K., & Hattori, N. (2018). Isolated nigral degeneration without pathological protein aggregation in autopsied brains with LRRK2 p.R1441H homozygous and heterozygous mutations. *Acta Neuropathologica Communications, 6*(1), 105. https://doi.org/10.1186/s40478-018-0617-y

Tang, L., Xu, N., Huang, M., Yi, W., Sang, X., Shao, M., Li, Y., Zhao-zhe, H., Liu, R., Shen, Y., Yue, F., Liu, X., Xu, C., & Liu, S. (2023). A primate nigrostriatal atlas of neuronal vulnerability and resilience in a model of Parkinson's disease. *Nature Communications, 14*(1). https://doi.org/10.1038/s41467-023-43213-2

Tay, T. L., Ronneberger, O., Ryu, S., Nitschke, R., & Driever, W. (2011). Comprehensive catecholaminergic projectome analysis reveals single-neuron integration of zebrafish ascending and descending dopaminergic systems. *Nature Communications, 2*(1). https://doi.org/10.1038/ncomms1171

Thomas Broome, S., & Castorina, A. (2022). Systemic rotenone administration causes extra-nigral alterations in C57BL/6 mice. *Biomedicines, 10*, 3174.

Tieu, K. (2011). A guide to neurotoxic animal models of parkinson's disease. *Cold Spring Harbor Perspectives in Medicine, 1*(1), Article a009316. https://doi.org/10.1101/cshperspect.a009316

Tolosa, E., Wenning, G., & Poewe, W. (2006). The diagnosis of parkinson's disease. *Lancet Neurology, 5*(1), 75–86.

Ullrich, C., & Humpel, C. (2009). Rotenone induces cell death of cholinergic neurons in an organotypic Co-Culture brain slice model. *Neurochemical Research, 34*(12), 2147–2153. https://doi.org/10.1007/s11064-009-0014-9

Vacchi, E., Senese, C., Chiaro, G., Disanto, G., Pinton, S., Morandi, S., Bertaina, I., Bianco, G., Staedler, C., Galati, S., Gobbi, C., Kaelin-Lang, A., & Melli, G. (2021). Alpha-synuclein oligomers and small nerve fiber pathology in skin are potential biomarkers of Parkinson's disease. *Npj Parkinson's Disease, 7*(1). https://doi.org/10.1038/s41531-021-00262-y

Van Der Heeden, J. F., Marinus, J., Martinez-Martin, P., Rodriguez-Blazquez, C., Geraedts, V. J., & Van Hilten, J. J. (2016). Postural instability and gait are associated with severity and prognosis of parkinson disease. *Neurology, 86*(24), 2243–2250. https://doi.org/10.1212/WNL.0000000000002768

Van Laar, A. D., Webb, K. R., Keeney, M. T., Van Laar, V. S., Zharikov, A., Burton, E. A., Hastings, T. G., Glajch, K. E., Hirst, W. D., Greenamyre, J. T., & Rocha, E. M. (2023). Transient exposure to rotenone causes degeneration and progressive parkinsonian motor deficits, neuroinflammation, and synucleinopathy. *Npj Parkinson's Disease, 9*(1). https://doi.org/10.1038/s41531-023-00561-6

Van Rompuy, A. S., Lobbestael, E., Van der Perren, A., Van den Haute, C., & Baekelandt, V. (2014). Long-term overexpression of human wild-type and T240R mutant parkin in rat substantia nigra induces progressive dopaminergic neurodegeneration. *Journal of neuropathology and experimental neurology, 73*(2), 159–174.

Vaz, R. L., Outeiro, T. F., & Ferreira, J. J. (2018). Zebrafish as an animal model for drug discovery in parkinson's disease and other movement disorders: A systematic review. *Frontiers in Neurology, 9*, 347.

Vaz, R. L., Sousa, S., Chapela, D., van der Linde, H. C., Willemsen, R., Correia, A. D., Outeiro, T. F., & Afonso, N. D. (2020). Identification of antiparkinsonian drugs in the 6-hydroxydopamine zebrafish model. *Pharmacology Biochemistry and Behavior, 189*. https://doi.org/10.1016/j.pbb.2019.172828

Verhave, P. S., Jongsma, M. J., Van Den Berg, R. M., Vis, J. C., Vanwersch, R. A. P., Smit, A. B., Van Someren, E. J. W., & Philippens, I. H. C. H. M. (2011). REM sleep behavior disorder in the marmoset MPTP model of early parkinson disease. *Sleep, 34*(8), 1119–1125. https://doi.org/10.5665/SLEEP.1174

Vilas, D., Gelpi, E., Aldecoa, I., Grau, O., Rodriguez-Diehl, R., Jaumà, S., Martí, M. J., & Tolosa, E. (2019). Lack of central and peripheral nervous system synuclein pathology in R1441G LRRK2 -associated Parkinson's disease. *Journal of Neurology, Neurosurgery & Psychiatry, 90*(7), 832–833. https://doi.org/10.1136/jnnp-2018-318473

Visanji, N. P., Brooks, P. L., Hazrati, L.-N., & Lang, A. E. (2013). The prion hypothesis in parkinson's disease: Braak to the future. *Acta Neuropathologica Communications, 1*, 2.

Vo, Q., Gilmour, T. P., Venkiteswaran, K., Fang, J., & Subramanian, T. (2014). Polysomnographic features of sleep disturbances and rem sleep behavior disorder in the unilateral 6-OHDA lesioned hemiparkinsonian rat. *Parkinson's Disease, 2014*. https://doi.org/10.1155/2014/852965

Vollstedt, E. J., Schaake, S., Lohmann, K., et al. (2023). Embracing monogenic Parkinson's disease: The MJFF global genetic PD cohort. *Movement Disorders, 38*(2), 286–303.

Volpicelli-Daley, L. A., Abdelmotilib, H., Liu, Z., Stoyka, L., Daher, J. P. L., Milnerwood, A. J., Unni, V. K., Hirst, W. D., Yue, Z., Zhao, H. T., Fraser, K., Kennedy, R. E., & West, A. B. (2016). G2019S-LRRK2 expression augments -Synuclein sequestration into inclusions in neurons. *Journal of Neuroscience, 36*(28), 7415–7427. https://doi.org/10.1523/jneurosci.3642-15.2016

von Coelln, R., & Shulman, L. M. (2016). Clinical subtypes and genetic heterogeneity: Of lumping and splitting in parkinson disease. *Current Opinion in Neurology, 29*(6), 727–734.

Walker, L., Stefanis, L., & Attems, J. (2019). Clinical and neuropathological differences between parkinson's disease, parkinson's disease dementia and dementia with lewy bodies-current issues and future directions. *Journal of Neurochemistry, 150*(5), 467–474.

Wang, Q., Liu, Y., & Zhou, J. (2015). Neuroinflammation in parkinson's disease and its potential as therapeutic target. *Translational Neurodegeneration, 4*, 19.

Wang, A., Zhong, G., Ying, M., Fang, Z., Chen, Y., Wang, H., Wang, C., Liu, C., & Guo, Y. (2024). Inhibition of NLRP3 inflammasome ameliorates LPS-induced neuroinflammatory injury in mice via PINK1/Parkin pathway. *Neuropharmacology, 257*, Article 110063. https://doi.org/10.1016/j.neuropharm.2024.110063

Wasel, O., & Freeman, J. L. (2020). Chemical and genetic zebrafish models to define mechanisms of and treatments for dopaminergic neurodegeneration. *International Journal of Molecular Sciences, 21*(17), 5981. https://doi.org/10.3390/ijms21175981

Wider, C., Dickson, D. W., & Wszolek, Z. K. (2010). Leucine-rich repeat kinase 2 gene-associated disease: Redefining genotype-phenotype correlation. *Neurodegenerative Diseases, 7*(1–3), 175–179.

Xia, N., Cabin, D. E., Fang, F., & Reijo Pera, R. A. (2022). Parkinson's disease: Overview of transcription factor regulation, genetics, and cellular and animal models. *Frontiers in Neuroscience, 16*, Article 894620.

Xie, H., Hu, H., Chang, M., Huang, D., Gu, X., Xiong, X., Xiong, R., Hu, L., & Li, G. (2016). Identification of chaperones in a MPP+-induced and ATRA/TPA-differentiated SH-SY5Y cell PD model. *American Journal of Translational Research, 8*(12), 5659–5671.

Xu, L., Hao, L. P., Yu, J., Cheng, S. Y., Li, F., Ding, S. M., & Zhang, R. (2023). Curcumin protects against rotenone-induced parkinson's disease in mice by inhibiting microglial NLRP3 inflammasome activation and alleviating mitochondrial dysfunction. *Heliyon, 9*(5). https://doi.org/10.1016/j.heliyon.2023.e16195

Yamamoto, N., Sawada, H., Izumi, Y., Kume, T., Katsuki, H., Shimohama, S., & Akaike, A. (2007). Proteasome inhibition induces glutathione synthesis and protects cells from oxidative stress: Relevance to parkinson disease. *Journal of Biological Chemistry, 282*(7), 4364–4372. https://doi.org/10.1074/jbc.M603712200Japan

Yang, L., Zhou, R., Tong, Y., Chen, P., Shen, Y., Miao, S., & Liu, X. (2020). Neuroprotection by dihydrotestosterone in LPS-induced neuroinflammation. *Neurobiology of Disease, 140*, Article 104814. https://doi.org/10.1016/j.nbd.2020.104814

Yu, H., Sun, T., He, X., Wang, Z., Zhao, K., An, J., Wen, L., Li, J. Y., Li, W., & Feng, J. (2022). Association between parkinson's disease and diabetes mellitus: From epidemiology, pathophysiology and prevention to treatment. *Aging and Disease, 13*(6), 1591–1605. https://doi.org/10.14336/AD.2022.0325

Zeng, X.-S., Geng, W.-S., & Jia, J.-J. (2018). Neurotoxin-induced animal models of parkinson disease: Pathogenic mechanism and assessment. *ASN Neuro, 10*, 1759091418777438.

Zhang, H., Yang, J., Guo, Y., Lu, P., Gong, X., Chen, K., Li, X., & Tang, M. (2024). Rotenone-induced PINK1/Parkin-mediated mitophagy: Establishing a silkworm model for Parkinson's disease potential. *Frontiers in Molecular Neuroscience, 17*. https://doi.org/10.3389/fnmol.2024.1359294

Zhao, F., Li, C., Zhuang, Y., Yan, Y., Gao, Y., & Behnisch, T. (2024). Apoptosis signal-regulating kinase 1 (Ask1) deficiency alleviates MPP+-induced impairment of evoked dopamine release in the mouse hippocampus. *Frontiers in Cellular Neuroscience, 18*. https://doi.org/10.3389/fncel.2024.1288991

Zheng, Y., Yu, Z., Zhao, J., Cai, H., Wang, Z., Wang, X., & Feng, T. (2022). Oral mucosa derived α−Synuclein as a potential diagnostic biomarker for parkinson's disease. *Frontiers in Aging Neuroscience*, 14. https://doi.org/10.3389/fnagi.2022.867528

Further reading

Breen, D. P., & Lang, A. E. (2017). Tracking the course of prodromal parkinson's disease. *Brain, 140*, 259–262.

Caproni, S., & Colosimo, C. (2020). Diagnosis and differential diagnosis of parkinson disease. *Clinics in Geriatric Medicine, 36*, 13–24.

Hirano, S. (2021). Clinical implications for dopaminergic and functional neuroimage research in cognitive symptoms of parkinson's disease. *Molecular Medicine, 27*, 40.

Kalia, L. V., & Lang, A. E. (2015). Parkinson's disease. *Lancet, 386*, 896–912.

Klingelhoefer, L., & Reichmann, H. (2015). Pathogenesis of parkinson disease-the gut-brain axis and environmental factors. *Nature Reviews Neurology, 11*, 625–636.

Liang, L., DeLong, M. R., & Papa, S. M. (2008). Inversion of dopamine responses in striatal medium spiny neurons and involuntary movements. *Journal of Neuroscience, 28*, 7537–7547.

Moretti, R., Torre, P., & Antonello, R. M. (2013). *Parkinson's disease: Behavioural and cognitive aspects: Behavioural & cognitive aspects* (1st ed.). New York, NY, USA: Nova Biomedical.

Nieoullon, A. (2002). Dopamine and the regulation of cognition and attention. *Progress in Neurobiology, 67*, 53–83.

Noyce, A. J., Lees, A. J., & Schrag, A.-E. (2016). The prediagnostic phase of parkinson's disease. *Journal of Neurology Neurosurgery and Psychiatry, 87*, 871–878.

Sanfeliu, C., Bartra, C., Suol, C., & Rodr, guez-F. (2023). E. New insights in animal models of neurotoxicity-induced neurodegeneration. *Frontiers in Neuroscience, 17*, Article 1248727.

Savica, R., Rocca, W. A., & Ahlskog, J. E. (2010). When does parkinson disease start? *Archives of Neurology, 67*, 798–801.

Schrag, A., Horsfall, L., Walters, K., Noyce, A., & Petersen, I. (2015). Prediagnostic presentations of parkinson's disease in primary care: A case-control study. *Lancet Neurology, 14*, 57–64.

Surmeier, D. J., Obeso, J. A., & Halliday, G. M. (2017). Selective neuronal vulnerability in parkinson disease. *Nature Reviews Neuroscience, 18*, 101–113.

CHAPTER

Parkinson's disease pathogenesis: From molecular insights to novel therapies

2

Muhammad Danial Bin Che Ramli[1], Zakirah Zainal Abidin[2], Blaire Okunsai[2], Genevieve Simboh Anak Umbar[1] and Tumelo Elina Mauta[1]

[1]*Management and Science University, Department of Diagnostic and Allied Health Science, Faculty of Health and Life Sciences, Shah Alam, Malaysia;* [2]*School of Graduate Studies, Management and Science University, Shah Alam, Malaysia*

2.1 Molecular and cellular mechanisms underlying Parkinson's disease (PD)

PD is a progressive neurodegenerative disorder primarily characterized by the loss of dopaminergic neurons in the substantia nigra pars compacta (SNpc) (Airavaara et al., 2020). Although its clinical manifestations are well documented, the underlying molecular and cellular mechanisms remain incompletely understood. Mounting evidence supports multifactorial pathogenesis involving α-synuclein aggregation, mitochondrial dysfunction, oxidative stress, and chronic neuroinflammation (Gunawardena, 2025; Khvastunov et al., 2024). These pathological processes are not only interdependent but also contribute to a self-perpetuating cycle of neuronal injury. Below, we detail the major mechanistic contributors to PD pathology.

2.1.1 Mechanisms of α-synuclein misfolding and neuronal toxicity

α-Synuclein is a 140-amino acid protein predominantly localized at presynaptic terminals, where it plays a critical role in modulating synaptic plasticity, vesicle trafficking, and neurotransmitter release, particularly dopamine (Gómez-Benito et al., 2020; Man et al., 2020). Under physiological conditions, α-synuclein exists in a dynamic equilibrium between unfolded monomers and α-helical conformers associated with lipid membranes. However, in PD, this balance is disrupted, leading to pathological misfolding and aggregation of α-synuclein into β-sheet-rich structures that accumulate as insoluble fibrils (Liu et al., 2025). These fibrils constitute the core components of Lewy bodies and Lewy neurites, which are neuropathological hallmarks of PD.

The aggregation process follows a nucleation-dependent polymerization model, where α-synuclein monomers misfold and form oligomeric intermediates that serve as seeds for fibril elongation (Singh et al., 2025). Soluble oligomers are now recognized as the most neurotoxic species, even more deleterious than mature fibrils. These oligomers can insert into cellular membranes, forming pore-like

Pharmacological Foundations of Parkinson's Disease. https://doi.org/10.1016/B978-0-443-27702-3.00027-3

structures that disrupt ion homeostasis and lead to calcium dysregulation. In addition, they impair vesicle dynamics, inhibit soluble N-ethylmaleimide-sensitive fusion protein attachment protein receptors (SNARE) complex assembly, and interfere with synaptic vesicle recycling, ultimately compromising neurotransmission and neuronal survival (Burré et al., 2015; Dewitt & Rhoades, 2013).

Moreover, multiple post-translational modifications (PTMs) have been implicated in accelerating α-synuclein aggregation and toxicity. Phosphorylation at serine 129 (Ser129), which is detected in over 90% of α-synuclein in Lewy bodies, has been shown to enhance aggregation and inhibit clearance mechanisms (Fayyad et al., 2020; Jiao et al., 2025). Additionally, ubiquitination and nitration of α-synuclein further contribute to its structural instability and reduced proteasomal degradation (Liu, Balaraman, et al., 2021). On the other hand, truncation, particularly at the C-terminal domain, increases the protein's hydrophobicity and aggregation kinetics, exacerbating cellular stress (Suthar & Lee, 2023). Hence, the accumulation of misfolded α-synuclein imposes a heavy burden on the cell's proteostasis network, leading to dysfunction of both the ubiquitin-proteasome system (UPS) and the autophagy-lysosomal pathway (ALP). Normally, these systems work cooperatively to clear damaged or misfolded proteins. However, α-synuclein aggregates can block proteasomal pores, inhibit chaperone-mediated autophagy, and destabilize lysosomal membranes, resulting in a positive feedback loop where impaired clearance promotes further aggregation.

Moreover, intracellular α-synuclein aggregates have been shown to associate with mitochondrial membranes, where they impair mitochondrial respiration, reduce adenosine triphosphate (ATP) production, and increase reactive oxygen species (ROS) generation (Ludtmann et al., 2018; Perfeito et al., 2014). This mitochondrial dysfunction further amplifies oxidative stress and activates apoptotic cascades, contributing to dopaminergic neuronal degeneration. Besides, emerging evidence also suggests that α-synuclein can interfere with nuclear processes by translocating into the nucleus and interacting with histones and DNA, potentially affecting gene expression and chromatin remodeling (Jos et al., 2025). In parallel, α-synuclein aggregates can induce endoplasmic reticulum (ER) stress, activate the unfolded protein response (UPR), and trigger pro-inflammatory signaling in glial cells (Zeng et al., 2024).

In summary, α-synuclein misfolding initiates a cascade of toxic events encompassing membrane disruption, synaptic dysfunction, mitochondrial damage, oxidative stress, impaired proteostasis, and inflammation. The multifaceted nature of α-synuclein toxicity underscores its central role in PD pathogenesis and highlights the importance of targeting multiple nodes in this pathway for therapeutic intervention.

2.1.2 Prion-like propagation of α-synuclein aggregates and disease progression

One of the most transformative insights in PD research is the discovery that misfolded α-synuclein exhibits prion-like properties, enabling it to act as a pathological seed that induces misfolding of native α-synuclein molecules in adjacent cells (Schwarzman et al., 2019). This template-directed misfolding and cell-to-cell transmission of α-synuclein aggregates form the basis of a self-perpetuating cycle of neurodegeneration. Several routes of propagation have been proposed, including exosome-mediated transport, tunneling nanotubes, and trans-synaptic spread via synaptic connections (Table 2.1).

Table 2.1 Propagation mechanisms of α-Synuclein in Parkinson's disease.

Mechanism	Description	References
Exosome-mediated transport	Exosomes carry α-syn between neurons, facilitated by NOD-, LRR-, and pyrin domain-containing protein 3 (NLRP3) inflammasome.	Si et al. (2021)
Tunneling nanotubes	Direct transfer of α-syn through actin-based nanotubes connecting cells.	De Cecco and Legname (2018)
Trans-synaptic spread	Prion-like propagation through synaptically connected neurons.	Jan et al. (2021) Wang et al. (2021)
Endocytosis/Macropinocytosis	Internalization of α-syn fibrils via endocytic pathways, involving cellular prion protein (PrPC).	De Cecco and Legname (2018)
Autophagy/Exo-Endocytosis	Modulation affects α-syn transfer, indicating involvement in propagation.	Tyson et al. (2017)

This concept is in line with Braak's hypothesis, which proposes a sequential anatomical progression of Lewy pathology. According to this model, the disease may originate in the enteric nervous system or olfactory bulb and subsequently ascend to the dorsal motor nucleus of the vagus nerve, midbrain, and eventually the neocortex (Rietdijk et al., 2017). This progression reflects the clinical transition from non-motor symptoms (e.g., anosmia, constipation) to motor dysfunction and cognitive impairment. Experimental models lend strong support to this gut-origin theory. For example, peripheral administration of synthetic α-synuclein preformed fibrils (PFFs) into the intestinal wall or vagus nerve leads to α-synuclein pathology in the central nervous system (CNS) via retrograde transport (Kim et al., 2019; Liu, Guo, et al., 2021). Furthermore, truncal vagotomy has been associated with reduced PD risk, highlighting the vagus nerve as a potential conduit for disease initiation (Liu et al., 2017).

This prion-like model also underscores the role of environmental factors, gut microbiota-derived metabolites, and peripheral immune activation in modulating α-synuclein conformation and transmissibility. These findings open new avenues for early diagnostics (e.g., peripheral α-synuclein biomarkers) and preventive strategies targeting the gut-brain interface.

2.1.3 Impaired mitophagy and mitochondrial DNA mutations in dopaminergic neurons

As discussed, mitochondrial dysfunction is a central pathological feature of PD, particularly in dopaminergic neurons of the SNpc, which are highly susceptible due to their intense bioenergetic demands, pacemaking activity, and exposure to oxidative stress from dopamine metabolism. One key mechanism underlying this vulnerability is the impairment of mitophagy, a selective form of autophagy responsible for the clearance of dysfunctional mitochondria.

Mitophagy is regulated by the phosphatase and TENsin homolog (PTEN)-induced kinase 1 (PINK1) and Parkin (encoded by PRKN) pathway. Under stress conditions, PINK1 accumulates on the outer mitochondrial membrane, recruiting Parkin to ubiquitinate mitochondrial surface proteins, which signals their degradation via autophagosomes (Sekine, 2020). Loss-of-function mutations in PINK1, Parkin, and related mitophagy genes result in incomplete mitochondrial turnover, leading to the accumulation of damaged mitochondria, reduced complex I activity, and increased production of ROS (Li, Yang, et al., 2023). Additionally, somatic mitochondrial DNA (mtDNA) mutations, which accumulate with age, contribute to defective oxidative phosphorylation and further compromise cellular energy metabolism (Li et al., 2019). In PD, these mutations are found at elevated levels within dopaminergic neurons, leading to heteroplasmy, respiratory chain defects, and cell death.

Furthermore, the substantia nigra also contains neuromelanin, which binds redox-active metals like iron and copper. In the context of impaired mitophagy, the metal-neuromelanin complexes can catalyze Fenton-like reactions. These reactions involve the reduction of hydrogen peroxide (H_2O_2) by iron or copper, producing highly reactive hydroxyl radicals (•OH) (Xiao et al., 2024). The presence of these radicals can lead to significant oxidative damage to cellular components such as lipids, proteins, and DNA (Zecca et al., 2008). Collectively, mitophagy failure, mtDNA instability, and iron dysregulation form a metabolic-toxic axis that accelerates dopaminergic neuronal degeneration in PD.

2.1.4 Oxidative stress and its role in neurodegeneration

Oxidative stress represents both a driver and consequence of PD pathology, stemming primarily from mitochondrial dysfunction, dopamine metabolism, and inflammatory responses. Dopamine itself is an inherently unstable molecule that undergoes auto-oxidation, producing dopamine quinones, H_2O_2, and superoxide anions, all of which contribute to neuronal toxicity.

An imbalance between ROS generation and antioxidant defense systems leads to cumulative oxidative damage to key cellular components: (i) Lipids: Lipid peroxidation products such as 4-hydroxynonenal (4-HNE) disrupt membrane integrity and signal transduction. (ii) Proteins: Oxidative modifications impair protein folding and function. (iii) DNA: Oxidized nucleotides such as 8-hydroxydeoxyguanosine (8-OHdG) compromise genome integrity and mitochondrial function. The antioxidant response mediated by enzymes like glutathione peroxidase, superoxide dismutase (SOD), and catalase is insufficient in PD, especially with advancing age, contributing to a pro-oxidative cellular environment (Ludtmann et al., 2018; Perfeito et al., 2014). This environment facilitates α-synuclein aggregation, cytoplasmic calcium dysregulation, mitochondrial permeability transition pore (mPTP) opening, and the activation of caspase-dependent and -independent cell death pathways. Thus, oxidative stress acts as a central convergence point linking mitochondrial dysfunction, protein misfolding, and neuroinflammation in PD.

2.1.5 Role of microglial activation and peripheral immune cell infiltration

Chronic neuroinflammation is a hallmark of PD and plays a dual role as both initiator and amplifier of neurodegeneration. In response to pathological stimuli, including extracellular α-synuclein aggregates, mitochondrial debris, and oxidized molecules, microglia, the CNS-resident immune cells, undergo activation and secrete a plethora of pro-inflammatory cytokines such as TNF-α, IL-1β, IL-6, and nitric oxide. Sustained microglial activation promotes a neurotoxic phenotype (M1-like) that not only exacerbates neuronal injury but also impairs adult neurogenesis and synaptic remodeling (Tang & Le, 2016). Importantly, α-synuclein acts as a damage-associated molecular pattern (DAMP) that activates pattern recognition receptors (PRRs), including TLR2, TLR4, and NLRP3 inflammasome, thereby perpetuating the inflammatory cascade (Gąssowska-Dobrowolska et al., 2024; Haque et al., 2020; Li et al., 2019) (Kou).

Moreover, the blood–brain barrier (BBB) disruption, often observed in PD, permits peripheral immune cell infiltration, including $CD4^+$ and $CD8^+$ T lymphocytes, monocytes, and natural killer cells, further intensifying neuroinflammation (Goleij et al., 2025; Li et al., 2015). In postmortem PD brains, major histocompatibility complex (MHC) molecule class II (or a type of protein found on the surface of antigen-presenting cells like dendritic cells, macrophages, and B cells) is upregulated on microglia, indicating enhanced antigen presentation and adaptive immune involvement (Imamura et al., 2003). Overall, crosstalk between central and peripheral immunity creates a feed-forward loop of neuroinflammation, contributing to progressive dopaminergic cell loss and non-motor symptoms such as depression and fatigue.

2.1.6 Gut–brain axis and its emerging role in neuroinflammation

The gut-brain axis (GBA) has emerged as a compelling framework for understanding the peripheral origins of PD. Epidemiological data suggest that gastrointestinal disturbances, particularly constipation, precede motor symptoms by up to 2 decades, hinting at early enteric nervous system involvement (Menozzi et al., 2021). Studies have consistently shown dysbiosis in the gut microbiota of PD patients, with a shift toward pro-inflammatory bacterial strains (e.g., Enterobacteriaceae) and a reduction in butyrate-producing, anti-inflammatory commensals (e.g., *Faecalibacterium prausnitzii*) (Alam et al., 2024; Shen et al., 2021). This imbalance weakens the intestinal epithelial barrier, facilitating the translocation of microbial products such as lipopolysaccharide (LPS) into systemic circulation.

Furthermore, LPS and other endotoxins can prime microglia, stimulate peripheral immune responses, and may even trigger α-synuclein misfolding within enteric neurons (Reinert et al., 2014). Experimental evidence supports that gut-derived α-synuclein can travel retrogradely to the CNS via the vagus nerve, and interventions such as vagotomy, probiotics, or fecal microbiota transplantation (FMT) can modulate disease phenotypes in animal models (Breen et al., 2019; Kim et al., 2019). The GBA thus acts as a bidirectional conduit where gut inflammation, microbial metabolites, and peripheral immunity intersect with central neurodegenerative processes, opening novel preventive and therapeutic possibilities.

In summary, visualizing the multifactorial nature of PD pathogenesis, Fig. 2.1 illustrates the interconnected molecular and cellular mechanisms driving neurodegeneration, emphasizing the central role of α-synuclein pathology and its interplay with mitochondrial dysfunction, oxidative stress, neuroinflammation, and gut-brain axis disruption.

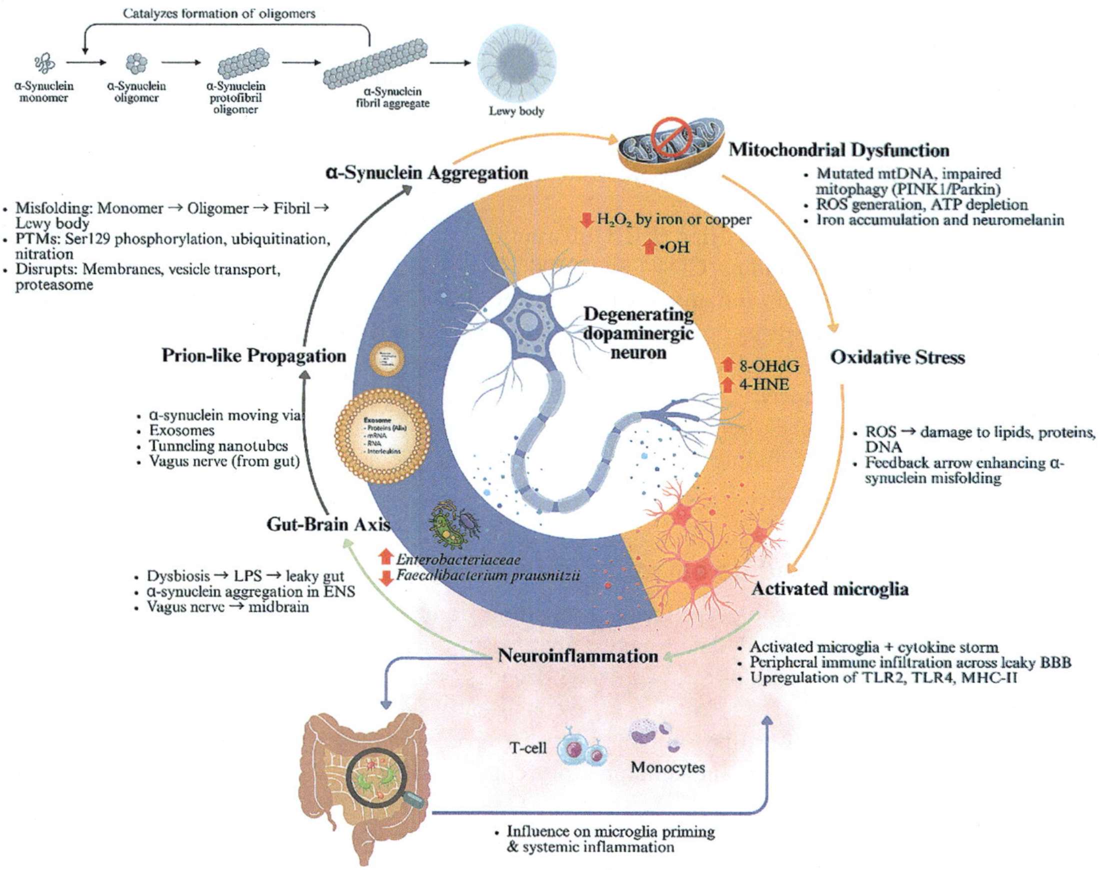

FIGURE 2.1

Integrated molecular and cellular mechanisms underlying Parkinson's disease (PD) pathogenesis. PD involves interconnected pathological processes including α-synuclein misfolding and aggregation, impaired mitochondrial dynamics and mitophagy, oxidative stress, chronic neuroinflammation, and gut-brain axis dysfunction. Misfolded α-synuclein aggregates into oligomers and fibrils, forming lewy bodies and propagating in a prion-like manner via neural and extracellular pathways. Mitochondrial dysfunction and oxidative stress exacerbate neuronal injury and promote further α-synuclein misfolding. Chronic microglial activation, peripheral immune cell infiltration, and gut-derived inflammation further perpetuate neurodegeneration. These processes form a self-sustaining cycle leading to progressive dopaminergic neuronal loss in the substantia nigra.

2.2 Genetic and epigenetic modulators of Parkinson's disease

Parkinson's disease (PD) is a multifaceted neurodegenerative disease characterized by a gradual degeneration of dopaminergic neurones in the substantia nigra pars compacta, a critical part of the brain that regulates movement (Cacabelos, 2017). Neuronal loss is often accompanied by the formation of abnormal protein clumps known as Lewy bodies, mostly made up of α-synuclein protein. This disorder is classified as a multisystemic α-synucleinopathy because it affects both the central and peripheral nervous systems through α-synuclein misfolding and aggregation (Cacabelos, 2017).

There are both genetic and epigenetic components to the multifactorial etiology of Parkinson's disease (PD), which is often triggered by environmental exposures (Ghosh & Saadat, 2023). A number of genetic mutations have been identified as being directly associated to hereditary Parkinson's disease. These include mutations in genes like SNCA (PARK1), LRRK2 (PARK8), PINK1 (PARK6), PRKN/Parkin (PARK2), and DJ-1 (PARK7) (Ghosh & Saadat, 2023). Mutations in SNCA and LRRK2 are related to autosomal dominant inheritance, whereas mutations in PINK1, PRKN, and DJ-1 are associated with autosomal recessive disorders (Paccosi & Proietti-De-Santis, 2023).

Mutations in the SNCA gene, which encodes the α-synuclein protein, play a crucial role. These mutations are hypothesized to result in a "gain-of-function", in which the abnormal protein aggregates, causing cellular damage and eventual neuronal death (Paccosi & Proietti-De-Santis, 2023). Similarly, mutations in the LRRK2 gene, which encodes a multi-domain kinase enzyme, have been identified as a substantial hereditary cause of familial and sporadic Parkinson's disease. The mutations have been shown to increase kinase activity and autophosphorylation of the enzyme, which are considered to contribute to neurodegeneration (Paccosi & Proietti-De-Santis, 2023). However, inherited genetic alterations do not account for all cases of Parkinson's disease. In fact, the substantial amount of Parkinson's disease cases is sporadic, caused by epigenetic changes, inheritable but reversible changes in gene expression that do not involve alterations to the DNA sequence (Ghosh & Saadat, 2023). These changes include DNA methylation, histone modifications, and regulation through non-coding RNAs. Together, they control how genes are turned on or off in response to signals from both inside and outside the cell, including stress, aging, nutrition, and toxins (Ghosh & Saadat, 2023).

Epigenetic modifications in Parkinson's disease have been shown to influence the expression of important genes, including SNCA. This suggests that environmental influences can influence α-synuclein synthesis and aggregation through epigenetic mechanisms (Ghosh & Saadat, 2023). For example, exposure to toxic agents such as insecticides, heavy metals, and air pollution can cause epigenetic modifications that, over time, lead to neuronal death. Such environmental cues can interact with an individual's genetic composition, increasing the likelihood of disease (a scenario known as gene-environment interaction) (Ghosh & Saadat, 2023).

Furthermore, aging, the main risk factor for Parkinson's disease, can cause progressive epigenetic dysregulation (Ghosh & Saadat, 2023). Lifestyle variables such as diet, cigarette smoking, lack of physical activity, and bad eating habits, have been found to cause epigenome modifications, affecting neurone viability and functionality. Although epigenetic modifications do not pass on to future generations, they can have a negative impact on neuronal cells by inducing protein misfolding, oxidative stress, and mitochondrial dysfunction abnormalities (Ghosh & Saadat, 2023). Such chemical disturbances eventually affect the ubiquitin-proteasome system, a critical cellular function that promotes the breakdown of abnormally folded or damaged proteins, exacerbating neurodegeneration (Ghosh & Saadat, 2023).

Finally, the development and progression of Parkinson's disease involve a complex combination of genetic mutations, epigenetic alterations, and environmental variables. Understanding how the components interact opens the door to the identification of biomarkers, early diagnostic indicators, and personalized therapy strategies that target both genetic and epigenetic pathways.

2.2.1 Monogenic forms of PD: Lessons from genetics

While the exact cause of Parkinson's disease (PD) is unknown in most cases, accumulating evidence suggests that hereditary factors play an essential role in the disease's susceptibility and progression. Those who have a first-degree relative with Parkinson's disease are two to three times more likely to develop the disorder than the general population (Tysnes & Storstein, 2017). Although the bulk of Parkinson's disease is sporadic, a tiny proportion, estimated to be between 5%–10%, can be traced to mutations in a single gene, known as monogenic or Mendelian varieties (Tysnes & Storstein, 2017).

Monogenic Parkinson's disease can emerge in a variety of inheritance pathways. Mutations in the SNCA, LRRK2, VPS35, and RAB32 genes have been related to autosomal dominant illnesses, which require only one copy of the gene mutation to induce disease (Lim & Klein, 2024). Autosomal recessive forms, which need two changed alleles (one from each parent), are associated with mutations in the PRKN (Parkin), PINK1, and DJ-1 (PARK7) genes. Importantly, mutations in the LRRK2 gene, which are particularly prevalent in some populations, can account for up to 40% of Parkinson's disease in certain communities (Tysnes & Storstein, 2017).

Though rare, monogenic variants of Parkinson's disease are extremely important for a variety of reasons. First, identifying a mutation in a single gene allows for a conclusive diagnosis within the patient's lifetime. Second, the discovery has important implications for family counseling, particularly in terms of inheritance patterns and risk to relatives (Bloem et al., 2021). Third, research into these genetic variants has helped us understand the pathophysiology of Parkinson's disease by revealing molecular pathways involving protein misfolding, mitochondrial malfunction, and cellular stress responses. Finally, monogenic PD serves as a model for the development of gene-targeted medicines, which are currently being developed and offer a step advance in personalized precision medicine for Parkinson's disease patients (Bloem et al., 2021).

Historically, researchers employed two main techniques to identify PD-related genes. Linkage analysis studies examine the inheritance of disease features and genetic markers in multigenerational families with many affected individuals. This method has proven useful for detecting rare, high-penetrance mutations (Shulman et al., 2011).

Most recently, association studies, mostly genome-wide association studies (GWAS), have been used to look at genetic variance between large groups of patients and controls. GWAS has been particularly successful in discovering common genetic variants that contribute somewhat to risk yet have incomplete penetrance (Ye et al., 2022). Nonetheless, the distinction between sporadic (non-familial) and monogenic (familial) Parkinson's disease is becoming less clear.

The majority of known sporadic cases are likewise predicted to have a genetic foundation, but with the usage of common variations with lesser penetrance or gene-environment interactions (Ye et al., 2022). For example, a person with an uncommon variation may not develop Parkinson's disease, a condition known as incomplete penetrance. Furthermore, patients with the same gene mutation may experience varying symptoms, onset ages, and progression rates. This heterogeneity implies that, even in monogenic PD, other genetic, epigenetic, or environmental variables influence disease manifestation. Importantly, because the underlying genetic changes are so clearly documented, monogenic variants of Parkinson's disease are especially accessible to study in cell culture and animal models (Blauwendraat et al., 2019).

While monogenic Parkinson's disease accounts for a small proportion of all cases, research into the disorder has produced critical insights into disease causes, diagnostic accuracy, treatment advancements, and genetic counseling (Blauwendraat et al., 2019). As we learn more about the genetic architecture of Parkinson's disease, it becomes clear that rare and common mutations account for a range of illness risk, and that familial and sporadic forms of Parkinson's disease are inextricably linked.

2.2.1.1 Key mutations in SNCA, LRRK2, PINK1, and PARKIN

Parkinson's disease (PD) has a variety of causes, including genetic traits, environmental exposures, and aging. In terms of genetic reasons, multiple major genes have been identified that, when mutated, result in monogenic Parkinson's disease. These include the autosomal dominant genes SNCA and LRRK2, as well as the autosomal recessive genes PINK1 and PARKIN (PRKN) (Cacabelos, 2017). Although these mutations account for just a small proportion of all cases of Parkinson's disease, they give invaluable information about disease causes and the development of targeted treatment strategies.

2.2.1.1.1 SNCA (alpha-synuclein)

The SNCA gene was the first to be linked to familial Parkinson's disease, and it encodes the protein alpha-synuclein, which is important to the disorder. Autosomal dominant Parkinson's disease is caused by SNCA mutations, which include missense mutations (e.g., A53T, E46K, A30P) and gene multiplicationsn (Jia et al., 2022). These mutations result in alpha-synuclein overexpression or misfolding, abnormal aggregation inside neurones, and the creation of Lewy bodies, which are the neuropathological hallmarks of Parkinson's disease (Morris et al., 2024).

Clinically, SNCA-associated Parkinson's disease can be diagnosed by an early onset in the 40s or 50s, as well as asymmetric motor characteristics such as bradykinesia and stiffness. While patients respond initially to dopamine replacement medication, the disease often progresses rapidly, with the appearance of non-motor symptoms such as dementia and autonomic dysfunction (Shulman et al., 2011). The identification of alpha-synuclein as the major component of Lewy bodies established a direct molecular relationship between familial and sporadic PD (Shulman et al., 2011).

2.2.1.1.2 LRRK2 (Leucine-rich repeat kinase 2)

Mutations in the LRRK2 gene are the most common cause of familial Parkinson's disease, although they can occur in sporadic cases in particular ethnic groups (Xiong & Yu, 2024). The LRRK2 gene encodes a large, multi-domain protein with kinase and GTPase activities that are involved in a variety of cellular processes, including autophagy, mitochondrial function, and microtubule dynamics. The most common disease-causing mutation, G2019S, is identified in up to 4% of familial PD and 1% of sporadic PD cases globally (Hur & Lee, 2021).

LRRK2-PD typically begins around the 50s age range and is clinically indistinguishable from idiopathic Parkinson's disease, with tremor-predominant presentation, bradykinesia, and rigidity that responds to L-DOPA. In some cases, incomplete penetrance has been seen in particular mutation carriers, which means that not all people with the mutation get Parkinson's disease (Day & Mullin, 2021). Mutant LRRK2 proteins typically exhibit enhanced kinase activity, making LRRK2 an attractive therapeutic target (Hur & Lee, 2021). Indeed, pharmacological suppression of LRRK2 is being investigated as a possible treatment.

2.2.1.1.3 PINK1 (PTEN-induced kinase 1)

Mutations in the PINK1 gene are the second most common autosomal recessive cause of early-onset Parkinson's disease (EOPD), behind PARKIN mutations (Borsche et al., 2021). PINK1 encodes a mitochondrial kinase, which is critical in recognizing and labeling defective mitochondria for disintegration by a quality-control process known as mitophagy. It cooperates with Parkin by promoting its recruitment to damaged mitochondria (Vizziello et al., 2021). PINK1-related PD Patients often appear in their 30s with classic motor symptoms such as tremor, bradykinesia, and stiffness (Vizziello et al., 2021). They may, however, exhibit specific characteristics such as hyperreflexia, early L-DOPA-induced dyskinesias, and occasional psychiatric disorders. The condition progresses slowly and improves with dopamine replacement, albeit with a higher risk of treatment-related side effects (Vizziello et al., 2021). The majority of PINK1 mutations are found in the gene's kinase domain, and while biallelic mutations are usually the cause of disease, there is some evidence that heterozygous variants can also predispose to it (Vizziello et al., 2021).

2.2.1.1.4 PARKIN (PRKN)

PARKIN mutations are the most common genetic cause of autosomal recessive early-onset Parkinson's disease, which typically appears before the age of 40. PARKIN is a gene that encodes an E3 ubiquitin ligase, a critical enzyme that marks damaged or misfolded proteins for destruction (Wahabi et al., 2018). It is essential for mitochondrial quality control, namely promoting mitophagy in conjunction with PINK1. PARKIN mutations cause loss of function, the accumulation of defective mitochondria, increased oxidative stress, and neuronal degeneration, particularly in the substantia nigra's dopaminergic neurones (Wahabi et al., 2018). PARKIN-related Parkinson's disease patients typically have moderate progression, an effective and persistent response to L-DOPA, and relatively modest non-motor symptoms. PARKIN-related PD, unlike sporadic PD, usually lacks Lewy bodies, but this can vary. Preclinical studies have demonstrated that Parkin has neuroprotective characteristics, defending neurones against a variety of cellular stresses such as toxins, oxidative damage, and protein buildup. As a result, knowing the mechanisms causing PARKIN malfunction provides critical insights into the pathophysiology of Parkinson's disease and informs therapy options (Wahabi et al., 2018).

Mutations in the SNCA, LRRK2, PINK1, and PARKIN genes are widely known genetic risk factors for Parkinson's disease. Although the mechanism of inheritance, age of symptom onset, and clinical characteristics differ, all these mutations have an impact on critical biological processes such as protein aggregation, mitochondrial malfunction, and disruption of the cellular clearance pathway (Wahabi et al., 2018). The study of these genetic variants improves our understanding of familial Parkinson's disease while also informing the pathogenic mechanisms of the more prevalent sporadic types (Wahabi et al., 2018). These findings pave the path for gene-based diagnostics, biomarker identification, and tailored therapy, which have the potential to change Parkinson's disease treatment in the years ahead.

2.2.2 Epigenetic changes driving PD pathogenesis

The word "epigenetics" was first used by Waddington in the 1940s to describe the complex link between an organism's phenotypic and its genetic expression. Currently, this field of study is being defined more precisely as heritable and reversible alterations in gene expression that occur without changes in the DNA sequence (Rathore et al., 2021). Epigenetic alterations control how genes are activated and deactivated, which can cause cells to behave and function differently. DNA methylation, histone changes, chromatin remodeling, and non-coding RNA activity, such as microRNAs and long non-coding RNAs, are among the most important epigenetic control mechanisms (Rathore et al., 2021).

Epigenetic alterations are now widely regarded as critical to the development and progression of Parkinson's disease. While specific gene mutations have long been linked to Parkinson's disease, epigenetic alterations either turn off or turn on the activities of these and other neurodegeneration-related genes (Song et al., 2023). For example, DNA methylation or changes in histone structure may reduce or raise the quantities of mRNAs and proteins that regulate critical activities such as mitochondrial function, oxidative stress response, and protein breakdown.

Epigenetic regulation controls brain development, neurogenesis, and neural plasticity. Given that the brain requires very fine-tuned gene expression, it is unsurprising that epigenetic disruptions could contribute to neurodegenerative illnesses like Parkinson's (Rathore et al., 2021). Indeed, studies have demonstrated that environmental factors such as nutrition, toxins, and stress can cause epigenetic changes that increase one's susceptibility to Parkinson's disease or exacerbate its course. Because these alterations are reversible, the epigenetic mechanism presents a viable alternative as a therapeutic target (Rathore et al., 2021).

2.2.2.1 DNA methylation, histone modifications, and non-coding RNAs in neurodegeneration

Epigenetic modification refers to any change that affects gene expression but does not directly alter the DNA sequence. Such changes are brought about through DNA methylation, histone modifications, and non-coding RNA control. These systems are critical for maintaining normal brain activities such as neurogenesis, synaptic plasticity, memory, and learning (Ghosh & Saadat, 2023). When disrupted, the alterations may promote the development of neurodegenerative diseases and play a role in the pathogenesis of Parkinson's disease (PD), which is characterized by disturbances in molecular processes within neurones.

2.2.2.1.1 DNA methylation in parkinsonism

One of the most well researched epigenetic alterations is DNA methylation. It is caused by the covalent addition of a methyl (-CH3) group to cytosine residues at their fifth carbon, primarily when cytosine is followed by guanine in the sequence (CpG), by an enzyme known as DNA methyltransferase, which has three major forms: DNMT1, DNMT3A, and DNMT3B (Ghosh & Saadat, 2023; Younesian et al., 2022). DNA methylation typically results in gene silence, making it critical for neuronal development, differentiation, and plasticity. Methylation patterns in the brain are quite dynamic and can be influenced by environmental factors, age, and stress (Younesian et al., 2022).

Abnormal DNA methylation has been linked to altered gene expression in Parkinson's disease (PD), particularly in genes involved in protein aggregation, oxidative stress, and mitochondrial function (Younesian et al., 2022). Elevated expression of α-synuclein, the primary protein component of Lewy bodies, has been associated with hypomethylation of CpG islands in intron one of the SNCA gene. Excessive α-synuclein aggregation causes neuronal damage and death. Furthermore, α-synuclein mislocalizes DNMT1 from the nucleus to the cytoplasm, disrupting global DNA methylation patterns and potentially leading to overexpression of additional PD-related genes such as CYP2E1 (Younesian et al., 2022).

DNA methylation is a possible diagnostic for early diagnosis since these changes can occur early in the disease's progression. According to current research, methylation patterns in the SNCA gene detected in peripheral blood samples could serve as a non-invasive diagnostic tool. Importantly, because it is reversible, DNA methylation is being studied as a potential therapeutic target.

2.2.2.1.2 Histone modifications and chromatin remodeling

The primary structural component of chromosomes, chromatin, is created by DNA looping around histone proteins. The N-terminal tails of histones can undergo a variety of post-translational modifications (PTMs), such as acetylation, methylation, phosphorylation, ubiquitylation, and SUMOylation. These alterations are critical for regulating gene expression because they alter chromatin structure, increasing or decreasing DNA accessibility for transcription (Fisher & Torrente, 2024).

Histone alterations have been linked to neuronal dysfunction in Parkinson's disease. Parkinson's disease (PD) can produce decreased histone H3 acetylation due to α-synuclein accumulation, which binds to histones and inhibits histone acetyltransferase (HAT) function (Fisher & Torrente, 2024). This decrease in histone acetylation, which also has an effect on gene transcription, exacerbates neurodegeneration. In Parkinson's disease models, histone deacetylase inhibitors (HDACi) can reduce α-synuclein toxicity and improve neuronal survival by increasing acetylation levels (Fisher & Torrente, 2024; Lardenoije et al., 2015).

Other histone marks, like as H2AK119ub, have been identified in PD settings and associated to transcriptional regulation. Enzymes responsible for these alterations, known as "writers" (e.g., HATs, HMTs), "erasers" (e.g., HDACs, demethylases), and "readers" (e.g., bromodomain-containing proteins), are increasingly being studied for their roles in neurodegeneration and as prospective therapeutic targets (Lardenoije et al., 2015).

2.2.2.1.3 Non-coding RNAs in gene regulation

Non-coding RNAs (ncRNAs) make up a large component of the transcriptome and do not encode proteins but play key regulatory roles at the transcriptional and post-transcriptional level. The two most common forms of ncRNAs are small ncRNAs (sncRNAs), also known as microRNAs (miRNAs), and long ncRNAs (lncRNAs). Each plays a distinct role in controlling genes (Lardenoije et al., 2015).

MiRNAs are the most characterized ncRNAs. They work by binding to complementary sequences in the $3'$ untranslated regions (UTRs) of target mRNAs, preventing translation or promoting mRNA degradation. This is performed through a multi-step process involving the Drosha and Dicer enzymes. Certain miRNAs regulate α-synuclein expression in Parkinson's disease. MiR-7 and miR-153 inhibit SNCA mRNA, reducing α-synuclein protein levels and providing neuroprotection (Lardenoije et al., 2015). Exposure to MPP^+, a neurotoxic used to imitate Parkinson's disease, causes downregulation of miR-7, resulting in increased α-synuclein production and neuronal death (Lardenoije et al., 2015).

MiR-433 indirectly influences SNCA expression by regulating FGF20, which increases α-synuclein levels. An increased incidence of Parkinson's disease has been linked to genetic variants in FGF20's $3'$ UTR that interfere with miR-433 binding. Overexpression of α-synuclein can alter miRNA profiles, leading to a feedback loop that exacerbates neurodegenerative effects (Lardenoije et al., 2015).

2.2.3 Gene-environment interactions in PD risk

It is becoming increasingly obvious that Parkinson's disease (PD) is caused by intricate interplay between environmental exposures and genetic predisposition. Even while rigorous genome-wide association studies (GWAS) have identified over 90 unique genetic markers connected to Parkinson's disease (PD), these account for just about 16% of the disease's total liability (Jacobs et al., 2020). Similarly, the effects of particular environmental risk factors are usually moderate. This means that the "missing heritability" of Parkinson's disease is most likely heavily influenced by gene-environment interactions.

Although 5%–10% of Parkinson's disease cases are familial, the majority are sporadic, indicating non-genetic reasons such as lifestyle decisions, environmental pollutants, and epigenetic changes (Vidović & Rikalovic, 2022). For example, different single-nucleotide polymorphisms (SNPs) within the SNCA gene, which encodes α-synuclein, are regarded as genetic risk variants, and epigenetic changes in this gene have been detected in sporadic PD cases. These SNPs may interact with environmental factors to influence Parkinson's disease development and progression (Vidović & Rikalovic, 2022).

The combination of genetic predisposition and environmental exposures has a major impact on the pathophysiology of Parkinson's disease. Some individuals may have genetic variants that render them more vulnerable to environmental shocks, particularly those that generate oxidative stress and disrupt proteostasis (Jacobs et al., 2020). Understanding these relationships is essential for designing targeted preventative methods, identifying biomarkers for early detection, and developing tailored risk prediction models.

2.2.3.1 Pesticides, heavy metals, and epigenetic alterations leading to sporadic PD

Approximately 90% of Parkinson's disease (PD) cases are sporadic, which means there is no known hereditary basis (Ascherio & Schwarzschild, 2016). Even though genetic research has helped us better understand the variety of Parkinson's disease and discovered a number of mutations associated with the condition, the majority of cases are caused by a combination of environmental and epigenetic influences. Long-term exposure to neurotoxic chemicals, particularly pesticides and heavy metals, is a key risk factor for Parkinson's disease (PD), particularly in genetically susceptible individuals, according to growing epidemiological and toxicological evidence (Yan et al., 2018).

Pesticides such as rotenone, paraquat, organophosphates, and organochlorines are the most commonly associated with Parkinson's disease (PD) among environmental contaminants. These compounds, which are widely used in agriculture, have been shown to generate PD-like disease in cellular and animal models (Simon et al., 2020). These compounds promote dopaminergic neuronal loss, α-synuclein aggregation, oxidative stress, and mitochondrial dysfunction, all of which contribute to Parkinson's disease pathology. Chronic pesticide exposure, whether occupational or passive environmental (e.g., living near treated agricultural fields), is significantly linked to an increased prevalence of Parkinson's disease (PD).

The historical discovery that MPTP, a contaminant found in synthetic opioids, might cause acute parkinsonism by selectively killing dopaminergic neurones raised the potential of pesticide-induced Parkinson's disease. Since then, multiple studies have confirmed that pesticides with structural similarities can reproduce this neurotoxicity (Yan et al., 2018). Epidemiological research has focused on gene-environment interactions and dose-response connections, implying that individuals with deficient detoxification genes may be more vulnerable to pesticide-induced neurotoxicity (Goldman, 2014).

Heavy metal exposure is another environmental risk that has been associated to sporadic Parkinson's disease. Iron, manganese, copper, and zinc are some of the metals that are required for normal cellular processes but, in excess, can be neurotoxic. These metals damage biological macromolecules like proteins and DNA and catalyze the generation of reactive oxygen species (ROS) (Doroszkiewicz et al., 2023). They also interfere with redox balance. Because of its high metabolic rate and poor antioxidant defenses, the brain is particularly sensitive to oxidative assaults. Heavy metals can alter metal ion transport, neurotransmission, and mitochondrial function, all of which are closely linked to Parkinson's disease pathology, as well as promote neuronal death (Doroszkiewicz et al., 2023).

Pesticides and heavy metals may also have an effect on epigenetic regulation, which is an important layer of gene expression control that does not involve changes in the DNA sequence. Environmental contaminants have the ability to alter chromatin structure, histone modifications, and DNA methylation patterns, potentially leading to the dysregulation of PD-related genes (Yan et al., 2018). For example, metal-induced oxidative stress can disrupt DNA repair pathways and epigenetically activate genes associated with cell death and neuroinflammation. When combined with inherited susceptibility or age-related epigenetic drift, these changes have the potential to accelerate disease progression.

Regardless of how intricate these interactions are, the overall epidemiological evidence clearly implies that environmental toxins play a role in sporadic Parkinson's disease. Animal and in vitro models that mimic critical characteristics of Parkinson's disease following exposure to specific drugs provide additional support (Goldman, 2014). Better exposure assessment tools, more precise identification of at-risk groups, and a better understanding of the pathways linking environmental exposure to neurodegeneration are just a few of the many challenges that remain to be solved.

The etiology of sporadic Parkinson's disease cannot be explained solely by genetics. Long-term exposure to pesticides and heavy metals significantly increases the risk of Parkinson's disease (PD), particularly when combined with genetic predispositions and epigenetic alterations (Yan et al., 2018). Future research should focus on untangling these complex linkages in order to discover the optimal techniques for disease prevention, early intervention, and public health regulation.

2.3 Neurotransmitter imbalance and circuitry dysfunction in parkinson's disease

Parkinson's disease (PD) is characterized as a progressive neurodegenerative disorder that predominantly impairs motor functions, while also encompassing a broad array of non-motor symptoms. A hallmark pathological feature of PD is the selective degeneration of dopaminergic neurons within the substantia nigra pars compacta (SNpc), which results in extensive neurochemical disruptions affecting various neurotransmitter systems (Kalia & Lang, 2015). These neurochemical alterations interfere with the complex circuitry of the basal ganglia, thereby contributing to both motor and non-motor impairments (Calabresi et al., 2014). This chapter aims to explore the primary neurotransmitter disturbances associated with PD, with particular emphasis on progressive loss of dopamine neurons, glutamatergic excitotoxicity, and the roles of serotonergic, noradrenergic, and cholinergic systems and their compensatory plasticity.

2.3.1 Dopaminergic neurodegeneration in the nigrostriatal pathway

This pathway, which extends from the substantia nigra pars compacta (SNc) to the dorsal striatum, plays a critical role in the fine regulation of voluntary movement through the basal ganglia-thalamo-cortical motor circuit. The cardinal motor symptoms of Parkinson's disease (PD)—namely bradykinesia, rigidity, resting tremor, and postural instability—manifest only after a threshold level of dopaminergic neuronal loss has been surpassed. Specifically, clinical symptoms typically emerge when striatal dopamine levels decline by approximately 70%–80% and when about 50%–60% of SNc neurons are degenerated (Airavaara et al., 2020; Kalia & Lang, 2015).

2.3.1.1 Underlying pathogenic mechanisms

Dopaminergic neurons exhibit heightened vulnerability to oxidative stress, primarily due to the autoxidation of dopamine, which generates reactive oxygen species (ROS) and toxic quinones. These oxidative byproducts inflict damage on essential cellular components, including mitochondrial DNA, proteins, and lipids, ultimately contributing to neuronal degeneration (Burbulla et al., 2017; He et al., 2023; Surmeier et al., 2017). Increased expression of the dopamine transporter (DAT) in surviving neurons, particularly under conditions of impaired autophagy-lysosomal function, may exacerbate dopamine reuptake and promote the accumulation of cytosolic dopamine, thereby intensifying susceptibility to oxidative injury and neurodegeneration (Harraz, 2023; Liu et al., 2025). Dysfunction of mitochondrial complex I is a consistent pathological feature in PD, leading to impaired oxidative phosphorylation, reduced ATP synthesis, and elevated ROS production. This mitochondrial dysfunction is proposed to act both as a causative factor and a downstream consequence of dopaminergic neuronal loss, as demonstrated in neurotoxin-induced models (e.g., MPTP, rotenone) and supported by postmortem analyses of PD brains (Lucchesi et al., 2025; Yang, 2025). Additionally, chronic activation of microglia and astrocytes in the substantia nigra pars compacta (SNc) results in sustained release of pro-inflammatory cytokines, further exacerbating neuronal damage and perpetuating a deleterious cycle of neuroinflammation and neurodegeneration (Rim et al., 2024; Kam et al., 2020).

2.3.1.2 Compensatory and maladaptive plasticity

During the preclinical phase of Parkinson's disease, surviving dopaminergic neurons initiate compensatory mechanisms to maintain motor function. These include upregulation of dopamine synthesis and release, increased dopamine turnover, and enhanced expression of dopamine receptors—particularly D2 receptors—in the striatum (Kalia & Lang, 2015; Pa*β* et al., 2024; Stokholm et al., 2021). While initially effective, these adaptations serve to mask clinical symptoms despite progressive neuronal loss. As dopaminergic depletion progresses, it disrupts the functional balance between the direct (facilitatory) and indirect (inhibitory) pathways within the basal ganglia. This disruption leads to hyperactivity of the subthalamic nucleus (STN) and globus pallidus internus (GPi), which in turn suppresses thalamocortical excitatory output, manifesting in motor symptoms such as bradykinesia and rigidity (Milosevic et al., 2018; Obeso et al., 2008). Over time, however, these compensatory mechanisms may become maladaptive. Postsynaptic dopamine receptor supersensitivity and aberrant synaptic remodeling are implicated in the emergence of motor complications, including levodopa-induced dyskinesias and motor fluctuations (Cerasa et al., 2014; Chase & Oh, 2000).

2.3.1.3 Clinical and experimental evidence

Positron emission tomography (PET) and single-photon emission computed tomography (SPECT) imaging studies have consistently revealed a progressive reduction in striatal dopamine transporter (DAT) binding, a biomarker that strongly correlates with disease severity (Kerstens & Varrone, 2020; Kraemmer et al., 2014). Additionally, animal models utilizing neurotoxins such as 6-hydroxydopamine (6-OHDA) and 1-methyl-4-phenyl-1,2,3,6-tetrahydropyridine (MPTP) in rodents and non-human primates recapitulate the selective degeneration of substantia nigra pars compacta (SNc) neurons and the resulting motor impairments, further substantiating the critical role of nigrostriatal pathway degeneration in Parkinson's disease (PD) pathogenesis (Fox & Brotchie, 2010).

2.3.2 Glutamate and excitotoxicity: A double-edged sword

2.3.2.1 Dysregulated NMDA receptor signaling and synaptic dysfunction

As the principal excitatory neurotransmitter of the central nervous system, glutamate plays a pivotal role in modulating synaptic transmission and plasticity within the basal ganglia circuitry. In PD, however, glutamatergic signaling becomes dysregulated, which contributes to both neurodegeneration and aberrant motor circuit function (Iovino et al., 2020).

2.3.2.1.1 Mechanisms of glutamate-mediated excitotoxicity

The compromised function of microglial and astrocytic glutamate transporters results in elevated extracellular glutamate concentrations, consequently leading to sustained activation of postsynaptic glutamate receptors (Haroon et al., 2017). The subsequent overstimulation of NMDA (N-methyl-D-aspartate) and AMPA (α-amino-3-hydroxy-5-methyl-4-isoxazolepropionic acid) receptors drives increased intracellular calcium influx. This critical event triggers cascades encompassing oxidative stress, mitochondrial dysfunction, and the activation of proteases and endonucleases, which ultimately culminate in neuronal apoptosis or necrosis (Verma et al., 2018). Furthermore, in PD, evidence indicates upregulated NMDA receptor expression and altered subunit composition within the striatum and other basal ganglia nuclei, thus increasing neuronal vulnerability to excitotoxic injury (Capó et al., 2025; Sitzia et al., 2020).

2.3.2.1.2 Impact on basal ganglia circuitry and motor symptoms

Normal synaptic plasticity in the striatum, including long-term potentiation (LTP) and long-term depression (LTD), relies on a finely tuned equilibrium between glutamatergic and dopaminergic signaling (Lerner & Kreitzer, 2012; Lisman et al., 2017). In PD, dopaminergic degeneration disrupts this balance, resulting in aberrant synaptic plasticity and deficits in motor learning. Although chronic levodopa treatment restores dopamine levels, it may paradoxically exacerbate glutamatergic dysregulation, increasing susceptibility to levodopa-induced dyskinesias (LID) (di Biase et al., 2023; Calabresi et al., 2015). Notably, excessive NMDA receptor-mediated signaling contributes to LID pathogenesis, and NMDA receptor antagonists such as amantadine have shown therapeutic potential in mitigating dyskinesias (Isaacson & Jenner, 2025; Riederer et al., 2025).

2.3.3 Beyond dopamine: Role of serotonergic, noradrenergic, and cholinergic systems

2.3.3.1 Contribution to non-motor symptoms (depression, cognitive impairment, autonomic dysfunction)

Although the dopaminergic system has long been the central focus of PD research and treatment, it is now widely recognized that PD is a multisystem neurodegenerative disorder characterized by extensive neurotransmitter dysregulation. The degeneration of serotonergic, noradrenergic, and cholinergic neurons plays a critical role in the non-motor symptoms of PD, which frequently emerge before motor impairments and significantly impair patients' quality of life (Hussein et al., 2023; Müller & Bohnen, 2013).

2.3.3.1.1 Serotonergic system

Serotonergic neurons, which primarily originate in the raphe nuclei, exhibit widespread projections throughout the brain and play a key modulatory role in mood, cognition, sleep, and autonomic functions (Ligneul & Mainen, 2023). In PD, the loss of serotonergic neurons and dysregulation of serotonin receptor expression are well-documented neuropathological features. Furthermore, these alterations are clinically linked to depression, anxiety, psychosis, sleep disturbances (including REM sleep behavior disorder), and the modulation of L-DOPA-induced dyskinesias (Li, 2023; McManus et al., 2025). Additionally, serotonin deficiency disrupts mood regulation and emotional processing, while serotonergic terminals in the striatum may ectopically convert exogenous L-DOPA to dopamine, leading to unregulated dopamine release and exacerbating motor complications.

2.3.3.1.2 Noradrenergic system

Noradrenergic neurons, primarily located in the locus coeruleus (LC), innervate numerous brain regions and play crucial roles in regulating arousal, attention, the stress response, and autonomic function. Notably, early and severe degeneration of LC neurons represents a pathological hallmark of PD that frequently precedes substantia nigra pars compacta (SNc) degeneration. These noradrenergic deficits significantly contribute to cognitive impairment (particularly affecting attention and executive function), mood disorders, and various autonomic disturbances, including orthostatic hypotension, urinary dysfunction, and gastrointestinal dysmotility (Ligneul & Mainen, 2023). Moreover, noradrenaline exerts important anti-inflammatory and neuroprotective effects in the brain; understanding these actions may lead to the development of new therapeutic strategies (Giri et al., 2024; Paredes-Rodriguez et al., 2020).

2.3.3.1.3 Cholinergic system

Cholinergic neurons in the basal forebrain (e.g., nucleus basalis of Meynert) and brainstem (e.g., pedunculopontine nucleus) are critical for cognitive processes, attention, learning, and motor control. Degeneration of these neurons is closely linked to cognitive decline, dementia, gait and balance disturbances, falls, and autonomic dysfunction (e.g., urinary incontinence, constipation) (Pasquini et al., 2021). Cholinergic deficits can manifest early in the disease course, sometimes preceding motor symptoms. Cholinesterase inhibitors have shown modest benefits in treating cognitive impairment and dementia in PD (Chen et al., 2020; Slater et al., 2024).

The interplay between dopaminergic, serotonergic, noradrenergic, and cholinergic systems creates a complex neurochemical environment in PD. Disruption of these interconnected networks underlies both the motor and non-motor symptoms of the disease (Hussein et al., 2023). Non-motor symptoms, including depression, anxiety, cognitive impairment, sleep disturbances, and autonomic dysfunction, often dominate the clinical picture as PD progresses and are major determinants of disability and caregiver burden (Lesley et al., 2025).

In conclusion, neurotransmitter imbalance and circuitry dysfunction are central to the pathogenesis and clinical presentation of PD. While dopaminergic degeneration in the nigrostriatal pathway is the cornerstone of motor symptoms, glutamatergic excitotoxicity and disruptions in serotonergic, noradrenergic, and cholinergic systems significantly contribute to non-motor symptoms and disease progression. Understanding these complex neurochemical interactions offers a more holistic view of PD and opens up avenues for targeted therapies beyond traditional dopamine replacement strategies.

2.4 Standard pharmacotherapy: Advances, challenges, and optimization

2.4.1 Levodopa and dopaminergic replacement therapy

2.4.1.1 Mechanisms, motor complications (dyskinesia, wearing-off phenomena)

As a precursor to dopamine, levodopa (L-DOPA) can be changed into dopamine in the brain (Riederer et al., 2025). An enzyme known as dopamine decarboxylase (DDC) converts L-DOPA into dopamine after it passes through the blood-brain barrier (BBB), unlike dopamine itself (Shebl & Salama, 2025). Because PD is brought on by the progressive loss of dopaminergic neurons in the substantia nigra, levodopa is used to treat the disorder (Antonini et al., 2023). The striatum has a severe dopamine shortage as a result of this cell death, which directly contributes to the hallmark motor symptoms of PD, including bradykinesia, stiffness, and tremor (Riederer et al., 2025). Levodopa aids in restoring this dopamine. Restoring dopamine signaling in the brain is the goal of dopaminergic replacement therapy, or DRT (Wu et al., 2024). This treatment's primary ingredients are levodopa (often in combination with a DDC inhibitor like benserazide or carbidopa), dopamine agonists (pramipexole and ropinirole), and enzyme inhibitors like COMT inhibitors (entacapone) and MAO-B inhibitors (selegiline) (Riederer et al., 2025).

Dopamine is produced from levodopa both inside and outside the brain (Kwon et al., 2022). Although the brain's conversion is medicinal, the peripheral reaction may result in undesirable side effects like nausea (Zhong et al., 2021). A medicine like carbidopa, which prevents this peripheral conversion and increases the amount of the drug that reaches the brain, is usually taken in conjunction with levodopa to counteract this (van Vliet et al., 2023). Once in the striatum, the freshly generated dopamine acts on D1 and D2 receptors to normalize the function of the direct and indirect motor pathways and restore normal signaling (Gerfen, 2023). This function restoration aids in reducing PD's motor symptoms.

Levodopa use over an extended period of time, usually 5 years, might result in motor problems such as dyskinesias and motor fluctuations (Julien et al., 2021). The "wearing-off" phenomenon, in which Parkinson's symptoms reappear before ethe next dose is due, is a frequent problem (Farzanehfar et al., 2022). Levodopa's brief half-life of about 1.5 h is the reason for this (Demailly et al., 2024). The brain's capacity to buffer dopamine is lost when the disease worsens and the patient's remaining dopamine-producing neurons are destroyed. At first, these neurons can store and release dopamine to maintain stable levels (Di Battista & Hey-Hawkins, 2022). Dopamine levels thus start to change with each dosage, resulting in observable "on" periods of improved motor control and "off" periods when symptoms reappear (Lee et al., 2025). Doctors may use extended-release levodopa formulations or dpamine agonists to treat this, increase the frequency of doses, or add drugs like COMT or MAO-B inhibitors to prolong the effects of the therapy (Regensburger et al., 2023).

The involuntary, uncontrollable motions that resemble writhing or twisting are known as levodopa-induced dyskinesia (LID) (Yoon et al., 2022). They are more prevalent in younger individuals or those taking large dosages of the drug, and they usually manifest when levodopa levels in the blood are at their peak (Fabbri et al., 2023). The pulsatibe, or "on-off," characteristic of dopamine stimulation from repeated dosages is the mechanism underlying LID, causing aberrant alterations in striatal neurons (di Biase et al., 2023). This can lead to an imbalance in the signaling pathways of the motor cortex and basal ganglia and make dopamine receptors, especially D1 receptors, excessively responsive (Kawahata et al., 2024). Using the lowest effective dose of levodopa, switching to continuous administration systems like a duodenal infusion, or adding drugs like amantadine, which is proven to lessen dyskinesia, are the goals of clinicians while managing LID (Kumar L. et al., 2024). Deep brain stimulation (DBS) may also be taken into consideration in some situations (Hariz & Blomstedt, 2022).

2.4.1.2 Strategies to optimize levodopa efficacy

Long-term usage of levodopa can result in motor problems such as "wearing-off" and dyskinesia, however it is the most effective treatment for PD symptoms (Lenka et al., 2022). Optimizing its efficacy, stability, and patient tolerance is therefore crucial. Several pharmaceutical techniques are frequently used to accomplish this, most commonly the combination of levodopa and enzyme inhibitors (Popławska-Domaszewicz et al., 2025). DDC inhibitor like benserazide or carbidogpa prevent the body from converting levodopa into dopamine (Qiu et al., 2025). This is important because it increases the amount of medication that reaches the brain and lessens peripheral adverse effects like nausea (Silva et al., 2021). COMT inhibitors, such as entacapone and opicapone, prolong the half-life of levodopa and lessen "wearing-off" symptoms by preventing its breakdown (St. Onge et al., 2021). Last but not least, MAO-B inhibitors like rasagiline and selegiline prolong the patient's "on" period, increase dopamine availability, and improve motor performance by preventing its breakdown in the brain (Chew et al., 2023).

Changing the levodopa dosage schedule is a popular tactic to control variations in a patient's motor symptoms (Saranza & Lang, 2021). This can be accomplished by administering smaller, more regular dosages to keep the body's medication levels more consistent, which helps to reduce motor fluctuations. For the same reason, doctors may also recommend formulations with controlled or extended release (Livingston & Monroe-Duprey, 2024). Dosage schedules can be also be changed to better suit each patient's unique symptom patterns throughout the day (Gutowski et al., 2023). Levodopa is frequently used in conjunction with medications such as pramipexole, ropinirole, and rotigotine as adjunct therapy (Richmond et al., 2023). As dopamine agonists, these medications directly activate dopamine receptors without requiring the body to convert them (Lees et al., 2023). By activating these receptors, they can assist lower the dosage of Levodopa needed and are useful in treating "wearing-off" symptoms and akinesia, or stiffness in the morning (Majali et al., 2021). One drug that functions as an NMDA receptor antagonist is amantadine, which is especially helpful because of its anti-dyskinetic properties (Rascol et al., 2021). It specifically aids in the reduction of levodopa-induced dyskinesia (LID) and provides some minor advantages in the direct treatment of Parkinson's disease symptoms (Bandopadhyay et al., 2022).

Levodopa efficacy optimization involves non-pharmacological strategies including dietary changes and continuous drug delivery in addition to pharmaceutical ones (Muleiro Alvarez et al., 2024). Because levodopa can compete with amino acids in protein for intestinal absorption and blood-brain barrier trafficking, dietary changes are crucial (O'Leary et al., 2025). Therefore, it is frequently recommended that patients refrain from eating high-protein meals right before their Levodopa dosages. A protein redistribution diet is a popular tactic that involves consuming more protein in the evening and less throughout the day (Rusch et al., 2023). In order to enhance gastrointestinal absorption, a number of techniques can be used. Prokinetic drugs such as domperidone may be used to treat gastroparesis, or delayed stomach emptying, in an individual (Sanger & Andrews, 2023). Levodopa should also normally be taken 30–60 min prior to meals, according to patient guidelines (Agnieszka et al., 2022). Orally disintegrating tablets (ODTs) or liquid versions of levodopa may be an option for people who have ongoing problems with absorption (Qin et al., 2024). To keep medication levels more consistent in patients with severe Parkinson's disease who have noticeable motor swings, Continuous Dopaminergic Delivery (CDD) techniques are used (Rota et al., 2022). Levodopa-Carbidopa Intestinal Gel (LCIG), which is administered by a jejunal infusion pump and offers steady plasma levels of the drug, is one such choice (Jost, 2023). Other examples include apomorphine infusion, a subcutaneous dopamine agonist, and the rotigotine transdermal patch, which continually distributes a dopamine agonist through the skin (Sharma & Burré, 2023).

Surgery, such as DBS, may be a possibility when drugs are no longer enough to manage symptoms. DBS reduces dyskinesia and motor fluctuations by targeting particular brain regions, such as the globus pallidus internus (GPi) or the subthalamic nucleus (STN) (Au et al., 2021). Levodopa dosage reductions are frequently possible with this treatment. DBS is most suited for individuals who exhibit poor response to previous therapy, have substantial "on-off" swings, and retain intact cognitive function (T. K Lee & Yankee, 2022).

2.4.2 Non-dopaminergic approaches: Beyond dopamine replacement

2.4.2.1 Adenosine A2A receptor antagonists and glutamate modulators

Over time, levodopa's efficiency decreases due to the increasing loss of dopamine neurons in PD. Furthermore, dyskinesia and "wearing-off" are two common motor problems associated with long-term levodopa treatment. Because they are unrelated to dopamine, many non-motor symptoms of PD, like fatigue and cognitive deterioration, are not alleviated by conventional dopamine replacement treatments (Saini et al., 2024). Glutamate, adenosine, acetylcholine, and serotonin are among the other neurotransmitter systems that are known to be implicated in the pathophysiology of the disease, and these considerations underscore the necessity of investigating them (Teleanu et al., 2022).

Adenosine A2A receptors are widely distributed throughout the striatum, particularly in the basal ganglia's indirect pathway, where they interact with and block dopamine D2 receptors to help reduce motor function (Franco et al., 2023). Without directly raising dopamine levels, these antagonists work by blocking the A2A receptors, which lessens the indirect pathway's overactivity and aids in restoring motor balance (Teymourian et al., 2022). Additionally, this strategy might shorten patients' "off" period and increase the effects of levodopa (Antonini et al., 2021). As the first A2A receptor antagonist authorized for use in conjunction with levodopa, Istradefylline aims to reduce "off" episodes in patients with advanced PD (Jenner et al., 2021). Although usually well tolerated, adverse symptoms like sleeplessness, hallucinations, or dyskinesia can occur in some people (Dressler & Pan, 2022).

The main excitatory neurotransmitter in the central nervous system is glutamate (Pal, 2021). Neurotoxicity, dyskinesia, and the onset of motor symptoms are all associated with an overabundance of glutamatergic activity in PD, especially in the motor cortex and subthalamic nucleus (STN) (Campanelli et al., 2022). To improve motor control and minimize Levodopa-induced dyskinesia (LID), it is possible to reduce aberrant neuronal firing by carefully controlling this glutamatergic transmission (Di Luca et al., 2022). By inhibiting NMDA-type glutamate receptors, amantadine helps to lessen excitotoxicity and aberrant striatal alterations (Beaurain et al., 2024). In particular, this technique works well for treating dyskinesia brought on by levodopa. Amantadine comes in immediate-release and extended-release formulations, including Gocovri, and is clinically regarded as the most effective treatment for dyskinesia in PD (Müller, 2022). Hallucinations, disorientation, ankle edema, and a skin condition known as livedo reticularis are possible adverse effects, despite the fact that it is usually beneficial (Sharma et al., 2024). Beyond Amantadine, other glutamate modulators are currently being investigated, primarily in preclinical or early clinical trials. For instance, mGluR5 antagonists target metabotropic glutamate receptors, which are implicated in neuroinflammation and dyskinesia (Budgett et al., 2022). Additionally, AMPA/kainate receptor antagonists are being explored for their potential to help control motor complications in PD (Rafe et al., 2024).

2.4.3 Adjunct therapies for non-motor symptoms

2.4.3.1 Antidepressants, cognitive enhancers and autonomic symptom management

Although motor symptoms are the hallmark of PD, non-motor symptoms such as depression, cognitive impairment, and autonomic dysfunction can be equally, if not more, incapacitating. Additional treatments are necessary for the efficient management of these non-motor symptoms because dopamine replacement therapy frequently does not alleviate them. Up to 50% of people with PD experience depression, which can occasionally even manifest before motor signs (Berg et al., 2021). This is probably caused by changes in the chemistry of dopamine, serotonin, and norepinephrine in the brain (Khushboo et al., 2022). Although they are commonly administered and typically well-tolerated, selective serotonin reuptake inhibitors (SSRIs), such as sertraline or escitalopram, may occasionally exacerbate tremors or induce apathy in individuals with PD (Moreira et al., 2025, pp. 143–176). An alternative that can help with both mood disorders and chronic pain is to use serotonin-norepinephrine reuptake inhibitors (SNRIs), such as venlafaxine or duloxetine (Bonilla-Jaime et al., 2022). Nortriptyline and desipramine are examples of tricyclic antidepressants (TCAs) that can be useful, but older people should use them with caution because they may cause anticholinergic adverse effects like dry mouth or disorientation (Bishara, 2023; Reinert et al., 2023). There are also minor antidepressant benefits from MAO-B inhibitors, including rasagiline or selegiline, which are used to alleviate motor symptoms (Galli et al., 2025).

Cognitive impairment can develop into PD dementia and is a common problem in PD, especially in its later stages (Gonzalez-Latapi et al., 2021). Problems with attention, executive function, and visuospatial skills are common symptoms of this illness. A cholinesterase inhibitor called rivastigmine, which raises acetylcholine levels in the brain, is the main treatment for PD dementia (Walczak-Nowicka & Herbet, 2021). It has been demonstrated to be effective in enhancing behavior and cognition, and it is currently the only drug specifically approved for PD dementia (Phillips et al., 2023). Galantamine and donepezil are two more cholinesterase inhibitors that are occasionally used off-label for PD dementia (Sun & Armstrong, 2021). In more severe cases, memantine, an NMDA receptor antagonist, has demonstrated limited advantages; nevertheless, these drugs might exacerbate tremors or induce adverse effects such as bradycardia, nausea, or dizziness, which calls for close patient monitoring (Devanand & Fremont, 2024).

The autonomic nervous system is often affected by PD, which can result in a variety of non-motor symptoms such as constipation, urine problems, sexual dysfunction, and orthostatic hypotension (Radad et al., 2023). Initially, non-pharmacological methods are used to treat orthostatic hypotension, which is defined as a sharp decrease in blood pressure while standing that results in light-headedness or fainting (Ko & Huh, 2021, pp. 303–316). These include encouraging patients to stand up gradually, employing compression stockings, and boosting their diet of salt and fluids (Kim, 2024). Drugs like fludrocortisone, which aids in fluid retention, or midodrine, a vasopressor, may be administered if these steps prove insufficient (Srinivas et al., 2024). In certain nations, droxidopa, a precursor to norepinephrine, is also an option. Increasing dietary fibber and fluid intake helps cure constipation, which is frequently caused by slow intestinal movement in PD and may be made worse by decreased physical activity or medication (Han et al., 2023). Prokinetic drugs like domperidone and mild laxatives like polyethylene glycol (PEG) may also be employed (Maheshwari & Sood, 2022). Bladder overactivity can lead to urinary issues such as urgency, frequency, or incontinence (Scarneciu et al., 2021). Mirabegron, a more recent beta-3 agonist, provides a safer option with less cognitive adverse effects than medications like oxybutynin or solifenacin, which can lessen these symptoms but should be used carefully because they may impair cognition (Chen, Chuang, et al., 2022; Chen, Qin, et al., 2022). Lastly, both psychological and physical factors can contribute to sexual dysfunction. Phosphodiesterase-5 inhibitors, like sildenafil, can be used to treat erectile dysfunction in men (Dong et al., 2021). Counseling and treating co-occurring anxiety or depression may also be helpful for both men and women (Johnstone et al., 2023).

2.5 Disease-modifying and neuroprotective strategies

2.5.1 Targeting α-synuclein aggregation and clearance

Mitigating intracellular and extracellular α-Synuclein accumulation or enhancing its clearance are viable therapeutic strategies for Parkinson's disease (PD) and related diseases that target synucleinopathies (Menon et al., 2022). These strategies include immunization, reducing α-synuclein expression, inhibiting oligomerization, limiting intracellular or extracellular aggregate accumulation, enhancing clearance, targeting genes or proteins involved in aggregation (such as silencing *SNCA*), promoting proteolytic degradation, and reducing posttranslational modifications like oxidation, nitration, phosphorylation, and C-terminal cleavage (Knecht et al., 2022; Vidović & Rikalovic, 2022) (Fig. 2.1). Immunotherapy targeting the modulation of extracellular α-Syn transmission holds therapeutic significance. Antibody-based therapies are considered the most effective treatments for targeting pathogenic proteins, especially those present in the extracellular environment (Nimmo et al., 2023). Various preclinical and clinical studies have developed alternative targeting strategies such as active and passive immunization to decrease the spread of α-Syn indirectly.

2.5.1.1 Small molecules and immunotherapy strategies (passive and active vaccination)

2.5.1.1.1 Small molecules

While nucleic acid-based treatment methods are becoming more widely used, using small molecules to target RNA for changing protein expression is seen as a new area in therapy development (Table 2.2). For instance, Anle138b, found through high-throughput screening for chemicals that block prion protein clumping, was shown to inhibit α-Syn oligomer formation in vitro. It also protects from rotenone and 1-methyl-4-phenyl-1,2,3,6-tetrahydropyridine (MPTP) in murine models, as well as against motor impairments and pathological alterations in A30P α-Syn transgenic mice (Wagner et al., 2013). Subsequent testing showed that Anle138b therapy slowed PD progression in the A30P α-Syn transgenic mouse model, even when given after onset (Levin et al., 2014). The protective effect of Anle138b includes the MI2 murine model of PD. This model expresses human, aggregation-prone, truncated 1–120 α-Syn, which is controlled by the tyrosine hydroxylase promoter, that also covers the motor impairments in models of MSA (Wegrzynowicz et al., 2019). Although there are no published results from this phase 1 trial (NCT04685265), the company has demonstrated that the drug is safe,

Table 2.2 Target α-Syn aggregation in small molecules.

Agent	Mechanism of action	Phase of development	Clinical trial number	Status/ Findings	References
Anle138b	Inhibit α-Syn oligomerization.	Phase 1	NCT04685265	No results publicly available	Wegrzynowicz et al. (2019)
NPT200-11	Displaces α-Syn from membranes, inhibits aggregation	Phase 1	NCT04875962	Demonstrates satisfactory safety and tolerability.	Smit et al. (2022)
		Phase 2	NCT04658186	Currently underway	
ENT-01 (squalamine salt)	Displaces α-Syn from lipid membranes	Phase 2	NCT03047629	Improved constipation in PD patients with minimal systemic absorption	Hauser et al. (2019)
NPT088	Fusion protein binds misfolded aggregates (α-syn, amyloid)	Preclinical in PD patients, however, phase 1 in ALZ patients.	NCT03008161	Demonstrates satisfactory safety and tolerability in ALZ patients, but shows no effect on clinical progression markers	Michelson et al. (2019)

tolerable, and has enough plasma concentrations for its effectiveness. It can prevent the development of α-Syn oligomers in vitro.

NPT200 11 is also known as minzasolmin (UCB0599). It is a second-generation oral small molecule designed to penetrate the blood-brain barrier (BBB). Minzasolmin blocks the oligomerization of α-Syn which help reduce the misfolding and buildup of this protein in vital neural structures (Price et al., 2018). The first phase of the clinical trial (NCT04875962) implemented a fixed dosage scheme with placebo controls for both groups. Researchers evaluated participants for safety throughout the duration of the study period. The primary endpoint evaluated treatment-induced adverse effects that occurred in comparison to initial baseline measurements. Secondary endpoints consisted of measuring the peak plasma concentration level alongside the time it took to reach this peak concentration during days 1 and 28 (Smit et al., 2022). The research demonstrated excellent safety and tolerability results. The current trial phase 2 (NCT04658186) evaluates the safety and tolerability of NPT200–11 compared to a placebo. The main objectives involve assessing the safety profile along with the tolerability characteristics of NPT200–11 against a placebo. This study aims to evaluate the progression of clinical symptoms develop during a period of 12–18 months among patients who have early-stage PD.

Squalamine functions as a disaggregator by removing α-Syn from lipid membrane surfaces. This therapy currently under investigation for PD symptom treatment because oral administration improves gut motility in A53T α-Syn transgenic mice (West et al., 2020). The synthetic salt of squalamine that known as ENT-01 underwent testing in PD patients following its initial preclinical evaluation (NCT03047629). During the phase 2 trial, patients obtained single ascending doses of ENT-01 every 3–7 days which ranged between 25 and 200 mg. ENT-01 treatment demonstrated low systemic absorption together with effective constipation reduction (Hauser et al., 2019).

NPT088 is a fusion protein molecule that helps in inhibiting α-Syn aggregation. This is a human immunoglobulin conjugated to a phage-derived capsid protein that identified as g3p, which possesses a universal amyloid-association motif that interacts with aggregated forms of various misfolded proteins including α-Syn, and alters the amyloid structure (Levenson et al., 2016). A completed multiple-dose safety trial of intravenously administered NPT088 has taken place in individuals with Alzheimer's disease (ALZ) (NCT03008161). This investigation showed good safety and acceptability. Nevertheless, it did not affect markers of disease progression, such as amyloid plaques, τ aggregates, or clinical symptoms (Michelson et al., 2019).

2.5.1.1.2 Immunotherapy strategies

Immunization is currently the primary treatment approach against α-Syn (Table 2.3). The aggregation of α-synuclein outside the cells causes the binding of the antibodies; however, with advances in technology that allow antibodies to enter cells, immunization may also help clear α-synuclein aggregates from inside the cells. In murine models of PD, research in both active and passive immunization has shown potential in providing neuroprotection. These studies collectively show that immunization strategies that target different α-Syn epitopes can result in decreased α-Syn oligomer accumulation, decreased neurodegeneration, including in dopaminergic neurons that are tyrosine hydroxylase (TH)-positive, and improved motor phenotype in a variety of mouse models of α-synucleinopathies (Lemos et al., 2020). Active immunotherapy aims to stimulate the patient's immune system to produce antibodies against α-syn by introducing synthetic peptides that mimic parts of the protein (Zheng et al., 2021).

Table 2.3 Immunotherapeutic agents in clinical trials for PD.

Type	Agent	Type of therapy	Phase of development	Clinical trial number	Status/Findings	References
Active	AFFITOPE PD01A	Synthetic peptide (C-terminal α-syn 110–130)	Phase 1	NCT01568099	Induced a specific antibody response; safe and well tolerated	Volc et al. (2020)
			Phase 1a	NTC01885494	An extension study of NCT01568099 and found to be safe	
	AFFITOPE PD03A	A similar platform to PD01A	Phase 1	NCT02267434	Generated lower antibody titers than those observed in the PD01A	
	UB-312	Synthetic peptide (C-terminal 12-a sequence)	Phase 1	NCT04075318	Not recruiting	Nimmo et al. (2020)
Passive	Prasinezumab (PRX002)	Humanized IgG1 mAb (C-terminal epitope)	Phase 1	NCT02095171	Reduced serum-free α-Syn and immunogenicity-free.	Schenk et al. (2016)
			Phase 1	NCT02157714	No change in the concentration of free α-syn in the cerebral fluid was observed.	Jankovic et al. (2018)
			Phase 2	NCT03100149	Prasinezumab did not significantly affect global or imaging measures of PD progression compared to placebo.	Pagano et al. (2022)

Continued

Table 2.3 Immunotherapeutic agents in clinical trials for PD.—cont'd

Type	Agent	Type of therapy	Phase of development	Clinical trial number	Status/Findings	References
			Phase 2b	NCT04777331	Currently underway	
	Cinpanemab (BIIB054)	Human IgG1 mAb (N-terminal epitope)	Phase 1	NCT02459886	Demonstrated favorable safety and tolerability.	Brys et al. (2019)
			Phase 1	NCT03716570	No results publicly available	Brys et al. (2019)
			Phase 2	NCT03318523	Did not provide any clinical benefit over placebo after 52 weeks	Lang et al. (2022)
	MEDI1341	Human mAb (C-terminal α-syn 103–129)	Phase 1 Phase 2	NCT03272165 NCT04449484	No results have been made publicly available	Schofield et al. (2019)
	Lu AF82422	Human mAb targeting soluble α-Syn	Phase 1	NCT03611569	No results have been made publicly available	Lindström et al. (2014)
	BAN0805 (ABBV-0805)	Humanized mAb targeting aggregated α-Syn	Phase 1	NCT04127695	Withdrawn	Nordström et al. (2021)

Clinical trials involving α-Syn antigens include the vaccines AFFITOPE PD01A, AFFITOPE PD03A, and UB312. AFFITOPE PD01A is a synthetic peptide made from the C-terminal amino acids 110 to 130 of α-Synuclein. The phase 1 trial (NCT01568099) tested different dosing schedules, ranging from one dose to four doses of 15 μg or 75 μg given every 4 weeks. Some trials also included a booster shot 36 weeks after the first shot (Volc et al., 2020). Along with good safety and tolerability, the dosage regimens produced an apparent immune response. The most common side effects were headache, fatigue, and injection-site reactions. The study originally lasted 12 months but was extended by another 9 months. During this extension, the remaining 24 patients were randomly assigned to either the 15 μg or 75 μg dose, and they were followed for 24 weeks (NCT01885494). PD01A treatment showed long-term safety and tolerability along with targeted active immunotherapy, resulting in a significant immune response and target engagement. AFFITOPE PD03A is a second antibody that was developed using the same technology as AFFITOPE PD01A. In the first trial (NCT02267434), the trial went similarly with PD01A. However, throughout the trial, it demonstrated PD03A generated lower antibody titers than those observed in the PD01A. In addition, UB-312 is another synthetic type of peptide-based immunization that targets the 12-amino-acid sequence in the α-Syn C terminus (Nimmo et al., 2023). A study demonstrated that the production of antibodies through UB-312 vaccination in guinea pigs interacted specifically with α-Syn oligomers and fibrils present in the brain tissue of post-mortem PD patients. The preclinical evaluation of UB-312 lacked any assessment of its protective effects in animal models that represent these diseases. The first phase clinical trial (NCT04075318) testing this immunization approach for PD continues to be in progress.

Passive immunization involves the administration of exogenous monoclonal antibodies that specifically bind extracellular α-syn aggregates to inhibit their aggregation while enabling microglia for clearance. Prasinezumab (PRX002/RO7046015) exists as a humanized IgG1 monoclonal antibody, which currently undergoes advanced evaluation. The monoclonal 9E4 antibody, which targets mouse α-Sy at amino acid 118–126, forms the base for this humanized version. Research showed passive immunization through 9E4 as an α-Syn C-terminus target effectively reached the CNS and inhibit α-Syn buildup. The administration of 9E4 successfully lowered the amount of α-Syn that built up in axons and synapses linked to neurodegenerative diseases. The first phase of human trial (NCT02095171) demonstrated that a single dose ascending maintained a positive safety profile. The treatment resulted in a dose-dependent decline of "free" a-Syn levels in the serum. The maximum effect was observed at a dosage of 30 mg/kg (Schenk et al., 2016). To measure its safety, the addition phase 1 (NCT02157714) trial was held, where the multiple ascending doses of it were administered to the PD patients. Consequently, no improvements or modifications were observed in the levels of free α-Syn in the cerebral spinal fluid (Jankovic et al., 2018). The trial in stage 2 (NCT03100149) consisted of monthly injection using low or high doses of prasinezumab (1500 or 4500 mg) in addition to an extension of 52 weeks. The results demonstrated that prasinezumab medication produced no significant difference in global and imaging analysis regarding the measurement of PD progression with placebo (Pagano et al., 2022). Based on the results of the extension trial (NCT04777331), it is expected to assess efficacy and safety of prasinezumab in early PD patients on steady treatment relative to a placebo. The research is in progress and will reach a completion in December 2026.

Cinpanemab is a human monoclonal antibody which bind to the N-terminal epitope in PD patients. Therapy with BIIB054 in three distinct mouse models, one with wild-type and with two alpha-Syn A53T transgenes, inhibits alpha-synuclein neuropathology and motor impairments after injections of preformed fibrils of alpha-Syn (Weihofen et al., 2019). The drug was seen to be well tolerated in a phase 1 (NCT02459886) clinical study in a single-ascending dose trial up to 45 mg/kg. There was little penetration of the drug to the cerebrospinal fluid as they demonstrated to only 0.13 to 0.56% of plasma concentration (Brys et al., 2019). The clinical examination of BIIB054 at 13 doses remains unpublished from the NCT03716570 trial. The Phase 2 (NCT03318523) evaluation of cinpanemab demonstrated no clinical advantage compared to placebo after 52 weeks of treatment (Lang et al., 2022). This led to the discontinuation of its further development.

Current research in MEDI1341 as the potential third monoclonal antibody is under development. MEDI1341 binds to the C terminus of α-Syn by interacting with an epitope between amino acids 103–129 based on its binding capacity to multiple α-Syn mutants (Schofield et al., 2019). The antibody binds specifically to aggregated α-synuclein but does not interact with β- or γ-synuclein while showing binding to Lewy bodies and Lewy neurites from post-mortem patient tissue. The initial trial phase (NCT03272165) involved a single ascending dose given to healthy volunteers over 1 hour. The final assessment took place after 13 weeks. The second trial (NCT04449484) aimed to assess multiple ascending doses over 8 weeks, with infusions every 4 weeks. Results from both studies are still unpublished.

Lu AF82422 functions as an agent that prevents α-Syn aggregation while undergoing evaluation for its potential therapeutic applications. Research on a single dose ranging from 1 to 30 mg/kg in a cynomolgus monkey showed that the pharmacokinetic parameters of Lu AF82422 fell within the expected range for a monoclonal antibody (mAb) targeting a soluble antigen (Lindström et al., 2014). The results of the first trial (NCT03611569) were the safety and tolerability of a single intravenous administration of Lu AF82422, including its pharmacokinetics, and pharmacodynamics. However, the study's results are still unpublished. Another substance that targets α-Synuclein aggregation is BAN0805, also known as ABBV-080. In a murine model of PD, mAB47 (a murine variant of ABBV-0805) showed a strong preference for binding to pathogenic soluble aggregated α-Syn and inhibits the buildup of α-Syn pathology. The trial was withdrawn for strategic reasons (NCT04127695) (Nordström et al., 2021)

2.5.2 Gene therapy for Parkinson's disease

Gene therapy encompasses treatments that involve the introduction of DNA into cells to modify protein production, thereby alleviating symptoms or potentially curing diseases. For decades, researchers have endeavored to refine gene therapy interventions for numerous diseases. Certain uncommon genetic diseases characterized by a specific, well-defined mutation in a particular gene have achieved notable advancements. A healthy gene is delivered into the cells of these patients in this scenario. The cellular apparatus utilizes the functional gene to synthesize a viable protein, hence potentially curing the patient. Some viruses can integrate their genetic material into the host cell's genetic material and researcher adeptly utilize these processes to advance gene therapy. The damaging DNA segments are removed from the virus, and the selected gene is integrated into the viral framework. The modified virus is subsequently injected into a designated area of the body, facilitating its ability to "infect" cells. Provided that everything proceeds as intended, the DNA segment incorporated into the altered virus is utilized by the cellular machinery to synthesize the desired protein. Adeno-associated virus (AAV) is frequently used in gene therapy due to its characteristic of not eliciting symptoms upon cellular introduction.

2.5.2.1 AAV-mediated dopamine biosynthesis and neuroprotective gene delivery

Adeno-associated virus (AAV) vectors are a common method for gene delivery in neuronal transduction in the brain because of their safety, effectiveness, and long-lasting expression. To address this imbalance, new gene therapies using AAV have been developed that mainly focus on three stages (Fig. 2.2): (1) introducing the enzyme aromatic L-amino acid decarboxylase (AADC) to increase dopamine levels in the substantia nigra, (2) reducing overactive glutamatergic output to the subthalamic nucleus (STN) through glutamic acid decarboxylase (GAD) by converting it into the inhibitory neurotransmitter GABA, and (3) integrating neurotrophic factors like Glial Cell Line Derived Neurotrophic Factor (GDNF) and Neurturin (NRTN) to improve neuronal functions in the substantia nigra and striatum.

The injection of AADC using AAV vectors, specifically AAV2-hAADC, has shown promising results in both preclinical and clinical studies. AADC is an enzyme essential for producing dopamine from its precursor, L-DOPA. In mouse models of PD directly injecting AAV2-hAADC into the striatum significantly increased the conversion of L-DOPA to dopamine. This resulted in improved motor function and noticeable behavioral changes (Sánchez-Pernaute et al., 2001). AAV2-hAADC is a neuroprotective drug and is injected into the brain of patients to reverse symptoms of PD as observed through Unified Parkinson's Disease Rating Scale (UPDRS).

The second GAD-based technique includes ferrying GAD to the subthalamic nucleus (STN). This is a method employed to treat enhanced glutamate in substantia nigra and this is achieved by transforming it into GABA to restore inhibition in an area that has experienced loss of dopamine and dysfunction of its circuits. AAV-GAD gene therapy targeting PD has been promising in preclinical studies both in rodent models and non-human primate (NHP) (Ye et al., 2024). In addition, the injection of AAV2-GAD into the substantia nigra led to significant motor improvements.

This third strategy consists of injecting the neurotrophic factors and these are molecules that assist the growth, survival and differentiation of the neurons. Preclinical research reveals the potential of direct injection of AAV vectors expressing neurotrophic factors (including GDNF and NRTN) into the substantia nigra and the striatum in NHP models. Injection of AAV2-GDNF in striatum of NHP was capable in protecting dopaminergic neurons in the substantia nigra. This probably occurred because of the relationship between such regions (Espinoza et al., 2020). Administering AAV that encodes human NRTN (AAV2-hNRTN) to the substantia nigra and striatum in NHP mice significantly reduced motor issues caused by MPTP (Fig. 2.3).

2.5.3 Stem cell and regenerative medicine approaches

The search for new treatments that tackle the underlying cause of PD is becoming increasingly important because current options have limitations. Cell therapy is one promising method. During cell therapy, dopaminergic neurons and other healthy, functional cells are transplanted into the brain. This process replaces the damaged cells and may prevent further nerve damage. By creating a lasting source of dopamine, this approach tries to address the root cause of PD in a more personalized way.

2.5.3.1 iPSC-derived dopaminergic neurons and transplantation strategies

Induced pluripotent stem cells (iPSCs) are somatic cells that are genetically reprogrammed of other cells to acquire stem cell characteristics (Biehl & Russell, 2009). The reprogramming process shows great potential in gene editing in which it enables the insertion of regulatory genes into the cell

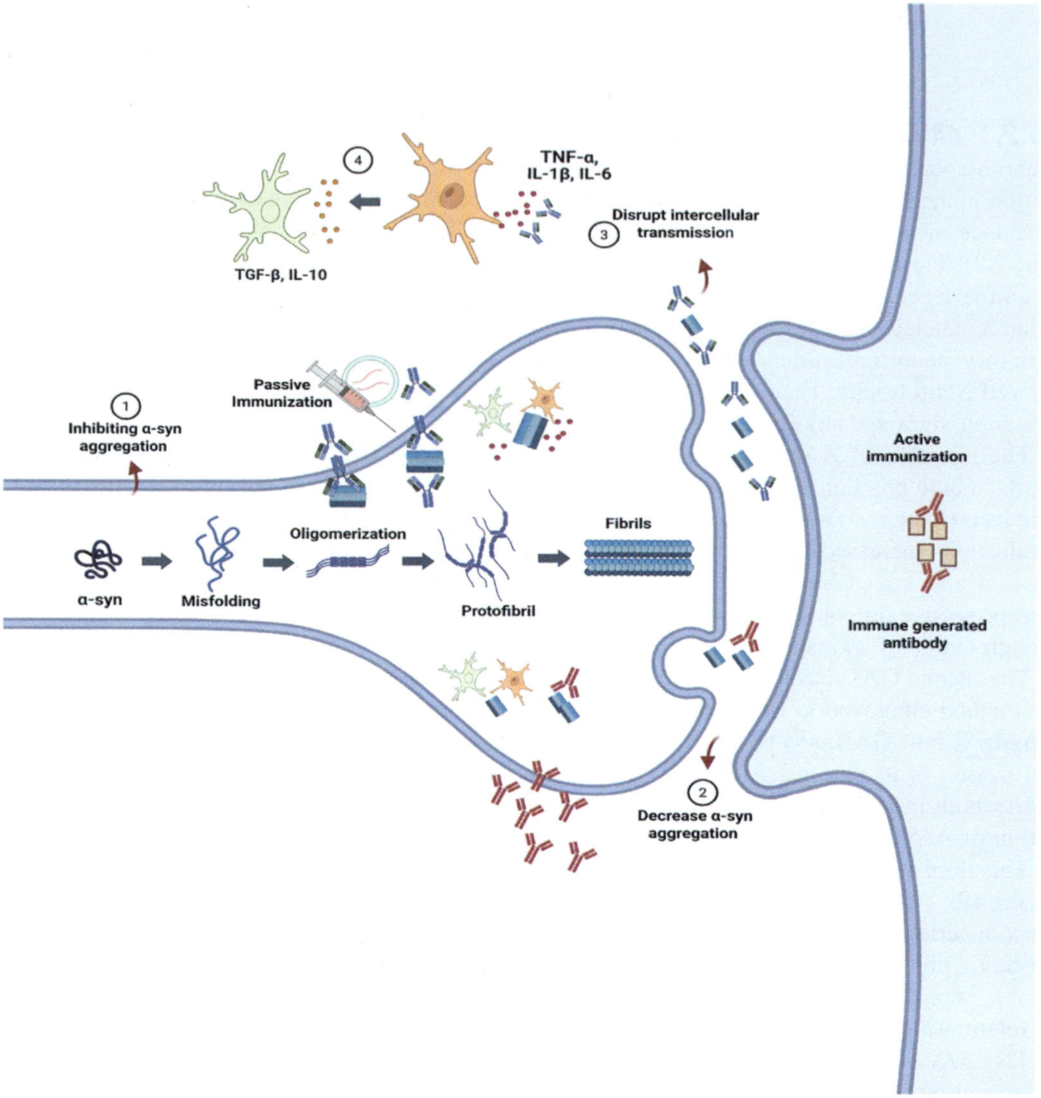

FIGURE 2.2

Alpha-synuclein (α-syn) begins its polymerization through individual molecules which transform into progressively larger structures, including oligomers and protofibrils, before forming fibrils that result in toxic inclusions. The accumulated forms trigger neuroinflammation through their ability to stimulate microglial and astrocytic cells. This activation leads to the release of pro-inflammatory cytokines like tumor necrosis factor-α (TNF-α), interleukin-1β (IL-1β), interleukin-6 (IL-6), and interferon-β (IFN-β). To address the toxicity linked to α-Syn, several immunotherapy strategies have been suggested. These strategies include: (1) preventing the aggregation of α-syn, (2) reducing the amount of α-syn released into the extracellular space, (3) blocking its transmission between cells, and (4) adjusting immune responses to promote an anti-inflammatory state. In active immunization, a small fragment of the α-syn protein is introduced into the body to activate an immune response. This response leads to the production of antibodies that help clearing α-Syn through phagocytosis. In contrast, passive immunization involves providing antibodies that can recognize different structural forms of α-Syn, assisting the immune system in identifying and removing them.

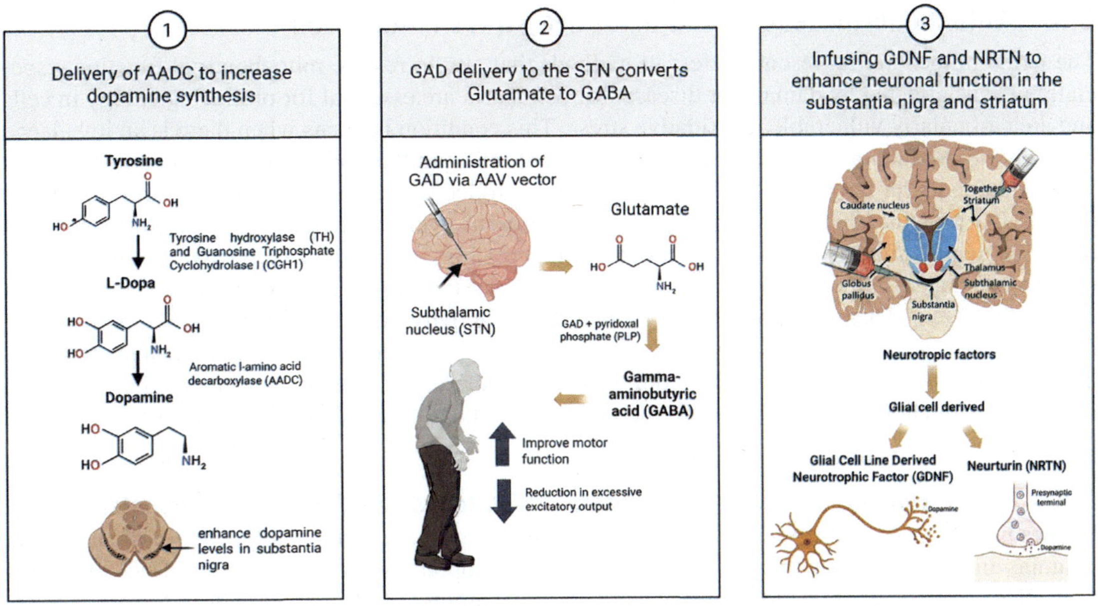

FIGURE 2.3

Presents three gene therapy approaches using AAV vectors for treating PD. (1) introducing the AADC gene increases dopamine production in the striatum by improving the conversion of l-DOPA. This results in better motor performance. (2) Delivering the GAD gene to the STN aids in converting excess glutamate into GABA. This helps restore inhibitory signaling and reduce motor impairments. (3) AAV-mediated delivery of neurotrophic factors like GDNF and NRTN supports the survival and function of dopaminergic neurons in the substantia nigra and striatum. This leads to significant recovery from motor deficits in experimental models.

genome. Induced pluripotent stem cells (iPSCs) are a feasible alternative to conventional pluripotent stem cells because they represent few ethical concerns. Due to the possibility of autologous production, induced pluripotent stem cell (iPSC) grafts are preferred over embryonic stem cell (ESC) grafts (Schweitzer et al., 2020). The process is used to produce neural products through grafting in their somatic cells thus, this eliminates the need to immunosuppress which usually accompanies graft with the embryonic origin of stem cells. Autologous transplantation of patient-specific iPSC-derived neurons is a promising method for treating neurological conditions. Autologous stem cell transplantation uses the patient's cells while allogeneic transplants are derived from another person, either a matched related or unrelated donor. This approach carries the risk of immunological rejection. Individual risk factors, such as specific genetic influences on PD development and relevant environmental exposures, highlight the potential benefits of adjusting a patient's genetic profile to tailor treatment strategies. Current study shows that neurons start to lose their normal functions and morphologies before they die, suggesting that just preventing neuronal death might not be an effective treatment approach (Fan et al., 2020). Therefore, cell transplantation appears to be a promising strategy for treating PD by addressing the root cause through the replacement of missing dopaminergic neurons.

2.5.4 Mitochondrial rescue and oxidative stress modulation

The term "mitochondrial rescue" refers to methods that aim to restore mitochondrial function, especially in cells affected by damage or disease. Mitochondria are essential for producing energy in cells and are particularly vulnerable to oxidative stress. This condition happens when there is an imbalance between the production of reactive oxygen species (ROS) and the body's ability to neutralize them. When mitochondria failed to function properly, they produce excessive ROS which harm mitochondrial DNA, proteins, and lipids; thus, creating a harmful cycle of cellular damage. Mitochondrial rescue strategies, such as stimulating mitochondrial creation, improving mitophagy (the process that removes damaged mitochondria), and using antioxidants that target mitochondria are important to disrupt this cycle. These therapies boost mitochondrial activity, reduce oxidative stress, and support overall cellular health. Managing oxidative stress is vital in neurodegenerative diseases and metabolic disorders where mitochondrial dysfunction plays a major role. Therefore, treatments that focus on improving mitochondrial health not only aid energy production but also protect against the harmful effects of oxidative stress.

2.5.4.1 Antioxidants, mitophagy enhancers and mitochondrial biogenesis boosters

Studies has highlighted the potential of natural antioxidants which include polyphenols, phenolic and vitamins in preventing and managing of PD. These compounds show promising effect of neuroprotective against oxidative stress and enhance the functioning of the mitochondria. Natural antioxidants possessed a neuroprotective effect since these compounds can neutralize ROS, inhibit their causes of oxidative damage to lipids, proteins and DNA, and enhance the overall resistance of the dopaminergic neurons (Mittal et al., 2023). Polyphenols, particularly flavonoids, are widely recognized for their antioxidant and neuroprotective properties. Grape seed extract, that is rich in polyphenols, such as proanthocyanidins and resveratrol has demonstrated some potential in preventing and reducing the symptoms of PD, as it possesses powerful antioxidant effects (Fandy, 2022). The presence of flavonoid isoquercitrin and quercetin protects against oxidative stress within the dopaminergic neurons as a form of potential treatment of PD (Magalingam et al., 2014). Further, it has been shown that the flavonoids have the possibility of enhancing neuroplasticity and stimulating cognitive activities which are normally impaired in conditions of neurodegenerative disorders.

Vitamins A, C, and E have shown protective effects against neuron damage caused by oxidative stress in Parkinson's disease (PD). These vitamins act by neutralizing harmful reactive species of nitrogen and oxygen and by inhibiting the accumulation of proteins that can contribute to reducing oxidative stress. Coenzyme Q10 (CoQ10) may serve as one of the potential agents in alleviating the progression of PD due to the deficiency of mitochondrial complex-1 and the production of free radicals (Sutachan et al., 2012). Furthermore, another compound such as α-lipoic acid has shown promising potential in treating PD models particularly in improving motor and behavioral symptoms induced by 6- hydroxydopamine. It helps in restoring ATP levels in the midbrain and improves on the structure of the mitochondria by reducing fragmentation and vacuolization. Phenolic compounds as Piceatannol, Thymoquinone, and Esculetin have been shown to be effective kinase inhibitors, which reducing oxidative stress and neuronal death in models of PD (Angeles et al., 2016). In addition, essential minerals like zinc and selenium play vital roles in the body's antioxidant defense systems. Zinc, for example, has been shown to enhance the activity of several antioxidant enzymes, offering neuroprotective effects in experimental PD models (Mbiydzenyuy et al., 2018). Urate is a naturally occurring antioxidant compound (low level of urate is linked to the reduced probability of PD), and it could provide neuroprotective properties such as able to scavenge free radicals. Moreover, artemisinin has demonstrated neuroprotective effect in reducing neurological damage by 6-OHDA and MPP+ in in vitro and in vivo assays. The drug mobilizes the ERK1/2 signaling pathway that reduce oxidative stress, enhances the activity of mitochondria and inhibits cell death. This is an indication of a potential therapy of artemisinin in preserving the mitochondrial function (Li, Yang, et al., 2023).

The role of regulating mitophagy to enhance mitochondrial biogenesis is important since both processes interactively to increase the status of mitochondrial health and functioning. Mitophagy refers to the selective removal of damaged or dysfunctional mitochondria, a process essential for cellular health and efficient energy production (Hurtado & Schnellmann, 2024; Palikaras et al., 2015). A proper balance between the formation of new mitochondria (biogenesis) and the clearance of damaged ones (mitophagy) is vital to prevent the buildup of malfunctioning mitochondria. The key controllers of this interaction are the PGC-1 alpha responsible of increased production of mitochondria, and other mitophagy receptors such as Parkin and PINK1, that identify damaged mitochondria for elimination. activating mitophagy not only eliminates harmful mitochondria but also facilitates the production of healthier ones by reducing cellular stress. This balance becomes especially important during periods of metabolic stress or physical exertion, when mitophagy is naturally upregulated to maintain mitochondrial quality. This method assists in facilitating the synthesis of the new mitochondria in the form of signaling that involves AMPK and SIRT1 (Chen, Chuang, et al., 2022; Chen, Qin, et al., 2022). In recent study, the mitophagy drugs are used to demonstrate that they can boost the mitochondrial biogenesis potential. This observation may result in the development of new interventions regarding the treatment of age-associated diseases and metabolic disorders that are related to mitochondrial dysfunction.

2.6 Emerging technologies and future perspectives

Parkinson's disease (PD) is a multifactorial neurodegenerative disorder characterized by a progressive loss of dopaminergic neurons. Lewy body pathology, and a range of motor and non-motor clinical manifestations. While progress has been made in symptomatic management, early recognition of PD and disease-modifying treatments remain largely still a distant reality. Recent advances in sciences and technology offer an important opportunity for advances in diagnosis, treatment, and possibly even prevention of PD.

2.6.1 Biomarker discovery for early and accurate diagnosis

Early and accurate PD diagnosis is necessary to initiate early treatment and improve clinical outcomes. Recent biomarker research has focused on cerebrospinal fluid (CSF) and blood-based biomarkers of underlying neuropathology.

2.6.1.1 CSF and blood biomarker for α-synuclein, DJ-1 and neurofilament light chain

Both phosphorylated (p-α-syn) and oligomeric (o-α-syn) forms of α-synuclein (α-syn) in CSF are potential diagnostic biomarkers in PD. A number of meta-analyses support the finding that PD patients have significantly lower total CSF α-syn levels compared to healthy controls (Zhou et al., 2015). Oosterveld et al. (2019), found that combining α-syn species may improve sensitivity and specificity in distinguishing PD from atypical parkinsonism syndromes. Additionally, PD patients had higher o-α-syn and p-S129-α-syn levels, with o-α-syn providing a high level of diagnostic accuracy (AUC $\approx$ 0.86–0.95%; 75%–89% sensitivity, 87%–91% specificity) (Majbour et al., 2020).

DJ-1, an oxidoreductase chaperone protein involved in oxidative stress and antioxidant defense has shown inconsistent results as a PD biomarker. Mutations in the DJ-1 gene (PARK7) can lead to inherited PD and oxidized DJ-1 (oxDJ-1) signifies oxidative stress that likely contributes to the PD disease process, but total DJ-1 concentrations in blood or CSF often shows little or no difference between PD and control (Chahine et al., 2013; Saito, 2017). That said, there have been several oxidized forms or evolving post-translational modifications of DJ-1 such as 4-hydroxy-2-nonenal modified DJ-1) that have been found to change in PD, especially in later stages, suggesting these may be more sensitive biomarkers for the disease (Lin et al., 2012). Current studies suggest that the market value of DJ-1 is greater in relation to other markers in multi-marker panels than with its use as a single marker, because confounding factors such as blood cell contamination and age my have an impact on plasma levels. Future development of sensitive tests for oxidized DJ-1 forms and antibodies against these variants enhance DJ-1 in its role as a biomarker for the onset and progression of PD (Chahine et al., 2013; Saito, 2017). Therefore, DJ-1 exists as a relevant marker because of its oxidized forms, and its utility in multi-marker schemes, rather than as an individual diagnostic marker.

Neurofilament light chain (Nfl), a cytoskeletal protein that is released after neuroaxonal injury, has rapidly emerged as well-validated biomarker with reproducible correlations to disease severity, motor decline, and cognitive impairment. Both elevated Nfl levels in serum and CSF have been shown to measure global progression markers and additionally revealed postural instability and gait disorder (PIGD) phenotype in early PD, as plasma Nfl was previously shown to differentiate PIGD from tremor-dominant subtypes and predicted poorer motor and cognitive outcomes at 2-year follow up (Ng et al., 2020). Buhmann et al. (2023) established that blood Nfl is a valid measure of neuroaxonal disruption and is associated with motor and cognitive decline and PIGD symptoms over time. Blood Nfl was also negatively correlated with cognitive function in Alzheimer's and other like dementias, with plasma levels independently correlating with more rapid cognitive decline (Bäckström et al., 2020). Consequently, blood Nfl has progressed from a candidate biomarker to a realistic, less invasive progression diagnostic in clinical and research settings.

2.6.2 Nanotechnology-driven drug delivery systems

The treatment of PD is notoriously challenging because of the highly selective blood-brain barrier (BBB), which restricts therapeutic access to and action in the central nervous system (CNS). Nevertheless, nanotechnology offers unprecedented solutions.

2.6.2.1 Nanocarriers for targeted therapy and BBB penetration

Between 2020 and 2025, lipid-based nanocarriers such as liposomes, solid lipid nanoparticles (SLNs) and nanostructured lipid carriers (NLCs) were increasingly embraced as novel drug delivery platforms for PD due primarily to enhanced CNS bioavailability targeting the BBB while mitigating peripheral side effects. Their amphiphilic composition facilitates the encapsulation and maintenance of both hydrophilic and lipophilic drugs, including dopamine and levodopa, protecting drugs from plasma enzymatic degradation, while allowing them to have sustained release properties that provides optimal therapeutic indices. In a review in 2024, Cai et al. reported that liposomal and SLN/NLC formulations robustly increase CNS levodopa concentration in preclinical PD models and increased behavioral or motor functions while decreasing systemic side effects. Surface-functionalization of lipid-based nanocarriers with ligands like apolipoprotein E or targeting peptides is beneficial to receptor-mediated transcytosis across the BBB. It optimizes the targeting of the brain (Teixeira et al., 2022). Moreover, systematic reviews prepared in 2023–24 showed specific drug-loaded lipid carriers particularly SLNs and NLCs compared to organic or in aqueous dispersion with LNPs enhanced attributes including overall stability, scalability, and payload capacity delivered as well as being compatible with the intranasal route of administration to bypass the BBB which reduced first pass effect of metabolism and lessen peripheral distribution (Agosti et al., 2024). In the case of PD, engineered NLCs containing neuroprotective phytochemicals delivered intranasally and characterized by neuroprotective phytochemicals showed a great improvement in motor behavior neuroinflammation and pathological markers in rotenone rodent models as compared to free drug suspensions (Hassan et al., 2023). Taken together, these studies suggest lipid-based nanocarriers may represent a potential, less intrusive approach to the next generation of PD medicines, with enhanced pharmacokinetics, targeting to brain, and safety profiles compared to traditional drugs.

Polymeric nanoparticles, especially from biocompatible polymers like PLGA and chitosan, have become extremely promising delivery mechanisms for levodopa, and antioxidant therapy for PD. The target delivery features of these nanocarriers can achieve regulated release, protection from enzyme breakdown, and bulk delivery to the brain-capitalizing on one of the significant issues faced by levodopa and other dopaminergic medicines, including BBB permeability and the rapid plasma half-life. The characteristics of PLGA-based systems were highlighted by (Alabrahim & Azzazy, 2022), who particularly discussed their advantages in increasing levodopa stability and maintaining levodopa release in a controlled or delayed pattern, which improves the duration of therapy and efficacy of treatment. The primary outcome of this method of drug delivery will be to lessen systemic side effects associated with all conditioning dopaminergic medications (Alabrahim & Azzazy, 2022). Ahmad et al. (2022) also used chitosan-based nanoparticles for intranasal levodopa delivery in male Wistar rats. The authors found that a formulation of chitosan C2 (553 ± 52 nm, zeta potential +46.2 mV, encapsulation efficiency ~82%) approximately doubled brain levodopa bioavailability compared to unformulated levodopa, but the levodopa drug structure was unaltered (Ahmad et al., 2022). In 2022, Mogharbel et al. demonstrated that biodegradable NH_2 PEO-PCL nanoparticles with levodopa and curcumin crossed in-vitro BBB models, had low cytotoxicity, and had potential as neuroprotective carriers (Mogharbel et al., 2022).

Within the new technology of nanomedicine for PD, there have been new smart nanocarriers developed, including gold nanorods (AuNRs) functionalised with Angiopep-2 (Au-PCBLD-ANG), which were designed to traverse the BBB, and release levodopa after it was exposed to oxidative stress, a feature of PD pathology AuNRs are sensitive in the second near-infrared (NIR-II) window according to (Liang et al., 2024) and were surface-modulated with Angiopep-2 since it is capable of recognizing low-density lipoprotein receptor-related protein 1 (LRP-1) to facilitate receptor-mediated transcytosis. The photothermal properties of gold nanorods may facilitate the relaxation of tight junctions, thereby augmenting paracellular permeability. Specifically, levodopa is conjugated via a diselenide bond that may be cleaved under conditions of reactive oxygen species (ROS) enrichment. This allows for site-specific release in the oxidative environment seen within the PD brain, whilst providing antioxidant effects via the scavenging of ROS. In-vivo experiments using MPTP-induced PD mice models showed that treatment with Au-PCBLD-ANG led to strong enhancement of motor functions, as indicated by enhancements in both locomote activity, and in the rotarod and pole tests, compared to free levodopa. Additionally, biochemical tests showed significant reductions in oxidative stress markers in brain tissues, including decreased levels of ROS and lipid peroxidation, and increased levels of SOD (superoxide dismutase) activity. Taken together, these findings suggests that Au-PCBLD-ANG is a potential dual-function nanoplatform for drug delivery and neuroprotection in a timely manner for the treatment of PD (Liang et al., 2024).

2.6.3 Artificial intelligence and precision medicine in PD

Artificial intelligence (AI) has fundamentally transformed biomedical research providing robust tools for data integration, biomarker identification, and drug development. AI now contributes to predictive diagnosis and personalized therapeutic interventions in PD (Valerio et al., 2025).

2.6.3.1 AI-driven drug repurposing and predicitve modeling for personalized therapy

Drug discovery research using AI algorithms for CNS drugs increasingly makes use of graph convolutional networks (GCNs) and deep learning technologies to predict BBB permeability which a useful filter for CNS drug candidates. Kong et al. (2021) published work on a relational GCN that combined drug-protein interaction graphs with molecular descriptors and were able to achieve an AUROC of 0.926, which outperformed conventional LightGBM methods designing a scalable solution to exponentially speed BBB permeability predictions in drug pipelines (Ding et al., 2022). There are also convolutional GNN architectures that have classified BBB-permeable molecules quite well, with around 1900 compound testing providing useful screening methods for early-stage CNS drug discovery (Jing et al., 2025), with accuracy and recall values around 0.94 and 0.96, respectively. All of these models will not only speed up pre-clinical testing but also help discover existing drugs with favorable CNS drug-like characteristics.

In PD, drug repurposing, AI-based models interrogating multi-omic, gene expression, and cheminformatic databases are finding unexpected neuroprotective options at an astonishing pace (Guo et al., 2025). developed a drug target network model to rank drug priorities with 28 FDA-approved medicines for PD based on their effectiveness and novelty. Cyproheptadine and Omaveloxolone have been shown to protect dopaminergic SH-SY5Y cell against MPP^+-induced cytotoxicity in-vitro and in-vivo MPTP-inhibited IL-6 expression and stabilized levels of tyrosine hydroxylase (TH) by blocking the MAPK/NF kB pathway, while Omaveloxolone stimulated the Nrf2/ARE pathway, and inhibited lipid peroxidation and neuronal loss (Guo et al., 2025). These findings extend past typical drug discovery practices and showcase the potential for AI to efficiently bridge drug-target interactions with PD-specific molecular networks and animal model data, rapidly generating hypothesis-driven repurposing leads with real therapeutic potential.

In addition to drug discovery, predictive modeling with multimodal AI is changing personalized therapy for PD using clinical, imaging and omics data. For instance, in a multimodal framework called RACF created by (Cao & Long, 2025), they fused SNP profiles with MRI data using deep cross-modal alignment and attention mechanisms to identify PD accurately. Another example, with nature-like experiments using RNNs on longitudinal RNA-seq and MDS-UPDRS scores achieved a strong prediction of phases of progression ($r = 0.83$) (Ahmed et al., 2022). Other models integrated functional/structural connectomes with genomes and used graph convolution and attention fusion and obtained correlation coefficients >0.8 in PD categorization (Chan et al., 2022). Together, these AI networks support precision neurology goals of predicting individual journeys and creating treatment plans that are based on comprehensive phenotypic and genotypic profiles so that disease may be managed in a more predictive, proactive, and individualized manner.

2.6.4 Gut microbiome modulation in PD: A novel therapeutic avenue

The gut-brain axis (GBA) and its effects on neuroinflammation, α-syn aggregation, and motor symptoms are new areas of study in PD. Now it is thought that the gastrointestinal (GI) system is the source of early PD pathology.

2.6.4.1 Probiotics, fecal microbiota transplantation, and microbiome-targeted interventions

Changes in gut microbiota composition are often noted in PD, many studies reported decreased abundance of SCFA-producers (e.g., *Faecalibacterium*, *Roseburia*) and increased pro-inflammatory taxa (e.g., Enterobacteriaceae) in PD cases compared to controls (Cheng et al., 2023). Sampson et al. (2016) found that transplantation of fecal microbiota from PD patients into α-synuclein-overexpressing mice caused motor dysfunction, microglial activation, and α-synuclein pathology promotion; intact fecal samples from healthy donors and did not cause the observed deficits. This landmark study demonstrated that dysbiotic gut microbiota can promote neurodegeneration associated with PD in the GBA from correlation to a causative (Sampson et al., 2016). In Yang et al. (2024) follow-up work published in CNS Neuroscience & Therapeutics, they duplicated the observed findings by transplanting feces from individuals with diagnosed PD into A53T α-synuclein transgenic mice. Also, they observed motor deficits, increased microglial and astrocyte activation, and α-synuclein aggregates in the brain and the gut (Feng et al., 2024). In contrast, when the mice were transplanted with fecal samples from healthy individuals, their pathology induced was not observed (Feng et al., 2024).

Probiotic supplementation has gained clinical momentum in the allevation of GI symptoms and systemic inflammation related to PD. For example, a 2023 randomized controlled trial of multistrain *Lactobacillus* and *Bifidobacterium* compared to placebo in 72 patients with PD, observed great increase in spontaneous bowl movements and stool consistency (Bristol Stool Scale) at 4 weeks (Ghalandari et al., 2023; Tan et al., 2020). In a 2023 meta-analysis of 11 RCTs (840 subjects), they found probiotics improved constipation outomes, lower laxative use, and a lower motor score (mean UPDRS III reduction -6.58, 96% CI -12.02 to -1.14) likely mediated by the modulation of inflammatory cytokines (e.g., IL-1β, TNF-α) and enhancement of gut barrier integrity (Xie et al., 2023). These changes were also reported with reduced fecal calprotectin and increased SCFAs (e.g., butyrate), indicating that changes in microbiota have fair contributions to the systemic anti-inflammatory benefits obtained (Kawahata et al., 2024).

Fecal microbiota transplantation (FMT) is becoming a potential disease-modifying intervention for PD. In 2023 pilot RCT of $n = 12$ PD patients, recipients of donor-derived FMT noted subjective improvements in motor function, constipation, and sleep. On the primary endpoint of the study (defined as UPDRS-III 'OFF' state score), there was a mean decrease of ~37.5% in 4 months (DuPont et al., 2023). A Chinese Phase 2 trial planned for 2023–24 ($n = 56$) reported improved UPDRS-total scores (mean group x time effect -6.56, $P < .05$), with restored gut microbial diversity but without serious side effects (Cheng et al., 2023). In a meta-analysis published in Neurology in 2025, researchers synthesized three placebo-controlled RCTs with 145 PD patients examining effectiveness of FMT interventions through September 2024. The meta-analysis showed no significant differences in the MDS UPDRS Parts I-IV, IBS-SSS, PDQ-39, or MoCA outcomes measures between FMT (MDS UPDRS Parts I-IV, $P > .999$; IBD-SSS, $P > .999$; PDQ-39, $P > .999$; MoCA, $P = .568$) and placebo (all outcomes $P > .5$ with minimal heterogeneity ($I^2 < 17\%$). There were more mild adverse gastrointestinal events reported with FMT (RR 3.32 [95% CI 1.01–10.87], $P = .05$) (Khowdiary et al., 2025)

In addition to probiotics and FMT, microbiome-targeted drugs intend to restore microbial balance and provide neuroprotection. Postbiotics such as sodium butyrate, which are non-viable microbial metabolites have been show to have neuroprotective effects in rodents displayed PD symptoms induced by MPTP through modifying microglial activation (an immune response), specifically reducing gut permeability and motor symptoms. Researchers found that butyrate therapy preserved dopaminergic neurons and improved motor function, while also supporting the integrity of the intestinal barrier (Missiego- Beltrán et al., 2024). Also, SCFA-enhacing dietary strategies like resistant starch supplements or high-fiber diets are being evaluated as methods to raise endogenous SCFA levels and reduce systemic inflammation. In a 2025 pilot interventional trial, PD patients on a 4-week high fiber diet (rich in lactulose and resistant starch) showed elevated fecal SCFA levels, specifically butyrate as well as reduced GI symptoms (Bedarf et al., 2025). Similarly, an open-label trial of prebiotic fiber bar reported no adverse effects and decreased intestinal inflammation, improvements in SCFs, and mild improvements in motor symptoms (Hall et al., 2023). Finally, a few phage treatments specifically targeting pathogenic bacteria (e.g., Enterobacteriaceae) are in early pre-clinical phases of development, by using bacteriophage to specifically inhibit gut populations while maintaining beneficial commensals. A 2024 study in Scientific Reports was able to show that bacteriophage targeting *Enterococcus faecalis*, a gut bacteria decarboxylates levodopa which will restore the effectiveness of levodopa and motor behaviors in MPTP-PD mice, by selectively inhibiting the *E. faecalis* without inhibiting beneficial gut microbiota (Hong et al., 2024). Combining the above approaches which are postbiotics, SCFA enhancers, and phage therapy, all provide novel and complementary approaches for rebalancing GBA signaling and potentially slowing the development of PD.

The convergence of biomarker science, nanotechnology, AI and microbiome investigations is changing how people manage PD moving forward. Ultimately, the development of reliable peripheral biomarkers may enable us to establish diagnosis before the clinical manifestation of disease. Likewise, smart nanocarriers and AI-directed treatment techniques are expanding capacity for targeted treatment. Research on microbiome modulation has found potential which not just for symptom management, but possibly with respect to altering the progression of the disease. This makes multidisciplinary, integrative approaches particularly important for translating new science and practice to clinical and thereby better outcomes for patients.

References

Agnieszka, W., Paweł, P., & Małgorzata, K. (2022). How to optimize the effectiveness and safety of Parkinson's disease therapy? - A systematic review of drugs interactions with food and dietary supplements. *Current Neuropharmacology, 20*(7), 1427–1447.

Agosti, E., Zeppieri, M., Antonietti, S., Battaglia, L., Ius, T., Gagliano, C., Fontanella, M. M., & Panciani, P. P. (2024). Navigating the nose-to-brain route: A systematic review on lipid-based nanocarriers for central nervous system disorders. *Pharmaceutics, 16*(3). https://doi.org/10.3390/pharmaceutics16030329

Ahmad, M. Z., Sabri, A. H. B., Anjani, Q. K., Domínguez-Robles, J., Abdul Latip, N., & Hamid, K. A. (2022). Design and development of levodopa loaded polymeric nanoparticles for intranasal delivery. *Pharmaceuticals, 15*(3). https://doi.org/10.3390/ph15030370

Ahmed, S., Komeili, M., & Park, J. (2022). Predictive modelling of Parkinson's disease progression based on RNA-sequence with densely connected deep recurrent neural networks. *Scientific Reports, 12*(1).

Airavaara, M., Parkkinen, I., Konovalova, J., Albert, K., Chmielarz, P., & Domanskyi, A. (2020). Back and to the future: From neurotoxin-induced to human parkinson's disease models. *Current Protocols in Neuroscience, 91* (1). https://doi.org/10.1002/cpns.88

Alabrahim, O. A. A., & Azzazy, H. M. E. S. (2022). Polymeric nanoparticles for dopamine and levodopa replacement in parkinson's disease. *Nanoscale Advances, 4*(24), 5233–5244. https://doi.org/10.1039/d2na00524g

Alam, M., Abbas, K., Mustafa, M., Usmani, N., & Habib, S. (2024). Microbiome-based therapies for Parkinson's disease. *Frontiers in Nutrition, 11*. https://doi.org/10.3389/fnut.2024.1496616

Angeles, D. C., Ho, P., Dymock, B. W., Lim, K. L., Zhou, Z. D., & Tan, E. K. (2016). Antioxidants inhibit neuronal toxicity in Parkinson's disease-linked LRRK2. *Annals of Clinical and Translational Neurology, 3*(4), 288–294. https://doi.org/10.1002/acn3.282

Antonini, A., Emmi, A., & Campagnolo, M. (2023). Beyond the dopaminergic system: Lessons learned from levodopa resistant symptoms in parkinson's disease. *Movement Disorders Clinical Practice, 10*(Suppl. 2), Article S50.

Antonini, A., Odin, P., Pahwa, R., Aldred, J., Alobaidi, A., Jalundhwala, Y. J., Kukreja, P., Bergmann, L., Inguva, S., Bao, Y., & Chaudhuri, K. R. (2021). The long-term impact of levodopa/carbidopa intestinal gel on 'Off'-time in patients with advanced parkinson's disease: A systematic review. *Advances in Therapy, 38*(6), 2854–2890. https://doi.org/10.1007/s12325-021-01747-1

Ascherio, A., & Schwarzschild, M. A. (2016). The epidemiology of parkinson's disease: Risk factors and prevention. *The Lancet Neurology, 15*(12), 1257–1272. https://doi.org/10.1016/S1474-4422(16)30230-7

Au, K. L. K., Wong, J. K., Tsuboi, T., Eisinger, R. S., Moore, K., Lemos Melo Lobo Jofili Lopes, J., Holland, M. T., Holanda, V. M., Peng-Chen, Z., Patterson, A., Foote, K. D., Ramirez-Zamora, A., Okun, M. S., & Almeida, L. (2021). Globus pallidus internus (GPi) deep brain stimulation for parkinson's disease: Expert review and commentary. *Neurology and Therapy, 10*(1), 7–30. https://doi.org/10.1007/s40120-020-00220-5

Bäckström, D., Linder, J., Jakobson Mo, S., Riklund, K., Zetterberg, H., Blennow, K., Forsgren, L., & Lenfeldt, N. (2020). NfL as a biomarker for neurodegeneration and survival in parkinson disease. *Neurology, 95*(7), Article E827. https://doi.org/10.1212/WNL.0000000000010084

Bandopadhyay, R., Mishra, N., Rana, R., Kaur, G., Ghoneim, M. M., Alshehri, S., Mustafa, G., Ahmad, J., Alhakamy, N. A., & Mishra, A. (2022). Molecular mechanisms and therapeutic strategies for levodopa-induced dyskinesia in parkinson's disease: A perspective through preclinical and clinical evidence. *Frontiers in Pharmacology, 13*. https://doi.org/10.3389/fphar.2022.805388

Beaurain, M., Salabert, A.-S., Payoux, P., Gras, E., Talmont, F., & Receptors, N. M. D. A. (2024). Distribution, role, and insights into neuropsychiatric disorders. *Pharmaceuticals, 17*(10), 1265. https://doi.org/10.3390/ph17101265

Bedarf, J. R., Romano, S., Heinzmann, S. S., Duncan, A., Traka, M. H., Ng, D., Segovia-Lizano, D., Simon, M. C., Narbad, A., Wüllner, U., & Hildebrand, F. (2025). A prebiotic dietary pilot intervention restores faecal metabolites and may be neuroprotective in Parkinson's Disease. *Npj Parkinson's Disease, 11*(1). https://doi.org/10.1038/s41531-025-00885-5

Berg, D., Borghammer, P., Fereshtehnejad, S. M., Heinzel, S., Horsager, J., Schaeffer, E., & Postuma, R. B. (2021). Prodromal Parkinson disease subtypes — Key to understanding heterogeneity. *Nature Reviews Neurology, 17*(6), 349–361. https://doi.org/10.1038/s41582-021-00486-9

Biehl, J. K., & Russell, B. (2009). Introduction to stem cell therapy. *Journal of Cardiovascular Nursing, 24*(2), 98–103. https://doi.org/10.1097/JCN.0b013e318197a6a5

Bishara, D. (2023). Managing drugs with anticholinergic activity. *Drug and Therapeutics Bulletin, 61*(9), 135–139. https://doi.org/10.1136/dtb.2022.000066

Blauwendraat, C., Nalls, M. A., & Singleton, A. B. (2019). The genetic architecture of Parkinson's disease. *The Lancet. Neurology, 19*(2), 170. https://doi.org/10.1016/S1474-4422(19)30287-X

Bloem, B. R., Okun, M. S., & Klein, C. (2021). Parkinson's disease. *The Lancet, 397*(10291), Article 22842303. https://doi.org/10.1016/S0140-6736(21)00218-X

Bonilla-Jaime, H., Sánchez-Salcedo, J. A., Estevez-Cabrera, M. M., Molina-Jiménez, T., Cortes-Altamirano, J. L., & Alfaro-Rodríguez, A. (2022). Depression and pain: Use of antidepressants. *Current Neuropharmacology, 20* (2), 384–402. https://doi.org/10.2174/1570159X19666210609161447

Borsche, M., Pereira, S. L., Klein, C., & Grünewald, A. (2021). Mitochondria and Parkinson's disease: Clinical, molecular, and translational aspects. *Journal of Parkinson's Disease, 11*(1), 45–60. https://doi.org/10.3233/JPD-201981

Breen, D. P., Halliday, G. M., & Lang, A. E. (2019). Gut-brain axis and the spread of α-synuclein pathology: Vagal highway or dead end? *Movement disorders: Official Journal of the Movement Disorder Society, 34*(3), 307–316.

Brys, M., Fanning, L., Hung, S., Ellenbogen, A., Penner, N., Yang, M., Welch, M., Koenig, E., David, E., Fox, T., Makh, S., Aldred, J., Goodman, I., Pepinsky, B., Liu, Y. T., Graham, D., Weihofen, A., & Cedarbaum, J. M. (2019). Randomized phase I clinical trial of anti–α-synuclein antibody BIIB054. *Movement Disorders, 34*(8), 1154–1163. https://doi.org/10.1002/mds.27738

Budgett, R. F., Bakker, G., Sergeev, E., Bennett, K. A., & Bradley, S. J. (2022). Targeting the type 5 metabotropic glutamate receptor: A potential therapeutic strategy for neurodegenerative diseases? *Frontiers in Pharmacology, 13*. https://doi.org/10.3389/fphar.2022.893422

Buhmann, C., Magnus, T., & Choe, C. (2023). Blood neurofilament light chain in Parkinson's disease. *Journal of Neural Transmission, 130*(6), 755–762.

Burbulla, L. F., Song, P., Mazzulli, J. R., Zampese, E., Wong, Y. C., Jeon, S., Santos, D. P., Blanz, J., Obermaier, C. D., Strojny, C., Savas, J. N., Kiskinis, E., Zhuang, X., Krüger, R., Surmeier, D. J., & Krainc, D. (2017). Dopamine oxidation mediates mitochondrial and lysosomal dysfunction in Parkinson's disease. *Science, 357*(6357), 1255–1261. https://doi.org/10.1126/science.aam9080

Burré, J., Sharma, M., & Südhof, T. C. (2015). Definition of a molecular pathway mediating α-synuclein neurotoxicity. *Journal of Neuroscience: The Official Journal of the Society for Neuroscience, 35*(13), 5221–5232.

Cacabelos, R. (2017). Parkinson's disease: From pathogenesis to pharmacogenomics. *International Journal of Molecular Sciences, 18*(3), 551. https://doi.org/10.3390/ijms18030551

Calabresi, P., Ghiglieri, V., Mazzocchetti, P., Corbelli, I., & Picconi, B. (2015). Levodopa-induced plasticity: A double-edged sword in Parkinson's disease? *Philosophical Transactions of the Royal Society B: Biological Sciences, 370*(1672), Article 20140184.

Calabresi, P., Picconi, B., Tozzi, A., Ghiglieri, V., & Di Filippo, M. (2014). Direct and indirect pathways of basal ganglia: a critical reappraisal. *Nature Neuroscience, 17*(8), 1022–1030. https://doi.org/10.1038/nn.3743. Epub 2014 Jul 28. PMID: 25065439.

Campanelli, F., Natale, G., Marino, G., Ghiglieri, V., & Calabresi, P. (2022). Striatal glutamatergic hyperactivity in Parkinson's disease. *Neurobiology of Disease, 168*, Article 105697. https://doi.org/10.1016/j.nbd.2022.105697

Cao, J., & Long, X. (2025). RACF: A multimodal deep learning framework for parkinson's disease diagnosis using SNP and MRI data. *Applied Sciences, 15*(8), 4513. https://doi.org/10.3390/app15084513

Capó, T., Biel Rebassa, J., Raïch, I., Lillo, J., Badia, P., Navarro, G., & Reyes-Resina, I. (2025). Future perspectives of NMDAR in CNS disorders. *Molecules, 30*(4), 877. https://doi.org/10.3390/molecules30040877

Cerasa, A., Fasano, A., Morgante, F., Koch, G., & Quattrone, A. (2014). Maladaptive plasticity in levodopa-induced dyskinesias and tardive dyskinesias: Old and new insights on the effects of dopamine receptor pharmacology. *Frontiers in Neurology, 5*. https://doi.org/10.3389/fneur.2014.00049

Chahine, L. M., Stern, M. B., & Chen-Plotkin, A. (2013). Blood-based biomarkers for Parkinson's disease. *Parkinsonism & Related Disorders, 20*, S99–S103.

Chan, Y. H., Wang, C., Soh, W. K., & Rajapakse, J. C. (2022). Combining neuroimaging and omics datasets for disease classification using graph neural networks. *Frontiers in Neuroscience, 16*. https://doi.org/10.3389/fnins.2022.866666

Chase, T. N., & Oh, J. D. (2000). Striatal mechanisms and pathogenesis of Parkinsonian signs and motor complications. *Annals of Neurology, 47*(4).

Chen, S. F., Chuang, Y. C., Wang, C. C., Liao, C. H., & Kuo, H. C. (2022b). Therapeutic efficacy and cognitive adverse events of overactive bladder medication in patients with central nervous system Disorders—A cohort study. *Journal of the Formosan Medical Association, 121*(10), 2101–2108. https://doi.org/10.1016/j.jfma.2022.04.004

Chen, Z., Li, G., & Liu, J. (2020). Autonomic dysfunction in Parkinson's disease: Implications for pathophysiology, diagnosis, and treatment. *Neurobiology of Disease, 134*, Article 104700.

Chen, L., Qin, Y., Liu, B., Gao, M., Li, A., Li, X., & Gong, G. (2022a). PGC-1α-Mediated mitochondrial quality control: Molecular mechanisms and implications for heart failure. *Frontiers in Cell and Developmental Biology, 10*(3), 500–800.

Cheng, Y., Tan, G., Zhu, Q., Wang, C., Ruan, G., Ying, S., Qie, J., Hu, X., Xiao, Z., Xu, F., Chen, L., Chen, M., Pei, Y., Zhang, H., Tian, Y., Chen, D., Liu, X., Huang, H., & Wei, Y. (2023). Efficacy of fecal microbiota transplantation in patients with Parkinson's disease: Clinical trial results from a randomized, placebo-controlled design. *Gut Microbes, 15*(2). https://doi.org/10.1080/19490976.2023.2284247

Chew, Z. X., Lim, C. L., Ng, K. Y., Chye, S. M., Ling, A. P. K., & Koh, R. Y. (2023). The role of monoamine oxidase B inhibitors in the treatment of parkin-son's Disease-An update. *CNS & Neurological Disorders - Drug Targets, 22*(3), 329–352. https://doi.org/10.2174/1871527321666211231100255

Day, J. O., & Mullin, S. (2021). The genetics of parkinson's disease and implications for clinical practice. *Genes, 12*(7), 1006. https://doi.org/10.3390/genes12071006

De Cecco, E., & Legname, G. (2018). The role of the prion protein in the internalization of α-synuclein amyloids. *Prion, 12*(1), 23–27. https://doi.org/10.1080/19336896.2017.1423186

Demailly, A., Moreau, C., & Devos, D. (2024). Effectiveness of continuous dopaminergic therapies in Parkinson's disease: A review of L-DOPA pharmacokinetics/pharmacodynamics. *Journal of Parkinson's Disease, 14*(5), 925–939.

Devanand, D. P., & Fremont, R. (2024). In A. Tasman, et al. (Eds.), *Cognitive enhancers and treatments for alzheimer's disease*. Cham: Tasman's Psychiatry. Springer.

Dewitt, D. C., & Rhoades, E. (2013). α-synuclein can inhibit SNARE-mediated vesicle fusion through direct interactions with lipid bilayers. *Biochemistry, 52*(14), 2385–2387. https://doi.org/10.1021/bi4002369

Di Battista, V., & Hey-Hawkins, E. (2022). Development of prodrugs for treatment of Parkinson's disease: New inorganic scaffolds for blood–brain barrier permeation. *Journal of Pharmaceutical Sciences, 111*(5), 1262–1279. https://doi.org/10.1016/j.xphs.2022.02.005

di Biase, L., Pecoraro, P. M., Carbone, S. P., Caminiti, M. L., & Di Lazzaro, V. (2023). Levodopa-Induced Dyskinesias in parkinson's disease: An overview on pathophysiology, clinical manifestations, therapy management strategies and future directions. *Journal of Clinical Medicine, 12*(13). https://doi.org/10.3390/jcm12134427

Di Luca, D. G., Reyes, N. G. D., & Fox, S. H. (2022). Newly approved and investigational drugs for motor symptom control in Parkinson's Disease. *Drugs, 82*(10), 1027–1053.

Ding, Y., Jiang, X., Kim, Y., & Wren, J. (2022). Relational graph convolutional networks for predicting blood–brain barrier penetration of drug molecules. *Bioinformatics, 38*(10), 2826–2831. https://doi.org/10.1093/bioinformatics/btac211

Dong, L., Zhang, X., Yan, X., Shen, Y., Li, Y., & Yu, X. (2021). Effect of Phosphodiesterase-5 inhibitors on the treatment of Male infertility: A systematic review and meta-analysis. *The World Journal of Men's Health, 39* (4), 776. https://doi.org/10.5534/wjmh.200155

Doroszkiewicz, J., Farhan, J. A., Mroczko, J., Winkel, I., Perkowski, M., & Mroczko, B. (2023). Common and trace metals in alzheimer's and parkinson's diseases. *International Journal of Molecular Sciences, 24*(21). https://doi.org/10.3390/ijms242115721

Dressler, D., & Pan, L. (2022). In *Clinical problems of drugs used to treat movement disorders Neuro-Psychopharmacotherapy* (pp. 4457–4466). Germany: Springer International Publishing. https://doi.org/10.1007/978-3-030-62059-2_456

DuPont, H. L., Suescun, J., Jiang, Z. D., Brown, E. L., Essigmann, H. T., Alexander, A. S., DuPont, A. W., Iqbal, T., Utay, N. S., Newmark, M., & Schiess, M. C. (2023). Fecal microbiota transplantation in Parkinson's disease—A randomized repeat-dose, placebo-controlled clinical pilot study. *Frontiers in Neurology, 14*. https://doi.org/10.3389/fneur.2023.1104759

Espinoza, S., Scarpato, M., Damiani, D., Managò, F., Mereu, M., Contestabile, A., Peruzzo, O., Carninci, P., Santoro, C., Papaleo, F., Mingozzi, F., Ronzitti, G., Zucchelli, S., & Gustincich, S. (2020). SINEUP non-coding RNA targeting GDNF rescues motor deficits and neurodegeneration in a mouse model of parkinson's disease. *Molecular Therapy, 28*(2), 642–652. https://doi.org/10.1016/j.ymthe.2019.08.005

Fabbri, M., Barbosa, R., & Rascol, O. (2023). Off-time treatment options for Parkinson's disease. *Neurology and therapy, 12*(2), 391–424.

Fan, Y., Winanto, & Ng, S.-Y. (2020). Replacing what's lost: A new era of stem cell therapy for Parkinson's disease. *Translational Neurodegeneration, 9*(1), 15–20.

Fandy, S. J. (2022). Grape seed extract's neuroprotective effect and parkinson's disease: A systematic review. *MNJ (Malang Neurology Journal), 9*(1), 44–51. https://doi.org/10.21776/ub.mnj.2023.009.01.9

Farzanehfar, P., Woodrow, H., & Horne, M. (2022). Sensor measurements can characterize fluctuations and wearing off in Parkinson's disease and guide therapy to improve motor, non-motor and quality of life scores. *Frontiers in Aging Neuroscience, 14*, Article 852992.

Fayyad, M., Majbour, N. K., Vaikath, N. N., Erskine, D., El-Tarawneh, H., Sudhakaran, I. P., Abdesselem, H., & El-Agnaf, O. M. A. (2020). Generation of monoclonal antibodies against phosphorylated α-Synuclein at serine 129: Research tools for synucleinopathies. *Neuroscience Letters, 725*. https://doi.org/10.1016/j.neulet.2020.134899

Feng, M., Zou, Z., Shou, P., Peng, W., Liu, M., & Li, X. (2024). Gut microbiota and Parkinson's disease: Potential links and the role of fecal microbiota transplantation. *Frontiers in Aging Neuroscience, 16*. https://doi.org/10.3389/fnagi.2024.1479343

Fisher, R. M. A., & Torrente, M. P. (2024). Histone post-translational modification and heterochromatin alterations in neurodegeneration: Revealing novel disease pathways and potential therapeutics. *Frontiers in Molecular Neuroscience, 17*. https://doi.org/10.3389/fnmol.2024.1456052

Fox, S. H., & Brotchie, J. M. (2010). The MPTP-Lesioned non-human primate models of parkinson's disease. Past, present, and future. *Progress in Brain Research, 184*, 133–157. https://doi.org/10.1016/S0079-6123(10)84007-5

Franco, R., Navarro, G., & Martínez-Pinilla, E. (2023). The adenosine A2A receptor in the basal ganglia: Expression, heteromerization, functional selectivity and signalling. *International Review of Neurobiology, 170*, 49–71.

Gąssowska-Dobrowolska, M., Olech-Kochańczyk, G., Culmsee, C., & Adamczyk, A. (2024). Novel insights into parkin–mediated mitochondrial dysfunction and Mito-Inflammation in α-Synuclein toxicity. The role of the cGAS–STING signalling pathway. *Journal of Inflammation Research, 17*, 4549–4574. https://doi.org/10.2147/JIR.S468609

Gómez-Benito, Granado, García-Sanz, Michel, Dumoulin, & Moratalla. (2020). Modeling parkinson's disease with the alpha-synuclein protein. *Frontiers in Pharmacology, 11*.

Galli, S., Pacilio, P., Bianchini, E., Alborghetti, M., De Carolis, L., Lombardo, P., Garramone, F., Salvetti, M., & Rinaldi, D. (2025). The role of MAO-B inhibitors in fatigue in parkinson's disease: A narrative review. *Journal of Clinical Medicine, 14*(8), 2598. https://doi.org/10.3390/jcm14082598

Gerfen, C. R. (2023). Segregation of D1 and D2 dopamine receptors in the striatal direct and indirect pathways: An historical perspective. *Frontiers in Synaptic Neuroscience, 14*. https://doi.org/10.3389/fnsyn.2022.1002960

Ghalandari, N., Assarzadegan, F., Habibi, S. A. H., Esmaily, H., & Malekpour, H. (2023). Efficacy of probiotics in improving motor function and alleviating constipation in parkinson's disease: A randomized controlled trial. *Iranian Journal of Pharmaceutical Research, 22*(1). https://doi.org/10.5812/ijpr-137840

Ghosh, P., & Saadat, A. (2023). Neurodegeneration and epigenetics: A review. *Neurologia, 38*(6), e62. https://doi.org/10.1016/j.nrl.2021.01.016

Giri, P. M., Banerjee, A., Ghosal, A., & Layek, B. (2024). Neuroinflammation in neurodegenerative disorders: Current knowledge and therapeutic implications. *International Journal of Molecular Sciences, 25*(7), 3995. https://doi.org/10.3390/ijms25073995

Goldman, S. M. (2014). Environmental toxins and parkinson's disease. *Annual Review of Pharmacology and Toxicology, 54*, 141–164. https://doi.org/10.1146/annurev-pharmtox-011613-135937

Goleij, P., Amini, A., Tabari, M. A. K., Hadipour, M., Sanaye, P. M., Alsharif, K. F., Daglia, M., Larsen, D. S., & Khan, H. (2025). The role of interleukin (IL)-2 cytokine family in parkinson's disease. *Cytokine, 191*. https://doi.org/10.1016/j.cyto.2025.156954

Gonzalez-Latapi, Bayram, Litvan, & Marras. (2021). Cognitive impairment in parkinson's disease: Epidemiology, clinical profile, protective and risk factors. *Behavioral Sciences, 11*(5).

Gunawardena, S. (2025). Alpha-synuclein in mitochondrial dysfunction: Opportunities or obstacles. *Neural Regeneration Research, 20*(1), 197–198. https://doi.org/10.4103/nrr.nrr-d-23-01966

Guo, X., Wang, J., Fan, H., Tao, W., Ren, Z., Li, X., Liu, S., Zhou, P., & Chen, Y. (2025). Computational drug repurposing in Parkinson's disease: Omaveloxolone and cyproheptadine as promising therapeutic candidates. *Frontiers in Pharmacology, 16*. https://doi.org/10.3389/fphar.2025.1539032

Gutowski, T., Antkiewicz, R., Szlufik, S., & Bacanin, N. (2023). Machine learning with optimization to create medicine intake schedules for Parkinson's disease patients. *PLoS One, 18*(10), Article e0293123. https://doi.org/10.1371/journal.pone.0293123

Hall, D. A., Voigt, R. M., Cantu-Jungles, T. M., Hamaker, B., Engen, P. A., Shaikh, M., Raeisi, S., Green, S. J., Naqib, A., Forsyth, C. B., Chen, T., Manfready, R., Ouyang, B., Rasmussen, H. E., Sedghi, S., Goetz, C. G., & Keshavarzian, A. (2023). An open label, non-randomized study assessing a prebiotic fiber intervention in a small cohort of Parkinson's disease participants. *Nature Communications, 14*(1). https://doi.org/10.1038/s41467-023-36497-x

Han, K., Kim, B., Lee, S. H., & Kim, M. K. (2023). A nationwide cohort study on diabetes severity and risk of Parkinson disease. *npj Parkinson's Disease, 9*(1), 11. https://www.nature.com/articles/s41531-023-00462-8.

Haque, M. E., Akther, M., Jakaria, M., Kim, I. S., Azam, S., & Choi, D. K. (2020). Targeting the microglial NLRP3 inflammasome and its role in parkinson's disease. *Movement Disorders, 35*(1), 20–33. https://doi.org/10.1002/mds.27874

Hariz, M., & Blomstedt, P. (2022). Deep brain stimulation for parkinson's disease. *Journal of Internal Medicine, 292*(5), 764–778. https://doi.org/10.1111/joim.13541

Haroon, E., Miller, A. H., & Sanacora, G. (2017). Inflammation, glutamate, and glia: A trio of trouble in mood disorders. *Neuropsychopharmacology, 42*(1), 193–215.

Harraz, M. M. (2023). Selective dopaminergic vulnerability in Parkinson's disease: New insights into the role of DAT. *Frontiers in Neuroscience, 17.* https://doi.org/10.3389/fnins.2023.1219441

Hassan, D. M., El-Kamel, A. H., Allam, E. A., Bakr, B. A., & Ashour, A. A. (2023). Chitosan-coated nanostructured lipid carriers for effective brain delivery of tanshinone IIA in Parkinson's disease: Interplay between nuclear factor-kappa β and cathepsin B. *Drug Delivery and Translational Research, 14*(2), 400–417.

Hauser, R. A., Sutherland, D., Madrid, J. A., Rol, M. A., Frucht, S., Isaacson, S., Pagan, F., Maddux, B. N., Li, G., Tse, W., Walter, B. L., Kumar, R., Kremens, D., Lew, M. F., Ellenbogen, A., Oguh, O., Vasquez, A., Kinney, W., Lowery, M., … Barbut, D. (2019). Targeting neurons in the gastrointestinal tract to treat parkinson's disease. *Clinical Parkinsonism and Related Disorders, 1,* 2–7. https://doi.org/10.1016/j.prdoa.2019.06.001

He, T., Lin, X., Su, A., Zhang, Y., Xing, Z., Mi, L., Wei, T., Li, Z., & Wu, W. (2023). Mitochondrial dysfunction-targeting therapeutics of natural products in Parkinson's disease. *Frontiers in Pharmacology, 14.* https://doi.org/10.3389/fphar.2023.1117337

Hong, J. P., Shin, S., Chung, S. H., Song, M. C., Shim, J. G., Kim, Y., Lee, B., Yeom, M., Park, H. J., Jung, K., Hong, J., & Hahm, D. H. (2024). Bacteriophages targeting Enterococcus faecalis enhance the therapeutic efficacy of levodopa in an MPTP-induced Parkinson's disease mouse model with E. faecalis gut colonization. *Scientific Reports, 14*(1). https://doi.org/10.1038/s41598-024-77038-w

Hur, E. M., & Lee, B. D. (2021). Lrrk2 at the crossroad of aging and parkinson's disease. *Genes, 12*(4). https://doi.org/10.3390/genes12040505

Hurtado, K. A., & Schnellmann, R. G. (2024). Mitophagy regulates mitochondrial number following pharmacological induction of mitochondrial biogenesis in renal proximal tubule cells. *Frontiers in Pharmacology, 15* (3), 22–35.

Hussein, A., Guevara, C. A., Del Valle, P., Gupta, S., Benson, D. L., & Huntley, G. W. (2023). Non-Motor symptoms of parkinson's disease: The neurobiology of early psychiatric and cognitive dysfunction. *The Neuroscientist, 29*(1), 97–116. https://doi.org/10.1177/10738584211011979

Imamura, K., Hishikawa, N., Sawada, M., Nagatsu, T., Yoshida, M., & Hashizume, Y. (2003). Distribution of major histocompatibility complex class II-positive microglia and cytokine profile of Parkinson's disease brains. *Acta Neuropathologica, 106*(6), 518–526. https://doi.org/10.1007/s00401-003-0766-2

Iovino, L., Tremblay, M., & Civiero, L. (2020). Glutamate-induced excitotoxicity in Parkinson's disease: The role of glial cells. *Journal of pharmacological sciences, 144*(3), 151–164.

Isaacson, S. H., & Jenner, P. (2025). Moving to a non-dopaminergic approach for the treatment of OFF fluctuations in Parkinson's disease. *Clinical Parkinsonism and Related Disorders, 12.* https://doi.org/10.1016/j.prdoa.2025.100303

Jacobs, B. M., Belete, D., Bestwick, J., Blauwendraat, C., Bandres-Ciga, S., Heilbron, K., Dobson, R., Nalls, M. A., Singleton, A., Hardy, J., Giovannoni, G., Lees, A. J., Schrag, A. E., & Noyce, A. J. (2020). Parkinson's disease determinants, prediction and gene-environment interactions in the UK Biobank. *Journal of Neurology, Neurosurgery and Psychiatry, 91*(10), 1046–1054. https://doi.org/10.1136/jnnp-2020-323646

Jan, A., Pereira Gonçalves, N., Bjerggaard Vaegter, C., Jensen, P. H., & Ferreira, N. (2021). The prion-like spreading of Alpha-Synuclein in parkinson's disease: Update on models and hypotheses. *International Journal of Molecular Sciences, 22*(15), 8338. https://doi.org/10.3390/ijms22158338

Jankovic, J., Goodman, I., Safirstein, B., Marmon, T. K., Schenk, D. B., Koller, M., Zago, W., Ness, D. K., Griffith, S. G., Grundman, M., Soto, J., Ostrowitzki, S., Boess, F. G., Martin-Facklam, M., Quinn, J. F., Isaacson, S. H., Omidvar, O., Ellenbogen, A., & Kinney, G. G. (2018). Safety and tolerability of multiple ascending doses of PRX002/RG7935, an Anti-α-Synuclein monoclonal antibody, in patients with parkinson disease. *JAMA Neurology, 75*(10), 1206. https://doi.org/10.1001/jamaneurol.2018.1487

Jenner, P., Mori, A., Aradi, S. D., & Hauser, R. A. (2021). Istradefylline–a first generation adenosine A2A antagonist for the treatment of Parkinson's disease. *Expert Review of Neurotherapeutics, 21*(3), 317–333. https://doi.org/10.1080/14737175.2021.1880896

Jia, F., Fellner, A., & Kumar, K. R. (2022). Monogenic parkinson's disease: Genotype, phenotype, pathophysiology, and genetic testing. *Genes, 13*(3), 471. https://doi.org/10.3390/GENES13030471

Jiao, J., Liu, W., Gao, G., & Yang, H. (2025). Serine-129 phosphorylated α-synuclein drives mitochondrial dysfunction and calcium dysregulation in Parkinson's disease model. *Frontiers in Aging Neuroscience, 17.* https://doi.org/10.3389/fnagi.2025.1538166

Jing, Y., Zhao, G., Xu, Y., McGuire, T., Hou, G., Zhao, J., Chen, M., Lopez, O., Xue, Y., & Xie, X.-Q. (2025). GCN-BBB: Deep learning blood-brain barrier (BBB) permeability PharmacoAnalytics with Graph Convolutional Neural (GCN) network. *The AAPS Journal, 27*(3). https://doi.org/10.1208/s12248-025-01059-0

Johnstone, S., Dela Cruz, G. A., Kalb, N., Tyagi, S. V., Potenza, M. N., George, T. P., & Castle, D. J. (2023). A systematic review of gender-responsive and integrated substance use disorder treatment programs for women with co-occurring disorders. *American Journal of Drug and Alcohol Abuse, 49*(1), 21–42. https://doi.org/10.1080/00952990.2022.2130348

Jos, S., Kambaru, A., Prasad, T. K., Parthasarathi, S., Kamariah, N., Nath, S., Padmanabhan, B., & Padavattan, S. (2025). Structural and functional insights into the nuclear role of Parkinson's disease-associated α-synuclein as a histone chaperone. *Communications Biology, 8*(1). https://doi.org/10.1038/s42003-025-08138-0

Jost, W. H. (2023). A novel treatment option for intrajejunal levodopa administration. *Expert Review of Neurotherapeutics, 23*(1), 9–13. https://doi.org/10.1080/14737175.2023.2176222

Julien, C., Hache, G., Dulac, M., Dubrou, C., Castelnovo, G., Giordana, C., Azulay, J.-P., & Fluchère, F. (2021). The clinical meaning of levodopa equivalent daily dose in Parkinson's disease. *Fundamental & Clinical Pharmacology, 35*(3), 620–630. https://doi.org/10.1111/fcp.12646

Kalia, L. V., & Lang, A. E. (2015). Parkinson's disease. *The Lancet, 386*(9996), 896–912. https://doi.org/10.1016/S0140-6736(14)61393-3

Kam, T. I., Hinkle, J. T., Dawson, T. M., & Dawson, V. L. (2020). Microglia and astrocyte dysfunction in parkinson's disease. *Neurobiology of Disease, 144*, 105028. https://doi.org/10.1016/j.nbd.2020.105028. Epub 2020 Jul 28. PMID: 32736085; PMCID: PMC7484088.

Kawahata, I., Finkelstein, D. I., & Fukunaga, K. (2024). Dopamine D1–D5 receptors in brain nuclei: Implications for Health and Disease. *Receptors, 3*(2), 155–181.

Kerstens, V. S., & Varrone, A. (2020). Dopamine transporter imaging in neurodegenerative movement disorders: PET vs. SPECT. *Clinical and Translational Imaging, 8*(5), 349–356. https://doi.org/10.1007/s40336-020-00386-w

Khowdiary, M. M., Al-kuraishy, H. M., Al-Gareeb, A. I., Albuhadily, A. K., Elhenawy, A. A., Babalghith, A. O., Shokr, M. M., Alexiou, A., Papadakis, M., & El-Saber Batiha, G. (2025). Dysregulation of serotonergic neurotransmission in Parkinson disease: A key duet. *European Journal of Pharmacology, 995.* https://doi.org/10.1016/j.ejphar.2025.177419

Khushboo, Siddiqi, N. J., de Lourdes Pereira, M., & Sharma, B. (2022). Neuroanatomical, biochemical, and functional modifications in brain induced by treatment with antidepressants. *Molecular Neurobiology, 59*(6), 3564–3584. https://doi.org/10.1007/s12035-022-02780-z

Khvastunov, V. O., Goleva, T. N., Epremyan, K. K., & Rogov, A. G. (2024). α-Synuclein expression causes Mitochondria fragmentation and increased sensitivity to oxidative stress in the yeast Yarrowia lipolytica. *Federation Nanobiotechnology Reports, 19*(6), 1016–1022. https://doi.org/10.1134/S2635167624602377

Kim, H. A. (2024). Treatment of hemodynamic orthostatic dizziness/vertigo. *Research in Vestibular Science, 23* (3), 79–88. https://doi.org/10.21790/rvs.2024.017

Kim, S., Kwon, S. H., Kam, T. I., Panicker, N., Karuppagounder, S. S., Lee, S., Lee, J. H., Kim, W. R., Kook, M., Foss, C. A., Shen, C., Lee, H., Kulkarni, S., Pasricha, P. J., Lee, G., Pomper, M. G., Dawson, V. L.,

Dawson, T. M., & Ko, H. S. (2019). Transneuronal propagation of pathologic α-Synuclein from the gut to the brain models Parkinson's Disease. *Neuron, 103*(4), 627. https://doi.org/10.1016/j.neuron.2019.05.035

Knecht, L., Folke, J., Dodel, R., Ross, J. A., & Albus, A. (2022). Alpha-synuclein immunization strategies for synucleinopathies in clinical studies: A biological perspective. *Neurotherapeutics, 19*(5), 1489–1502. https://doi.org/10.1007/s13311-022-01288-7

Ko, H.-Y., & Huh, S. (2021). *Orthostatic hypotension and associated supine hypertension*. Springer Science and Business Media LLC. https://doi.org/10.1007/978-981-16-3679-0_17

Kong, D., Chen, Y., & Ding, X. (2021). Parkinson's disease diagnosis and severity prediction with machine learning techniques. In *Proceedings of the 2021 International Conference on Intelligent Medicine and Health* (pp. 35–39). https://dl.acm.org/doi/fullHtml/10.1145/3484377.3484383.

Kraemmer, J., Kovacs, G. G., Perju-Dumbrava, L., Pirker, S., Traub-Weidinger, T., & Pirker, W. (2014). Correlation of striatal dopamine transporter imaging with post mortem substantia nigra cell counts. *Movement Disorders, 29*(14), 1767–1773. https://movementdisorders.onlinelibrary.wiley.com/doi/abs/10.1002/mds.25975.

Kumar, L., Malhotra, M., Sharma, A., Singh, A. P., & Singh, A. P. (2024). A holistic approach to Parkinson's Disease: Integrating advances in pathophysiology, diagnosis, and therapy. *Journal of Drug Delivery and Therapeutics, 14*(5).

Kwon, DK., Kwatra, M., Wang, J., & Ko, H. S. (2022). Levodopa-induced dyskinesia in Parkinson's disease: pathogenesis and emerging treatment strategies. *Cells, 11*(23), 3736. https://www.mdpi.com/2073-4409/11/23/3736.

Lang, A. E., Siderowf, A. D., Macklin, E. A., Poewe, W., Brooks, D. J., Fernandez, H. H., Rascol, O., Giladi, N., Stocchi, F., Tanner, C. M., Postuma, R. B., Simon, D. K., Tolosa, E., Mollenhauer, B., Cedarbaum, J. M., Fraser, K., Xiao, J., Evans, K. C., Graham, D. L., … Dam, T. (2022). Trial of Cinpanemab in early Parkinson's Disease. *New England Journal of Medicine, 387*(5), 408–420. https://doi.org/10.1056/NEJMoa2203395

Lardenoije, R., Iatrou, A., Kenis, G., Kompotis, K., Steinbusch, H. W. M., Mastroeni, D., Coleman, P., Lemere, C. A., Hof, P. R., van den Hove, D. L. A., & Rutten, B. P. F. (2015). The epigenetics of aging and neurodegeneration. *Progress in Neurobiology, 131*, 21–64. https://doi.org/10.1016/j.pneurobio.2015.05.002

Lee, T. K., & Yankee, E. L. (2022). A review on Parkinson's disease treatment. *Neuroimmunology and Neuroinflammation, 8*, 222–244. https://doi.org/10.20517/2347-8659.2020.58

Lee, B., Young, C. B., Cai, W., Yuan, R., Ryman, S., Kim, J., Yang, L., Henderson, V. W., Poston, K. L., & Menon, V. (2025). Dopaminergic modulation and dosage effects on brain state dynamics and working memory component processes in Parkinson's disease. *Nature Communications, 16*(1). https://doi.org/10.1038/s41467-025-56660-w

Lees, A., Tolosa, E., Stocchi, F., Ferreira, J. J., Rascol, O., Antonini, A., & Poewe, W. (2023). Optimizing levodopa therapy, when and how? Perspectives on the importance of delivery and the potential for an early combination approach. *Expert Review of Neurotherapeutics, 23*(1), 15–24. https://doi.org/10.1080/14737175.2023.2176220

Lemos, M., Venezia, S., Refolo, V., Heras-Garvin, A., Schmidhuber, S., Giese, A., Leonov, A., Ryazanov, S., Griesinger, C., Galabova, G., Staffler, G., Wenning, G. K., & Stefanova, N. (2020). Targeting α-synuclein by PD03 AFFITOPE® and Anle138b rescues neurodegenerative pathology in a model of multiple system atrophy: Clinical relevance. *Translational Neurodegeneration, 9*(1). https://doi.org/10.1186/s40035-020-00217-y

Lenka, A., Di Maria, G., Lamotte, G., Bahroo, L., & Jankovic, J. (2022). Practical pearls to improve the efficacy and tolerability of levodopa in Parkinson's disease. *Expert Review of Neurotherapeutics, 22*(6), 489–498. https://doi.org/10.1080/14737175.2022.2091436

Lerner, T. N., & Kreitzer, A. C. (2012). RGS4 is required for dopaminergic control of striatal LTD and susceptibility to parkinsonian motor deficits. *Neuron, 73*(2), 347–359. https://www.sciencedirect.com/science/article/pii/S0896627311010518.

Lesley, R., Simpson, J., Dale, M., Eccles, F., Lock, S., & Gunn, S. (2025). Predictors of informal caregiver burden in parkinson's disease: A systematic review. *Western Journal of Nursing Research, 47*(6), 524–543. https://doi.org/10.1177/01939459251327968

Levenson, J. M., Schroeter, S., Carroll, J. C., Cullen, V., Asp, E., Proschitsky, M., Chung, C. H. Y., Gilead, S., Nadeem, M., Dodiya, H. B., Shoaga, S., Mufson, E. J., Tsubery, H., Krishnan, R., Wright, J., Solomon, B., Fisher, R., & Gannon, K. S. (2016). NPT088 reduces both amyloid-β and tau pathologies in transgenic mice. *Alzheimer's and Dementia: Translational Research and Clinical Interventions, 2*(3), 141–155. https://doi.org/10.1016/j.trci.2016.06.004

Levin, J., Schmidt, F., Boehm, C., Prix, C., Bötzel, K., Ryazanov, S., Leonov, A., Griesinger, C., & Giese, A. (2014). The oligomer modulator anle138b inhibits disease progression in a Parkinson mouse model even with treatment started after disease onset. *Acta Neuropathologica, 127*(5), 779–780. https://doi.org/10.1007/s00401-014-1265-3

Li, J. (2023). Role of 5-HT receptors and transporters in psychiatric disorders. In *Proceedings of SPIE - The international Society for optical engineering, 12611*United States: SPIE. https://doi.org/10.1117/12.2668997

Li, J.y., Ma, S.s., Huang, Q.y., & Li, M.t. (2015). The function of neuroinflammation in parkinson disease. *Sheng li ke xue jin zhan [Progress in physiology], 46*(3), 175–179.

Li, H., Slone, J., Lin, F., & Huang, T. (2019). Mitochondrial DNA variants and common diseases: A mathematical model for the diversity of age-related mtDNA mutations. *Cells, 8*(6), 608. https://doi.org/10.3390/cells8060608

Li, J., Yang, D., Li, Z., Zhao, M., Wang, D., Sun, Z., Wen, P., Dai, Y., Gou, F., Ji, Y., Zhao, D., & Yang, L. (2023). PINK1/Parkin-mediated mitophagy in neurodegenerative diseases. *Ageing Research Reviews, 84*, Article 101817.

Liang, K., Yang, L., Kang, J., Liu, B., Zhang, D., Wang, L., Wang, W., & Wang, Q. (2024). Improving treatment for Parkinson's disease: Harnessing photothermal and phagocytosis-driven delivery of levodopa nanocarriers across the blood-brain barrier. *Asian Journal of Pharmaceutical Sciences, 19*(6).

Ligneul, R., & Mainen, Z. F. (2023). Serotonin. *Current Biology, 33*(23), Article R1216. https://doi.org/10.1016/j.cub.2023.09.068

Lim, S. Y., & Klein, C. (2024). Parkinson's Disease is predominantly a genetic disease. *Journal of Parkinson's Disease, 14*(3), 467–482. https://doi.org/10.3233/JPD-230376

Lin, X., Cook, T. J., Zabetian, C. P., Leverenz, J. B., Peskind, E. R., Hu, S. C., Cain, K. C., Pan, C., Edgar, J. S., Goodlett, D. R., Racette, B. A., Checkoway, H., Montine, T. J., Shi, M., & Zhang, J. (2012). DJ-1 isoforms in whole blood as potential biomarkers of Parkinson disease. *Scientific Reports, 2*. https://doi.org/10.1038/srep00954

Lindström, V., Fagerqvist, T., Nordström, E., Eriksson, F., Lord, A., Tucker, S., Andersson, J., Johannesson, M., Schell, H., Kahle, P. J., Möller, C., Gellerfors, P., Bergström, J., Lannfelt, L., & Ingelsson, M. (2014). Immunotherapy targeting α-synuclein protofibrils reduced pathology in (Thy-1)-h[A30P] α-synuclein mice. *Neurobiology of Disease, 69*, 134–143. https://doi.org/10.1016/j.nbd.2014.05.009

Lisman, J., Buzsáki, G., Eichenbaum, H., Nadel, L., Ranganath, C., & Redish, A. D. (2017). Viewpoints: how the hippocampus contributes to memory, navigation and cognition. *Nature Neuroscience, 20*(11), 1434–1447. https://doi.org/10.1038/nn.4661

Liu, X., Balaraman, K., Lynch, C. C., Hebron, M., Wolf, C., & Moussa, C. (2021). Novel ubiquitin specific Protease-13 inhibitors alleviate neurodegenerative pathology. *Metabolites, 11*(9), 622.

Liu, B., Fang, F., Pedersen, N. L., Tillander, A., Ludvigsson, J. F., Ekbom, A., Svenningsson, P., Chen, H., & Karin, W. (2017). Vagotomy and Parkinson disease A Swedish register-based matched-cohort study). *Neurology, 88*(21), 1996–2002. https://doi.org/10.1212/WNL.0000000000003961

Liu, D., Guo, J. J., Su, J. H., Svanbergsson, A., Yuan, L., Haikal, C., Li, W., Gouras, G., & Li, J. Y. (2021). Differential seeding and propagating efficiency of α-synuclein strains generated in different conditions. *Translational Neurodegeneration, 10*(1). https://doi.org/10.1186/s40035-021-00242-5

Liu, M., Liu, S., Lin, Z., Chen, X., Jiao, Q., Du, X., & Jiang, H. (2025). Targeting the interplay between autophagy and the Nrf2 pathway in parkinson's disease with potential therapeutic implications. *Biomolecules, 15*(1), 149. https://doi.org/10.3390/biom15010149

Livingston, C., & Monroe-Duprey, L. (2024). A review of levodopa formulations for the treatment of parkinson's disease available in the United States. *Journal of Pharmacy Practice, 37*(2), 485–494. https://doi.org/10.1177/08971900221151194

Lucchesi, M., Biso, L., Bonaso, M., Longoni, B., Buchignani, B., Battini, R., Santorelli, F. M., Doccini, S., & Scarselli, M. (2025). Mitochondrial dysfunction in genetic and non-genetic parkinson's disease. *International Journal of Molecular Sciences, 26*(9), 4451. https://doi.org/10.3390/ijms26094451

Ludtmann, M. H. R., Angelova, P. R., Horrocks, M. H., Choi, M. L., Rodrigues, M., Baev, A. Y., Berezhnov, A. V., Yao, Z., Little, D., Banushi, B., Al-Menhali, A. S., Ranasinghe, R. T., Whiten, D. R., Yapom, R., Dolt, K. S., Devine, M. J., Gissen, P., Kunath, T., Jaganjac, M., … Gandhi, S. (2018). α-synuclein oligomers interact with ATP synthase and open the permeability transition pore in Parkinson's disease. *Nature Communications, 9*(1). https://doi.org/10.1038/s41467-018-04422-2

Müller, T. (2022). GOCOVRI ® (amantadine) extended-release Capsules in Parkinson's Disease. *Neurodegenerative Disease Management, 12*(1), 15–28. https://doi.org/10.2217/nmt-2021-0028

Müller, M. L. T. M., & Bohnen, N. I. (2013). Cholinergic dysfunction in parkinson's disease. *Current Neurology and Neuroscience Reports, 13*(9). https://doi.org/10.1007/s11910-013-0377-9

Magalingam, K. B., Radhakrishnan, A., & Nagaraja, H. (2014). Protective effects of flavonol isoquercitrin, against 6-hydroxy dopamine (6-OHDA) - Induced toxicity in PC12 cells. *BMC Research Notes, 7*(49).

Maheshwari, A., & Sood, M. R. (2022). Drugs acting on the gut: Prokinetics, antispasmodics, laxatives. In C. Faure, N. Thapar, & C. Di Lorenzo (Eds.), *Pediatric neurogastroenterology*. Cham: Springer.

Majali, M. A., Sunnaa, M., & Chand, P. (2021). Emerging pharmacotherapies for motor symptoms in Parkinson's Disease. *Journal of Geriatric Psychiatry and Neurology, 34*(4), 263–273.

Majbour, N. K., Aasly, J. O., Hustad, E., Thomas, M. A., Vaikath, N. N., Elkum, N., Van De Berg, W. D. J., Tokuda, T., Mollenhauer, B., Berendse, H. W., & El-Agnaf, O. M. A. (2020). CSF total and oligomeric α-Synuclein along with TNF-α as risk biomarkers for Parkinson's disease: A study in LRRK2 mutation carriers. *Translational Neurodegeneration, 9*(1). https://doi.org/10.1186/s40035-020-00192-4

Man, W. K., De Simone, A., Barritt, J. D., Vendruscolo, M., Dobson, C. M., & Fusco, G. (2020). A role of cholesterol in modulating the binding of α-Synuclein to synaptic-like vesicles. *Frontiers in Neuroscience, 14*. https://doi.org/10.3389/fnins.2020.00018

Mbiydzenyuy, N. E., Ninsiima, H. I., Valladares, M. B., & Pieme, C. A. (2018). Zinc and linoleic acid pre-treatment attenuates biochemical and histological changes in the midbrain of rats with rotenone-induced parkinsonism. *BMC Neuroscience, 19*(1). https://doi.org/10.1186/s12868-018-0429-9

McManus, G., Galfano, A., Budrow, C., Lipari, N., Tseng, K. Y., Manfredsson, F. P., & Bishop, C. (2025). Effects of genetic knockdown of the serotonin transporter on established L-DOPA-induced dyskinesia and gene expression in hemiparkinsonian rats. *Neuropharmacology, 266*. https://doi.org/10.1016/j.neuropharm.2024.110227

Menon, S., Armstrong, S., Hamzeh, A., Visanji, N. P., Sardi, S. P., & Tandon, A. (2022). Alpha-Synuclein targeting therapeutics for Parkinson's Disease and related synucleinopathies. *Frontiers in Neurology, 13*. https://doi.org/10.3389/fneur.2022.852003

Menozzi, E., Macnaughtan, J., & Schapira, A. H. V. (2021). The gut-brain axis and Parkinson disease: Clinical and pathogenetic relevance. *Annals of Medicine, 53*(1), 611–625.

Michelson, D., Grundman, M., Magnuson, K., Fisher, R., Levenson, J. M., Aisen, P., Marek, K., Gray, M., & Hefti, F. (2019). Randomized, placebo controlled trial of NPT088, A Phage-Derived, amyloid-targeted treatment for Alzheimer's Disease. *The Journal of Prevention of Alzheimer's Disease, 6*(4), 228–231. https://doi.org/10.14283/jpad.2019.37

Milosevic, L., Kalia, S. K., Hodaie, M., Lozano, A. M., Fasano, A., Popovic, M. R., & Hutchison, W. D. (2018). Neuronal inhibition and synaptic plasticity of basal ganglia neurons in Parkinson's disease. *Brain, 141*(1), 177–190. https://doi.org/10.1093/brain/awx296

Missiego-Beltrán, J., Olalla-Álvarez, E. M., González-Brugera, A., & Beltrán-Velasco, A. I. (2024). Implications of butyrate signaling pathways on the motor symptomatology of parkinson's disease and neuroprotective Effects—Therapeutic approaches: A systematic review. *International Journal of Molecular Sciences, 25*(16), 8998.

Mittal, P., Dhankhar, S., Chauhan, S., Garg, N., Bhattacharya, T., Ali, M., Chaudhary, A. A., Rudayni, H. A., Al-Zharani, M., Ahmad, W., Khan, S. U. D., Singh, T. G., & Mujwar, S. (2023). A review on natural antioxidants for their role in the treatment of parkinson's disease. *Pharmaceuticals, 16*(7). https://doi.org/10.3390/ph16070908

Mogharbel, B. F., Cardoso, M. A., Irioda, A. C., Stricker, P. E. F., Slompo, R. C., Appel, J. M., de Oliveira, N. B., Perussolo, M. C., Saçaki, C. S., da Rosa, N. N., Dziedzic, D. S. M., Travelet, C., Halila, S., Borsali, R., & de Carvalho, K. A. T. (2022). Biodegradable nanoparticles loaded with levodopa and curcumin for treatment of parkinson's disease. *Molecules, 27*(9). https://doi.org/10.3390/molecules27092811

Moreira, C. V. L., Ayobami, O. J., Ogbu, J. I., Rosemberg, D. B., & Fajemiroye, J. O. (2025). *Drugs and interaction attributes fundamentals of drug and non-drug interactions: Physiopathological perspectives and clinical approaches*. Brazil: Springer Nature. https://doi.org/10.1007/978-3-031-80107-5_6

Morris, H. R., Spillantini, M. G., Sue, C. M., & Williams-Gray, C. H. (2024). The pathogenesis of Parkinson's disease. *The Lancet, 403*(10423), 293–304. https://doi.org/10.1016/S0140-6736(23)01478-2

Muleiro Alvarez, Cano-Herrera, Osorio Martínez, Vega Gonzales-Portillo, Monroy, Murguiondo Pérez, Torres-Ríos, van Tienhoven, Garibaldi Bernot, Esparza Salazar, & Ibarra. (2024). A comprehensive approach to Parkinson's Disease: Addressing its molecular, clinical, and therapeutic aspects. *International Journal of Molecular Sciences, 25*(13).

Ng, A. S. L., Tan, Y. J., Yong, A. C. W., Saffari, S. E., Lu, Z., Ng, E. Y., Ng, S. Y. E., Chia, N. S. Y., Choi, X., Heng, D., Neo, S., Xu, Z., Keong, N. C. H., Tay, K. Y., Au, W. L., Tan, L. C. S., & Tan, E. K. (2020). Utility of plasma Neurofilament light as a diagnostic and prognostic biomarker of the postural instability gait disorder motor subtype in early Parkinson's disease. *Molecular Neurodegeneration, 15*(1). https://doi.org/10.1186/s13024-020-00385-5

Nimmo, C., Brien, K., Millard, J., Grant, A. D., Padayatchi, N., Pym, A. S., O'Donnell, M., Goldstein, R., Breuer, J., & Balloux, F. (2020). Dynamics of within-host Mycobacterium tuberculosis diversity and heteroresistance during treatment. *EBioMedicine, 55*, 102747. https://doi.org/10.1016/j.ebiom.2020.102747

Nimmo, J. T., Verma, A., Dodart, J.-C., Wang, C. Y., Savistchenko, J., Melki, R., Carare, R. O., & Nicoll, J. A. R. (2023). Correction: Novel antibodies detect additional α-synuclein pathology in synucleinopathies: Potential development for immunotherapy. *Alzheimer's Research & Therapy, 15*(1). https://doi.org/10.1186/s13195-022-01156-8

Nordström, E., Eriksson, F., Sigvardson, J., Johannesson, M., Kasrayan, A., Jones-Kostalla, M., Appelkvist, P., Söderberg, L., Nygren, P., Blom, M., Rachalski, A., Nordenankar, K., Zachrisson, O., Amandius, E., Osswald, G., Moge, M., Ingelsson, M., Bergström, J., Lannfelt, L., … Fälting, J. (2021). ABBV-0805, a novel antibody selective for soluble aggregated α-synuclein, prolongs lifespan and prevents buildup of α-synuclein pathology in mouse models of Parkinson's disease. *Neurobiology of Disease, 161*, Article 105543. https://doi.org/10.1016/j.nbd.2021.105543

O'Leary, E., Jiang, Y., Kristensen, L. S., Hansen, T. B., & Kjems, J. (2025). The therapeutic potential of circular RNAs. *Nature Reviews Genetics*, 1–15.

Obeso, J. A., Rodríguez-Oroz, M. C., Benitez-Temino, B., Blesa, F. J., Guridi, J., Marin, C., & Rodriguez, M. (2008). Functional organization of the basal ganglia: Therapeutic implications for Parkinson's disease. *Movement Disorders, 23*(3), Article S548. https://doi.org/10.1002/mds.22062

Oosterveld, L. P., Verberk, I. M., Majbour, N. K., El-Agnaf, O. M., Weinstein, H. C., Berendse, H. W., Teunissen, C. E., & Van De Berg, W. D. (2019). CSF or serum neurofilament light added to A-Synuclein panel discriminates Parkinson's from controls. *Movement Disorders, 35*(2), 288–295.

Paß, T., Ricke, K. M., Hofmann, P., Chowdhury, R. S., Nie, Y., Chinnery, P., Endepols, H., Neumaier, B., Carvalho, A., Rigoux, L., Steculorum, S. M., Prudent, J., Riemer, T., Aswendt, M., Liss, B., Brachvogel, B., & Wiesner, R. J. (2024). Preserved striatal innervation maintains motor function despite severe loss of nigral dopaminergic neurons. *Brain, 147*(9), 3189–3203. https://doi.org/10.1093/brain/awae089

Paccosi, E., & Proietti-De-Santis, L. (2023). Parkinson's disease: From genetics and epigenetics to treatment, a miRNA-Based strategy. *International Journal of Molecular Sciences, 24*(11), 9547. https://doi.org/10.3390/ijms24119547

Pagano, G., Taylor, K. I., Anzures-Cabrera, J., Marchesi, M., Simuni, T., Marek, K., Postuma, R. B., Pavese, N., Stocchi, F., Azulay, J. P., Mollenhauer, B., López-Manzanares, L., Russell, D. S., Boyd, J. T., Nicholas, A. P., Luquin, M. R., Hauser, R. A., Gasser, T., Poewe, W., … Bonni, A. (2022). Trial of prasinezumab in early-stage Parkinson's Disease. *New England Journal of Medicine, 387*(5), 421–432. https://doi.org/10.1056/NEJMoa2202867

Pal, M. M. (2021). Glutamate: The master neurotransmitter and its implications in chronic stress and mood disorders. *Frontiers in Human Neuroscience, 15*. https://doi.org/10.3389/fnhum.2021.722323

Palikaras, K., Lionaki, E., & Tavernarakis, N. (2015). Balancing mitochondrial biogenesis and mitophagy to maintain energy metabolism homeostasis. *Cell Death & Differentiation, 22*(9), 1399–1401.

Paredes-Rodriguez, E., Vegas-Suarez, S., Morera-Herreras, T., De Deurwaerdere, P., & Miguelez, C. (2020). The noradrenergic System in parkinson's disease. *Frontiers in Pharmacology, 11*. https://doi.org/10.3389/fphar.2020.00435

Pasquini, J., Brooks, D. J., & Pavese, N. (2021). The cholinergic brain in Parkinson's Disease. *Movement Disorders Clinical Practice, 8*(7), 1012–1026.

Perfeito, R., Lázaro, D. F., Outeiro, T. F., & Rego, A. C. (2014). Linking alpha-synuclein phosphorylation to reactive oxygen species formation and mitochondrial dysfunction in SH-SY5Y cells. *Molecular and Cellular Neuroscience, 62*, 51–59. https://doi.org/10.1016/j.mcn.2014.08.002

Phillips, O., Ghosh, D., & Fernandez, H. H. (2023). Parkinson disease dementia management: An update of Current evidence and future directions. *Current Treatment Options in Neurology, 25*, 93–119.

Popławska-Domaszewicz, K., Metta, V., Odin, P., & Chaudhuri, K. R. (2025). The device-aided intrajejunal delivery of levodopa–entacapone–carbidopa intestinal gel the treatment of Parkinson's disease: Overview of efficacy and safety. *Expert Review of Medical Devices, 22*(6), 533–544. https://doi.org/10.1080/17434440.2025.2499153

Price, D. L., Koike, M. A., Khan, A., Wrasidlo, W., Rockenstein, E., Masliah, E., & Bonhaus, D. (2018). The small molecule alpha-synuclein misfolding inhibitor, NPT200-11, produces multiple benefits in an animal model of Parkinson's disease. *Scientific Reports, 8*(1). https://doi.org/10.1038/s41598-018-34490-9

Qin, F., Wan, C., & Zhang, Y. (2024). Computer-aided optimization of carbidopa/levodopa orally disintegrating tablets. *Drug development and industrial pharmacy, 50*(4), 331–340.

Qiu, H., Liu, C., & Wang, Z. (2025). Levodopa-induced motor complications associated with benserazide and carbidopa in Parkinson's disease: A disproportionality analysis of the FAERS database. *Frontiers in Pharmacology, 16*, Article 1529932.

Radad, K., Moldzio, R., Krewenka, C., Kranner, B., & Rausch, W. D. (2023). Pathophysiology of non-motor signs in Parkinson's disease: Some recent updating with brief presentation. *Exploration of Neuroprotective Therapy, 3*(1), 24–46. https://doi.org/10.37349/ent.2023.00036

Rafe, M. R., Saha, P., & Bello, S. T. (2024). Targeting NMDA receptors with an antagonist is a promising therapeutic strategy for treating neurological disorders. *Behavioural Brain Research, 472*, Article 115173.

Rascol, O., Fabbri, M., & Poewe, W. (2021). Amantadine in the treatment of Parkinson's disease and other movement disorders. *The Lancet. Neurology, 20*(12), 1048–1056.

Rathore, A. S., Birla, H., Singh, S. S., Zahra, W., Dilnashin, H., Singh, R., Keshri, P. K., & Singh, S. P. (2021). Epigenetic modulation in parkinson's disease and potential treatment therapies. *Neurochemical Research, 46* (7), 1618–1626. https://doi.org/10.1007/s11064-021-03334-w

Regensburger, M., Ip, C. W., Kohl, Z., Schrader, C., Urban, P. P., Kassubek, J., & Jost, W. H. (2023). Clinical benefit of MAO-B and COMT inhibition in Parkinson's disease: Practical considerations. *Journal of Neural Transmission, 130*(6), 847–861. https://doi.org/10.1007/s00702-023-02623-8

Reinert, K. R. S., Umphlet, C. D., Quattlebaum, A., & Boger, H. A. (2014). Short-term effects of an endotoxin on substantia nigra dopamine neurons. *Brain Research, 1557*, 164–170. https://doi.org/10.1016/j.brainres.2014.02.005

Reinert, J. P., Veronin, M. A., & Medina, C. (2023). Tricyclic antidepressants in nociceptive and neuropathic pain: A review of their analgesic properties in combination with opioids. *The Journal of pharmacy technology: jPT: official publication of the Association of Pharmacy Technicians, 39*(1), 35–40.

Richmond, A. M., Lyons, K. E., & Pahwa, R. (2023). Safety review of current pharmacotherapies for levodopa-treated patients with Parkinson's disease. *Expert Opinion on Drug Safety, 22*(7), 563–579.

Riederer, P., Strobel, S., Nagatsu, T., Watanabe, H., Chen, X., Löschmann, P. A., … Monoranu, C. M. (2025). Levodopa treatment: impacts and mechanisms throughout Parkinson's disease progression: P. Riederer et al. *Journal of Neural Transmission, 132*(6), 743–779. https://link.springer.com/article/10.1007/s00702-025-02893-4.

Rietdijk, C. D., Perez-Pardo, P., Garssen, J., van Wezel, R. J. A., & Kraneveld, A. D. (2017). Exploring braak's hypothesis of Parkinson'S disease. *Frontiers in Neurology, 8*. https://doi.org/10.3389/fneur.2017.00037

Rim, C., You, M. J., Nahm, M., & Kwon, M. S. (2024). Emerging role of senescent microglia in brain aging-related neurodegenerative diseases. *Translational Neurodegeneration, 13*(1). https://doi.org/10.1186/s40035-024-00402-3

Rota, Urso, van Wamelen, Leta, Boura, Odin, Espay, Jenner, & Chaudhuri. (2022). Why do 'OFF' periods still occur during continuous drug delivery in Parkinson's disease? *Translational Neurodegeneration, 11*(1).

Rusch, C., Flanagan, R., Suh, H., & Subramanian, I. (2023). To restrict or not to restrict? Practical considerations for optimizing dietary protein interactions on levodopa absorption in Parkinson's disease. *Npj Parkinson's Disease, 9*(1). https://doi.org/10.1038/s41531-023-00541-w

Sánchez-Pernaute, R., Harvey-White, J., Cunningham, J., & Bankiewicz, K. S. (2001). Functional effect of adeno-associated virus mediated gene transfer of aromatic L-amino acid decarboxylase into the striatum of 6-OHDA-lesioned rats. *Molecular Therapy, 4*(4), 324–330. https://doi.org/10.1006/mthe.2001.0466

Saini, N., Singh, N., Kaur, N., Garg, S., Kaur, M., Kumar, A., Verma, M., Singh, K., & Singh Sohal, H. (2024). Motor and non-motor symptoms, drugs, and their mode of action in Parkinson's disease (PD): A review. *Medicinal Chemistry Research, 33*(4), 580–599. https://doi.org/10.1007/s00044-024-03203-5

Saito, Y. (2017). DJ-1 as a biomarker of Parkinson's disease. *Advances in Experimental Medicine and Biology, 1037*, 149–171. https://doi.org/10.1007/978-981-10-6583-5_10

Sampson, T. R., Debelius, J. W., Thron, T., Janssen, S., Shastri, G. G., Ilhan, Z. E., Challis, C., Schretter, C. E., Rocha, S., Gradinaru, V., Chesselet, M. F., Keshavarzian, A., Shannon, K. M., Krajmalnik-Brown, R., Wittung-Stafshede, P., Knight, R., & Mazmanian, S. K. (2016). Gut Microbiota regulate motor deficits and neuroinflammation in a model of Parkinson's Disease. *Cell, 167*(6), 1469. https://doi.org/10.1016/j.cell.2016.11.018

Sanger, G. J., & Andrews, P. L. R. (2023). Review article: An analysis of the pharmacological rationale for selecting drugs to inhibit vomiting or increase gastric emptying during treatment of gastroparesis. *Alimentary Pharmacology and Therapeutics, 57*(9), 962–978. https://doi.org/10.1111/apt.17466

Saranza, G., & Lang, A. E. (2021). Levodopa challenge test: Indications, protocol, and guide. *Journal of Neurology, 268*(9), 3135–3143. https://doi.org/10.1007/s00415-020-09810-7

Scarneciu, I., Lupu, S., Bratu, O., Teodorescu, A., Maxim, L., Brinza, A., Laculiceanu, A., Rotaru, R., Lupu, A.-M., & Scarneciu, C. (2021). Overactive bladder: A review and update. *Experimental and Therapeutic Medicine, 22*(6). https://doi.org/10.3892/etm.2021.10879

Schenk, D. B., Koller, M., Ness, D. K., Griffith, S. G., Grundman, M., Zago, W., Soto, J., Atiee, G., Ostrowitzki, S., & Kinney, G. G. (2016). First-in-human assessment of PRX002, an anti-α-synuclein monoclonal antibody, in healthy volunteers. *Movement Disorders, 32*(2), 211–218.

Schofield, D. J., Irving, L., Calo, L., Bogstedt, A., Rees, G., Nuccitelli, A., Narwal, R., Petrone, M., Roberts, J., Brown, L., Cusdin, F., Dosanjh, B., Lloyd, C., Dobson, C., Gurrell, I., Fraser, G., McFarlane, M., Rockenstein, E., Spencer, B., … Perkinton, M. S. (2019). Preclinical development of a high affinity α-synuclein antibody, MEDI1341, that can enter the brain, sequester extracellular α-synuclein and attenuate α-synuclein spreading in vivo. *Neurobiology of Disease, 132*, Article 104582. https://doi.org/10.1016/j.nbd.2019.104582

Schwarzman, A. L., Senkevich, K. A., Emelyanov, A. K., & Pchelina, S. N. (2019). Prion properties of Alpha-Synuclein. *Molekuliarnaia Biologiia, 53*(3), 380–387. https://doi.org/10.1134/S0026898419030182

Schweitzer, J. S., Song, B., Herrington, T. M., Park, T. Y., Lee, N., Ko, S., Jeon, J., Cha, Y., Kim, K., Li, Q., Henchcliffe, C., Kaplitt, M., Neff, C., Rapalino, O., Seo, H., Lee, I. H., Kim, J., Kim, T., Petsko, G. A., … Kim, K. S. (2020). Personalized iPSC-derived dopamine progenitor cells for Parkinson's disease. *New England Journal of Medicine, 382*(20), 1926–1932. https://doi.org/10.1056/NEJMoa1915872

Sekine, S. (2020). PINK1 import regulation at a crossroad of mitochondrial fate: The molecular mechanisms of PINK1 import. *Journal of Biochemistry, 167*(3), 217–224.

Sharma, M., & Burré, J. (2023). α-Synuclein in synaptic function and dysfunction. *Trends in neurosciences, 46*(2), 153–166.

Sharma, K., Chib, S., Gupta, A., Singh, R., & Chalotra, R. (2024). Interplay between α-synuclein and parkin genes: Insights of Parkinson's disease. *Molecular Biology Reports, 51*(1). https://doi.org/10.1007/s11033-024-09520-7

Shebl, N., & Salama, M. (2025). Exploring dopa decarboxylase as an ideal biomarker in Parkinson's disease with focus on regulatory mechanisms, cofactor influences, and metabolic implications. *Npj Biomedical Innovations, 2*(1). https://doi.org/10.1038/s44385-024-00005-7

Shen, T., Yue, Y., He, T., Huang, C., Qu, B., Lv, W., & Lai, H. Y. (2021). The Association between the Gut Microbiota and Parkinson's Disease, a meta-analysis. *Frontiers in Aging Neuroscience, 13*. https://doi.org/10.3389/fnagi.2021.636545

Shulman, J. M., De Jager, P. L., & Feany, M. B. (2011). Parkinson's disease: Genetics and pathogenesis. *Annual Review of Pathology: Mechanisms of Disease, 6*, 193–222. https://doi.org/10.1146/ANNUREV-PATHOL-011110-130242/CITE/REFWORKS

Si, X. L., Fang, Y. J., Li, L. F., Gu, L. Y., Yin, X. Z., Jun-Tian, Yan, Y. P., Pu, J. L., & Zhang, B. R. (2021). From inflammasome to Parkinson's disease: Does the NLRP3 inflammasome facilitate exosome secretion and exosomal alpha-synuclein transmission in Parkinson's disease? *Experimental Neurology, 336*. https://doi.org/10.1016/j.expneurol.2020.113525

Silva, S., Almeida, A. J., & Vale, N. (2021). Importance of nanoparticles for the delivery of antiparkinsonian drugs. *Pharmaceutics, 13*(4), 508.

Simon, D. K., Tanner, C. M., & Brundin, P. (2020). Parkinson disease epidemiology, pathology, Genetics, and pathophysiology. *Clinics in Geriatric Medicine, 36*(1), 1–12. https://doi.org/10.1016/j.cger.2019.08.002

Singh, K. S., Verma, R., Singh, N., Singh, L. R., & Gupta, A. (2025). Factors responsible for alpha-Synuclein aggregation. *Progress in Molecular Biology and Translational Science, 211*, 271–292. https://doi.org/10.1016/bs.pmbts.2024.11.004

Sitzia, G., Mantas, I., Zhang, X., Svenningsson, P., & Chergui, K. (2020). NMDA receptors are altered in the substantia nigra pars reticulata and their blockade ameliorates motor deficits in experimental parkinsonism. *Neuropharmacology, 174*, Article 108136. https://doi.org/10.1016/j.neuropharm.2020.108136

Slater, N. M., Melzer, T. R., Myall, D. J., Anderson, T. J., & Dalrymple-Alford, J. C. (2024). Cholinergic basal forebrain integrity and cognition in Parkinson's Disease: A reappraisal of magnetic resonance imaging evidence. *Movement Disorders, 39*(12), 2155–2172. https://doi.org/10.1002/mds.30023

Smit, J. W., Basile, P., Prato, M. K., Detalle, L., Mathy, F. X., Schmidt, A., Lalla, M., Germani, M., Domange, C., Biere, A. L., Bani, M., Carson, S., & Genius, J. (2022). Phase 1/1b studies of UCB0599, an oral inhibitor of α-Synuclein misfolding, including a randomized Study in Parkinson's Disease. *Movement Disorders, 37*(10), 2045–2056. https://doi.org/10.1002/mds.29170

Song, H., Chen, J., Huang, J., Peng, S., Liu, Y., Xu, L., Wei, C., Mu, X., Lu, X., Wang, W., Zhang, N., Shang, M., Mei, Mo, Zhang, W., Zhao, H., & Han, F. (2023). Epigenetic modification in Parkinson's disease. *Frontiers in Cell and Developmental Biology, 11*. https://doi.org/10.3389/fcell.2023.1123621

Srinivas, V., Choubey, U., Kapparath, S., Shaik, T., Singh, B., Mahmood, R., Garg, N., Aggarwal, P., & Jain, R. (2024). Age-Related orthostatic hypotension: A comprehensive analysis of prevalence, mechanisms, and management in the geriatric population. *Cardiology in Review.* https://doi.org/10.1097/crd.0000000000000636

St Onge, E., Vanderhoof, M., & Miller, S. (2021). Opicapone (Ongentys): A new COMT inhibitor for the treatment of Parkinson's Disease. *The Annals of pharmacotherapy, 55*(9), 1159–1166.

Stokholm, K., Thomsen, M. B., Phan, J. A., Møller, L. K., Bay-Richter, C., Christiansen, S. H., Woldbye, D. P. D., Romero-Ramos, M., & Landau, A. M. (2021). α-Synuclein overexpression increases dopamine D2/3 receptor binding and immune activation in a model of early parkinson's disease. *Biomedicines, 9*(12). https://doi.org/10.3390/biomedicines9121876

Sun, & Armstrong. (2021). Treatment of Parkinson's Disease with cognitive impairment: Current approaches and future directions. *Behavioral Sciences, 11*(4).

Surmeier, D. J., Obeso, J. A., & Halliday, G. M. (2017). Selective neuronal vulnerability in Parkinson disease. *Nature Reviews Neuroscience, 18*(2), 101–113. https://doi.org/10.1038/nrn.2016.178. PMID: 28104909; PMCID: PMC5564322.

Sutachan, J. J., Casas, Z., Albarracin, S. L., Stab, B. R., Samudio, I., Gonzalez, J., Morales, L., & Barreto, G. E. (2012). Cellular and molecular mechanisms of antioxidants in Parkinson's disease. *Nutritional Neuroscience, 15*(3), 120–126. https://doi.org/10.1179/1476830511Y.0000000033Colombia

Suthar, S. K., & Lee, S. Y. (2023). Truncation or proteolysis of α-synuclein in Parkinsonism. *Ageing Research Reviews, 90*. https://doi.org/10.1016/j.arr.2023.101978

Tan, A. H., Lim, S., Chong, K. K., Manap, M.a. a. A., Hor, J. W., Lim, J. L., Low, S. C., Chong, C. W., Mahadeva, S., & Lang, A. E. (2020). Probiotics for constipation in Parkinson disease. *Neurology, 96*(5).

Tang, Y., & Le, W. (2016). Differential roles of M1 and M2 microglia in neurodegenerative diseases. *Molecular Neurobiology, 53*(2), 1181–1194. https://doi.org/10.1007/s12035-014-9070-5

Teixeira, M. I., Lopes, C. M., Amaral, M. H., & Costa, P. C. (2022). Surface-modified lipid nanocarriers for crossing the blood-brain barrier (BBB): A current overview of active targeting in brain diseases. *Colloids and Surfaces B Biointerfaces, 221*, Article 112999.

Teleanu, Niculescu, Roza, Vladâcenco, Grumezescu, & Teleanu. (2022). Neurotransmitters-Key factors in neurological and neurodegenerative disorders of the central nervous System. *International Journal of Molecular Sciences, 23*(11).

Teymourian, H., Tehrani, F., Longardner, K., Mahato, K., Podhajny, T., Moon, J. M., Kotagiri, Y. G., Sempionatto, J. R., Litvan, I., & Wang, J. (2022). Closing the loop for patients with Parkinson disease: Where are we? *Nature Reviews Neurology, 18*(8), 497–507. https://doi.org/10.1038/s41582-022-00674-1

Tysnes, O. B., & Storstein, A. (2017). Epidemiology of Parkinson's disease. *Journal of Neural Transmission, 124*(8), 901–905. https://doi.org/10.1007/s00702-017-1686-y

Tyson, T., Senchuk, M., Cooper, J. F., George, S., Van Raamsdonk, J. M., & Brundin, P. (2017). Novel animal model defines genetic contributions for neuron-to-neuron transfer of α-synuclein. *Scientific Reports, 7*(1). https://doi.org/10.1038/s41598-017-07383-6

Valerio, J. E., Aguirre Vera, G.d. J., Fernandez Gomez, M. P., Zumaeta, J., & Alvarez-Pinzon, A. M. (2025). AI-Driven advances in parkinson's disease neurosurgery: Enhancing patient selection, trial efficiency, and therapeutic outcomes. *Brain Sciences, 15*(5). https://doi.org/10.3390/brainsci15050494

van Vliet, E. F., Knol, M. J., Schiffelers, R. M., Caiazzo, M., & Fens, M. H. A. M. (2023). Levodopa-loaded nanoparticles for the treatment of Parkinson's disease. *Journal of Controlled Release, 360*, 212–224. https://doi.org/10.1016/j.jconrel.2023.06.026

Verma, M., Wills, Z., & Chu, C. T. (2018). Excitatory dendritic mitochondrial calcium toxicity: Implications for Parkinson's and other neurodegenerative diseases. *Frontiers in Neuroscience, 12*, 523.

Vidović, M., & Rikalovic, M. G. (2022). Alpha-Synuclein aggregation pathway in parkinson's disease: Current status and novel therapeutic approaches. *Cells, 11*(11), 1732. https://doi.org/10.3390/cells11111732

Vizziello, M., Borellini, L., Franco, G., & Ardolino, G. (2021). Disruption of mitochondrial homeostasis: The role of PINK1 in parkinson's disease. *Cells, 10*(11), 3022. https://doi.org/10.3390/cells10113022

Volc, D., Werner, P., Kutzelnigg, A., Lührs, P., Thun-Hohenstein, C., Schneeberger, A., Galabova, G., Majbour, N., Vaikath, N., El-Agnaf, O., Winter, D., Mihailovska, E., Mairhofer, A., Schwenke, C., Staffler, G., & Medori, R. (2020). Safety and immunogenicity of the α-synuclein active immunotherapeutic PD01A in patients with Parkinson's disease: A randomised, single-blinded, phase 1 trial. *The Lancet Neurology, 19*(7), 591–600. https://doi.org/10.1016/s1474-4422(20)30136-8

Wagner, J., Ryazanov, S., Leonov, A., Levin, J., Shi, S., Schmidt, F., Prix, C., Pan-Montojo, F., Bertsch, U., Mitteregger-Kretzschmar, G., Geissen, M., Eiden, M., Leidel, F., Hirschberger, T., Deeg, A. A., Krauth, J. J., Zinth, W., Tavan, P., Pilger, J., … Giese, A. (2013). Anle138b: A novel oligomer modulator for disease-modifying therapy of neurodegenerative diseases such as prion and Parkinson's disease. *Acta Neuropathologica, 125*(6), 795–813. https://doi.org/10.1007/s00401-013-1114-9

Wahabi, K., Perwez, A., & Rizvi, M. A. (2018). Parkin in parkinson's disease and cancer: A double-edged sword. *Molecular Neurobiology, 55*(8), 6788–6800. https://doi.org/10.1007/S12035-018-0879-1

Walczak-Nowicka, Ł. J., & Herbet, M. (2021). Acetylcholinesterase inhibitors in the treatment of neurodegenerative diseases and the role of acetylcholinesterase in their pathogenesis. *International Journal of Molecular Sciences, 22*(17). https://doi.org/10.3390/ijms22179290

Wang, X., Shinkai, Y., & Doi, M. (2021). Retrogradely transmitted α-synuclein is taken up by the endophilin-independent endocytosis in the C. elegans neural circuit. *Biochemical and biophysical research communications, 552*, 176–182.

Wegrzynowicz, M., Bar-On, D., Calo', L., Anichtchik, O., Iovino, M., Xia, J., Ryazanov, S., Leonov, A., Giese, A., Dalley, J. W., Griesinger, C., Ashery, U., & Spillantini, M. G. (2019). Depopulation of dense α-synuclein aggregates is associated with rescue of dopamine neuron dysfunction and death in a new Parkinson's disease model. *Acta Neuropathologica, 138*(4), 575–595. https://doi.org/10.1007/s00401-019-02023-x

Weihofen, A., Liu, Y. T., Arndt, J. W., Huy, C., Quan, C., Smith, B. A., Baeriswyl, J. L., Cavegn, N., Senn, L., Su, L., Marsh, G., Auluck, P. K., Montrasio, F., Nitsch, R. M., Hirst, W. D., Cedarbaum, J. M., Pepinsky, R. B., Grimm, J., & Weinreb, P. H. (2019). Development of an aggregate-selective, human-derived α-synuclein antibody BIIB054 that ameliorates disease phenotypes in Parkinson's disease models. *Neurobiology of Disease, 124*, 276–288. https://doi.org/10.1016/j.nbd.2018.10.016

West, C. L., Mao, Y. K., Delungahawatta, T., Amin, J. Y., Farhin, S., McQuade, R. M., Diwakarla, S., Pustovit, R., Stanisz, A. M., Bienenstock, J., Barbut, D., Zasloff, M., Furness, J. B., & Kunze, W. A. (2020). Squalamine restores the function of the enteric nervous System in mouse models of Parkinson's Disease. *Journal of Parkinson's Disease, 10*(4), 1477–1491. https://doi.org/10.3233/JPD-202076

Wu, C., Wu, H., Zhou, C., Guo, T., Guan, X., Cao, Z., Wu, J., Liu, X., Chen, J., Wen, J., Qin, J., Tan, S., Duanmu, X., Gu, L., Song, Z., Zhang, B., Huang, P., Xu, X., & Zhang, M. (2024). The effect of dopamine replacement therapy on cortical structure in Parkinson's disease. *CNS Neuroscience & Therapeutics, 30*(4). https://doi.org/10.1111/cns.14540

Xiao, J., Guo, S., Wang, D., & An, Q. (2024). Fenton-Like reaction: Recent advances and new trends. *Chemistry - A European Journal, 30*(24). https://doi.org/10.1002/chem.202304337

Xie, L., Chen, D., Zhu, X., & Cheng, C. (2023). Efficacy and safety of probiotics in Parkinson's constipation: A systematic review and meta-analysis. *Frontiers in Pharmacology, 13.* https://doi.org/10.3389/fphar.2022.1007654

Xiong, Y., & Yu, J. (2024). LRRK2 in Parkinson's disease: Upstream regulation and therapeutic targeting. *Trends in Molecular Medicine, 30*(10), 982–996. https://doi.org/10.1016/j.molmed.2024.07.003

Yan, D., Zhang, Y., Liu, L., Shi, N., & Yan, H. (2018). Pesticide exposure and risk of Parkinson's disease: Dose-response meta-analysis of observational studies. *Regulatory Toxicology and Pharmacology, 96*, 57–63. https://doi.org/10.1016/j.yrtph.2018.05.005

Yang, H. M. (2025). Mitochondrial dysfunction in neurodegenerative diseases. *Cells, 14*(4). https://doi.org/10.3390/cells14040276

Yang, H., Shao, Y., Hu, Y., Qian, J., Wang, P., Tian, L., … Le, W. (2024). Fecal microbiota from patients with Parkinson's disease intensifies inflammation and neurodegeneration in A53T mice. *CNS Neuroscience & Therapeutics, 30*(8), Article e70003. https://onlinelibrary.wiley.com/doi/full/10.1111/cns.70003.

Ye, D., Chukwu, C., Yang, Y., Hu, Z., & Chen, H. (2024). Adeno-associated virus vector delivery to the brain: Technology advancements and clinical applications. *Advanced Drug Delivery Reviews, 211*, Article 115363. https://doi.org/10.1016/j.addr.2024.115363

Ye, H., Robak, L. A., Yu, M., Cykowski, M., & Shulman, J. M. (2022). Genetics and pathogenesis of parkinson's syndrome. *Annual Review of Pathology, 18.* https://doi.org/10.1146/ANNUREV-PATHMECHDIS-031521-034145

Yoon, W., Min, S., Ryu, H. S., Chung, S. J., & Chung, J. (2022). Discovery of levodopa-induced dyskinesia-associated genes using genomic studies in patients and Drosophila behavioral analyses. *Communications Biology, 5*(1). https://doi.org/10.1038/s42003-022-03830-x

Younesian, S., Yousefi, A. M., Momeny, M., Ghaffari, S. H., & Bashash, D. (2022). The DNA methylation in neurological diseases. *Cells, 11*(21). https://doi.org/10.3390/cells11213439

Zecca, L., Casella, L., Albertini, A., Bellei, C., Zucca, F. A., Engelen, M., Zadlo, A., Szewczyk, G., Zareba, M., & Sarna, T. (2008). Neuromelanin can protect against iron-mediated oxidative damage in system modeling iron overload of brain aging and Parkinson's disease. *Journal of Neurochemistry, 106*(4), 1866–1875. https://doi.org/10.1111/j.1471-4159.2008.05541.x

Zeng, H., Liu, Y., Liu, X., Li, J., Lu, L., Xue, C., Wu, X., Zhang, X., Zheng, Z., & Lu, G. (2024). Interplay of α-Synuclein oligomers and endoplasmic reticulum stress in Parkinson'S Disease: Insights into cellular dysfunctions. *Inflammation.* https://doi.org/10.1007/s10753-024-02156-6

Zheng, H., Xie, Z., Zhang, X., Mao, J., Wang, M., Wei, S., Fu, Y., Zheng, H., He, Y., Chen, H., & Xu, Y. (2021). Investigation of α-Synuclein species in plasma exosomes and the oligomeric and phosphorylated α-Synuclein as potential peripheral biomarker of Parkinson's disease. *Neuroscience, 469*, 79–90. https://doi.org/10.1016/j.neuroscience.2021.06.033

Zhong, W., Shahbaz, O., Teskey, G., Beever, A., Kachour, N., Venketaraman, V., & Darmani, N. A. (2021). Mechanisms of nausea and vomiting: Current knowledge and recent advances in intracellular emetic signaling systems. *International Journal of Molecular Sciences, 22*(11), 5797. https://doi.org/10.3390/ijms22115797

Zhou, B., Wen, M., Yu, W.-F., Zhang, C.-L., & Jiao, L. (2015). The diagnostic and differential diagnosis utility of cerebrospinal fluid α -Synuclein levels in parkinson's disease: A meta-analysis. *Parkinson's Disease, 2015*, 1–11. https://doi.org/10.1155/2015/567386

CHAPTER

Cultural and regional considerations in Parkinson's pharmacotherapy

3

Adejoke Elizabeth Memudu[1], Kenechukwu Emmanuel Nwanama[2], Esther Abosede Adewumi[3], Baliqis Adejoke Olukade[4], Gideon S. Alex[5], Abayomi Oyeyemi Ajagbe[6], Ibilola Funsho Itiolu[7] and Kenneth Chiedozie Oparaji[8]

[1]*Anatomy Department, Faculty of Basic Medical Sciences Edo State University, Iyamho, Edo State, Nigeria;* [2]*Sancta Maria Catholic College of Nursing Sciences, Uzairue, Edo State, Nigeria;* [3]*School of Science, Environment and Engineering, University of Salford, Manchester, United Kingdom;* [4]*Department of Molecular Medicine, Morsani College of Medicine, University of South Florida, Tampa, FL, United States;* [5]*University of Port Harcourt, Rivers State, Nigeria;* [6]*Department of Anatomy, Nile University of Nigeria, Abuja, Nigeria;* [7]*Pharmacology and Therapeutics Department, Faculty of Basic Clinical Sciences University of Ilorin, Ilorin, Kwara State, Nigeria;* [8]*Department of Physiology, Faculty of Basic Medical Sciences, Alex Ekwueme Federal University Ndufu-Alike (AE-FUNAI), Abakaliki, Ebonyi State, Nigeria*

Parkinson disease (PD) is a global prevalent progressive neurodegenerative disorder that impacts quality of life. Pharmacotherapy is a cornerstone of PD management, but its effectiveness can be influenced by various cultural and regional factors creating disparities in treatment outcomes across diverse populations. There is need to explore the relationship between cultural practices, regional healthcare infrastructure, and pharmacotherapy strategies for PD management. This cultural consideration will highlight the impact or influence of traditional medicine and cultural attitudes toward modern pharmacotherapy that may affect PD treatment in evidence-based practices. Regional differences in dietary habits, lifestyle factors, and environmental exposures can also influence the course of PD and the response to treatment. For example, diets rich in antioxidants and certain nutrients may have neuroprotective effects, while exposure to environmental toxins may increase the risk of developing PD. By addressing cultural and regional barriers, that may influence the efficacy, accessibility, and adherence to PD pharmacological interventions, healthcare providers can enhance the effectiveness of PD pharmacotherapy and improve the quality of life for individuals with this debilitating disease across diverse populations. This chapter also indicates the importance of personalized pharmacotherapy in PD management through global collaboration in research and policy-making to ensure equitable and effective treatment for PD patients worldwide. Additionally, patient education and support programs can empower patients to make informed decisions about their treatment and improve medication adherence. By addressing cultural and regional barriers, healthcare providers can enhance the effectiveness of PD pharmacotherapy and improve the quality of life for individuals with this debilitating disease.

Pharmacological Foundations of Parkinson's Disease. https://doi.org/10.1016/B978-0-443-27702-3.00010-8

3.1 Introduction

Parkinson disease, the second most prevalent neurodegenerative disease globally, is typified by physical manifestations of motor symptoms including bradykinesia, tremor, and stiffness associated with the death of dopaminergic neurons in the substantia nigra pars compacta (Ayano, 2016; Kouli et al., 2018). PD symptoms also include loss of smell, sleep dysfunction, mood disorders, excessive salivation, constipation, and extensive periodic limb movements during sleep (Mirpour et al., 2018). Early-onset PD can happen before the age of 50, although it usually develops between the ages of 55 and 65 (Schwamborn, 2018). The exact cause of PD is still mostly unclear, environmental and genetic variables both have a role in its development (Kouli et al., 2018). Dopaminergic cell death has been linked to several cellular processes, such as protein misfolding, compromised autophagy, endoplasmic reticulum stress, mitochondrial malfunction, and alteration of calcium homeostasis (Michel et al., 2016). Lewy bodies are intracellular α-synuclein aggregates that are the pathogenic characteristic of PD (Kouli et al., 2018). Neuroinflammation, defective protein degradation pathways, and α-syn toxicity interact intricately in the pathophysiology of PD (Minchev et al., 2022). Both the central and peripheral nervous systems exhibit neuroinflammation, which is characterized by glial cell activation and is essential to the development of illness (Joshi & Singh, 2018). Neuronal injury is caused by mitochondrial malfunction and oxidative stress (Minchev et al., 2022).

Motor symptoms are a hallmark of PD; nevertheless, nonmotor symptoms have a substantial influence on patients' quality of life and may occur years before motor manifestations (Jones et al., 2020; Schapira et al., 2017). Sleep issues, cognitive decline, depression, hyposmia, pain, and autonomic dysfunction are some of these nonmotor characteristics (Schapira et al., 2017; Suzuki et al., 2014). Motor symptoms are caused by the death of dopaminergic neurons in the substantia nigra pars compacta, whereas nonmotor symptoms are caused by disruptions in nondopaminergic systems (Radad et al., 2023). The pathophysiology of PD and the specific sensitivity of midbrain dopaminergic neurons have been extensively studied using animal models, both genetic and toxin-based (Blesa & Przedborski, 2014). A key factor in the pathophysiology of PD is mitochondrial dysfunction, which connects environmental toxins and genetic abnormalities (Helley et al., 2017; Park et al., 2018). In the majority of PD patients, the interaction of environmental variables and genetic predisposition probably causes the illness to start (Polito et al., 2016).

The clinical presentation, development, and response to therapy for PD vary greatly, which makes standardized treatments difficult to implement (Giladi et al., 2016; Payami, 2017). To address this variability, precision medicine customizes treatments according to each patient's unique genetic, biochemical, and clinical characteristics (Reed et al., 2021). Although precision medicine for PD is still in its infancy, it has enormous promise to enhance treatment results and patients' quality of life (Bu et al., 2016; Reed et al., 2021). The variety of PD progression and cognitive impairment has been clarified by recent genetic research. GBA mutations are linked to worse cognitive outcomes and a quicker rate of illness development (Dulski et al., 2024; Fagan & Pihlstrøm, 2017). In contrast to idiopathic PD, LRRK2 mutations could result in a milder cognitive impairment (Fagan & Pihlstrøm, 2017). PD patients with LRRK2 and GBA mutations showed diverse network connection patterns in metabolic brain imaging, which may account for their disparate clinical trajectories (Schindlbeck et al., 2020). These results emphasize how genetic variables play a significant role in PD heterogeneity and should help with patient categorization for clinical trials and individualized treatment plans

(Dulski et al., 2024). Additionally, studies on biomarkers have greatly advanced our knowledge of how PD develops and possible therapeutic outcomes. Biomarkers of cerebrospinal fluid (CSF), such as tau pathology indicators, neurofilament light chain, and α-synuclein species, have the potential to indicate chronic pathological processes (Kwon et al., 2022). Furthermore, imaging methods including MRI, SPECT, and PET have shed light on the structural and functional alterations in PD patients' brains (Niccolini, 2017). The most effective strategy for early identification and tracking the course of a disease is now provided by these neuroimaging techniques, especially functional imaging (Algarni & Stoessl, 2016).

Despite its potential to improve healthcare, personalized medicine (PM) has several implementation issues. The high expenses of genetic testing and analysis are significant obstacles (Fodor & Karnieli, 2016; Misra & Bisui, 2014). There are additional challenges due to ethical concerns about the privacy and preservation of genetic data (Al-Eitan & Tarkhan, 2016). According to Knowles et al. (2017), proving effectiveness still requires extensive validation research and clinical trials. Realizing the full potential of customized medicine in enhancing patient care and healthcare efficiency requires addressing these issues.

The therapy of PD and patient results are greatly impacted by cultural and geographical variations. Sociocultural differences in PD knowledge and healthcare access were highlighted by research conducted in Turkey by Sayan et al. (2020), which discovered differences in education levels, family history, and cognitive ability between the northwest and southeast areas. Cross-cultural research by Achen et al. (2023) highlights the need for culturally appropriate support services by revealing variations in caregiver experiences and views across different nations. While certain characteristics, such as motor disability, have an impact on stigma regardless of culture, others, such as sex, education, and occupation, may have a culturally specific effect (Karacan et al., 2023). According to Branson et al. (2016), there are racial differences in the prevalence of PD, treatment accessibility, and research participation. African Americans have lower prevalence and incidence rates than Caucasians. These results highlight how crucial it is to take regional and cultural aspects into account while managing and studying PD.

Treatment for PD is greatly influenced by cultural beliefs and traditional medical practices, especially in Asian and African populations where acupuncture and herbal medicines are frequently utilized in addition to mainstream therapy (Bega & Zadikoff, 2014). Levodopa from *Mucuna pruriens*, a natural source, has demonstrated promise in treating PD symptoms (Panova et al., 2020). Particularly in low-income nations where traditional medicines are frequently unavailable or prohibitively expensive, this plant-based strategy may provide a sustainable, economical option for the management of PD (Fothergill-Misbah et al., 2020). However, questions concerning the safety and effectiveness of herbal remedies are raised by the absence of regulatory control and standardization (Hamood et al., 2024). The care of PD, a complicated neurological illness, necessitates a multidisciplinary approach. By customizing treatments according to genetic, biochemical, and clinical profiles, personalized medicine integration presents the possibility of better patient outcomes (Bu et al., 2016; Titova et al., 2017). Personalized medicine for PD is still in its infancy, though, and implementation is fraught with difficulties. To obtain more customized and comprehensive treatment plans, future PD management should concentrate on combining various techniques (Reed et al., 2021; Titova et al., 2017).

3.2 Global epidemiology of Parkinson disease

Parkinson disease incidence and prevalence are influenced medical conditions, genetic, and environmental factors which differs across regions. PD affects 1%–2% of adults over 60 and rises to 3.5% by the age of 85–89, making it the second most prevalent neurodegenerative illness after Alzheimer disease (Rizek et al., 2016); hence, it is considered the fastest growing neurological disorder (Osborne et al., 2022). According to statistics, there are over six million cases of PD globally, this is predicted to increase in the next 30 years; hence, the prevalence of PD has increased by 2.5 times in the last generation, making it one of the main causes of neurological impairment (GBD 2016 Neurology Collaborators, 2019; Tolosa et al., 2021).

a) **Prevalence and incidence in different regions:** As of 2023, the global prevalence of PD was estimated at 1.51 per 1000 individuals, with projections indicating a rise to over 12 million cases by 2040. This increase is primarily attributed to aging populations and it is notably 40% more common in men than in women (Ben-Shlomo et al., 2024). Geographically, the prevalence and incidence of PD exhibit considerable variation. For instance, North America and Europe have higher prevalence rates potentially due to longer life expectancies and comprehensive healthcare systems that facilitate diagnosis and reporting. Asia has a relatively lower prevalence rates. However, China is projected to account for nearly half of the global PD population by 2030, reflecting both demographic shifts and increased recognition of the disease (Ben-Shlomo et al., 2024). In Africa, a lower prevalence rates have been reported, which may result from under diagnosis, limited access to healthcare, and shorter life expectancies (Ben-Shlomo et al., 2024). In a very recent study by Su et al. (2025), it was predicted that there would be about 25.2 million cases of PD worldwide in 2050. This rise in the prevalence of PD can be correlated with changes in the environment, people's lifestyle, and healthcare service brought about by growing population, technological advancement, social, and economic progress. According to studies, contaminants from the environment such particulate matter, naphtha and its derivatives, job-related exposure, and the use of insecticides and pest control chemicals increase the risk of PD in areas that are rapidly growing (Aravindan et al., 2024).

b) **Genetic and environmental contributors:** The etiology of PD reveals that the interactions between the genes and the environment are recognized as the root cause of its pathogenesis, which explains the complex interplay between genetic predispositions and exposure to environmental factors which also differs in individual due to variation in human genotype thereby leading to a range of disease manifestations (Ball et al., 2019). Approximately 5%–10% of PD cases are familial, with mutations in genes such as SNCA, LRRK2, GBA, and MAPT identified as contributors; however, the majority of cases are sporadic, with heritability estimates around 30%, suggesting significant environmental influences (Morris et al., 2024). Studies have shown that alterations in the α-synuclein (α-syn) protein encoding *SNCA* gene are the main component of Lewy bodies, a hallmark of PD. Following the identification of the mutation in the *SNCA* as the main cause of autosomal dominant PD, further genetic studies have also established the mutations of other genes relating to autosomal dominant PD such as *LRRK2, VSP35, and CHCHD2* and other mutated genes such as *Parkin, PINK1, DJ-1, ATP13A2, FBXO7, and PLA2G6* relating to autosomal recessive pattern of PD (Pang et al., 2019). Several research have identified toxins present in the environment that can be linked to an increased risk of PD. Exposure to toxins in the environment, including herbicides, pesticides, industrial solvents such as trichlorethylene, and air pollution, has been strongly linked to an increased risk of PD (Tsalenchuk et al., 2023). The pesticides such as the rotenone and herbicides such as paraquat have structural characteristics common with 1-methyl-4-phenylpyridinium (MPP), a metabolite of MPTP in the brain that induces parkinsonism (Elmorsy et al., 2023). Rotenone and paraquat are known mitochondrial toxins which may contribute to dopaminergic neuronal degeneration (Elmorsy et al., 2023; Tsalenchuk et al., 2023). Urban regions reported to have high levels of air pollution put dwellers at risk of developing PD, while rural environment invested in agricultural activities have also been linked to increased risk of developing PD primarily due to constant use of herbicides and pesticides (Sakowski et al., 2024).

c) **Regional healthcare disparities:** Disparities in healthcare access and quality significantly impact the diagnosis, treatment, and management of PD across different regions. In developed countries, there are advanced healthcare infrastructures which enables early diagnosis and comprehensive management of PD, leading to possible improved patient outcomes. In developing countries, there are limited healthcare resources, lack of specialized medical professionals, and inadequate access to medications result in delayed diagnoses and suboptimal management of PD. Additionally, cultural factors and stigma associated with neurological disorders may further hinder individuals from seeking medical attention (Deliz et al., 2024).

3.3 Cultural factors in pharmacotherapy

3.3.1 Beliefs and stigma around PD

The stigma associated with PD adversely affects both patients and carers, leading to reduces quality of life, increased emotional stress or anxiety and feeling of loneliness (Karacan et al., 2023). Though a great deal of study has been done on the clinical manifestations of PD, little is known about the social and or psychological side effects, such as the stereotypes attached and the stigma. There is need to focus on the stigma that affects a patient's willingness to seek treatment. There have been reports and observations of PD stigma worldwide, and stigma seems to have a significant impact on PD sufferers' health-related quality of life (HRQoL) (Fothergill-Misbah, 2023; Karacan et al., 2023; Maffoni et al., 2017). In a recent publication byCrooks et al. (2025), it was stated that participants in research study emphasized how typical it is for the general public to be bias and have discriminating beliefs and views about PD. Due to these beliefs, people living with PD and their carers regularly experience hostile discrimination and sometimes isolation. The participants were frustrated about how most people commonly misperceive the only symptom of PD to the tremors and knowing very little about other symptoms, especially the non-motor-related ones. For example, in a study done on PD patients from Israeli, participants highlighted how people's lack of knowledge about nonmotor symptoms including stiffness in muscles and impairment of speech undermines the complex characteristics of PD (Abo-Jabel et al., 2021). Henry et al. (2021) conducted a multinational study to investigate whether the clinical manifestation of PD correlated with the attached stigma, and these varied from place to place; their report revealed that the stigma is associated with the specific clinical symptoms of PD. For instance, the stigma relating to bowel/bladder illness was significantly higher in US than it was in Mexico, and this is because the PD symptoms relating to bowel and bladder incontinence was also higher in US Henry et al. (2021).The complicated social phenomenon of stigma, which includes exclusion, discrimination, prejudice, and stereotypes, has a big impact on the lives of people with PD (Crooks et al., 2025). A well-established deterrent to seeking medical attention, stigma can have a detrimental impact on one's mental and physical health, social standing, and worsen existing conditions (Fothergill-Misbah, 2023; McDaniels et al., 2023). It is distinct from shame, an emotional reaction marked by a profound feeling of one's own inadequacy or dishonor(Crooks et al., 2025). Although stigma is the unfavorable social impression that others place on a person because of a specific illness, shame is more intimate and results from internalized ideas about one's own value or conduct(Crooks et al., 2025; Fothergill-Misbah, 2023).

Tremor, slowed speech, or dyskinesias are examples of visible or physical signs of PD that can "discredit" and "devalue" people by making them appear "different." This causes people to become alarmed, avoid, and be labeled by others (enacted stigma)(Fothergill-Misbah, 2023; Maffoni et al., 2017). The awareness of one's clumsiness and incapacity to carry out routine tasks at work as well as basic motor motions can lead to stigma. A decline in physical functioning leads to a decrease in social participation and activity, which is associated with the experience of stigma(Maffoni et al., 2017). In addition to being a patient experience, stigma may also be a sentiment that defines family caregivers. PD is an undesired trait that affects the entire family, causing problems in public places as well as an unwelcome sense of guilt and sympathy(Crooks et al., 2025; Maffoni et al., 2017).

Cultural notions like witchcraft and curses made stigma even worse(Crooks et al., 2025). According to participants in Fothergill-Misbah's (2023) study, stigma is influenced by cultural beliefs, and some of them attribute PD to supernatural origins. These ideas, which are frequently associated with guilt and punishment, have a significant effect on people with PD, resulting in prejudice and social exclusion(Crooks et al., 2025).

3.4 Traditional medicine versus modern pharmacotherapy

The use of traditional medicine has become increasingly popular in the treatment of an array of diseases globally including PD, resulting in various laboratory research over the last decade to test the efficacy of natural product or plant-based medicine nutritional value alleviate the symptoms of PD with minimal negative side effects (Kumari et al., 2023). Natural substances produced from Chinese plant-based remedies such as curcumin, gambogic acid, emodin, cepharanthine, berberine, β-elemene, ursolic acid, oridonin, and wogonin have been reported to show positive neuroprotective actions against PD neuropathology, this has translated to application in modern pharmacotherapy through the use of their active ingredients in medicinal herbs (such Acanthopanax, Alpinia, and Astragalus) seen to be beneficial in PD models through their potentials to have antiaging properties, reverse free radical generation, reduce oxidative stress, and improve the secretion of dopamine (Yin et al., 2021). Modern pharmacotherapy involve two primary drug therapy which are dopaminergic (DAergic) and non-DAergic therapy targeted to treat PD motor symptoms. DAergic medications include catechol-O-methyl transferase (COMT) inhibitors, monoamine oxidase type B (MAO-B) inhibitors, levodopa or levodopa with dopa-decarboxylase inhibitors (DDC-I), and dopamine (DA) agonists. These medications, which have been around for decades, effectively treat PD's motor symptoms(Dong et al., 2016; Schapira, 2007).

Since ancient times, people have utilized herbal remedies, and new research indicates that some of them may help reduce the symptoms of PD (Dong et al., 2016). Numerous substances derived from herbs have demonstrated anti-PD properties in experiments. In the meanwhile, attempts have been undertaken to figure out how they work, either in vivo or in vitro as well as their bioavailability and blood-brain barrier penetration (Li et al., 2013). For example, saponins and phenolics are often poorly absorbed, conjugated, or devoid of their sugar ornamentation; as a result, their blood concentrations would be low, and their in vivo antioxidant activities would be minimal(Chen et al., 2022; Li et al., 2013).

3.5 Adherence and perception of treatment in diverse cultures

The term "adherence" is thought to be more appropriate as it acknowledges the patient's autonomy and calls for his or her consent to the advice provided by the medical expert(Hughes, 2004). In PD, cultural views, social level, background in education, emotional well-being, and features of the healthcare system interact in a complex way that impacts adherence to prescribed medications (James et al., 2024). Medication use is a psychological, social, and interpersonal process in addition to a pharmacological one(Hughes, 2004). As with any group, measuring adherence in the elderly has been a significant difficulty and idiopathic PD is still most commonly associated with aging(Hughes, 2004; Reeve et al., 2014). The concept of nonadherence to PD treatment includes both skipping medicine doses and taking all required doses at a different time of day than set time, as timing is crucial while taking PD medication (James et al., 2024). Studies have also proven that socio-economic factors significantly affect adherence to treatment in PD. Additionally, several studies demonstrated that there is a lower adherence to treatment among African Americans. Comparing families with lower incomes versus family with higher income, the former was also thought to be potential indicators of lower adherence to treatment. In many African countries, the availability of antiparkinsonian medications is still a major issue (Gil et al., 2024).

3.6 Regional variations in drug availability

a. **Accessibility of PD medications (e.g., levodopa and dopamine agonists)** Among the pharmacological management of early-stage PD typically employs levodopa, dopamine agonists, or monoamine oxidase B (MAO-B) inhibitors. Levodopa, the most efficacious, directly replenishes depleted dopamine. Dopamine agonists act by stimulating dopamine receptors, while MAO-B inhibitors prolong dopamine's synaptic availability by inhibiting its degradation (Binde et al., 2020). These drugs mitigate motor symptoms and enhance patient quality of life. According to World Health Organization (WHO), levodopa is recognized as one of the most efficacious and readily available pharmacological agents for the management of PD, and it has been shown to provide significant relief from various motor symptoms associated with this debilitating condition (WHO, 2022). In primary healthcare, the proportion of patients who have access to levodopa ranges from an estimated 34%–58%, indicating a significant variation in accessibility that may have profound implications for patient outcomes and quality of life. This disparity in availability emphasizes the urgent need for enhanced healthcare policies and strategies aimed at improving access to this critical medication, ensuring that a larger segment of the population suffering from PD can benefit from its therapeutic effects. In an observation letter to the International Parkinson and Movement Disorder Society (MDS), Yang et al. (2020) reported findings from 50 U.S. states, indicating that neurologists prescribed 12.4 million standardized 30-day PD medication classes. The proportion of L-dopa prescriptions varied across states, ranging from 23.6% to 57.0%, while the percentage of prescribers issuing prescriptions ranged from 16.5% to 72.5%.

b. **Regulatory approvals and pricing disparities:** PD necessitates long-term pharmacological intervention due to its progressive state. However, disparities in regulatory approval processes and medication pricing create significant barriers, limiting equitable access to essential treatments for affected individuals (DeMaagd & Philip, 2015; Binde et al., 2020). Regulatory agencies, such as the U.S. Food and Drug Administration (FDA), the European Medicines Agency (EMA), and their international counterparts, follow distinct and often intricate approval pathways (Joppi et al., 2020), which can lead to significant delays and inconsistencies in the availability of essential medications for managing PD symptoms. Furthermore, disparities in drug pricing stem from various factors, including patent protections, differences in healthcare policies, insurance coverage, and pharmaceutical manufacturing costs, all of which contribute to significant price variations across regions. In the United States, PD medications are often considerably more expensive than in European and Asian markets, where the availability of generic alternatives helps reduce costs and improve patient access. To these disparities requires a coordinated effort to harmonize regulatory frameworks, encourage the adoption of generic medications, and enhance transparency in pharmaceutical pricing. These measures are essential to expanding access to critical PD treatments.

c. **Challenges in rural versus urban settings:** In the contest of a part of African country in the year 2024, an esteemed society, the International Parkinson and Movement Disorder Society (MDS), with contribution from the author Zewde (2024), compiled the list of challenges in the onset of PD due to aging process while also highlighted the notably low prevalence of this neurodegenerative disorder in Ethiopia, which is classified as one of the nations situated on the African continent. Zewde emphasized on the regions where PD is more frequent as observed tend to be urban areas where affected individuals have greater access to essential medical attention and specialized care. Despite, the presence of these urban medical facilities, the availability and accessibility of PD medications remain severely constrained, a situation that can be traced back to a multitude of factors, which include and not limited to the inadequacy of infrastructure and the lack of advanced healthcare equipment, which are critical elements still requiring substantial improvement, particularly in the more remote rural locales of the country. All these underscores the urgent need for comprehensive strategies and interventions aimed at enhancing the overall healthcare framework, ensuring that individuals suffering from PD, regardless of their geographical location, have equitable access to the necessary medical treatments and resources essential for managing their condition effectively (Zewde, 2024).

3.6.1 Genetic and ancestral influences

Genetic heterogeneity can influence the response to treatment and drug metabolism in PD. Medication responses in patients can be very diverse, and it is critical to have an understanding of the pharmacokinetic and pharmacodynamic drug properties when assessing ethnic diversity of outcome to treatment. Genetic factors play a significant role, with 20%–95% of patient variation being accounted for (Belle & Singh, 2008). Discovery of polymorphism of drug-metabolizing enzymes and receptors has paved the way for pharmacogenetic testing. High-throughput sequencing of 60,706 human exomes revealed rare genetic variants in drug-related genes that affect patient risk across drugs and geographic ancestries. 44% Of the population carries germline variants in oncological drug targets, which affect response to disease therapy (Schärfe et al., 2017). Several common genetic variants involved in dopamine action and metabolism have been identified in recent studies, which affect the efficacy of medication and side effects in PD. Some of the genes implicated are dopamine receptor genes (DRD1-4), the dopamine transporter gene (SLC6A3) (Contin et al., 2005), and the catechol-O-methyltransferase gene (COMT).

Investigating the link between insulin resistance and PD severity, midbrain organoids from PD patients carrying the GBA1-N370S mutation were obtained. By modulating insulin levels, dysregulated insulin signaling in GBA-PD organoids was identified (Zagare et al., 2025). Transcriptomics revealed impaired insulin signaling pathways, identifying FOXO1 as a potential therapeutic target. Notably, FOXO1 downregulation rescued dopaminergic neuron loss in GBA-PD organoids (Zagare et al., 2025). Besides, antidiabetic drug therapy with metformin and pioglitazone showed promising benefits in controlling GBA-PD-related phenotypes, displaying insulin signaling as an important aspect of PD severity. Variations in the genes are of tremendous value in Africa, with respect to drug development and treatment. CYP variants study revealed distinct genetic predisposition, where several variants existed with potential clinical significance. Interestingly, CYP2B6*6, CYP2C8*2, CYP2D6*3, CYP2D6*17, CYP2D6*29, CYP3A5*6, and CYP3A5*7 variants were observed, which are recognized for potential contributions toward adverse drug reaction (Rajman et al., 2017). A study conducted large-scale genomic analysis of 1136 pharmacogenomic variants in 3714 individuals. The results showed that Admixed Americans and Europeans had an increased risk of drug toxicity, while East Asians and Oceanians had low risk. Polygenic risk scores identified distinct patterns and population-defining variation by drug class (Karamperis et al., 2024).

3.6.1.1 Case studies

The genetics of PD is intricate, with both Mendelian genes (e.g., PRKN, SNCA, LRRK2) and non-Mendelian components, such as single nucleotide polymorphisms (SNPs) (Nissar et al., 2022), significantly accounting for disease susceptibility and progression, with a final role in determining diagnosis and treatment strategies. The disease is also modulated by ancestral and ethnic aspects, with varying genetic variants and mutation having a role in its progression in various populations. Synuclein Alpha (SNCA) has been considered to be the lead causative gene in early FPD onset with five missense mutations identified to date viz., A30P, E46K, H50Q, G51D, and A53T (Siddiqui et al., 2016). A large-scale multiancestry meta-analysis of PD was conducted to clarify the genetics basis of the disease and meta-analyzing data from 49,049 cases, 18,785 proxy cases, and 2,458,063 controls from diverse populations (Kim et al., 2024). In the analysis, 78 independent genome-wide significant loci were identified, including 12 potentially novel loci: MTF2, PIK3CA, ADD1, SYBU, IRS2, USP8, PIGL, FASN, MYLK2, USP25, EP300, and PPP6R2. Additionally, highly penetrant mutations in SNCA, Parkin, and LRRK2 genes have been linked to rare, monogenic's disease (PD) types. LRRK2 and GBA rare variants also impart risk. Over 20 common variants with modest effect sizes alter PD risk. Investigations of Mendelian PD types have provided insight into pathophysiology, but treatments of efficacy have not been identified. The functional basis for the involvement of common risk alleles in PD risk is largely unclear, and additional work is warranted (Hernandez et al., 2016). A 2020 East Asian metagenome-wide association study (GWAS) of 6724 PD cases and 24,851 controls identified 11 genome-wide significant loci. Of these, nine loci (PARK16, ITPKB, MCCC1, SNCA, FAM47E,

SCARB2, DLG2, LRRK2, RIT2, and FYN) had been previously described in European populations, while two new loci (SV2C and WBSCR17) were population-specific. A replication study confirmed the association of SV2C (rs246814) with PD in both European and Japanese populations, while indicating possible genetic heterogeneity at the WBSCR17 locus (rs9638616) between the two populations (Foo et al., 2020). Moreover, a GWAS study of PD in African and African admixed populations identified a novel risk factor. The analysis of 197,918 participants found a significant association at the GBA1 locus (rs3115534-G) that is remarkably common among PD patients of African ancestry (Rizig et al., 2023). Notably, this intronic variant is distinct from the known GBA1 variants (p.E365K and p.N409S) in Europeans and Ashkenazi populations, highlighting the importance of population diversity studies in uncovering population-specific genetic risk factors.

3.7 Dietary and nutritional considerations

The well-established relationship between dietary protein and levodopa, the main drug used to treat PD, can have a substantial effect on how effectively a therapy works (Rusch et al., 2023; Virmani et al., 2016). PD is mostly treated with levodopa, a dopamine precursor that may pass across the blood-brain barrier (Stansley & Yamamoto, 2015). Levodopa is often taken orally, where it is absorbed in the small intestine and then circulated to the brain (Contributions of gut bacteria and diet to drug pharmacokinetics in the treatment of Parkinson's disease, 2019). The b0,+AT-rBAT exchanger is the primary mediator of intestinal absorption of levodopa, and the TAT1 uniporter is essential for its efflux from enterocytes (Camargo et al., 2014) since dopamine cannot pass across the blood-brain barrier (Pedrosa de Menezes et al., 2024). The "protein effect" refers to the motor fluctuations that occur when PD patients consume high-protein meals because they drastically lower the bioavailability of levodopa (Virmani et al., 2016; Wang et al., 2017). This impact affects 12.4% of patients who have fluctuations, and it is most noticeable in individuals with motor difficulties (Virmani et al., 2016). Low-protein and protein-redistribution diets are examples of protein-restricted diets (PRDs) that can enhance levodopa effectiveness and lessen motor fluctuations (Rusch et al., 2023; Wang et al., 2017). Levodopa's effectiveness and patient quality of life may be enhanced by optimizing dietary recommendations in terms of amount, content, and consumption timing (Guebila & Thiele, 2016; Rusch et al., 2023). It has also been demonstrated that PRDs, dietary fiber, vitamin C, and caffeine enhance the absorption of levodopa and lessen motor fluctuations (Keun et al., 2021). Hyperhomocysteinemia, a side effect of levodopa metabolism linked to several problems, can also be lessened by taking supplements of vitamins B6, B12, and folic acid (Keun et al., 2021). In PD patients, iron chelation treatment has demonstrated promise in lowering oxidative damage and enhancing motor function (Devos et al., 2014). Iron supplements, however, may hinder the absorption of levodopa, which might lessen its efficacy. Healthcare professionals should take into account the effects of iron supplements and gut flora on treatment results, and patients are recommended to take levodopa on an empty stomach or with a light, carbohydrate-based meal to maximize its effectiveness.

High levels of antioxidants, antiinflammatory substances, and omega-3 fatty acids (Franco et al., 2023) are thought to contribute to the protective effect of the Mediterranean diet (MD). These nutrients help combat oxidative stress and chronic neuroinflammation, two major causes of neuronal degeneration in PD (Bisaglia, 2023). Reduced probabilities of PD are linked to following a Mediterranean diet that is high in fruits, vegetables, whole grains, olive oil, and fish (Knight et al., 2022; Rees et al.,

2024). According to Gardener and Caunca (2018), plant polyphenols in the MD may contribute to neuroprotection by activating molecular pathways that are comparable to those of calorie-restriction diets.

Western-style diets heavy in red meat, processed foods, and saturated fats have been linked to a higher incidence of PD and a worsening of symptoms (Anwar et al., 2024; de Queiroz Cavalcanti et al., 2023). These diets may exacerbate PD by causing oxidative stress, inflammation, and dysbiosis of the gut microbiota (de Queiroz Cavalcanti et al., 2023). Worsening nonmotor symptoms, such as a worse quality of life and more severe constipation, are linked to higher sugar intake (Palavra et al., 2021). Increased sugar intake may momentarily improve dopamine deficit, but it may also exacerbate neurodegeneration in PD by causing insulin resistance and diabetes (Haas et al., 2022). PD patients may benefit from traditional Asian diets high in plant-based foods and fermented products because fermented soy products, which are popular in East Asian cuisines, contain bioactive compounds that may help manage neurodegenerative diseases (Jang et al., 2021). By reducing inflammation and oxidative stress, plant-based diets rich in phytochemicals may offer neuroprotection and PD symptom relief (Shah & Duda, 2015). According to recent studies, gut dysbiosis plays a crucial role in the pathophysiology of PD by inducing neuroinflammation and changing the balance of neurotransmitters, which both accelerate the course of PD (Alam et al., 2024). Evidence suggests that α-synuclein aggregation may start in the gut and extend to the central nervous system, highlighting the critical function of the gut-brain axis (Dutta et al., 2019; Rani & Mondal, 2021). The makeup of the gut microbiota may be positively influenced by dietary treatments such as Mediterranean and ketogenic diets, which may lower the risk of PD or halt its progression (Sobral et al., 2025). The possible neuroprotective benefits of soy and its phytoestrogens in PD have been investigated. According to certain studies, phytoestrogens generated from soy may provide neuroprotection by interacting with estrogen receptors and having antioxidant qualities (Goyal et al., 2021). However, there is a lack of long-term effectiveness and safety evidence, and beans contain many bioactive chemicals that can be hazardous when taken in excess (Rijntjes, 2019). As a result, care should be taken while thinking about using beans as a natural treatment for PD.

Traditional African diets are high in green vegetables, legumes, and whole grains, which provide vital nutrients and substances that promote health (Oluwole et al., 2021). Even though African diets are varied, they frequently lack vital micronutrients that are necessary for brain function. Many African nations have high rates of vitamin A, B, D, iron, zinc, and calcium deficiencies (White et al., 2021). Neurological illnesses are among the many health problems that can result from these impairments (Kerac et al., 2014). Furthermore, although direct connections to PD are still unclear, dependence on staple foods like cassava, which contains cyanogenic glycosides, has been linked to neurological diseases in certain groups (Kashala-Abotnes et al., 2019; Step et al., 2024). The significance of tailored, culturally aware dietary management strategies for PD is highlighted by recent studies. To enhance quality of life(Subramanian et al., 2023), suggest a holistic wellness paradigm that takes into account cultural context and customized lifestyle treatments, such as food. Noting the possible influence of economic and environmental variables(Navarro-Meza et al., 2015), draw attention to the socio-demographic factors that affect the dietary habits of PD patients living in rural areas. To maximize treatment success and quality of life, our findings highlight the need to include nutritional care in PD therapy, taking into account patients' cultural origins, socioeconomic considerations, and unique disease features.

3.8 Traditional and complementary therapies

The use of herbal medicine in the treatment of PD, a neurodegenerative condition marked by the death of dopaminergic neurons, has shown encouraging promise. Numerous natural substances and plants have been studied for their neuroprotective qualities, focusing on some harmful elements such as oxidative stress, protein aggregation, and mitochondrial dysfunction (Yin et al., 2021). Herbs with antioxidant, antiinflammatory, and antiapoptotic properties, including the levodopa-rich leguminous herb *Mucuna pruriens*, have been shown to have neuroprotective benefits (Srivastav et al., 2017). These natural compounds affect several signaling pathways linked to neuronal stress, including AMPK, NF-κB, and PI3K (Yin et al., 2021). According to research byPanova et al. (2020), *M. pruriens* may be superior to synthetic levodopa formulations because it contains extra bioactive components that boost dopaminergic and neuroprotective activity. High-dose *M. pruriens* has a more favorable tolerance profile than levodopa, but its clinical effects are similar (Panova et al., 2020). When used in conjunction with levodopa as an adjuvant therapy for advanced PD, *M. pruriens* has been shown to reduce the time to "on" state and lengthen the "on" time without aggravating dyskinesias; however, at high dosages, psychological side effects were seen (Botello-Villagrana & Martinez-Ramirez, 2022). Although encouraging, *M. pruriens* has to be shown as a long-term, controlled clinical study to be a viable supplemental treatment for PD (Panova et al., 2020).

Herbs that have been shown to have neuroprotective properties in PD include *Ginkgo biloba, Bacopa monnieri (Brahmi)*, and *Withania somnifera (Ashwagandha)* (Quasmi et al., 2024; Srivastav et al., 2017). These and other herbs, such as *Curcuma longa* and *Mucuna pruriens,* have antioxidant qualities and may enhance mitochondrial activity, which is essential for the best possible neural functioning (Srivastav et al., 2017). In animal models of PD, *Withania somnifera* in particular has demonstrated the capacity to preserve dopaminergic neurons (Singh et al., 2015). These natural compounds are thought to have neuroprotective properties because they can lower proinflammatory cytokines, remove α-synuclein aggregation, control oxidative stress, and raise dopamine levels (Singla et al., 2021). Through several methods, *bacopa monnieri* has demonstrated promise as a neuroprotective drug in PD. According to preclinical research, it can improve cognitive performance while lowering neuroinflammation, oxidative stress, and dopaminergic neuronal degeneration (Goyal et al., 2022; Singh et al., 2021). *Bacopa monnieri* extract improved behavioral measures and dopamine levels in a mouse model of PD, exhibiting both neuroprotective and neurorescue effects (Singh et al., 2021). Although more research is required to validate its effectiveness, a pilot clinical investigation indicated that *Bacopa monnieri* may help PD patients with their emotional function (Santos et al., 2023). Other herbs, such as *Ginkgo biloba,* have also been researched for possible PD benefits (Srivastav et al., 2017).

The potential health advantages of turmeric and its primary ingredient, curcumin, have been thoroughly investigated, especially in neurological illnesses. Curcumin has been shown to have neuroprotective, antioxidant, and antiinflammatory qualities (Abbas et al., 2020; Lopresti, 2017). According to in vitro research, pretreatment with curcumin may shield LRRK2-mutant PD cells from mitochondrial damage (Abrahams et al., 2021). Curcumin therapy alleviated behavioral changes, decreased oxidative damage, and increased mitochondrial enzyme complex activity in a mouse model of PD (Khatri & Juvekar, 2016). According toAbbas et al. (2020), these qualities make it a viable option for the treatment of neurodegenerative illnesses including Parkinson and Alzheimer.

Furthermore, Chinese herbal remedies with neuroprotective properties, such as *Uncaria rhynchophylla* and *Gastrodia elata,* are among the most widely utilized herbs for PD in Taiwan (Lin et al., 2021). According to Zeng (2017), Chinese herbal remedies can lessen dyskinesia, decrease the need for dopaminergic medications, and alleviate symptoms while slowing the course of PD. However, there are still issues with guaranteeing the safety, consistency, and bioavailability of herbal substances, especially when used with traditional PD drugs (Lin et al., 2021; Zeng, 2017).

Traditional treatments for PD are being supplemented with alternative therapies, which are gaining popularity. Tai Chi and dancing are examples of mind-body therapies that have been demonstrated to improve motor function and lessen impairment (Bega & Zadikoff, 2014). To manage nonmotor symptoms, acupuncture, cognitive therapy, and traditional Chinese medicine are being investigated; nevertheless, more high-quality randomized controlled studies are required (Liu & Wang, 2024). The potential of complementary treatments, such as yoga and cannabis, to reduce both motor and nonmotor symptoms is being investigated (Deuel & Seeberger, 2020). Tai Chi and yoga are beneficial for people with PD and stroke in recent research. Both yoga and Tai Chi helped PD patients with their postural stability, functional mobility, and balance (Gao et al., 2014; Khuzema et al., 2020; Van Puymbroeck et al., 2018). In PD patients, Tai Chi successfully lowered fall risk and occurrence (Gao et al., 2014). Although its benefits on balance, walking ability, and depression were not definitive, Tai Chi improved motor function and independence for stroke patients (García-Muñoz et al., 2023). According to Khuzema et al. (2020), home-based Tai Chi and yoga programs were discovered to be appealing and well-adhered solutions for PD patients. Even though these alternate methods seem promising, further study is needed to determine their safety and effectiveness in the treatment of PD.

Dance therapy and music therapy have become popular supplementary therapies for PD. Music therapy has been shown to improve movement fluidity and gait patterns in people with PD by providing rhythmic auditory stimulation (Ashoori et al., 2015; Pereira et al., 2019). According toMeulenberg et al. (2023), dance therapy has been shown to improve motor coordination and lessen stiffness, especially when it comes to Argentine tango. Beyond traditional rehabilitation activities, these treatments provide functional benefits by fostering neuroplasticity and stimulating sensory-motor integration (Meulenberg et al., 2023). Additionally, PD patients' quality of life, communication, cognitive abilities, and motor symptoms can all be enhanced by music and dance therapy (Machado Sotomayor et al., 2021). These affordable, noninvasive treatments have the potential to treat both motor and nonmotor symptoms of PD, even if the precise processes are still being studied (Machado Sotomayor et al., 2021; Pereira et al., 2019).

Patients with PD frequently employ massage treatment and other alternative therapies to reduce their symptoms. Numerous massage approaches can enhance quality of life and lessen motor and nonmotor symptoms in people with PD, according to a systematic review study (Angelopoulou et al., 2020). Anma massage was shown to significantly enhance motor function, discomfort, tiredness, stiffness, and difficulty moving following both one-time and ongoing sessions (Donoyama et al., 2014). A significant percentage of PD patients claim that complementary treatments, including massage, yoga, and meditation, are useful for both motor and nonmotor symptoms (Donley et al., 2019).

Ayurveda and other traditional medicine systems have long been used to treat PD. Herbal remedies, dietary adjustments, and lifestyle adjustments are all part of Ayurvedic practices (Pathak- Gandhi & Vaidya, 2017). According toBorah et al. (2017) and Quasmi et al. (2024), medicinal herbs including *Curcuma longa, Withania somnifera*, and *Mucuna pruriens* have demonstrated potential in the treatment of PD. Antioxidant-rich substances found in these plants may help treat oxidative stress in PD (Quasmi et al., 2024). *Panchakarma* and other Ayurvedic therapies have also been investigated for possible advantages (Pathak- Gandhi & Vaidya, 2017). Tai Chi and dancing are examples of mind-body therapies that have proven to be safe and effective in the treatment of PD (Bega & Zadikoff, 2014). However, many complementary and alternative treatments for PD still lack adequate clinical evidence, despite the Eastern countries' long history and extensive use of traditional medicines. This underscores the need for more thorough research to confirm the effectiveness of these treatments (Bega & Zadikoff, 2014).

Globally, traditional medical systems aid in the treatment of PD. In Japan, herbal remedies such as Yokukansan are used to treat PD symptoms in Kampo medicine, which is based on Traditional Chinese Medicine (Bega & Zadikoff, 2014). Yokukansan has demonstrated effectiveness in treating PD patients' cognitive deficits, sleep issues, and behavioral and psychological problems (Jang et al., 2018). By controlling neurotransmitters and cellular processes, it could also have neuroprotective benefits (Jang et al., 2018; Okamoto et al., 2014). Though there is no scientific proof, traditional African herbal treatments for neurological disorders have been derived from plants including *Kigelia africana* and *Mondia whitei* (Srivastav et al., 2017). Similarly, traditional healers in South America use botanicals from the Amazonian that may have neuroprotective qualities, but they have not yet been well studied in clinical settings (Srivastav et al., 2017). Even though complementary and alternative medicine is widely used to treat PD, more thorough clinical research is required to develop evidence-based recommendations for various therapies (Bega & Zadikoff, 2014).

3.9 Socioeconomic and political challenges

In the sub-Sahara Africa (SSA) region, the population of those with PD is known to be relatively small (Akinyemi, 2012). This low prevalence may possibly stem from several issues such as:

- the relatively youthful population in SSA, of less than 5% of the total population being above 65 years;
- the assumption that neurological diseases are part of normal aging; and
- the scarcity of epidemiological studies in SSA

This sparsity of epidemiological information on PD in SSA arises from the paucity of PD prevalence studies (most from several decades ago) as well as the absence of community-based incidence studies (Quarshie et al., 2021; Williams et al., 2018). This is quite challenging given that the causative factors in PD (mostly gene and the environment) can be quite heterogenous and this heterogeneity often dictates the kind of care, treatment, quality of life, outcome, and inadvertently, social impact across different cultures (Fothergill-Misbah, 2023).

Also, it is important to note that epidemiological patterns hugely depend on the rate of disease detection, which in turn is dependent on diagnostic factors and the accuracy of diagnosis in the general population (Dekker et al., 2020). Thus, in PD, the first and foremost infrastuctural and personnel challenge is the availability of neurological and auxillary services in the medical centers in Africa. In a few instances where these centers are found, accessibility to such services by the general population is greatly limited mostly due to significant financial constraints as well as the sociocultural perception of the disease (Bower & Zenebe, 2005). In many SSA countries, there are preconceived beliefs and misconceptions that exist among the communities about neurological conditions (Mokaya et al., 2017). Accusations of witchcraft, presumed mental illness, and even guilt all attribute to the stigmatization of the patients, ultimately contributing to the delay or prevention of the correct diagnosis or access to appropriate treatment for PD sufferers (Mokaya et al., 2017).

Tackling the major regional challenges and obstacles to PD pharmacotherapy mostly border on the recognition of these issues as follows:

- **Lack of awareness and wrong perception of the disease:** On the lack of awareness, the use of local languages and the media can be used to create awareness campaigns, and culture specific educational materials as well as disseminate information aimed at improving awareness in the populations and encourage them to seek care earlier than they currently do. According to Komolafe et al. (2020), quiz competitions, arts and cultural events among school learners can help to raise awareness on neurological disorders. PD support groups and clubs as well as organization of community-based rehabilitation can also help in the care of patients living in rural communities.
- **Dearth of neurological and ancillary services to provide healthcare for PD patients:** this is due to limited training facilities as well as the widespread emigration of skilled personnel to more economically developed countries. The paucity of health personnel, the training of multidisciplinary teams involved in the management of the disease should be strongly encouraged and adequately remunerated. On the nonavailability and unaffordability of drugs, a multisectorial approach involving governments, pharmaceutical organizations, and other key stakeholders is necessary. In addition, the enrollment of patients in health insurance programmes, increased access to neuroimaging, as well as the incorporation of PD care into health insurance systems will greatly impact the management of the disease (Okubadejo et al., 2019). Finally, it is important to buttress the need for a holistic approach in tackling the myriads of sociocultural challenges involved in the pharmacotherapy of PD in SSA. It is only through this approach that the huge disparity in the management of the disease in our region can be bridged and brought to par with that of the developed world.

3.10 Future directions and recommendations

Across cultural and regional landscapes there are challenges posed by PD and there is a need to address those challenges using multifactorial approaches, that is, advocating for equitable drug distribution, integration of cultural considerations into clinical guidelines, and active participation of consortia like the AfrAbia PD Genomic Consortium to mitigate disparities.

3.10.1 Advocacy for equitable drug distribution

Equitable drug distribution is important in addressing the disparities in PD treatment, particularly in low and middle—income countries (LMIC) where access to neurological care and essential medicines is limited (Okubadejo et al., 2019). The main factors affecting the disparities are because these essential neurological medications are unavailable and unaffordable across various regions of the Africa continent, this has led to delay in treatments and management of the diseases. To look into these disparities, it is imperative to advocate for policies that ensure the availability of affordable PD medications. Collaborative efforts between governments, nongovernmental organizations, and pharmaceutical companies can facilitate the introduction of strengthening health and social systems through the promotion of care models that are welcomed by the community's culture and socioeconomic reality and also creating systems of services that are affordable, accessible, and supports affected patients throughout their health journey (Schiess et al., 2022).

3.10.2 Integration of cultural considerations into clinical guidelines

Cultural beliefs and practices significantly influence patients' perceptions of PD and their adherence to prescribed treatments. In many diverse communities, traditional medicine plays a pivotal role in healthcare system. A study by Siddiqi & Koemeter-Cox, 2021, revealed that promoting diversity, equity, and inclusion in Parkinson care is crucial to addressing disparities and improving outcomes for all patients (Siddiqi & Koemeter-Cox, 2021). The outstanding factors for inclusion of cultural consideration in PD clinical guidelines should address variation in genetic and ethnic disposition to disease presentation and medication response, clinical studies that include diverse population, integration of indigenous medicine (Lau et al., 2022; Park et al., 2023; Wang et al., 2022), and others like social belief, stigmatization and care giver support system. The evaluation of the efficacy of indigenous in managing PD symptoms reveal that there were significant improvement indicating better symptom management compared to conventional Western medicine alone. Additionally, patients treated with indigenous medicine reported enhanced **quality of life** and experienced **fewer adverse reactions** than those receiving western medicine alone, highlighting both the clinical effectiveness and safety benefits of Indigeneous medicine in PD treatment. Inclusion of some population especially black minority is low in clinical studies, it is therefore imperative to incorporate diverse ethnic groups to generate data that reflects the broader population especially the underrepresented in PD research and clinical guidelines.

3.10.3 Role of consortia in addressing disparities (AfrAbia PD genomic consortium)

The AfrAbia PD Genomic Consortium (AAPDGC) is part of the **Global Parkinson Genetics Program (GP2)**, formed to address issues around underrepresentation of African and Arab populations in PD research. The AAPDGC aims at three major issues which include capacity building, genetics research and policy advocacy all in a bid to promote international collaborations and reduce health disparities across African and Arab populations (Mohamed, 2023). This will be achieved by mapping out the genetic loci associated with PD in diverse populations, which can lead to a more precise and effective treatments. The inclusion of a broader range of genetic backgrounds, will help the consortium to improve on its genetic research and development of therapeutic intervention geared toward individuals (Mohamed et al., 2024).

3.11 Conclusion

Parkinson disease, is a global prevalent neurodegenerative disorder best managed via pharmacotherapy, however effectiveness of pharmacotherapy in PD is influenced by various cultural and regional factors which creates disparities in treatment outcomes across diverse populations. By addressing these cultural and regional barriers in PD pharmacological interventions, healthcare providers can enhance the effectiveness of PD pharmacotherapy and improve the quality of life for individuals with PD across diverse populations.

References

Abbas, S., Latif, M.S., Shafie, N.S., Ghazali, M.I., Kormin, F., 2020. Neuroprotective expression of turmeric and curcumin. Food Research 4 (6), 2366–2381. https://doi.org/10.26656/fr.2017.4(6).363.

AboJabel, H., Argavan, E., Hassin-Baer, S., Inzelberg, R., Werner, P., 2021. Exploring the perceptions and stigmatizing experiences of Israeli family caregivers of people with Parkinson's disease. Journal of Aging Studies 56, 100910. https://doi.org/10.1016/j.jaging.2020.100910.

Abrahams, S., Miller, H.C., Lombard, C., van der Westhuizen, F.H., Bardien, S., 2021. Curcumin pre-treatment may protect against mitochondrial damage in LRRK2-mutant Parkinson's disease and healthy control fibroblasts. Biochemistry and Biophysics Reports 27. https://doi.org/10.1016/j.bbrep.2021.101035.

Achen, B., Chambi, C.T., Bruno, V., 2023. P. 022 Cross-cultural experiences and expectations from caregivers of people living with Parkinson's disease: A comprehensive review. Canadian Journal of Neurological Sciences 50 (s2), S63.

Akinyemi, R.O., 2012. Epidemiology of Parkinsonism and Parkinson's disease in Sub-Saharan Africa: Nigerian profile. Journal of Neurosciences in Rural Practice 3, 233–234. https://doi.org/10.4103/0976-3147.102586.

Al-Eitan, L., Tarkhan, H.A., 2016. Practical challenges and translational issues in pharmacogenomics and personalized medicine from 2010 onwards. Current Pharmacogenomics and Personalized Medicine 14 (1), 7–17.

Alam, M., Abbas, K., Mustafa, M., Usmani, N., Habib, S., 2024. Microbiome-based therapies for Parkinson's disease. Frontiers in Nutrition 11. https://doi.org/10.3389/fnut.2024.1496616.

Algarni, M.A., Stoessl, A.J., 2016. The role of biomarkers and imaging in Parkinson's disease. Expert Review of Neurotherapeutics 16 (2), 187–203. https://doi.org/10.1586/14737175.2016.1135056.

Angelopoulou, E., Anagnostouli, M., Chrousos, G.P., Bougea, A., 2020. Massage therapy as a complementary treatment for Parkinson's disease: A systematic literature review. Complementary Therapies in Medicine 49. https://doi.org/10.1016/j.ctim.2020.102340.

Anwar, L., Ahmad, E., Imtiaz, M., Ahmad, M., Aziz, M.F., ibad, T., 2024. The impact of diet on Parkinson's disease: A systematic review. Cureus 16 (9). https://doi.org/10.7759/cureus.70337.

Aravindan, A., Newell, M.E., Halden, R.U., 2024. Literature review and meta-analysis of environmental toxins associated with increased risk of Parkinson's disease. Science of the Total Environment 931, 172838. https://doi.org/10.1016/j.scitotenv.2024.172838.

Ashoori, A., Eagleman, D.M., Jankovic, J., 2015. Effects of auditory rhythm and music on gait disturbances in Parkinson's disease. Frontiers in Neurology 6, 234.

Ayano, G., 2016. Parkinson's disease: A concise overview of etiology, epidemiology, diagnosis, comorbidity and management. Journal of Neurological Disorders. 4 (6).

Ball, N., Teo, W.P., Chandra, S., Chapman, J., 2019. Parkinson's disease and the environment. Frontiers in Neurology 10, 218. https://doi.org/10.3389/fneur.2019.00218.

Bega, D., Zadikoff, C., 2014. Complementary &alternative management of Parkinson's disease: An evidence-based review of eastern influenced practices. Journal of Movement Disorders 7 (2), 57–66. https://doi.org/10.14802/jmd.14009.

Belle, D.J., Singh, H., 2008. Genetic factors in drug metabolism. American Family Physician 77 (11), 1553–1560.

Ben-Shlomo, Y., Darweesh, S., Llibre-Guerra, J., Marras, C., San Luciano, M., Tanner, C., 2024. The epidemiology of Parkinson's disease. Lancet (London, England) 403 (10423), 283–292. https://doi.org/10.1016/S0140-6736(23)01419-8.

Binde, C.D., Tvete, I.F., Gåsemyr, J.I., Natvig, B., Klemp, M., 2020. Comparative effectiveness of dopamine agonists and monoamine oxidase type-B inhibitors for Parkinson's disease: A multiple treatment comparison meta-analysis. European Journal of Clinical Pharmacology 76 (12), 1731–1743.

Bisaglia, M., 2023. Mediterranean diet and Parkinson's disease. International Journal of Molecular Sciences 24 (1), 42. https://doi.org/10.3390/ijms24010042.

Blesa, J., Przedborski, S., 2014. Parkinson's disease: Animal models and dopaminergic cell vulnerability. Frontiers in Neuroanatomy 8. https://doi.org/10.3389/fnana.2014.00155.

Borah, A., Choudhury, A., Paul, R., Mazumder, M.K., Chetia, S., 2017. Neuroprotective effect of ayurvedic preparations and natural products on Parkinson's disease neuroprotective natural products: Clinical aspects and mode of action. Wiley Blackwell, India. https://doi.org/10.1002/9783527803781.ch5.

Botello-Villagrana, F., Martinez-Ramirez, D., 2022. Mucuna pruriens as adjunct therapy to levodopa in advanced Parkinson's disease. Revista Mexicana de Neurociencia 22 (5). https://doi.org/10.24875/rmn.21000010.

Bower, J.H., Zenebe, G., 2005. Neurologic services in the nations of Africa. Neurology 64, 412–415.

Branson, C.O., Ferree, A., Hohler, A.D., Saint-Hilaire, M.-H., 2016. Racial disparities in Parkinson disease: A systematic review of the literature. Advances in Parkinson's Disease 5 (4), 87–96. https://doi.org/10.4236/apd.2016.54011.

Bu, L.L., Yang, K., Xiong, W.X., Liu, F.T., Anderson, B., Wang, Y., Wang, J., 2016. Toward precision medicine in Parkinson's disease. Annals of Translational Medicine 4 (2).

Camargo, S.M.R., Vuille-Dit-Bille, R.N., Mariotta, L., Ramadan, T., Huggel, K., Singer, D., Götze, O., Verrey, F., 2014. The molecular mechanism of intestinal levodopa absorption and its possible implications for the treatment of Parkinson's disease. Journal of Pharmacology and Experimental Therapeutics 351 (1), 114–123. https://doi.org/10.1124/jpet.114.216317.

Chen, J., Xu, J., Huang, P., Luo, Y., Shi, Y., Ma, P., 2022. The potential applications of traditional Chinese medicine in Parkinson's disease: A new opportunity. Biomedicine & Pharmacotherapy 149, 112866. https://doi.org/10.1016/j.biopha.2022.112866.

Contin, M., Martinelli, P., Mochi, M., Riva, R., Albani, F., Baruzzi, A., 2005. Genetic polymorphism of catechol-O-methyltransferase and levodopa pharmacokinetic-pharmacodynamic pattern in patients with Parkinson's disease. Movement Disorders 20, 734–739.

Contributions of gut bacteria and diet to drug pharmacokinetics in the treatment of Parkinson's disease. Frontiers in Neurology 10, 2019, 1087.

Crooks, S., Mitchell, G., Wynne, L., Carter, G., 2025. Exploring the stigma experienced by people affected by Parkinson's disease: A systematic review. BMC Public Health 25. https://doi.org/10.1186/s12889-024-21236-8.

de Queiroz Cavalcanti, S.A., de Almeida, L.A., Gasparotto, J., 2023. Effects of a high saturated fatty acid diet on the intestinal microbiota modification and associated impacts on Parkinson's disease development. Journal of Neuroimmunology 382, 578171.

Dekker, M.C.J., Coulibaly, T., Bardien, S., Ross, O.A., Carr, J., Komolafe, M., 2020. Parkinson's disease research on the African continent: Obstacles and opportunities. Frontiers in Neurology 11, 512. https://doi.org/10.3389/fneur.2020.00512.

Deliz, J.R., Tanner, C.M., Gonzalez-Latapi, P., 2024. Epidemiology of Parkinson's disease: An update. Current Neurology and Neuroscience Reports 24 (6), 163–179. https://doi.org/10.1007/s11910-024-01339-wm.

DeMaagd, G., Philip, A., 2015. Parkinson's disease and its management. Pharmacy and Therapeutics 40 (8), 504–532.

Deuel, L.M., Seeberger, L.C., 2020. Complementary therapies in Parkinson disease: A review of acupuncture, Tai Chi, Qi Gong, yoga, and Cannabis. Neurotherapeutics 17 (4), 1434–1455. https://doi.org/10.1007/s13311-020-00900-y.

Devos, D., Moreau, C., Devedjian, J.C., Kluza, J., Petrault, M., Laloux, C., Jonneaux, A., Ryckewaert, G., Garçon, G., Rouaix, N., Duhamel, A., Jissendi, P., Dujardin, K., Auger, F., Ravasi, L., Hopes, L., Grolez, G., Firdaus, W., Sablonnière, B., Strubi-Vuillaume, I., Zahr, N., Destée, A., Corvol, J.C., Pöltl, D., Leist, M., Rose, C., Defebvre, L., Marchetti, P., Cabantchik, Z.I., Bordet, R., 2014. Targeting chelatable iron as a therapeutic modality in Parkinson's disease. Antioxidants and Redox Signaling 21 (2), 195–210. https://doi.org/10.1089/ars.2013.5593.

Dong, J., Cui, Y., Song, L., Le, W., 2016. Current pharmaceutical treatments and alternative therapies of Parkinson's disease. Current Neuropharmacology 14 (4), 339–355. https://doi.org/10.2174/1570159X14666151120123025.

Donley, S., McGregor, S., Wielinski, C., Nance, M., 2019. Use and perceived effectiveness of complementary therapies in Parkinson's disease. Parkinsonism & Related Disorders 58, 46–49. https://doi.org/10.1016/j.parkreldis.2018.08.003.

Donoyama, N., Suoh, S., Ohkoshi, N., 2014. Effectiveness of Anma massage therapy in alleviating physical symptoms in outpatients with Parkinson's disease: A before-after study. Complementary Therapies in Clinical Practice 20 (4), 251–261.

Dulski, J., Ross, O.A., Wszolek, Z.K., 2024. Genetics of Parkinson's disease: State-of-the-art and role in clinical settings. Neurologia I Neurochirurgia Polska 58 (1), 38–46.

Dutta, S.K., Verma, S., Jain, V., Surapaneni, B.K., Vinayek, R., Phillips, L., Nair, P.P., 2019. Parkinson's disease: The emerging role of gut dysbiosis, antibiotics, probiotics, and fecal microbiota transplantation. Journal of Neurogastroenterology and Motility 25 (3), 363–376. https://doi.org/10.5056/jnm19044.

Elmorsy, E., Al-Ghafari, A., Al Doghaither, H., Hashish, S., Salama, M., Mudyanselage, A.W., Carter, W.G., 2023. Differential effects of Paraquat, Rotenone, and MPTP on cellular bioenergetics of undifferentiated and differentiated human neuroblastoma cells. Brain Sciences 13 (12), 1717.

Fagan, E.S., Pihlstrøm, L., 2017. Genetic risk factors for cognitive decline in Parkinson's disease: A review of the literature. European Journal of Neurology 24 (4), 561. https://doi.org/10.1111/ene.13258.

Fodor, A., Karnieli, E., 2016. Challenges of implementing personalized (precision) medicine: A focus on diabetes. Personalized Medicine 13 (5), 485–497. https://doi.org/10.2217/pme-2016-0022.

Foo, J.N., Chew, E.G., Chung, S.J., Peng, R., Blauwendraat, C., Nalls, M.A., Mok, K.Y., Satake, W., Toda, T., Chao, Y., Tan, L.C., 2020. Identification of risk loci for Parkinson disease in Asians and comparison of risk between Asians and Europeans: A genome-wide association study. JAMA Neurology 77 (6), 746–754.

Fothergill-Misbah, N., 2023. The lived experience of stigma and Parkinson's disease in Kenya: A public health challenge. BMC Public Health 23 (1), 364. https://doi.org/10.1186/s12889-023-15278-7.

Fothergill-Misbah, N., Maroo, H., Cham, M., Pezzoli, G., Walker, R., Cilia, R., 2020. Could Mucuna pruriens be the answer to Parkinson's disease management in sub-Saharan Africa and other low-income countries worldwide? Parkinsonism & Related Disorders 73, 3–7.

Franco, G.A., Interdonato, L., Cordaro, M., Cuzzocrea, S., Di Paola, R., 2023. Bioactive compounds of the mediterranean diet as nutritional support to fight neurodegenerative disease. International Journal of Molecular Sciences 24 (8), 7318. https://doi.org/10.3390/ijms24087318.

Gao, Q., Leung, A., Yang, Y., Wei, Q., Guan, M., Jia, C., He, C., 2014. Effects of Tai Chi on balance and fall prevention in Parkinson's disease: A randomized controlled trial. Clinical Rehabilitation 28 (8), 748–753. https://doi.org/10.1177/0269215514521044.

García-Muñoz, C., González-García, P., Casuso-Holgado, M.J., Martínez-Calderón, J., Heredia-Rizo, A.M., 2023. Are movement-based mindful exercises (QIGONG, TAI CHI, AND YOGA) beneficial for stroke and Parkinson's disease? A scoping review. Complementary Therapies in Medicine 72, 102912.

Gardener, H., Caunca, M.R., 2018. Mediterranean diet in preventing neurodegenerative diseases. Current Nutrition Reports 7, 10–20.

GBD 2016 Neurology Collaborators, 2019. Global, regional, and national burden of neurological disorders, 1990-2016: A systematic analysis for the global burden of disease study 2016. The Lancet Neurology 18 (5), 459–480. https://doi.org/10.1016/S1474-4422(18)30499-X.

Gil, G., Tosin, M.H.S., Ferraz, H.B., 2024. The impact of the socioeconomic factor on Parkinson's disease medication adherence: a scoping review. O impacto do fator socioeconômico na adesão à medicação na doença de Parkinson: uma revisão de escopo. Arquivos de neuro-psiquiatria 82 (2), 1–8. https://doi.org/10.1055/s-0044-1779608.

Giladi, N., Mirelman, A., Thaler, A., Orr-Urtreger, A., 2016. A personalized approach to Parkinson's disease patients based on founder mutation analysis. Frontiers in Neurology 7. https://doi.org/10.3389/fneur.2016.00071.

Goyal, A., Gopika, S., Kumar, A., Garabadu, D., 2022. A comprehensive review on preclinical evidence-based neuroprotective potential of Bacopa monnieri against Parkinson's disease. Current Drug Targets 23 (9), 889–901. https://doi.org/10.2174/1389450123666220316091734.

Goyal, A., Verma, A., Agrawal, N., 2021. Dietary phytoestrogens: Neuroprotective role in Parkinson's disease. Current Neurovascular Research 18 (2), 254–267.

Guebila, M.B., Thiele, I., 2016. Model-based dietary optimization for late-stage, levodopa-treated, Parkinson's disease patients. NPJ Systems Biology and Applications 2. https://doi.org/10.1038/npjsba.2016.13.

Haas, J., Berg, D., Bosy-Westphal, A., Schaeffer, E., 2022. Parkinson's disease and sugar intake—reasons for and consequences of a still unclear craving. Nutrients 14 (15), 3240. https://doi.org/10.3390/nu14153240.

Hamood, H.M., Alsaedi, M.A.Z., Al-Qrimli, A.F., Jawad, A.Q., 2024. Parkinson disease pharmacological and herbal management: A review. South Asian Research Journal of Applied Medical Sciences 6 (01), 1–9. https://doi.org/10.36346/sarjams.2024.v06i01.001.

Helley, M.P., Pinnell, J., Sportelli, C., Tieu, K., 2017. Mitochondria: A common target for genetic mutations and environmental toxicants in Parkinson's disease. Frontiers in Genetics 8. https://doi.org/10.3389/fgene.2017.00177.

Henry, R.S., Perrin, P.B., Lageman, S.K., Villaseñor, T., Cariello, A.N., Pugh, M., Smith, E.R., Arroyo, M., Zarate, A., Avila, J., Soto-Escageda, J.A., 2021. Parkinson's symptoms and caregiver affiliate stigma: A multinational study. Current Alzheimer Research 18 (3), 222–231. https://doi.org/10.2174/1567205018666210608100917.

Hernandez, D.G., Reed, X., Singleton, A.B., 2016. Genetics in Parkinson disease: Mendelian versus non-mendelian inheritance. Journal of Neurochemistry 139, 59–74.

Hughes, C.M., 2004. Medication non-adherence in the elderly: How big is the problem? Drugs & Aging 21 (12), 793–811. https://doi.org/10.2165/00002512-200421120-00004.

James, D., Smith, J., Lane, E., Thomas, R., Brown, S., Seage, H., 2024. Adherence to Parkinson's disease medication: A case study to illustrate reasons for non-adherence, implications for practice and engaging under-represented participants in research. Exploratory Research in Clinical and Social Pharmacy 14, 100450. https://doi.org/10.1016/j.rcsop.2024.100450.

Jang, J.H., Jung, K., Kim, J.S., Jung, I., Yoo, H., Moon, C., 2018. Potential application of Yokukansan as a remedy for Parkinson's disease. Evidence-Based Complementary and Alternative Medicine 2018. https://doi.org/10.1155/2018/1875928.

Jang, C.H., Oh, J., Lim, J.S., Kim, H.J., Kim, J.S., 2021. Fermented soy products: Beneficial potential in neurodegenerative diseases. Foods 10 (3). https://doi.org/10.3390/foods10030636.

Jones, S., Torsney, K.M., Scourfield, L., Berryman, K., Henderson, E.J., 2020. Neuropsychiatric symptoms in Parkinson's disease: Aetiology, diagnosis and treatment. BJPsych Advances 26 (6), 333–342. https://doi.org/10.1192/bja.2019.79.

Joppi, R., Bertele, V., Vannini, T., Garattini, S., Banzi, R., 2020. Food and Drug Administration vs European Medicines Agency: Review times and clinical evidence on novel drugs at the time of approval. British Journal of Clinical Pharmacology 86 (1), 170–174. https://doi.org/10.1111/bcp.14130.

Joshi, N., Singh, S., 2018. Updates on immunity and inflammation in Parkinson disease pathology. Journal of Neuroscience Research 96 (3), 379–390. https://doi.org/10.1002/jnr.24185.

Karacan, A.V., Kibrit, S.N., Yekedüz, M.K., Doğulu, N., Kayis, G., Unutmaz, E.Y., Abali, T., Eminoğlu, F.T., Akbostancı, M.C., Yilmaz, R., 2023. Cross-cultural differences in stigma associated with Parkinson's disease: A systematic review. Journal of Parkinson's Disease 13 (5), 699–715. https://doi.org/10.3233/JPD-230050.

Karamperis, K., Katz, S., Melograna, F., Ganau, F.P., Van Steen, K., Patrinos, G.P., Lao, O., 2024. Genetic ancestry in population pharmacogenomics unravels distinct geographical patterns related to drug toxicity. iScience 27 (10).

Kashala-Abotnes, E., Okitundu, D., Mumba, D., Boivin, M.J., Tylleskär, T., Tshala-Katumbay, D., 2019. Konzo: A distinct neurological disease associated with food (cassava) cyanogenic poisoning. Brain Research Bulletin 145, 87–91. https://doi.org/10.1016/j.brainresbull.2018.07.001.

Kerac, M., Postels, D.G., Mallewa, M., Alusine Jalloh, A., Voskuijl, W.P., Groce, N., Gladstone, M., Molyneux, E., 2014. The interaction of malnutrition and neurologic disability in Africa. Seminars in Pediatric Neurology 21 (1), 42–49. https://doi.org/10.1016/j.spen.2014.01.003.

Keun, J.T.B., Arnoldussen, I.A., Vriend, C., van de Rest, O., 2021. Dietary approaches to improve efficacy and control side effects of levodopa therapy in Parkinson's disease: A systematic review. Advances in Nutrition 12 (6), 2265–2287.

Khatri, D.K., Juvekar, A.R., 2016. Neuroprotective effect of curcumin as evinced by abrogation of rotenone-induced motor deficits, oxidative and mitochondrial dysfunctions in mouse model of Parkinson's disease. Pharmacology Biochemistry and Behavior 150–151, 39–47. https://doi.org/10.1016/j.pbb.2016.09.002.

Khuzema, A., Brammatha, A., Arul Selvan, V., 2020. Effect of home-based Tai Chi, yoga or conventional balance exercise on functional balance and mobility among persons with idiopathic Parkinson's disease: An experimental study. Hong Kong Physiotherapy Journal 40 (01), 39–49.

Kim, J.J., Vitale, D., Otani, D.V., Lian, M.M., Heilbron, K., Iwaki, H., Lake, J., Solsberg, C.W., Leonard, H., Makarious, M.B., 2024. Multi-ancestry genome-wide association meta-analysis of Parkinson's disease. Nature Genetics 56 (1), 27–36.

Knight, E., Geetha, T., Burnett, D., Ramesh Babu, J., 2022. The role of diet and dietary patterns in Parkinson's disease. Nutrients 14 (21), 4472. https://doi.org/10.3390/nu14214472.

Knowles, L., Luth, W., Bubela, T., 2017. Paving the road to personalized medicine: Recommendations on regulatory, intellectual property and reimbursement challenges. Journal of Law and the Biosciences 4 (3), 453–506.

Komolafe, M.A., Olorunmoteni, O.E., Fehintola, F.O., 2020. Effect of health education on level of awareness and knowledge of Nigerian in-school adolescents on stroke and its risk factors. Journal of Stroke and Cerebrovascular Diseases 29, 104757. https://doi.org/10.1016/j.jstrokecerebrovasdis.2020.104757.

Kouli, A., Torsney, K.M., Kuan, W.L., 2018. Parkinson's disease: Etiology, neuropathology, and pathogenesis. Exon Publications.

Kumari, N., Anand, S., Shah, K., Chauhan, N.S., Sethiya, N.K., Singhal, M., 2023. Emerging role of plant-based bioactive compounds as therapeutics in Parkinson's disease. Molecules 28 (22), 7588. https://doi.org/10.3390/molecules28227588.

Kwon, E.H., Tennagels, S., Gold, R., Gerwert, K., Beyer, L., Tönges, L., 2022. Update on CSF biomarkers in Parkinson's disease. Biomolecules 12 (2), 329. https://doi.org/10.3390/biom12020329.

Lau, Y.H., Podlewska, A., Ocloo, J., et al., 2022. Does ethnicity influence recruitment into clinical trials of Parkinson's disease? Journal of Parkinson's Disease 12 (3), 975–981.

Li, X.-zhao, Zhang, S.-nan, Liu, S.-min, Lu, F., 2013. Recent advances in herbal medicines treating Parkinson's disease. Fitoterapia 84 (1), 273–285. https://doi.org/10.1016/j.fitote.2012.12.009.

Lin, C.H., Chiu, H.E., Wu, S.Y., Tseng, S.T., Wu, T.C., Hung, Y.C., Hsu, C.Y., Chen, H.J., Hsu, S.F., Kuo, C.E., Hu, W.L., 2021. Chinese herbal products for non-motor symptoms of Parkinson's disease in Taiwan: A population-based study. Frontiers in Pharmacology 11. https://doi.org/10.3389/fphar.2020.615657.

Liu, H., Wang, X.P., 2024. Alternative therapies for non-motor symptoms in Parkinson's disease: A mini review. Neuropsychiatric Disease and Treatment 2585–2591.

Lopresti, A.L., 2017. Curcumin for neuropsychiatric disorders: A review of in vitro, animal and human studies. Journal of Psychopharmacology 31 (3), 287–302. https://doi.org/10.1177/0269881116686883.

Machado Sotomayor, M.J., Arufe-Giráldez, V., Ruíz-Rico, G., Navarro-Patón, R., 2021. Music therapy and parkinson's disease: A systematic review from 2015–2020. International Journal of Environmental Research and Public Health 18 (21), 11618. https://doi.org/10.3390/ijerph182111618.

Maffoni, M., Giardini, A., Pierobon, A., Ferrazzoli, D., Frazzitta, G., 2017. Stigma experienced by Parkinson's disease patients: A descriptive review of qualitative studies. Parkinson's Disease 2017, 1–7. https://doi.org/10.1155/2017/7203259.

McDaniels, B., Pontone, G.M., Mathur, S., Subramanian, I., 2023. Staying hidden: The burden of stigma in PD. Parkinsonism & Related Disorders 116, 105838. https://doi.org/10.1016/j.parkreldis.2023.105838.

Meulenberg, C.J.W., Rehfeld, K., Jovanović, S., Marusic, U., 2023. Unleashing the potential of dance: A neuroplasticity-based approach bridging from older adults to Parkinson's disease patients. Frontiers in Aging Neuroscience 15. https://doi.org/10.3389/fnagi.2023.1188855.

Michel, P.P., Hirsch, E.C., Hunot, S., 2016. Understanding dopaminergic cell death pathways in Parkinson disease. Neuron 90 (4), 675–691.

Minchev, D., Kazakova, M., Sarafian, V., 2022. Neuroinflammation and autophagy in Parkinson's disease—novel perspectives. International Journal of Molecular Sciences 23 (23), 14997.

Mirpour, S., Turkbey, E.B., Marashdeh, W., El Khouli, R., Subramaniam, R.M., 2018. Impact of DAT-SPECT on management of patients suspected of parkinsonism. Clinical Nuclear Medicine 43 (10), 710–714.

Misra, S.C., Bisui, S., 2014. Critical challenges for adopting personalized medicine system in healthcare management: Perspectives of clinicians and patients. International Journal of E-Health and Medical Communications 5 (2), 70–89. https://doi.org/10.4018/ijehmc.2014040104.

Mohamed, W., 2023. Parkinson's genetics research on underrepresented AfrAbia populations: Current state and future prospects. American Journal of Neurodegenerative Disease 12 (2), 23–41.

Mohamed, W., Eltantawi, M.A., Mecheri, Y., Zewde, Y.Z., Kamel, W.A., Al-Mubarak, B.R., Sassi, S.B., 2024. The AfrAbia+ plus Parkinson's disease genomic consortium. The Lancet Neurology 23 (2), 140–141.

Mokaya, J., Gray, W.K., Carr, J., 2017. Beliefs, knowledge and attitudes towards Parkinson's disease among a Xhosa speaking black population in South Africa: A cross-sectional study. Parkinsonism & Related Disorders 41, 51–57. https://doi.org/10.1016/j.parkreldis.2017.05.009.

Morris, H.R., Spillantini, M.G., Sue, C.M., Williams-Gray, C.H., 2024. The pathogenesis of Parkinson's disease. Lancet (London, England) 403 (10423), 293–304. https://doi.org/10.1016/S0140-6736(23)01478-2.

Navarro-Meza, M., Morales-Sánchez, E.W., Pacheco-Moisés, F., Ortiz, G.G., 2015. Hábitos alimentarios y factores sociodemográficos de pacientes con enfermedad de Parkinson en zonas rurales. Nutricion Hospitalaria 32 (6), 2783–2791. https://doi.org/10.3305/nh.2015.32.6.9742.

Niccolini, F., 2017. Imaging in Parkinson's Disease. Elsevier.

Nissar, S., Aga, S.S., Banday, M.Z., Majid, S., 2022. Single nucleotide polymorphisms and Parkinson's disease susceptibility. In: Genetic polymorphism and disease. CRC Press, pp. 217–231.

Okamoto, H., Iyo, M., Ueda, K., Han, C., Hirasaki, Y., Namiki, T., 2014. Yokukan-san: A review of the evidence for use of this Kampo herbal formula in dementia and psychiatric conditions. Neuropsychiatric Disease and Treatment 10, 1727–1742. https://doi.org/10.2147/NDT.S65257.

Okubadejo, N.U., Ojo, O.O., Wahab, K.W., Abubakar, S.A., Obiabo, O.Y., Salawu, F.K., Oshinaike, O.O., 2019. A nationwide survey of Parkinson's disease medicines availability and affordability in Nigeria. Movement Disorders Clinical Practice 16, 27–33. https://doi.org/10.1002/mdc3.12682.

Oluwole, O.B., Nicholas-Okpara, V.A.N., Gloria, E., Ibekwe, D., Eboagwu, I., Elemo, O., Adegboyega, M.O., 2021. Colorectal cancer in Africa: Causes, dietary inter-vention, and lifestyle change. International Journal of Nutrition 6, 21–34.

Osborne, J.A., Botkin, R., Colon-Semenza, C., DeAngelis, T.R., Gallardo, O.G., Kosakowski, H., Martello, J., Pradhan, S., Rafferty, M., Readinger, J.L., Whitt, A.L., 2022. Physical therapist management of Parkinson disease: A clinical practice guideline from the American physical Therapy Association. Physical Therapy 102 (4), pzab302.

Palavra, N.C., Lubomski, M., Flood, V.M., Davis, R.L., Sue, C.M., 2021. Increased added sugar consumption is common in Parkinson's disease. Frontiers in Nutrition 8. https://doi.org/10.3389/fnut.2021.628845.

Pang, S.Y.Y., Ho, P.W.L., Liu, H.F., Leung, C.T., Li, L., Chang, E.E.S., Ramsden, D.B., Ho, S.L., 2019. The interplay of aging, genetics and environmental factors in the pathogenesis of Parkinson's disease. Translational Neurodegeneration 8, 23. https://doi.org/10.1186/s40035-019-0165-9.

Panova, A.S., Dergachev, D.S., Subotyalov, M.A., Dergachev, V.D., 2020. Review of Mucuna pruriens L. therapeutic potential for Parkinson's disease. Meditsinskiy sovet = Medical Council 2020 (8), 82–87. https://doi.org/10.21518/2079-701x-2020-8-82-87.

Park, J.S., Davis, R.L., Sue, C.M., 2018. Mitochondrial dysfunction in Parkinson's disease: New mechanistic insights and therapeutic perspectives. Current Neurology and Neuroscience Reports 18, 1–11.

Park, K.W., Ryu, H.S., Shin, E., Park, Y., Jeon, S.R., Kim, S.Y., Chung, S.J., 2023. Ethnicity-and sex-specific genome wide association study on Parkinson's disease. NPJ Parkinson's Disease 9 (1), 141.

Pathak- Gandhi, N., Vaidya, A.D.B., 2017. Management of Parkinson's disease in ayurveda: Medicinal plants and adjuvant measures. Journal of Ethnopharmacology 197, 46–51. https://doi.org/10.1016/j.jep.2016.08.020.

Payami, H., 2017. The emerging science of precision medicine and pharmacogenomics for Parkinson's disease. Movement Disorders 32 (8), 1139–1146. https://doi.org/10.1002/mds.27099.

Pedrosa de Menezes, Bloem, B.R., Beckers, M., Piat, C., Benarroch, E.E., Savica, R., 2024. Molecular variability in Levodopa absorption and clinical implications for the management of Parkinson's disease. Journal of Parkinson's Disease 14 (7), 1353–1368.

Pereira, A.P.S., Marinho, V., Gupta, D., Magalhães, F., Ayres, C., Teixeira, S., 2019. Music therapy and dance as gait rehabilitation in patients with Parkinson disease: A review of evidence. Journal of Geriatric Psychiatry and Neurology 32 (1), 49–56. https://doi.org/10.1177/0891988718819858.

Polito, L., Greco, A., Seripa, D., 2016. Genetic profile, environmental exposure, and their interaction in Parkinson's disease. Parkinson's Disease 2016 (1), 6465793.

Quarshie, J.T., Mensah, E.N., Quaye, O., Aikins, A.R., 2021. The current state of Parkinsonism in West Africa: A systematic review. Parkinson's Disease 2021, 7479423.

Quasmi, M.N., Pooja, Kumar, S., 2024. Various herbal remedies for the management of Parkinson's disease: A review. Research Journal of Pharmacy and Technology 17 (2), 963–970.

Radad, K., Moldzio, R., Krewenka, C., Kranner, B., Rausch, W.D., 2023. Pathophysiology of non-motor signs in Parkinson's disease: Some recent updating with brief presentation. Exploration of Neuroprotective Therapy 3 (1), 24–46. https://doi.org/10.37349/ent.2023.00036.

Rajman, I., Knapp, L., Morgan, T., Masimirembwa, C., 2017. African genetic diversity: Implications for cytochrome P450-mediated drug metabolism and drug development. EBioMedicine 17, 67–74.

Rani, L., Mondal, A.C., 2021. Unravelling the role of gut microbiota in Parkinson's disease progression: Pathogenic and therapeutic implications. Neuroscience Research 168, 100–112.

Reed, X., Schumacher-Schuh, A., Hu, J., Bandres-Ciga, S., 2021. Advancing personalized medicine in common forms of Parkinson's disease through genetics: Current therapeutics and the future of individualized management. Journal of Personalized Medicine 11 (3), 169. https://doi.org/10.3390/jpm11030169.

Rees, J., Ryan, J., Laws, M., Devine, A., 2024. A comprehensive examination of the evidence for whole of diet patterns in Parkinson's disease: A scoping review. Nutritional Neuroscience 27 (6), 547–565.

Reeve, A., Simcox, E., Turnbull, D., 2014. Ageing and Parkinson's disease: Why is advancing age the biggest risk factor? Ageing Research Reviews 14, 19–30. https://doi.org/10.1016/j.arr.2014.01.004.

Rijntjes, M., 2019. Knowing your beans in Parkinson's disease: A critical assessment of current knowledge about different beans and their compounds in the treatment of Parkinson's disease and in animal models. Parkinson's Disease 2019, 1–9. https://doi.org/10.1155/2019/1349509.

Rizek, P., Kumar, N., Jog, M.S., 2016. An update on the diagnosis and treatment of Parkinson disease. Canadian Medical Association Journal 188 (16), 1157–1165.

Rizig, M., Bandres-Ciga, S., Makarious, M.B., et al., 2023. Identification of genetic risk loci and causal insights associated with Parkinson's disease in African and African admixed populations: A genome-wide association study. The Lancet Neurology 22, 1015–1025.

Rusch, C., Flanagan, R., Suh, H., Subramanian, I., 2023. To restrict or not to restrict? Practical considerations for optimizing dietary protein interactions on levodopa absorption in Parkinson's disease. NPJ Parkinson's Disease 9 (1). https://doi.org/10.1038/s41531-023-00541-w.

Sakowski, S.A., Koubek, E.J., Chen, K.S., Goutman, S.A., Feldman, E.L., 2024. Role of the exposome in neurodegenerative disease: Recent insights and future directions. Annals of Neurology 95 (4), 635–652. https://doi.org/10.1002/ana.26897.

Santos, A.F.D., Souza, M.M.Q., Amaral, E.C., Albuquerque, E.R., Bortoloti, D.S., Gasparotto Junior, A., Lourenco, E.L.B., Lovato, E.C.W., Livero, F.A.D.R., 2023. Bacopa monnieri in patients with Parkinson's disease: A pilot study. Journal of Medicinal Food 26 (2), 114–119. https://doi.org/10.1089/jmf.2022.0106.

Sayan, S., Degirmenci, Y., Kotan, D., 2020. A glance into regional Parkinson's disease characteristics: What differs from Northwest to Southeast of Turkey? Neuroscience & Medicine 11 (3), 63–73.

Schapira, A.H.V., 2007. Treatment options in the modern management of Parkinson disease. Archives of Neurology 64 (8), 1083–1088. https://doi.org/10.1001/archneur.64.8.1083.

Schapira, A.H., Chaudhuri, K.R., Jenner, P., 2017. Non-motor features of Parkinson disease. Nature Reviews Neuroscience 18 (7), 435–450.

Schärfe, C.P.I., Tremmel, R., Schwab, M., Kohlbacher, O., Marks, D.S., 2017. Genetic variation in human drug-related genes. Genome Medicine 9, 1–15.

Schiess, N., Cataldi, R., Okun, M.S., Fothergill-Misbah, N., Dorsey, E.R., Bloem, B.R., Dua, T., 2022. Six action steps to address global disparities in Parkinson disease: A World Health Organization priority. JAMA Neurology 79 (9), 929–936.

Schindlbeck, K.A., Vo, A., Nguyen, N., Tang, C.C., Niethammer, M., Dhawan, V., Eidelberg, D., 2020. LRRK2 and GBA variants exert distinct influences on Parkinson's disease-specific metabolic networks. Cerebral Cortex 30 (5), 2867–2878.

Schwamborn, J.C., 2018. Is Parkinson's disease a neurodevelopmental disorder and will brain organoids help us to understand it? Stem Cells and Development 27 (14), 968–975. https://doi.org/10.1089/scd.2017.0289.

Shah, S.P., Duda, J.E., 2015. Dietary modifications in Parkinson's disease: A neuroprotective intervention? Medical Hypotheses 85 (6), 1002–1005. https://doi.org/10.1016/j.mehy.2015.08.018.

Siddiqi, B., Koemeter-Cox, A., 2021. A call to action: Promoting diversity, equity, and inclusion in Parkinson's research and care. Journal of Parkinson's Disease 11 (3), 905–908.

Siddiqui, I., Pervaiz, N., Abbasi, A., 2016. The Parkinson disease gene SNCA: Evolutionary and structural insights with pathological implication. Scientific Reports 6, 24475. https://doi.org/10.1038/srep24475.

Singh, B., Pandey, S., Rumman, M., Kumar, S., Kushwaha, P.P., Verma, R., Mahdi, A.A., 2021. Neuroprotective and neurorescue mode of action of Bacopa monnieri (L.) Wettst in 1-methyl-4-phenyl-1,2,3,6-tetrahydropyridine-induced Parkinson's disease: An in silico and in vivo study. Frontiers in Pharmacology 12. https://doi.org/10.3389/fphar.2021.616413.

Singh, N., Rai, S.N., Singh, D., Singh, S.P., 2015. Withania somnifera shows ability to counter Parkinson's Disease: An update. SOJ Neurology 2, 1–4.

Singla, R.K., Agarwal, T., He, X., Shen, B., 2021. Herbal resources to combat a progressive & degenerative nervous system disorder-Parkinson's disease. Current Drug Targets 22 (6), 609–630.

Sobral, J., Empadinhas, N., Esteves, A.R., Cardoso, S.M., 2025. Impact of nutrition on the gut microbiota: Implications for Parkinson's disease. Nutrition Reviews 83 (4), 713–727. https://doi.org/10.1093/nutrit/nuae208.

Srivastav, S., Fatima, M., Mondal, A.C., 2017. Important medicinal herbs in Parkinson's disease pharmacotherapy. Biomedicine & Pharmacotherapy 92, 856–863.

Stansley, B.J., Yamamoto, B.K., 2015. L-dopa and brain serotonin system dysfunction. Toxics 3 (1), 75–88. https://doi.org/10.3390/toxics3010075.

Step, K., Eltaraifee, E., Elsayed, I., Rasaholiarison, N., Okubadejo, N., Walker, R., Periñan, M.T., 2024. Advancing Parkinson's disease research in Africa: A strategic training framework of the global Parkinson's genetics program. Movement Disorders 40 (1), 51.

Su, D., Cui, Y., He, C., Yin, P., Bai, R., Zhu, J., Lam, J.S.T., Zhang, J., Yan, R., Zheng, X., Wu, J., Zhao, D., Wang, A., Zhou, M., Feng, T., 2025. Projections for prevalence of Parkinson's disease and its driving factors in 195 countries and territories to 2050: Modelling study of Global Burden of Disease Study 2021. BMJ 388, e080952. https://doi.org/10.1136/bmj-2024-080952.

Subramanian, I., Perepezko, K., Stone, B., Chaudhuri, R.K., Pontone, G.M., 2023. Wellness in Parkinson's disease: A framework for management using a holistic culturally sensitive approach. touchREVIEWS in Neurology 19 (1), 8–13.

Suzuki, K., Miyamoto, T., Miyamoto, M., Numao, A., Sakuta, H., Fujita, H., Hirata, K., 2014. Sleep disturbances in patients with parkinson's disease. In: A synopsis of Parkinson's Disease. IntechOpen.

Titova, N., Jenner, P., Chaudhuri, K.R., 2017. The future of Parkinson's treatment–personalised and precision medicine. European Neurological Review 12 (1), 15–16.

Tolosa, E., Garrido, A., Scholz, S.W., Poewe, W., 2021. Challenges in the diagnosis of Parkinson's disease. The Lancet Neurology 20 (5), 385–397. https://doi.org/10.1016/S1474-4422(21)00030-2.

Tsalenchuk, M., Gentleman, S.M., Marzi, S.J., 2023. Linking environmental risk factors with epigenetic mechanisms in Parkinson's disease. NPJ Parkinson's Disease 9, 123. https://doi.org/10.1038/s41531-023-00568-z.

Van Puymbroeck, M., Walter, A., Hawkins, B.L., Sharp, J.L., Woschkolup, K., Urrea-Mendoza, E., Revilla, F., Adams, E.V., Schmid, A.A., Cherniack, E.P., 2018. Functional improvements in Parkinson's disease following a randomized trial of yoga. Evidence-Based Complementary and Alternative Medicine 2018 (1). https://doi.org/10.1155/2018/8516351.

Virmani, T., Tazan, S., Mazzoni, P., Ford, B., Greene, P.E., 2016. Motor fluctuations due to interaction between dietary protein and levodopa in Parkinson's disease. Journal of Clinical Movement Disorders 3 (1). https://doi.org/10.1186/s40734-016-0036-9.

Wang, Z., Wang, T., Sheng, B., Song, W., Ji, P., 2022. The effect of the integrated Chinese and Western medicine for the treatment of Parkinson's disease: A meta-analysis. Computational and Mathematical Methods in Medicine 2022, 1–11.

Wang, L., Xiong, N., Huang, J., Guo, S., Liu, L., Han, C., Zhang, G., Jiang, H., Ma, K., Xia, Y., Xu, X., Li, J., Liu, J.Y., Wang, T., 2017. Protein-restricted diets for ameliorating motor fluctuations in Parkinson's disease. Frontiers in Aging Neuroscience 9. https://doi.org/10.3389/fnagi.2017.00206.

White, J.M., Beal, T., Arsenault, J.E., Okronipa, H., Hinnouho, G.M., Chimanya, K., Matji, J., Garg, A., 2021. Micronutrient gaps during the complementary feeding period in 6 countries in Eastern and Southern Africa: A comprehensive nutrient gap assessment. Nutrition Reviews 79, 16–25. https://doi.org/10.1093/nutrit/nuaa142.

Williams, U., Bandmann, O., Walker, R., 2018. Parkinson's Disease in Sub-Saharan Africa: A review of epidemiology, genetics and access to care. Journal of Movement Disorders 11 (2), 53–64.

World Health Organization: WHO electronic essential, 2022. Google Scholar.

Yang, W., Hamilton, J.L., Kopil, C., Beck, J.C., Tanner, C.M., Albin, R.L.,… Thompson, T., 2020. Current and projected future economic burden of Parkinson's disease in the US. npj Parkinson's Disease 6 (1), 15.

Yin, R., Xue, J., Tan, Y., Fang, C., Hu, C., Yang, Q., Mei, X., Qi, D., 2021. The positive role and mechanism of herbal medicine in Parkinson's disease. Oxidative Medicine and Cellular Longevity, 9923331. https://doi.org/10.1155/2021/9923331.

Zagare, A., Hemedan, A., Almeida, C., Frangenberg, D., Gomez-Giro, G., Antony, P., Halder, R., Krüger, R., Glaab, E., Ostaszewski, M., Arena, G., 2025. Insulin resistance is a modifying factor for Parkinson's disease. Movement Disorders 40 (1), 67–76.

Zeng, B.Y., 2017. Effect and mechanism of Chinese herbal medicine on Parkinson's disease. International Review of Neurobiology 135, 57–76. https://doi.org/10.1016/bs.irn.2017.02.004.

Zewde, Y.Z., 2024. Improving access to Parkinson's medications in underserved regions in Ethiopia. International Parkinson and Movement Disorder. Society - Moving Along 28 (2). https://movementdisorders.org/Moving-Along/underserved-areas-Ethiopa-medication-access.

CHAPTER

The tango of Parkinson's treatment: Patients, science and the ryhthm of hope

4

Sara Omar[1,2]

[1]*John D. Dingell VA Medical Center, Detroit, MI, United States;* [2]*Wayne State University, Neurology Department, Detroit, MI, United States*

4.1 The opening step: ancient whispers and first moves

The narrative of Parkinson's disease (PD) threads back to 5000 BCE Ancient texts from Ayurvedic medicine hinted at a condition similar to PD. They described tremors, rigidity, and the slowed movement. Likewise, ancient Greek and Chinese texts whispered of similar symptoms, though cloaked in mystery (Manyam, 1990).

In 1817, the symphony of PD began with a single, trembling note—Dr. James Parkinson described the disorder in his pioneering work, "An Essay on the Shaking Palsy" (Parkinosn, 1817). From that point, the orchestra begins to gather: neurologists, patients, researchers—all taking their seats, tuning their instruments, uncertain of the melody but driven by the need to understand the rhythm. Certainty was exclusive to the knowledge that the rhythm would include tremors at rest, postural instability, bradykinesia (slower movement), and muscle rigidity, and the rest was about to unfold.

4.2 Finding the beat-naming the dance and early insights

The story of PD took a significant leap when French neurologist Jean-Martin Charcot engaged with it comprehensively. He distinguished it from other neurological disorders, coining the term "Parkinson's disease" in 1877- in homage to the visionary James Parkinson (Walusinski, 2018). The focus shifted from tremors to the rigidity and balance issues that characterized the disorder. Yet, defining PD wasn't fully concrete till the early 20th century, when researchers pinpointed the substantia nigra, a critical brain region, as the cornerstone of PD. Later the groundbreaking Frederic Lewy unveiled Lewy bodies, the protein aggregates regarded now as PD's pathological signatures (Lewy, 1912).

The first movement was hesitant-discordant notes in a minor key; during the transformative era of the 1950s and 60s, researchers Arvid Carlsson and Nils-Ake Hillarp first demonstrated that dopamine was a crucial neurotransmitter in the brain's motor pathways, specifically in the basal ganglia (Carlsson et al., 1957). Scientists unveiled the pivotal truth that a loss of dopaminergic neurons within the substantia nigra is a rooted cause of PD (Cotzias et al., 1967; Hornykiewicz, 2002; Olanow et al., 2009).

Pharmacological Foundations of Parkinson's Disease. https://doi.org/10.1016/B978-0-443-27702-3.00024-8

4.3 The dopamine waltz: revolutionizing the stage

The dopamine discovery, in the 20th century, was indeed a groundbreaking discovery that paved the way for dopamine replacement therapy, marking a significant shift in treatment methods. This work set the stage for the development of levodopa (L-DOPA) as a treatment for PD (the L-DOPA revolution). Clinical trials in the 1960s showcased the remarkable potential of L-DOPA to ease PD symptoms, providing dramatic improvements in motor function and quality of life for patients. L-DOPA, a precursor to dopamine, works by crossing the blood-brain barrier and converting it into dopamine in the brain, compensating for the loss of dopaminergic neurons. Today, it remains the gold standard for treatment, despite some complications (Rosenthal, 1980). Over time, patients may face challenges like motor fluctuations and dyskinesia that accompany this powerful ally. The violins strained toward harmony, but the melody slips through their fingers. Promising molecules fall flat, like dancers who miss a step mid-performance. The tempo slows, and for a moment, there's silence. But it's not the end.

In the late 1970s and early 1980s, trials showed that bromocriptine, a dopamine agonist, could ease motor symptoms in PD on its own. It was especially helpful for early-stage PD or for patients who couldn't tolerate L-DOPA. Trials confirmed that bromocriptine improved tremor, rigidity, and bradykinesia by stimulating dopamine receptors directly (Chen et al., 2022).

Further studies found that when bromocriptine was combined with L-DOPA, it boosted the therapeutic effect, especially in patients with "wearing-off" symptoms Combinatorial therapy also delayed the need for higher L-DOPA doses, reducing risks like motor fluctuations and dyskinesia; providing steadier dopamine stimulation, resulting in smoother symptom control. Bromocriptine was an early option, one of the first oral dopamine agonists available before newer drugs like pramipexole or ropinirole.

Despite newer dopamine agonists offering better tolerability, bromocriptine's early use and clinical value helped it remain relevant for many years. This was attributed to its established safety profile (side effects like hypotension and hallucinations were manageable for many patients).

4.4 Crescendo of care: MAO-B inhibitors and neuromodulation's rise

Then the second movement rises; triumphs of science step in like a sudden swell of brass and percussion. Monoamine oxidase-B (MAO-B) inhibitors represent the third major class of pharmacotherapy for PD, introduced after levodopa and dopamine agonists (Rascol et al., 2000). Deep brain stimulation (DBS) and stem cell therapy also enters like a sweeping crescendo later in this movement (Olanow et al., 2014). The tango begins, patients and doctors locked in step, moving through time with elegance and precision. Every medication, every discovery, is a graceful pivot, a daring dip into hope. The rhythm isn't perfect, but it's passionate. There's fire in the dance.

These MAO-B inhibitors broaden the treatment options for PD (Rascol et al., 2000). They provide early monotherapy choices and ways to enhance levodopa's effects while ensuring better safety profiles.

Adaptive deep brain stimulation (aDBS), on the other hand, represents a shift from continuous to closed-loop neuromodulation. Worthy to mention, a conceptual precursor to closed-loop DBS was first explored by Delgado's team in the 1960s, who developed feedback-triggered stimulation devices capable of detecting neural activity and delivering stimulation in response (Delgado, 1969).

Modern closed-loop DBS approaches later emerged through translational work in non-human primates. In 2011, Rosin and colleagues from Bergman's group demonstrated that closed-loop stimulation in macaque models improved motor outcomes more effectively than continuous stimulation, paving the way for adaptive neuromodulation strategies in humans (Rosin et al., 2011). Subsequently, early human applications of adaptive DBS were developed by Peter Brown's group at Oxford, demonstrating the feasibility of neural biomarker-guided stimulation in Parkinson's disease (Little et al., 2013; Little & Brown, 2014). Similar adaptive stimulation approaches were later explored by Alberto Priori's group in Italy, further supporting the safety and feasibility of sensing-guided neuromodulation in clinical settings (Arlotti et al., 2018; Oertel & Schulz, 2016; Schapira et al., 2020).

Medtronic's BrainSense Adaptive DBS system entered its pivotal ADAPT-PD trial in January 2021 and received FDA approval in February 2025, marking a new era of patient-specific therapy. Basically, BrainSense allows real-time adjustment of stimulation based on abnormal neural signals for better symptom control ("Deep-Brain Stimulation of the Subthalamic Nucleus or the Pars Interna of the Globus Pallidus in Parkinson's Disease," 2001).

Meanwhile Glovadalen (UCB-0022), a selective dopamine D_1 receptor modulator, progressed from preclinical development into its first-in-human Phase 1 study in April 2021 and entered Phase 2 (ATLANTIS) trials in November 2023, offering a new oral approach to enhance dopamine signaling in PD patients, with ongoing evaluations of efficacy, safety, and pharmacodynamics across multiple sites. Glovadalen, or UCB-0022, is a small molecule that enhances dopamine's effect at D_1 receptors without direct agonism, amplifying dopamine activity significantly in vitro (Little et al., 2013; *Medtronic Receives FDA Approval for BrainSense Adaptive DBS System. Medtronic Newsroom*, 2025; *UCB Announces First Patient Dosed in ATLANTIS Phase 2 Study of UCB0022 (Glovadalen) in Parkinson's Disease*, 2023).

4.5 Regenerative tango: stem cells and genetic choreography

These advancements; from real-time neuromodulation to receptor-targeted pharmacology, were enabled by the modern era research breakthroughs and genetics breakthroughs. For instance, Genetic discoveries, particularly mutations in LRRK2, PARKIN, and PINK1 guided neuromodulation in the sense of clarifying which circuits and pathways (e.g., mitochondrial deficits in PINK1/PARKIN or synaptic/inflammatory changes in LRRK2) are disrupted. Hence, researchers were able to select optimal DBS targets and develop adaptive DBS systems that adjust stimulation in real time based on mutation-specific electrophysiological biomarkers. This is also leading the way in the future to combining gene-corrective therapies with closed-loop neural modulation for best outcomes.

The stem cell therapy bemdaneprocel was designed in 2021, received FDA Fast Track and RMAT designations that same year as well as in 2024, completing its Phase 1 (exPDite trial) in September 2024, and began its registrational Phase 3 exPDite-2 study in early 2025 (Therapeutics, 2024). Phase 1 "exPDite" Trial enrolled 12 participants in 2022–23; 24-month safety and tolerability data were presented on September 27, 2024. exPDite-2 is a randomized, sham surgery-controlled double-blind trial assessing the efficacy and safety of bemdaneprocel in ~102 people living with moderate PD. Initiated in H1 2025, exPDite-2 is the first registrational Phase III clinical trial for an investigational allogeneic pluripotent stem cell-derived therapy to treat PD 025 (Therapeutics, 2024).

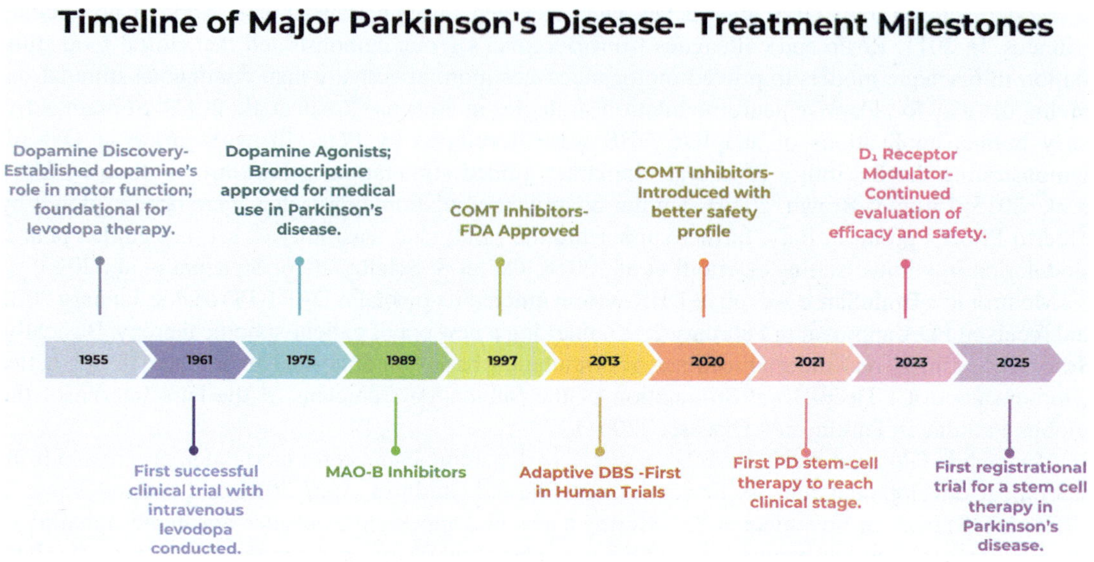

FIGURE 4.1

Timeline of major Parkinson's disease-treatment milestones.

Fig. 4.1 and Table 4.1 summarizing the major pharmacologic and therapeutic milestones in PD disease treatment (AAN 2025, 2025; BMJ Best Practice US, 2025; Cotzias et al., 1967; History of Parkinson's disease, 2024; Jankovic, 2011; Kalia and Lang, 2015; Little & Brown, 2014; Olanow et al., 2009, 2014; Pagano et al., 2022; Poewe, 2024; Rosin et al., 2011; The Story of Parkinson's Disease, 2025; U. Department of Veterans Affairs, 2025).

4.6 Illuminating the dance floor: biomarkers in the spotlight

On the topic of research breakthroughs, identifying biomarkers for early diagnosis and progression-tracking is a major research momentum. To begin with imaging biomarkers, this includes molecular and structural scans. Dopamine-related PET/SPECT remains the standard for confirming nigrostriatal degeneration. Even though it reliably shows reduced striatal uptake in PD, levels plateau after a few years, limiting their use to long-term progression. New MRI techniques are emerging: neuromelanin-sensitive MRI can detect loss of the pigmented neurons in the substantia nigra, and quantitative susceptibility mapping (QSM) highlights iron accumulation (Espay, Kalia, & Gan-Or, 2023). Other advanced imaging (diffusion MRI, functional connectivity, α-synuclein PET tracers in development) is under study, but not yet routine. At the same time, fluid biomarkers from CSF or blood focus on PD pathology, particularly α-synuclein seed amplification (RT-QuIC) assays showed promising results (Espay, Kalia, & Gan-Or, 2023). They could detect misfolded α-synuclein "seeds" in CSF with ~88% sensitivity and 95% specificity for PD versus controls (Iranzo et al., 2021; Mollenhauer et al., 2019). These assays can even identify prodromal cases (e.g., RBD patients) and distinguish PD from other dementias. Total α-syn levels by ELISA have been less reliable, given that α-synuclein is a small

Table 4.1 Major pharmacologic and therapeutic milestones in PD disease treatment.

Date	Class	Key development	Outcome
1957–60	Dopamine discovery	Arvid Carlsson demonstrated dopamine as a neurotransmitter; Nils-Ake Hillarp contributed to storage mechanisms.	Established dopamine's role in motor function; foundational for levodopa therapy.
1961	Levodopa (L-DOPA)	First successful clinical trial with intravenous levodopa conducted.	Became the gold standard for Parkinson's treatment.
1975	Dopamine agonists	Bromocriptine approved for medical use in Parkinson's disease.	Enabled dose-sparing therapy and reduced motor fluctuations.
1989	MAO-B inhibitors	Selegiline (Eldepryl) approved by FDA.	Offered early monotherapy or enhanced L-DOPA effects.
1997	COMT inhibitors	Tolcapone (Tasmar) approved; noted for liver toxicity concerns.	Improved levodopa efficacy but limited by safety issues.
1999	COMT inhibitors	Entacapone (Comtan) approved; better safety profile.	Enabled combination therapy (e.g., Stalevo), reduced "off" time.
2020	COMT inhibitors	Opicapone (Ongentys) approved as once-daily option.	Provided stable levodopa levels with less frequent dosing.
2011	Adaptive DBS (animal)	Closed-loop DBS tested in macaques by Bergman's group.	Validated real-time neural feedback for motor improvement.
2013	Adaptive DBS (human)	First in-human trials by Peter Brown and Alberto Priori.	Demonstrated feasibility and safety of sensing-guided DBS.
2021	Adaptive DBS (BrainSense™)	Medtronic launched ADAPT-PD trial.	Personalized DBS entered clinical testing; FDA approved in 2025.
2021	D_1 receptor modulator	Glovadalen (UCB-0022) entered Phase 1 clinical trials.	Novel oral drug enhancing dopamine D_1 signaling.
2023	D_1 receptor modulator	Glovadalen entered Phase 2 (ATLANTIS trial).	Continued evaluation of efficacy and safety.
2021	Stem cell therapy	Bemdaneprocel designed; received FDA Fast Track & RMAT status.	First PD stem-cell therapy to reach clinical stage.
2024	Stem cell therapy	Phase 1 exPDite trial completed.	Showed safety/tolerability; supported progression to Phase 3.
2025	Stem cell therapy	Phase 3 (exPDite-2) launched.	First registrational trial for a stem cell therapy in Parkinson's disease.

presynaptic protein with a partially unclear role in normal functions. In healthy neurons, α-synuclein binds synaptic vesicle membranes and is thought to regulate vesicle pools and neurotransmitter release; it likely modulates vesicle trafficking rather than being essential for baseline transmission (Braak et al., 2003; Jankovic & Tan, 2024; Mollenhauer et al., 2019). In pathological conditions, α-synuclein misfolds and aggregates into fibrils that accumulate as Lewy bodies and Lewy neurites—the histological hallmark of PD. These aggregates are enriched in phosphorylated, insoluble α-synuclein (typically at serine-129). There is abundant evidence that misfolded α-synuclein spreads in a prion-like manner: aggregated fibrils can be taken up by neurons and then template the misfolding of native α-synuclein. According to Braak's hypothesis, pathology may even start in the gut or olfactory bulb and ascend via connected pathways (e.g., the vagus nerve) to reach the substantia nigra over years. A side note, despite the failure of α-synuclein in clinical trials, therapeutic efforts strive to sequester, clear or silence the toxic protein species, reflecting its central role in PD pathogenesis. In a later section, we will be surveying some of the failed therapies in clinical trials.

Continuing with biomarkers, neurofilament light chain (NfL) is another key biomarker; elevated CSF or plasma NfL correlates with cognitive decline and is higher in atypical parkinsonian syndromes; thus it may help discriminate PD from conditions like Multiple System Atrophy and progressive Supranuclear Palsy. Blood NfL rises with disease severity and may predict dementia in PD, but is non-specific (also up in Alzheimer's, aging). Other fluid markers include CSF tau/Aβ (inform dementia risk), inflammatory cytokines, and exosomal proteins. For instance, neuronal exosomes carrying α-synuclein are under study as blood tests, one study reporting an AUC≈0.86 for distinguishing PD versus controls. Multiplex panels (e.g., Simoa) now measure NfL, tau, GFAP together. [31,32] In sum, α-synuclein seed assays stand out for PD diagnosis, while markers like NfL and GFAP help assess neurodegeneration and cognitive involvement.

Extended from that, as stated earlier, genetic biomarkers are also crucial in understanding PD pathogenesis and developing targeted therapies. They identify inherited risk factors and stratify patients based on their genetic makeup. Key PD genes include LRRK2 and GBA. LRRK2 G2019S mutation, autosomal dominant, occurs in 1%–3% of sporadic and up to 10% of familial cases. GBA mutations, autosomal recessive and associated with Gaucher's gene, affect 5%–10% of cases. Both mutations increase synuclein pathology and are therapeutic targets. Though not routinely used for diagnosis, genetic biomarkers are precious in understanding PD mechanisms and developing targeted therapies (Braak et al., 2003; Jankovic & Tan, 2024).

4.7 Keeping in sync: the dance of drug delivery

Moving forward to explore the role of drug delivery systems in this delicate dance of treatment. As every step in tango keeps the dance in sync, the successful drug delivery system ensures the right medications stay on track, hitting its mark at the right moment. maintain the rhythm of PD's treatment. Even Though, Novel infusion devices and nanocarriers are being engineered to overcome the blood-brain barrier. Preclinical studies are focused on non-invasive ultrasound and microbubbles to temporarily open the BBB and deliver genes or drugs to the brain, in this chapter we will remain focused on drug delivery systems that made it to clinical trials.

Table 4.2: PD Drug Delivery Therapies that have emerged over the last few years (from 2022 to 2025) (*AbbVie announces positive topline results for the Phase 3 TEMPO-2 trial evaluating*

Table 4.2 Recent drug delivery systems for PD.

Delivery method	Therapy (Sponsor)	Description	Clinical phase & outcomes	Status	Delivery platform/ Materials
Oral tablet	Tavapadon (Cerevel/ AbbVie)	Selective D_1/D_5 dopamine receptor partial agonist (once-daily).	Phase 3 (TEMPO-2) met primary & key secondary endpoints (MDS-UPDRS II +III). Positive topline (Dec 2024).	Phase 3 complete; NDA expected.	Oral pill (once-daily tablet).
Subcutaneous (SC) infusion	ND0612 (NeuroDerm/ Mitsubishi)	Continuous levodopa/carbidopa liquid infusion to reduce "OFF" fluctuations.	Phase 3 (BouNDless): +1.72 h "ON" time versus oral LD/CD ($P < .0001$). Data published Lancet Neurol. 2024.	FDA complete response letter (2023); resubmission planned.	Portable infusion pump with polymeric reservoir and cannula; aqueous LD/CD solution delivered 24 h/day.
SC infusion (wearable pump)	Onapgo (SPN-830, Supernus)	Continuous apomorphine infusion for advanced PD "OFF" episodes.	Phase 3 (TOLEDO): −1.89 h OFF time versus placebo. FDA Advisory panel positive (Sep 2024).	FDA approved Feb 2025.	Wearable subcutaneous infusion pump (non-invasive portable device).
Intracerebral injection	AB-1005 (AskBio/ Bayer)	AAV2-GDNF gene therapy (GDNF neurotrophic factor) delivered to putamen.	Phase 1b (36-mo): well tolerated; trends toward motor improvement. Phase 2 (REGENERATE-PD) started Jan 2025.	Phase 2 ongoing (2025); Fast Track & RMAT designations.	AAV2 viral vector via stereotactic infusion (convection-enhanced) into striatum.
Intracerebral infusion	CDNF (Herantis)	Recombinant Cerebral dopamine Neurotrophic factor protein.	Phase 1/2: direct brain infusion via implanted pump; met safety/ tolerability endpoints.	Phase 1/2 complete; 1-year follow-up ongoing; exploring less-invasive delivery.	Implantable intracranial infusion pump (CED device) delivering CDNF protein.
Surgical graft	Bemdaneprocel (BlueRock/Bayer)	Human ESC-derived midbrain	Phase 1 (exPDite): safe; significant UPDRS	Phase 3 enrolling (H1 2025).	Stem cell-derived neuron graft (surgical

Continued

Table 4.2 Recent drug delivery systems for PD.—cont'd

Delivery method	Therapy (Sponsor)	Description	Clinical phase & outcomes	Status	Delivery platform/ Materials
		dopaminergic neuron transplant.	improvements at 24 mo (high-dose: −21.9 points UPDRS III). Phase 3 (exPDite-2, n˜100) initiated 2025.		stereotactic transplantation into striatum).
Intracisternal injection	PR001 (Prevail/ AbbVie)	AAV9-based GBA1 gene-replacement therapy.	Phase 1/2a (PROPEL) recruiting (n˜20); no results reported yet. Focus on GBA-PD and Gaucher type 2.	Phase 1/2 ongoing (2022–29).	AAV9 viral vector delivered via intrathecal/ intracisternal injection.
Focused ultrasound (FUS)	LIFUS BBB opening (Sunnybrook)	Low-intensity focused ultrasound + microbubbles to open BBB for drug delivery.	Phase 1: safely opened BBB in PD patients to infuse man made enzyme (imiglucerase (Cerezyme)) into putamen. Improved brain enzyme levels. Larger trials planned.	Early clinical stage (proof-of-concept).	Low-intensity FUS system with microbubble contrast (temporary BBB disruption).
Intranasal (Nose-to-brain)	Nanoparticle approaches (various)	Intranasal administration of drugs/growth factors using nanocarriers (lipidic or polymeric).	Preclinical and early clinical research: studies show enhanced brain uptake of encapsulated dopamine/GDNF in animal models; no late-phase human data yet.	Experimental (preclinical/early-stage R&D).	Lipid or polymer nanoparticles (e.g., PLGA, liposomes) formulated for intranasal delivery.

Tavapadon as a monotherapy for Parkinson's disease. AbbVie Newsroom, 2024; "AAN 2025 highlights: game-changing research in neurology," 2025; "AbbVie's acquired Parkinson's disease drug shines in Phase III trial," 2024; *Mitsubishi Tanabe Pharma America presents open-label extension outcomes and additional data from Phase 3 BouNDless trial of investigational ND0612 in Parkinson's disease. Mitsubishi Tanabe Pharma America*, 2024; *Parkinson therapy ND0612 receives complete response letter. NeurologyLive*, 2024; *Phase 3 of ND0612 clinical trial initiated in the United States for Parkinson's disease*, 2025; "FDA approves apomorphine infusion device SPN-830 as new Parkinson treatment," 2025; "Onapgo (apomorphine hydrochloride) FDA approval history," 2025; Pharmaceutical Executive, 2025).

4.8 Stumbles and recoveries: lessons from trials off beat

While successful trials are the spotlight moments; filled with lifted hands, daring turns, and hopeful embraces, setbacks form the foundation, the creaking floorboards that bear the weight of progress. Failed trials may bring disappointment, but they offer essential insights that guide future research. Together, both success and failure are not dancing to a finished piece, but to a choreography still in the making.

Among the few notable unsuccessful trails are:

1. Prasinezumab (Roche/Prothena), a monoclonal antibody targeting alpha-synuclein aggregates, failed to show significant benefits in slowing PD progression during the Phase 2 PASADENA and PADOVA trials. Despite some positive trends in secondary outcomes, the primary endpoints were not met (Pagano et al., 2022).
2. Another antibody targeting alpha-synuclein, Cinpanemab (Biogen), also did not demonstrate efficacy in a Phase 2 trial, which led to the discontinuation of its development (Jankovic & Poewe, 2012; Kalia & Lang, 2015; Poewe et al., 2017; Schapira et al., 2017).
3. Aimed at reducing levodopa-induced motor complications, Foliglurax (Lundbeck) failed to achieve significant improvements in a Phase 2 trial, resulting in the termination of its development program.
4. Targeting GBA mutation-associated PD, Venglustat (Sanofi) did not show efficacy in a Phase 2 trial, leading Sanofi to halt its development for PD.
5. Intended to improve cognitive function in PD patients, SAGE-718 by Sage Therapeutics failed to show significant benefits in a Phase 2 trial, prompting the company to discontinue its development for PD (Jankovic & Poewe, 2012; Kalia & Lang, 2015; Poewe et al., 2017; Schapira et al., 2017).
6. Minzasolmin, an oral small molecule developed by UCB/Novartis and aimed at preventing alpha-synuclein aggregation, showed no effect on PD symptoms in the ORCHESTRA Phase 2 trial, leading to the cessation of its development.

The heterogeneous nature of PD symptoms across patients makes it challenging to achieve statistically significant improvements in diverse trial populations. It was also noted that Targeting alpha-Synuclein aggregates is among the common reasons for study failure. Several therapies aimed at reducing alpha-synuclein aggregates did not translate into clinical benefits, possibly due to the complexity of PD pathology or the timing of intervention. worthy also to include trial design and endpoints among the most common reasons some trials fail. Some trials have faced design limitations, short durations, insufficient sample sizes, or endpoints that failed to capture meaningful clinical change.

4.9 New moves and fresh beats: emerging therapies take the floor

On the flip side, recent breakthroughs in PD research are bringing new hope to patients and families, as innovative treatments begin to reshape what care looks like. Among these, tavapadon-a medication developed by AbbVie-is a selective partial agonist of the D1 and D5 dopamine receptors, designed to activate these receptors in the brain while avoiding overstimulation of the D2/D3 receptors, which are linked to many of the side effects seen with current dopamine therapies. In the Phase 3 (TEMPO-2 trial), tavapadon helped people with early-stage PD move more easily and manage daily activities. With a good safety record and the potential to be used alone or alongside other treatments, AbbVie is preparing to seek FDA approval in 2025 (Espay, Brundin, & Lang, 2023; *A Study to Evaluate the Efficacy and Safety of Tavapadon in Early Parkinson's Disease*, 2024).

Another encouraging option is lixisenatide, a medication originally developed for diabetes that belongs to the GLP-1 receptor agonist class. Lixisenatide works by targeting GLP-1 receptors, which are found in the pancreas and the brain. In the brain, activating these receptors is thought to boost dopamine function, reduce inflammation, and promote cell survival-effects that may help slow the progression of PD motor symptoms. In the Phase 2 (LixiPark trial), lixisenatide slowed the worsening of symptoms over a year in people newly diagnosed with PD, making it the second drug in its class to show potential disease-modifying effects (Athauda et al., 2024; *Parkinson's UK. LixiPark trial shows potential to slow Parkinson's progression. Parkinson's UK News*, 2024; *LixiPark: A Study of Lixisenatide in Early Parkinson's Disease. NCT03439943*, 2024).

In a different direction, early research at University of California, San Francisco has explored psilocybin, a naturally occurring psychedelic compound found in certain mushrooms. Psilocybin works by activating serotonin receptors in the brain, which can lead to profound changes in mood, perception, and cognition. A single dose led to weeks of improved mood, movement, and memory in PD patients, all without serious side effects. This marks the first time a psychedelic has been tested for a degenerative brain disease, opening up new possibilities for patient well-being (Flores-Torres et al., 2023; Francisco, 2023).

But it's not just new drugs making waves. Gene and cell therapies are now stepping into the spotlight. AB-1005, a gene therapy from AskBio and Bayer, delivers a gene designed to restore or enhance dopamine production in the brain. In Phase 1b trials, moderate-stage PD patients gained more than two extra hours of "good on" time each day and required less levodopa. The FDA recognized its potential by granting it Fast Track status in 2024 (*AskBio's AB-1005 Receives FDA Fast Track Designation for Parkinson's Disease. AskBio News*, 2024; *A Phase 1b Study of AB-1005 in Parkinson's Disease. NCT04167540*, 2024; Kordower et al., 2023; Schweitzer et al., 2023; Takahashi, 2023). Bemdaneprocel, a stem cell therapy, involves implanting dopaminergic progenitor cells-cells that can mature into dopamine-producing neurons-into the brain. It has proven safe and well-tolerated for up to 21 months after implantation, with no major side effects reported so far. NouvNeu001, another cell therapy, uses induced pluripotent stem cells (iPSCs), which are reprogrammed from a patient's own cells, to generate new dopamine neurons. Early data suggest safety and possible motor benefits for those in mid-to late-stage PD. These therapies aim to restore the dopamine-producing cells lost in PD,

Table 4.3 Recent breakthroughs in PD therapies.

Therapy	Type	Key outcome	Success factors
Tavapadon	Dopamine D1/D5 receptor agonist	Improved motor functions	Targeted mechanism, favorable safety profile
Lixisenatide	GLP-1 receptor agonist	Reduced motor disability progression	Repurposed drug, neuroprotective potential
Adaptive DBS (BrainSense)	Neuromodulation device	Dynamic symptom management	Real-time adaptation, reduced medication need
Bemdaneprocel	Stem cell therapy	Sustained dopaminergic activity	Innovative approach, long-term safety
Rasagiline (ADAGIO study)	MAO-B inhibitor	Slowed disease progression with early treatment	Early intervention, robust study design

offering a glimpse of what regenerative medicine might achieve in the future (*AskBio's AB-1005 Receives FDA Fast Track Designation for Parkinson's Disease. AskBio News*, 2024; *A Phase 1b Study of AB-1005 in Parkinson's Disease. NCT04167540*, 2024; Kordower et al., 2023; Schweitzer et al., 2023; Takahashi, 2023).

AS mentioned earlier, Medtronic's BrainSense system (aDBS) was approved by the FDA in 2024. Unlike conventional DBS, which delivers constant electrical stimulation, aDBS uses sensors to listen to the brain in real time and adjusts stimulation automatically, providing more precise symptom control and often reducing medication side effects. Many people report better quality of life and less need for pills (Medtronic, 2024; Little & Brown, 2014).

Taken together, these advances paint a picture of a hopeful future for PD care-one that tackles symptoms, aiming to slow the disease, and puts patients' needs at the center Table 4.3.

4.10 The veteran's tango: a unique and complex dance

These innovations are especially meaningful for veterans, who often face unique challenges with PD.

For veterans, their tango is unlike any other; measured not only by tremors or slowed steps, but by the invisible weight of war, trauma, and time. Each movement carries echoes of past missions, of environments touched by toxins, of wounds both seen and unseen.

This is a tango shaped by service that was deliberate and determined. The steps may be uncertain, but they are never aimless. Behind those steps are questions still searching for answers. Why does PD look and feel different in so many veterans? Could their exposures, their experiences, even their genes be part of the story? Scientists and clinicians are listening closely, working to understand the patterns that emerge from lives spent in service.

Indeed, PD is a complex neurodegenerative disorder affected by environmental as well as genetic influences via genetics. The emerging research suggests that the incidence is higher for certain populations such as military veterans because exposures are related to the service that potentially links to it. Several factors make veterans with PD a unique group. These factors/patterns matter to improve treatment and diagnosis (*Committee to Review the Health Effects in Vietnam Veterans of Exposure to Herbicides. Veterans and Agent Orange: Update*, 2012; Tanner et al., 2011; Gardner & Yaffe, 2015; Jafari et al., 2013).

Among these factors are age and military Service History: veterans are often older and may have a history of exposure to unique environmental factors such as toxins, combat stress, or physical trauma that may contribute to PD risk. Some studies suggest that veterans, particularly those exposed to Agent Orange in Vietnam, may have a higher risk of developing PD due to chemical exposure (*Committee to Review the Health Effects in Vietnam Veterans of Exposure to Herbicides. Veterans and Agent Orange: Update*, 2012; Tanner et al., 2011; Gardner & Yaffe, 2015; Jafari et al., 2013).

Veterans are indeed more likely to have experienced head injuries such as both concussions or even more severe traumatic brain injuries (TBI) and that these injuries have been found to link to an increased risk of them developing neurodegenerative diseases including PD.

Comorbidities such as PTSD, depression, and cardiovascular disease are the medical conditions that are more common in the veteran population and that veterans with PD often have. These comorbidities complicate management. These make managing PD harder in veterans (Jafari et al., 2013; Papoutsi et al., 2018; Weisskopf, 2012).

In response, several clinical trials-many led by the U.S. Department of Veterans Affairs-have turned their attention to veterans with PD. These studies do more than collect data; they aim to bring relief, improve care, and offer new hope to those whose service hasn't ended, but simply changed form.

1. CHAPS Trial—Nurse-Led Care Management

In the CHAPS (Care Coordination for Health Promotion and Activities in PD Disease) trial, 328 veterans across the southwestern U.S. received a more personalized kind of care—nurse-led management designed to better meet their daily needs. The results were magnificent, those in the intervention group adhered more closely to recommended care practices and reported fewer symptoms of depression. This showed that compassionate, coordinated care can make a measurable difference in veterans' lives (Connor et al., 2019).

2. Ketamine for Depression in Veterans with PD (NCT06231563)

Depression can be one of the most debilitating aspects of PD, especially in veterans. In an ongoing Phase 2 trial the San Francisco VA Medical Center is now testing intravenous ketamine for depression in veterans with PD, while also looking at its broader effects on the Ketamine acts on glutamate receptors in the brain, which may help restore neuroplasticity and reduce inflammation. Beyond symptom relief, researchers are also looking at how ketamine may influence the brain's plasticity and inflammation, pushing toward a deeper understanding of its potential benefits (*Ketamine for Depression in Veterans with Parkinson's Disease (NCT06231563)*, 2025; Zarate, 2017).

3. Telemedicine-Delivered Cognitive Behavioral Therapy (CBT)

Getting to a specialist isn't always easy, especially for older veterans or those in rural areas. That's why VA researchers explored how cognitive behavioral therapy, delivered entirely through telemedicine, could help. The results speak volumes: veterans receiving this care experienced significant, lasting relief from depression. It's a promising model for expanding access to mental health support without adding travel burdens (Dobkin et al., 2020; *Telehealth for Veterans with Parkinson's Disease*, 2025).

4. VA-NIH Deep Brain Stimulation (DBS) Study

For veterans with advanced PD who no longer respond well to medication, deep brain stimulation (DBS) offers new possibilities. In a major VA-NIH study, patients undergoing DBS gained an average of 4.6 extra hours of good motor function each day.

Adaptive DBS, with its personalized, AI-driven approach, is already improving lives for veterans across the country. The VA also runs six specialized centers (PADRECCs) that offer expert care, research, and support for veterans with PD. Recent studies have highlighted the importance of monitoring veterans who've experienced traumatic brain injury or PTSD, as both raise the risk of developing PD. Hearing loss is another factor, but early intervention with hearing aids may help lower that risk. Community support groups and partnerships, like the Michigan Veterans with PD Support Group and the VA's collaboration with the PD Foundation, provide friendship, resources, and advocacy for veterans and their caregivers (Weaver et al., 2009; Education and Clinical Centers (PADRECCs), 2025; Veterans and Parkinson's Disease, 2025; Michigan Veterans with Parkinson's Disease Support Group, 2025; U., 2025; Goldman and Tanner, no date; Foltynie et al., 2011).

4.11 An ever-flowing tango of hope

The final movement isn't an end, it's rather a turning point. A quiet bridge between what is and what could be. Beneath it all, the river of time keeps flowing, catching glimmers of every spotlight, every misstep, every breakthrough. Researchers become composers. Patients, the dancers. Each study is a rehearsal. Each trial, a chance to refine the rhythm.

And as the curtain lifts on what's next, one truth becomes clear: Parkinson's isn't a solo. It's an ensemble; a symphony of science and human strength, a dance of resilience and resolve, all moving to the steady rhythm of hope. The river keeps flowing, ever forward, toward a cure.

Then, just beyond the edge of the spotlight, a distant rhythm begins to rise. A new dance stirs in the wings. These dancers are younger, their movements vibrant, full of potential. Yet within their improvized steps is something undeniable: a raw, hopeful energy that is waiting to be seen, heard, understood.

AI disclosure

During the preparation of this work the author(s) used Grammarly in order to Readability. After using this tool/service, the author(s) reviewed and edited the content as needed and take(s) full responsibility for the content of the publication.

References

AAN 2025 highlights: Game-changing research in neurology. (2025). delveinsight.

AbbVie announces positive topline results for the Phase 3 TEMPO-2 trial evaluating Tavapadon as a monotherapy for Parkinson's disease. (2024). AbbVie Newsroom.

AbbVie's acquired Parkinson's disease drug shines in Phase III trial. (2024). Clinical Trials Arena.

Arlotti, M., Marceglia, S., Foffani, G., Volkmann, J., Lozano, A. M., Moro, E., Cogiamanian, F., Prenassi, M., Bocci, T., Cortese, F., Rampini, P., Barbieri, S., & Priori, A. (2018). Eight-hours adaptive deep brain stimulation in patients with Parkinson disease. *Neurrology, 90*(11), e971–e976.

AskBio's AB-1005 receives FDA fast track designation for Parkinson's disease. (2024). AskBio News.

Athauda, D., Maclagan, K., & Skene, S. S. (2024). Lixisenatide in early Parkinson's disease: A multicentre, randomised, double-blind, placebo-controlled trial. *New England Journal of Medicine, 390*(8), 742–753. https://doi.org/10.1056/NEJMoa2309307

BMJ best practice US.(2025).

Braak, H., Del Tredici, K., Rüb, U., De Vos, R. A. I., Jansen Steur, E. N. H., & Braak, E. (2003). Staging of brain pathology related to sporadic Parkinson's disease. *Neurobiology of Aging, 24*(2), 197–211. https://doi.org/10.1016/S0197-4580(02)00065-9

Carlsson, A., Lindqvist, M., & Magnusson, T. (1957). 3,4-Dihydroxyphenylalanine and 5-hydroxytryptophan as reserpine antagonists [16]. *Nature, 180*(4596), 1200. https://doi.org/10.1038/1801200a0

Chen, H., Wan, H., Zhang, M., Wardlaw, J. M., Feng, T., & Wang, Y. (2022). Perivascular space in Parkinson's disease: Association with CSF amyloid/tau and cognitive decline. *Parkinsonism & Related Disorders, 95*, 70–76. https://doi.org/10.1016/j.parkreldis.2022.01.002

Committee to Review the Health Effects in Vietnam Veterans of Exposure to Herbicides. (2012). *Veterans and agent Orange: Update*. National Academies Press.

Connor, K. I., Cheng, E. M., Barry, F., Siebens, H. C., Lee, M. L., Ganz, D. A., Mittman, B. S., Connor, M. K., Edwards, L. K., McGowan, M. G., & Vickrey, B. G. (2019). Randomized trial of care management to improve Parkinson disease care quality. *Neurology, 92*(16), E1831. https://doi.org/10.1212/WNL.0000000000007324

Cotzias, G. C., Van Woert, M. H., & Schiffer, L. M. (1967). Aromatic amino acids and modification of parkinsonism. *New England Journal of Medicine, 276*(7), 374–379. https://doi.org/10.1056/NEJM196702162760703

Deep-brain stimulation of the subthalamic nucleus or the pars interna of the globus pallidus in Parkinson's disease. *New England Journal of Medicine, 345*(13), (2001), 956–963. https://doi.org/10.1056/nejmoa000827

Delgado, J. M. R. (1969). *Physical control of the mind: Toward a pyschocvivlized society.* Harper and Row.

Dobkin, R. D., Mann, L., Interian, A., & Gara, M. A. (2020). Telephone-based cognitive-behavioral therapy for depression in Parkinson disease. *JAMA Neurology, 77*(5), 551–559. https://doi.org/10.1001/jamaneurol.2020.0021

Education and clinical centers (PADRECCs).(2025).

Espay, A. J., Brundin, P., & Lang, A. E. (2023a). Tavapadon for Parkinson's disease: Pharmacology and clinical development. *Movement Disorders, 38*(S1), 1. https://doi.org/10.1002/mds.29400

Espay, A. J., Kalia, L. V., & Gan-Or, Z. (2023b). Disease modification and biomarker development in Parkinson disease: Current status and future perspectives. *Nature Reviews Neurology, 19*(2), 91–110. https://doi.org/10.1038/s41582-022-00760-1

FDA approves apomorphine infusion device SPN-830 as new Parkinson treatment. In . *NeurologyLive*, (2025).

Flores-Torres, M. H., Bjornevik, K., Hung, A. Y., Healy, B. C., Schwarzschild, M. A., Blacker, D., & Ascherio, A. (2023). Subjective cognitive decline in women with features suggestive of prodromal Parkinson's disease. *Movement Disorders, 38*. https://doi.org/10.1002/mds.29503

Foltynie, T., Zrinzo, L., Martinez-Torres, I., Tripoliti, E., Petersen, E., Holl, E., Aviles-Olmos, I., Jahanshahi, M., Hariz, M., & Limousin, P. (2011). MRI-guided STN DBS in Parkinson's disease without microelectrode recording: Efficacy and safety. *Journal of Neurology, Neurosurgery & Psychiatry, 82*(4), 358–363. https://doi.org/10.1136/jnnp.2010.205542

Francisco, S. (2023). *Psilocybin shows promise for Parkinson's disease in early study.* UCSF News.

Gardner, R. C., & Yaffe, K. (2015). Epidemiology of mild traumatic brain injury and neurodegenerative disease. *Molecular and Cellular Neuroscience, 66*, 75–80. https://doi.org/10.1016/j.mcn.2015.03.001

JG Goldman, CM. Tanner, Etiology of Parkinson's disease. *Handbook of Clinical Neurology*. 147 59–89, doi: 10.1016/B978-0-444-64008-7.00005-2.

History of Parkinson's disease. (2024). Wikipedia.

Hornykiewicz, O. (2002). Dopamine miracle: From brain homogenate to dopamine replacement. *Movement Disorders, 17*(3), 501–508. https://doi.org/10.1002/mds.10115

Iranzo, A., Fairfoul, G., Ayudhaya, A. C. N., Serradell, M., Gelpi, E., Vilaseca, I., Sanchez-Valle, R., Gaig, C., Santamaria, J., Tolosa, E., Riha, R. L., & Green, A. J. E. (2021). Detection of α-synuclein in CSF by RT-QuIC in patients with isolated rapid-eye-movement sleep behaviour disorder: A longitudinal observational study. *The Lancet Neurology, 20*(3), 203–212. https://doi.org/10.1016/S1474-4422(20)30449-X

Jafari, S., Etminan, M., Aminzadeh, F., & Ali, S. (2013). Head injury and risk of Parkinson disease: A systematic review and meta-analysis. *Movement Disorders, 28*(9), 1222–1229. https://doi.org/10.1002/mds.25458

Jankovic, J. (2011). The history of Parkinson's disease: Early clinical descriptions and neurological therapies. *Handbook of Clinical Neurology, 100*, 1–18. https://doi.org/10.1016/B978-0-444-52014-2.00001-0

Jankovic, & Poewe, W. (2012). Therapies in Parkinson's disease: An update and review. *Current Opinion in Neurology, 259*, S367–S378. https://doi.org/10.1007/s00415-012-6547-4

Jankovic, J., & Tan, E. K. (2024). In *Parkinson's disease: Etiology, clinical features, and diagnosis*.

Kalia, L. V., & Lang, A. E. (2015). Parkinson's disease. *The Lancet, 386*(9996), 896–912. https://doi.org/10.1016/S0140-6736(14)61393-3

Ketamine for depression in veterans with Parkinson's disease (NCT06231563).(2025).

Kordower, J. H., Fiandaca, M. S., & Freeman, T. B. (2023). Gene therapy for Parkinson's disease: Recent advances. *Nature Reviews Neurology, 19*, 23–34. https://doi.org/10.1038/s41582-022-00745-6

Lewy, F. H. (1912). Paralysis agitans. Pathologische Anatomie. *Handbuch der Neurologie, 3*.

Little, S., & Brown, P. (2014). Focusing brain therpaeutic interventions in space and time for Parkinson's disease. *Current Biology, 24*(18), R898–R909.

Little, S., Pogosyan, A., Neal, S., Zavala, B., Zrinzo, L., Hariz, M., Foltynie, T., Limousin, P., Ashkan, K., FitzGerald, J., Green, A. L., Aziz, T. Z., & Brown, P. (2013). Adaptive deep brain stimulation in advanced Parkinson disease. *Annals of Neurology, 74*(3), 449–457. https://doi.org/10.1002/ana.23951

LixiPark. (2024). In *A study of lixisenatide in early Parkinson's disease*.

Manyam, B. V. (1990). Paralysis agitans and levodopa in "Ayurveda": Ancient Indian medical treatise. *Movement Disorders, 5*(1), 47–48. https://doi.org/10.1002/mds.870050112

Medtronic. (2024). *Medtronic receives FDA approval for BrainSense adaptive DBS system*. Medtronic News.

Medtronic receives FDA approval for BrainSense adaptive DBS system. (2025). Medtronic Newsroom.

Michigan veterans with Parkinson's disease support group.(2025).

Mitsubishi Tanabe Pharma America presents open-label extension outcomes and additional data from Phase 3 BouNDless trial of investigational ND0612 in Parkinson's disease. (2024). Mitsubishi Tanabe Pharma America.

Mollenhauer, B., Caspell-Garcia, C. J., Coffey, C. S., Taylor, P., Singleton, A., Shaw, L. M., Trojanowski, J. Q., Frasier, M., Simuni, T., Iranzo, A., Oertel, W., Siderowf, A., Weintraub, D., Seibyl, J., Toga, A. W., Tanner, C. M., Kieburtz, K., Chahine, L. M., Marek, K., & Galasko, D. (2019). Longitudinal analyses of cerebrospinal fluid α-Synuclein in prodromal and early Parkinson's disease. *Movement Disorders, 34*(9), 1354–1364. https://doi.org/10.1002/mds.27806

Oertel, W., & Schulz, J. B. (2016). Current and experimental treatments of Parkinson disease: A guide for neuroscientists. *Journal of Neurochemistry, 139*(S1), 325–337. https://doi.org/10.1111/jnc.13750

Olanow, C. W., Kieburtz, K., Odin, P., Espay, A. J., Standaert, D. G., Fernandez, H. H., Vanagunas, A., Othman, A. A., Widnell, K. L., Robieson, W. Z., Pritchett, Y., Chatamra, K., Benesh, J., Lenz, R. A., & Antonini, A. (2014). Continuous intrajejunal infusion of levodopa-carbidopa intestinal gel for patients with advanced Parkinson's disease: A randomised, controlled, double-blind, double-dummy study. *The Lancet Neurology, 13*(2), 141–149. https://doi.org/10.1016/S1474-4422(13)70293-X

Olanow, C. W., Stern, M. B., & Sethi, K. (2009). The scientific and clinical basis for the treatment of Parkinson disease (2009). *Neurology, 72*(21), S1. https://doi.org/10.1212/WNL.0b013e3181a1d44c

Onapgo (apomorphine hydrochloride) FDA approval history.(2025).

Pagano, G., Taylor, K. I., Anzures-Cabrera, J., Marchesi, M., Simuni, T., Marek, K., Postuma, R. B., Pavese, N., Stocchi, F., Azulay, J. P., Mollenhauer, B., López-Manzanares, L., Russell, D. S., Boyd, J. T., Nicholas, A. P., Luquin, M. R., Hauser, R. A., Gasser, T., Poewe, W., … Bonni, A. (2022). Trial of Prasinezumab in early-stage Parkinson's disease. *New England Journal of Medicine, 387*(5), 421–432. https://doi.org/10.1056/NEJMoa2202867

Parkinson's, U. K. (2024). *LixiPark trial shows potential to slow Parkinson's progression.* Parkinson's UK News.

Papoutsi, C., Poots, A., Clements, J., Wyrko, Z., Offord, N., & Reed, J. E. (2018). Improving patient safety for older people in acute admissions: Implementation of the Frailsafe checklist in 12 hospitals across the UK. *Age and Ageing, 47*(2), 311–317. https://doi.org/10.1093/ageing/afx194

Parkinosn, J. (1817). An essay on the Shaking Palsy. Whittingham and Rowland.

Parkinson therapy ND0612 receives complete response letter. In . *NeurologyLive*, (2024).

Pharmaceutical Executive. (2025). In *FDA approves Supernus Pharmaceuticals' Onapgo for managing motor fluctuations in Parkinson disease.* Pharmaceutical Executive.

A phase 1b Study of AB-1005 in Parkinson's disease. NCT04167540.(2024).

Phase 3 of ND0612 clinical trial initiated in the United States for Parkinson's disease.(2025).

Poewe, W. (2024). In *Parkinson's disease drug therapies in the clinical trial pipeline.*

Poewe, W., Seppi, K., Tanner, C. M., Halliday, G. M., Brundin, P., Volkmann, J., Schrag, A. E., & Lang, A. E. (2017). Parkinson disease. *Nature Reviews Disease Primers, 3*, 1–21. https://doi.org/10.1038/nrdp.2017.13

Rascol, O., Brooks, D. J., Korczyn, A. D., De Deyn, P. P., Clarke, C. E., & Lang, A. E. (2000). A five-year study of the incidence of dyskinesia in patients with early Parkinson's disease who were treated with ropinirole or levodopa. *New England Journal of Medicine, 342*(20), 1484–1491. https://doi.org/10.1056/NEJM200005183422004

Rosenthal, A. S. (1980). Regulation of the immune response — Role of the macrophage. *New England Journal of Medicine, 303*(20), 1153–1156. https://doi.org/10.1056/NEJM198011133032005

Rosin, B., Slovik, M., Mitelman, R., Rivlin-Etzion, M., Haber, S. N., Israel, Z., Vaadia, E., & Bergman, H. (2011). Closed-loop deep brain stimulation is superior in amerliorating parkinsonism. *Neuron, 72*(2), 370–384.

Schapira, A. H. V., Chaudhuri, K. R., & Jenner, P. (2017). Non-motor features of Parkinson disease. *Nature Reviews Neuroscience, 18*(7), 435–450. https://doi.org/10.1038/nrn.2017.62

Schapira, A. H. V., Fox, S. H., & Hauser, t a (2020). Novel therapies for Parkinson's disease. *Lancet Neurology, 19*(4), 340–350. https://doi.org/10.1016/S1474-4422(19)30431-6

Schweitzer, J. S., Song, B., & Herrington. (2023). Phase 1 trial of autologous iPSC-derived dopaminergic progenitor cells for Parkinson's disease. *Nature Medicine, 29*, 1120–1128. https://doi.org/10.1038/s41591-023-02408-7

The story of Parkinson's disease. ATrain education.(2025).

A study to evaluate the efficacy and safety of Tavapadon in early Parkinson's disease.(2024).

Takahashi, J. (2023). Cell therapy for Parkinson's disease with induced pluripotent stem cells. *Journal of Parkinson's Disease, 13*(s1), 79. https://doi.org/10.3233/JPD-223592

Tanner, C. M., Kame, F., Ross, G. W., Hoppin, J. A., Goldman, S. M., Korell, M., Marras, C., Bhudhikanok, G. S., Kasten, M., Chade, A. R., Comyns, K., Richards, M. B., Meng, C., Priestley, B., Fernandez, H. H., Cambi, F., Umbach, D. M., Blair, A., Sandler, D. P., & Langston, J. W. (2011). Rotenone, paraquat, and Parkinson's disease. *Environmental Health Perspectives, 119*(6), 866–872. https://doi.org/10.1289/ehp.1002839

Telehealth for veterans with Parkinson's disease. (2025). U.S. Department of Veterans Affairs Office of Research & Development.

Therapeutics. (2024). In *BlueRock therapeutics announces positive 24-Month data from phase 1 study of bemdaneprocel in Parkinson's disease.*

U., Department of Veterans Affairs. (2025). In *Parkinson's disease in veterans: Research and care.*
UCB announces first patient dosed in ATLANTIS phase 2 study of UCB0022 (Glovadalen) in Parkinson's disease. (2023). UCB Press Release.
Veterans and Parkinson's disease. (2025). Parkinson's Foundation.
Walusinski, O. (2018). Jean-Martin Charcot and Parkinson's disease: Teaching and teaching materials. *Revue Neurologique, 174*(7–8), 491–505. https://doi.org/10.1016/j.neurol.2017.08.005
Weaver, F. M., Follett, K., Stern, M., Hur, K., Harris, C., Marks, W. J., Rothlind, J., Sagher, O., Reda, D., Moy, C. S., Pahwa, R., Burchiel, K., Hogarth, P., Lai, E. C., Duda, J. E., Holloway, K., Samii, A., Horn, S., Bronstein, J., … Huang, G. D. (2009). Bilateral deep brain stimulation vs best medical therapy for patients with advanced Parkinson disease: A randomized controlled trial. *JAMA, 301*(1), 63–73. https://doi.org/10.1001/jama.2008.929
Weisskopf, M. G. (2012). Traumatic brain injury and posttraumatic stress disorder as risk factors for Parkinson's disease. *JAMA Neurology, 69*(8), 1015–1022. https://doi.org/10.1001/archneurol.2012.2064
Zarate, t a (2017). Ketamine for depression: Clinical and preclinical studies. *Annual Review of Neuroscience, 40,* 1–23. https://doi.org/10.1146/annurev-neuro-072116-031232

Further reading

Foreman, K. B., Addison, O., & Dibble, L. E. (2011). Testing balance and fall risk in persons with Parkinson disease, an argument for ecologically valid testing. *Parkinsonism & Related Disorders, 17*(3). https://doi.org/10.1016/j.parkreldis.2010.12.007
The Fox Foundation. (2024). In *Adaptive DBS: A new era for Parkinson's treatment.* MJFF News.

CHAPTER

5 Environmental neurotoxins, circadian rhythms and their pharmacological antagonists in Parkinson's disease

Maha Awan
Sulaiman Al Rajhi University, Al Bukayriyah, Saudi Arabia

5.1 Introduction

Parkinson's Disease (PD) is the second most common neurodegenerative disorder globally, characterized by a progressive loss of dopaminergic neurons in the substantia nigra pars compacta (SNpc) and the presence of intraneuronal proteinaceous inclusions known as Lewy bodies, primarily composed of aggregated alpha-synuclein (α-syn) (Subramaniam & Chesselet, 2013). This pathology leads to a deficiency of dopamine in the striatum, manifesting clinically as cardinal motor symptoms: bradykinesia, resting tremor, rigidity, and postural instability. Beyond motor impairments, PD encompasses a wide spectrum of non-motor symptoms (NMS), including olfactory dysfunction, sleep disturbances, autonomic dysfunction, cognitive impairment, and psychiatric issues, which significantly impact patients' quality of life and can precede motor onset by years (Tieu, 2011).

Current pharmacotherapies for PD, such as levodopa and dopamine agonists, primarily offer symptomatic relief by replenishing dopamine levels or mimicking dopamine activity (Armstrong & Okun, 2020). However, these treatments do not halt or reverse the underlying neurodegenerative process, and long-term use is often associated with motor complications like dyskinesias and "wearing-off" phenomena (Ntetsika et al., 2021). The quest for disease-modifying therapies remains a critical unmet need in PD research (Ntetsika et al., 2021).

While genetic factors contribute to a subset of PD cases (approximately 5%–10%) (Tieu, 2011), the majority are considered sporadic, arising from a complex interplay between genetic predisposition and environmental influences (Subramaniam & Chesselet, 2013). A growing body of evidence implicates exposure to various environmental neurotoxins—including certain pesticides, industrial solvents, heavy metals, and components of air pollution—as significant risk factors for PD (Dorsey & Bloem, 2024). These toxicants are thought to contribute to PD pathogenesis by inducing oxidative stress, mitochondrial dysfunction, neuroinflammation, and promoting α-syn aggregation, pathways that are central to the neurodegenerative cascade in PD (Dias et al., 2013).

Concurrently, disruptions in the circadian rhythm, the body's internal 24-hour clock, are increasingly recognized as an integral feature of PD, often manifesting as sleep-wake cycle

Pharmacological Foundations of Parkinson's Disease. https://doi.org/10.1016/B978-0-443-27702-3.00015-7

disturbances (e.g., REM sleep behavior disorder (RBD), insomnia, excessive daytime sleepiness (EDS)), altered hormonal profiles (e.g., melatonin, cortisol), and dysregulation of core body temperature (Chen et al., 2024). These circadian disturbances are not merely symptoms but are thought to have a bidirectional relationship with PD pathology: neurodegeneration can impair circadian control mechanisms, and conversely, chronic circadian dysfunction may exacerbate neuroinflammation, oxidative stress, and protein misfolding, thereby contributing to disease progression and symptom severity (Chen et al., 2024). Furthermore, emerging research suggests a potential interplay where environmental neurotoxins might induce or worsen circadian dysregulation, and a disrupted circadian system could increase vulnerability to these toxins (Asadpoordezaki et al., 2023).

This chapter aims to provide a comprehensive overview of the roles of environmental neurotoxins and circadian rhythm disruption in the pathophysiology of PD. It will delve into the mechanisms by which specific toxins contribute to neuronal damage and explore how circadian dysregulation interfaces with these processes. Critically, this chapter will review the current landscape and future prospects of pharmacological antagonists and therapeutic strategies designed to counteract the detrimental effects of these environmental and chronobiological factors, with the ultimate goal of identifying novel avenues for slowing disease progression and improving the lives of individuals with PD. The multifactorial nature of PD, involving genetic susceptibility, environmental exposures, and endogenous processes like circadian rhythmicity, underscores the need for a holistic understanding to develop effective, personalized therapeutic interventions.

5.2 Pathophysiology of Parkinson's disease

Parkinson's Disease (PD) is a complex neurodegenerative disorder with a multifaceted pathophysiology. Understanding the core pathological features and the intricate molecular mechanisms driving neuronal demise is crucial for developing effective therapeutic interventions.

5.2.1 Core pathological features

The cardinal pathological hallmarks of PD are the progressive loss of dopaminergic (DA) neurons, particularly in the substantia nigra pars compacta (SNpc), and the widespread presence of intracytoplasmic protein aggregates known as Lewy bodies and Lewy neurites (Subramaniam & Chesselet, 2013). The SNpc is a critical brain region involved in motor control, and its DA neurons project to the striatum. The degeneration of these neurons leads to a significant reduction in striatal dopamine levels, typically by 60%–80% at the time of motor symptom onset, which underlies the characteristic motor impairments of PD such as bradykinesia, resting tremor, rigidity, and postural instability (Tieu, 2011). While the SNpc is the most prominently affected region, neurodegeneration also occurs in other dopaminergic and non-dopaminergic areas of the central and peripheral nervous systems, contributing to the diverse array of non-motor symptoms observed in PD (Tieu, 2011) (Fig. 5.1).

Lewy bodies are primarily composed of misfolded and aggregated alpha-synuclein (α-syn), a presynaptic protein whose normal function is not fully elucidated but is thought to be involved in synaptic vesicle trafficking and neurotransmitter release (Subramaniam & Chesselet, 2013). The accumulation and aggregation of α-syn into insoluble fibrils are considered central to PD pathogenesis, leading to cellular dysfunction and eventual neuronal death (Dias et al., 2013).

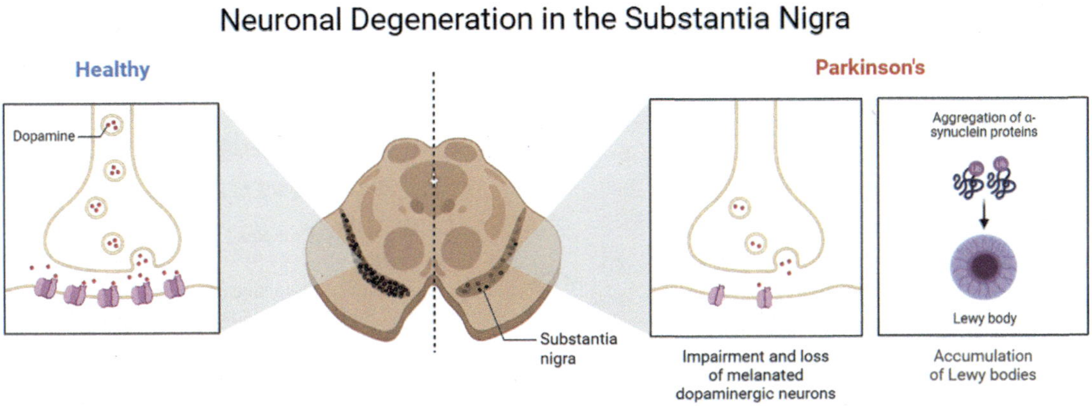

FIGURE 5.1

Neuronal degeneration in the substantia nigra.

Created with BioRender.com

5.2.2 Key molecular mechanisms

Several interconnected molecular mechanisms are believed to contribute to the neurodegenerative process in PD. These pathways often influence each other, creating a vicious cycle that perpetuates neuronal damage (Fig. 5.2).

5.2.2.1 Oxidative stress

Oxidative stress, resulting from an imbalance between the production of reactive oxygen species (ROS) and the brain's antioxidant defense mechanisms, is a prominent feature in PD (Dias et al., 2013). Dopaminergic neurons in the SNpc are particularly vulnerable due to several factors:

- **Dopamine Metabolism:** The enzymatic metabolism of dopamine by monoamine oxidase (MAO-B) and its auto-oxidation generate ROS, including hydrogen peroxide (H2O2) and superoxide anions (O2−). H2O2 can further react with ferrous iron (Fe2+) via the Fenton reaction to produce highly reactive hydroxyl radicals (OH) (Zhou et al., 2023). This inherent characteristic of dopamine metabolism creates a pro-oxidant environment within these neurons.
- **Mitochondrial Dysfunction:** Mitochondria are a major source of ROS. Impairment of the mitochondrial electron transport chain (ETC), particularly Complex I, leads to electron leakage and increased O2− production (Dias et al., 2013).
- **Elevated Iron Levels:** Increased levels of iron have been consistently found in the SNpc of PD patients. Iron can catalyze the formation of OH radicals, exacerbating oxidative damage (Dias et al., 2013).
- **Neuroinflammation:** Activated microglia and astrocytes release ROS and reactive nitrogen species (RNS), such as nitric oxide (NO), which can react with O2− to form peroxynitrite (ONOO−), a potent oxidant and nitrating agent (Dias et al., 2013).
- **Reduced Antioxidant Defenses:** Depletion of antioxidants like glutathione (GSH) further compromises the ability of neurons to neutralize ROS (Dias et al., 2013).

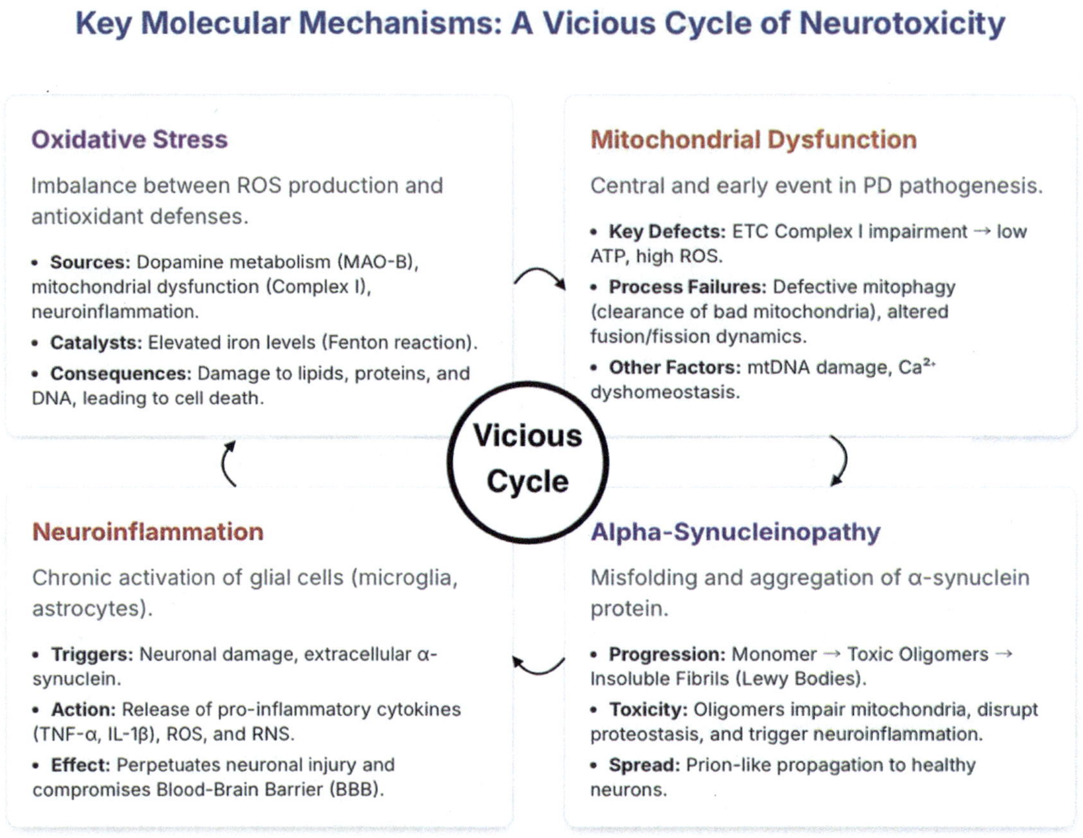

FIGURE 5.2

Key molecular mechanisms: a vicious cycle of neurotoxicity.

Oxidative stress leads to damage of critical cellular components, including lipids (lipid peroxidation), proteins (protein carbonylation and nitration), and nucleic acids (DNA and RNA oxidation), ultimately contributing to neuronal dysfunction and death (Dias et al., 2013).

5.2.2.2 Mitochondrial dysfunction

Mitochondrial dysfunction is a central and early event in both sporadic and familial forms of PD (Subramaniam & Chesselet, 2013). Key aspects include:

- **Complex I Impairment:** Reduced activity of mitochondrial ETC Complex I is a well-established finding in the SNpc of PD patients and can be induced by environmental toxins (e.g., MPTP, rotenone) and genetic mutations (e.g., *PINK1*, *LRRK2*) (Subramaniam & Chesselet, 2013). This defect leads to decreased ATP production, impaired calcium buffering, and increased ROS generation (Subramaniam & Chesselet, 2013).
- **Altered Mitochondrial Dynamics:** Mitochondria are dynamic organelles that undergo continuous fusion and fission. Imbalances in these processes, often linked to PD-associated genes

like *PINK1*, *Parkin*, and *LRRK2*, result in fragmented or overly fused mitochondria, impairing their function and distribution (Subramaniam & Chesselet, 2013).

- **Defective Mitophagy:** Mitophagy is a selective form of autophagy responsible for clearing damaged mitochondria. Mutations in *PINK1* and *Parkin* impair mitophagy, leading to the accumulation of dysfunctional mitochondria, which further generate ROS and release pro-apoptotic factors (Subramaniam & Chesselet, 2013).
- **Mitochondrial DNA (mtDNA) Damage:** mtDNA is particularly susceptible to oxidative damage due to its proximity to ROS production sites and limited repair mechanisms. Accumulation of mtDNA mutations can further compromise mitochondrial function (Subramaniam & Chesselet, 2013).
- **Calcium Dyshomeostasis:** Dysregulation of intracellular calcium (Ca2+) homeostasis can lead to mitochondrial Ca2+ overload, triggering the mitochondrial permeability transition pore (mPTP) opening, swelling, and release of apoptotic factors. SNpc neurons have a high reliance on L-type Ca2+ channels for pacemaking activity, making them susceptible to Ca2+-induced mitochondrial stress (Subramaniam & Chesselet, 2013).

The interplay between mitochondrial dysfunction and oxidative stress creates a detrimental feedback loop, where each exacerbates the other, driving neurodegeneration (Dias et al., 2013).

5.2.2.3 Neuroinflammation

Chronic neuroinflammation, characterized by the activation of glial cells (microglia and astrocytes), is another key contributor to PD pathology (Dias et al., 2013).

- **Microglial Activation:** In PD, microglia become activated by various stimuli, including neuronal damage, extracellular α-syn aggregates, and toxins. Activated microglia can adopt different phenotypes, with the M1 pro-inflammatory state being predominant in PD, releasing cytotoxic factors (Dias et al., 2013).
- **Release of Inflammatory Mediators:** Activated microglia and astrocytes release a plethora of inflammatory molecules, including pro-inflammatory cytokines (e.g., tumor necrosis factor-alpha (TNF-α), interleukin-1 beta (IL-1\beta), IL-6), chemokines, ROS, RNS (via inducible nitric oxide synthase, iNOS), and glutamate (Dias et al., 2013). These mediators perpetuate the inflammatory response and directly contribute to neuronal injury and death.
- **Blood-Brain Barrier (BBB) Dysfunction:** Neuroinflammation can compromise the integrity of the BBB, allowing peripheral immune cells and inflammatory molecules to infiltrate the brain, further amplifying the neuroinflammatory cascade (Rekatsina et al., 2020).

Neuroinflammation is not merely a consequence of neuronal death but an active contributor to the progressive nature of neurodegeneration in PD (Dias et al., 2013).

5.2.2.4 Alpha-synucleinopathy

The misfolding, aggregation, and accumulation of α-syn are central to the pathogenesis of PD and other synucleinopathies (Subramaniam & Chesselet, 2013).

- **Factors Promoting Aggregation:** Several factors can trigger or accelerate α-syn misfolding and aggregation, including genetic mutations in the *SNCA* gene (encoding α-syn), post-translational modifications (e.g., phosphorylation, nitration, ubiquitination), oxidative stress, dopamine and its oxidation products, metal ions (e.g., iron, copper), and interactions with lipid membranes (Ball et al., 2019).

- **Neurotoxic Species:** Small soluble oligomers and protofibrils of α-syn are considered the most neurotoxic species, rather than the large insoluble fibrils found in Lewy bodies. These oligomers can disrupt cellular homeostasis through various mechanisms (Dias et al., 2013).
- **Mechanisms of Toxicity:** Aggregated α-syn can:
  - Impair mitochondrial function by interacting with mitochondrial membranes and proteins, inhibiting Complex I activity, and inducing mPTP opening (Subramaniam & Chesselet, 2013).
  - Disrupt proteostasis by inhibiting the ubiquitin-proteasome system (UPS) and autophagic pathways, leading to the accumulation of misfolded proteins (Dias et al., 2013).
  - Interfere with synaptic vesicle trafficking and neurotransmitter release (Dias et al., 2013).
  - Induce endoplasmic reticulum (ER) stress.
  - Increase plasma membrane permeability and disrupt calcium homeostasis.
  - Activate microglia and astrocytes, triggering neuroinflammation (Dias et al., 2013).
- **Prion-like Propagation:** Misfolded α-syn can spread from affected neurons to healthy, interconnected neurons in a prion-like manner, contributing to the progressive and topographical spread of pathology in PD (Dias et al., 2013).

The interconnectedness of these pathological mechanisms—oxidative stress, mitochondrial dysfunction, neuroinflammation, and α-synucleinopathy—is a critical concept. Each process can initiate or exacerbate the others, creating a self-amplifying cascade of neurotoxicity that drives the relentless progression of PD. For instance, mitochondrial dysfunction generates ROS, which promotes α-syn aggregation and inflammation. Aggregated α-syn, in turn, can impair mitochondrial and proteasomal function and activate glia, further fueling oxidative stress and inflammation. Dopamine itself, while essential for neuronal function, also contributes to this vulnerability through its oxidative metabolism and interaction with α-syn (Zhou et al., 2023). Understanding these intricate interactions is paramount for developing therapies that can effectively target multiple points in this complex pathogenic network.

5.3 Environmental neurotoxins and Parkinson's disease

The etiology of Parkinson's Disease (PD) is increasingly understood as a complex interplay between genetic susceptibility and environmental factors. Among these, exposure to specific neurotoxins present in the environment has garnered significant attention as a potential contributor to PD development and progression (Dorsey & Bloem, 2024). These toxins, originating from various sources such as agricultural practices, industrial processes, and pollution, can induce pathological changes in the brain that mirror those seen in idiopathic PD.

5.3.1 Overview of environmental risk factors

A substantial body of epidemiological and experimental research supports the role of environmental toxicants in PD. These agents can enter the body through multiple routes, including ingestion, inhalation, and dermal contact, and subsequently reach the brain, where they can exert their neurotoxic effects (Dorsey & Bloem, 2024) (Table 5.1). Many of these toxins share common mechanisms of action, such as the induction of oxidative stress, impairment of mitochondrial function, promotion of neuroinflammation, and disruption of protein homeostasis, particularly affecting alpha-synuclein (α-syn) (Ball et al., 2019). The long latency period often observed between exposure and disease onset, coupled with variability in individual susceptibility (influenced by genetic makeup, duration and intensity of exposure, and concurrent exposures), complicates the definitive establishment of causal links but strengthens the argument for a significant environmental contribution to PD.

5.3.2 Specific neurotoxins and their mechanisms in PD pathogenesis

5.3.2.1 Pesticides and herbicides

Exposure to pesticides and herbicides has been consistently associated with an increased risk of PD in numerous epidemiological studies (Grotewold & Albin, 2024). Several specific compounds have been extensively studied for their ability to induce parkinsonian pathology in experimental models.

- **Rotenone:** This naturally derived pesticide is a potent inhibitor of mitochondrial Complex I, a key enzyme in the electron transport chain. By inhibiting Complex I, rotenone leads to ATP depletion, increased production of reactive oxygen species (ROS), and oxidative stress (Sherer et al., 2003). Experimental exposure to rotenone in animal models can replicate many features of PD, including selective dopaminergic neuron degeneration in the substantia nigra pars compacta (SNpc) and the formation of α-syn-positive cytoplasmic inclusions resembling Lewy bodies (Sherer et al., 2003). Beyond mitochondrial inhibition, rotenone has also been shown to impair microtubule dynamics and affect the RhoGTPase RhoA pathway, potentially disrupting axonal transport and neuronal polarity (Bisbal & Sanchez, 2019). Epidemiological studies have reported associations between rotenone exposure and increased PD risk, with some studies showing significantly elevated odds ratios, although the number of individuals with direct, high-level exposure may be limited (Greenamyre et al., 2010).
- **Paraquat:** This widely used herbicide is structurally similar to MPP+, the toxic metabolite of MPTP (1-methyl-4-phenyl-1,2,3,6-tetrahydropyridine). Paraquat's neurotoxicity is primarily mediated by its ability to undergo redox cycling, generating superoxide radicals and inducing oxidative stress (Rappold et al., 2011). Its entry into dopaminergic neurons is thought to be facilitated by transporters such as the dopamine transporter (DAT), particularly after its reduction to a monovalent cation (PQ+), and the organic cation transporter-3 (Oct3) may play a modulating role in its clearance from non-dopaminergic cells. Exposure to paraquat has been shown to cause dopaminergic cell loss and α-syn upregulation and aggregation in animal models (Rappold et al., 2011). Epidemiological studies, especially those considering co-exposure with other pesticides like the fungicide maneb (a dithiocarbamate), have frequently reported an increased risk of PD (Grotewold & Albin, 2024). However, some reviews of reviews suggest that a definitive causal link between paraquat alone (Richardson et al., 2019) and PD has not been unequivocally established, emphasizing the need for higher quality epidemiological data (Weed, 2021).
- **Other Pesticides (Maneb, Organochlorines, Benomyl):**
  - **Maneb:** This manganese-containing dithiocarbamate fungicide is often studied in conjunction with paraquat. Its neurotoxicity may involve mechanisms related to its manganese content and has been shown to induce PD-like phenotypes in mice, potentially involving asparagine endopeptidase (AEP) (Domico et al., 2006).

Table 5.1 Key environmental neurotoxins implicated in Parkinson's disease.

Neurotoxin class	Specific agent(s)	Key proposed mechanisms of neurotoxicity	Selected epidemiological evidence for PD risk association	References
Pesticides/ Herbicides	Rotenone	Mitochondrial complex I inhibition, ATP depletion, oxidative stress, microtubule disruption, α-syn aggregation	Animal models show PD pathology; human studies suggest risk	Sherer et al. (2003)
	Paraquat (often with Maneb)	Redox cycling, superoxide generation, oxidative stress, DAT-mediated uptake (as PQ+), α-syn upregulation/ aggregation	Increased risk, especially with Maneb co-exposure	Grotewold and Albin (2024)
	Maneb	Mn-containing dithiocarbamate, potential AEP involvement	Increased risk, often studied with paraquat	Grotewold and Albin (2024)
	Organochlorines (e.g., Dieldrin)	GABA-A receptor effects, oxidative stress, mitochondrial dysfunction, proteasomal impairment	Some studies suggest association	Grotewold and Albin (2024)
	Benomyl	ALDH inhibition, DOPAL accumulation, selective dopaminergic damage	Associated with increased PD risk	Fitzmaurice et al. (2013)
Industrial solvents	Trichlorethylene (TCE)	Mitochondrial dysfunction (complex I), TaClo metabolite formation, LRRK2 activation, oxidative stress	Occupational exposure, contaminated water (Camp Lejeune)	Dorsey et al. (2023)
	Perchlorethylene (PERC), carbon tetrachloride (CCl_4)	Oxidative stress, microglial activation, mitochondrial dysfunction	Trend toward increased risk in twin study	Goldman et al. (2012)

Table 5.1 Key environmental neurotoxins implicated in Parkinson's disease.—cont'd

Neurotoxin class	Specific agent(s)	Key proposed mechanisms of neurotoxicity	Selected epidemiological evidence for PD risk association	References
Heavy metals	Manganese (Mn)	Oxidative stress, mitochondrial dysfunction, neuroinflammation, disruption of dopamine/glutamate/GABA systems, transporter dysregulation (SLC30A10, SLC39A14)	Welders, contaminated water; Manganism shares features with PD	Magro et al. (2025)
	Lead (Pb)	Calcium dysregulation, oxidative stress, mitochondrial damage, genotoxicity, potential α-syn fibrillation	Occupational exposure associated with increased risk	Sanders et al. (2009)
Air pollution	PM2.5, NO2, ultrafine particles, CO, O3	Neuroinflammation, BBB disruption, oxidative stress, α-syn pathology, direct entry to brain via olfactory nerve	Long-term exposure to PM2.5, NO2 associated with risk	Xie et al. (2025)

- **Organochlorine Pesticides (e.g., Dieldrin):** Dieldrin, a persistent organochlorine, has been detected in post-mortem PD brains and is linked to neurotoxicity through mechanisms including GABAA receptor effects, severe oxidative stress, mitochondrial dysfunction, and proteasomal impairment (Richardson et al., 2019). Epidemiological studies have suggested an association between organochlorine exposure and PD risk (Grotewold & Albin, 2024).
- **Benomyl:** This fungicide has been shown to inhibit aldehyde dehydrogenase (ALDH), leading to the accumulation of the toxic dopamine metabolite 3,4-dihydroxyphenylacetaldehyde (DOPAL), which can cause selective dopaminergic neuronal damage. Higher exposure to benomyl has been associated with increased PD risk in epidemiological studies (Fitzmaurice et al., 2013). A study nested in the Agricultural Health Study found that PD was positively associated with groups of pesticides that impair mitochondrial function (overall OR = 1.7) or cause oxidative stress (overall OR = 2.0), supporting the role of these mechanisms in human PD. Specific pesticides like benomyl (mitochondrial inhibitor) and permethrin (both mitochondrial inhibitor and oxidative stressor) showed positive associations (Tanner et al., 2011).

5.3.2.2 Industrial solvents

Occupational and environmental exposure to certain industrial solvents has also been implicated in PD.

- **Trichlorethylene (TCE):** TCE is a common environmental contaminant found in groundwater and used in various industrial applications like metal degreasing and dry cleaning. Animal studies demonstrate that TCE can induce selective dopaminergic neurodegeneration and mitochondrial dysfunction (particularly Complex I inhibition), and activate LRRK2 kinase activity (Dorsey et al., 2023). Its metabolite, TaClo (1-trichloromethyl-1,2,3,4-tetrahydro-β-carboline), is also suspected to contribute to its neurotoxicity (Dorsey et al., 2023). Epidemiological evidence includes case reports, occupational studies showing increased PD risk (e.g., a 500% increased risk in one study), and notable clusters such as individuals exposed to contaminated water at Camp Lejeune who later developed PD (Dorsey et al., 2023).
- Other Solvents (Perchlorethylene - PERC, Carbon Tetrachloride - CCl_4): PERC (tetrachloroethylene) and CCl_4 are also ubiquitous environmental contaminants. A study in discordant twin pairs found that exposure to PERC (OR 10.5, trending toward significance) and CCl_4 (OR 2.3, trending toward significance) was associated with an increased risk of PD. These solvents are thought to share mechanisms with TCE, including the induction of oxidative stress, microglial activation, and mitochondrial dysfunction (Goldman et al., 2012).

5.3.2.3 Heavy metals

Exposure to certain heavy metals, through occupational settings or environmental contamination, is another area of concern for PD risk.

- **Manganese (Mn):** Chronic overexposure to manganese can lead to a neurological disorder known as manganism, which shares some motor features with PD (e.g., bradykinesia, rigidity, postural instability) but also has distinct characteristics (e.g., "cock-walk" gait, earlier cognitive/psychiatric symptoms, poor levodopa response, specific MRI findings). Mechanisms of Mn neurotoxicity include oxidative stress, mitochondrial dysfunction, neuroinflammation, and disruption of neurotransmitter systems (dopamine, glutamate, GABA) (Magro et al., 2025). Mn accumulation is particularly noted in the basal ganglia, especially the globus pallidus in classical manganism, though chronic lower-level exposure may also affect the SNpc (Lucchini & Tieu, 2023). Transporters like SLC30A10 and SLC39A14 play a crucial role in Mn homeostasis, and mutations in these genes lead to inherited forms of hypermanganesemia with parkinsonism-dystonia (Magro et al., 2025). Epidemiological studies have linked chronic Mn exposure, particularly in welders and those exposed to contaminated drinking water, to an increased risk of parkinsonism and a more rapid progression of motor symptoms (Lucchini & Tieu, 2023).
- **Lead (Pb):** Lead is a well-known neurotoxicant. Proposed mechanisms relevant to PD include interference with calcium regulation and signaling, induction of oxidative stress, mitochondrial damage, and genotoxic effects (Sanders et al., 2009). Lead can cross the blood-brain barrier and accumulate in the brain (Sanders et al., 2009). Epidemiological studies, particularly those using objective measures of chronic exposure like bone lead levels, have reported an association between occupational lead exposure and an increased risk of PD, with odds ratios greater than 2 for the highest exposure quartiles. Heavy metal cations like lead have also been suggested to stimulate free radical formation and promote α-syn fibrillation (Coon et al., 2006). However, specific pathways

linking lead directly to dopaminergic neurodegeneration in PD, beyond general neurotoxicity, are less clearly defined than for toxins like MPTP or rotenone (Sanders et al., 2009).

5.3.2.4 Air pollution

Ambient air pollution, a complex mixture of particulate matter (PM), gases, and chemicals, is increasingly recognized as a risk factor for neurodegenerative diseases, including PD (Dorsey & Bloem, 2024).

- **Components:** Key components implicated include fine particulate matter (PM2.5—particles with a diameter <2.5 μm), ultrafine particles (<0.1 μm), nitrogen dioxide (NO2), ozone (O3), and carbon monoxide (CO). These particles can carry various toxic substances, including heavy metals and organic compounds like polycyclic aromatic hydrocarbons (PAHs) (Xie et al., 2025).
- **Mechanisms:** Air pollutants are thought to contribute to PD pathogenesis via several mechanisms:
  - **Neuroinflammation:** PM2.5 can cross the compromised blood-brain barrier (BBB) or enter via the olfactory nerve, triggering microglial activation and the release of pro-inflammatory cytokines (Xie et al., 2025).
  - **Oxidative Stress:** Inhalation of pollutants induces systemic and central oxidative stress (Atterling Brolin et al., 2025).
  - **Blood-Brain Barrier Disruption:** Inflammation and oxidative stress can damage the BBB, increasing its permeability to neurotoxic agents (Xie et al., 2025).
  - **Alpha-Synuclein Pathology:** Animal models show that exposure to particulate matter can promote α-syn aggregation and propagation, potentially via the olfactory bulb. Autopsy studies have also found α-syn pathology in individuals exposed to high air pollution levels (Atterling Brolin et al., 2025).
- **Epidemiological Evidence:** Several epidemiological studies have reported associations between long-term exposure to PM2.5 and NO2 and an increased risk of PD, with odds ratios for PM2.5 around 1.10–1.34 per 5 $\mu g/m^3$ increase. However, results for other pollutants like PM10 and ozone are less consistent (Xie et al., 2025).

The diversity of these environmental neurotoxins, their ubiquitous presence, and their shared mechanistic themes—particularly the induction of oxidative stress and mitochondrial dysfunction—underscore the importance of environmental factors in PD. Furthermore, the concept of gene-environment interactions is crucial; genetic predispositions may render individuals more vulnerable to the neurotoxic effects of these environmental agents (Dorsey & Bloem, 2024). For example, variants in genes involved in dopamine transporter (*DAT*) have been linked to higher PD risk upon paraquat exposure (Rappold et al., 2011), and TCE exposure has been shown to activate LRRK2 kinase, a gene implicated in familial PD (Dorsey et al., 2023). Accurately assessing exposure over long latent periods and accounting for complex mixtures and interactions remain significant challenges in epidemiological research (Dorsey & Bloem, 2024).

5.4 Circadian rhythm disruption and Parkinson's disease

The circadian system, an endogenous biological pacemaker, governs a multitude of physiological and behavioral processes in a roughly 24-hour cycle. Disruptions to this intricate system are increasingly recognized as a significant, and often early, feature of Parkinson's Disease (PD), contributing to both non-motor and motor symptoms and potentially influencing disease progression.

5.4.1 The human circadian system: an overview

The master circadian clock in mammals resides in the suprachiasmatic nucleus (SCN) of the anterior hypothalamus (Chen et al., 2024). The SCN integrates environmental light cues, perceived by intrinsically photosensitive retinal ganglion cells (ipRGCs), to synchronize the body's internal rhythms with the external light-dark cycle (Baser et al., 2025). At the molecular level, this rhythmicity is driven by a complex network of transcriptional-translational feedback loops (TTFLs) involving core clock genes such as *CLOCK* (Circadian Locomotor Output Cycles Kaput) and *BMAL1* (Brain and Muscle ARNT-Like 1), which form a heterodimer to activate the transcription of *Period* (*Per1, Per2, Per3*) and *Cryptochrome* (*Cry1, Cry2*) genes (Chen et al., 2024). The PER and CRY proteins, in turn, translocate to the nucleus to inhibit CLOCK-BMAL1 activity, thus completing the negative feedback loop (Chen et al., 2024). The SCN orchestrates peripheral clocks located in virtually all body tissues through neural and hormonal signals, including the rhythmic secretion of melatonin from the pineal gland (promoting sleep and suppressed by light) and cortisol from the adrenal glands (peaking in the early morning). This hierarchical system ensures the temporal coordination of diverse functions like sleep-wake cycles, hormone release, metabolism, core body temperature, and immune responses (Chen et al., 2024).

5.4.2 Circadian disruption in Parkinson's disease patients

A wide array of circadian disruptions is highly prevalent in PD patients, often predating the onset of cardinal motor symptoms by years or even decades (Xu et al., 2024) (Table 5.2). These include:

- **Sleep-Wake Cycle Disturbances:** These are among the most common NMS in PD, affecting up to 90% of patients (Asadpoordezaki et al., 2023). Manifestations include:
- **REM Sleep Behavior Disorder (RBD):** Characterized by dream enactment behavior due to loss of normal muscle atonia during REM sleep. RBD is a strong prodromal marker for synucleinopathies, including PD (Xu et al., 2024).
- **Restless Legs Syndrome (RLS):** An urge to move the legs, typically accompanied by unpleasant sensations, often worsening at night (Xu et al., 2024).
- **Excessive Daytime Sleepiness (EDS):** Unintended episodes of sleepiness during the day (Xu et al., 2024).
- **Insomnia and Sleep Fragmentation:** Difficulty initiating or maintaining sleep and frequent nocturnal awakenings (Asadpoordezaki et al., 2023). Actigraphy studies often reveal reduced amplitude of rest-activity rhythms, increased nocturnal activity, and altered phasing (e.g., phase advance) in PD patients (Chen et al., 2024).
- **Altered Melatonin and Cortisol Profiles:** PD patients frequently exhibit dysregulated melatonin secretion, often characterized by reduced overall levels, blunted nocturnal peaks, or phase shifts in its rhythm. Cortisol rhythms can also be altered, with flattened diurnal profiles or phase shifts reported (Chen et al., 2024).
- **Dysregulation of Core Body Temperature:** The normal diurnal fluctuation in core body temperature can be blunted or phase-shifted in PD, particularly in patients with depression (Chen et al., 2024).

Table 5.2 Manifestations and mechanisms of circadian disruption in Parkinson's disease.

Circadian manifestation in PD	Common symptoms/ Signs	Underlying mechanisms/ Contributors in PD	References
Sleep-wake cycle disturbances	RBD, RLS, EDS, insomnia, sleep fragmentation, altered rest-activity rhythms (actigraphy)	Dopaminergic degeneration, α-synucleinopathy in sleep-regulating brainstem nuclei, SCN dysfunction, altered melatonin/cortisol, medication side effects, motor symptoms interfering with sleep.	Chen et al. (2024)
Hormonal rhythm alterations	Reduced/blunted/phase-shifted melatonin secretion, altered cortisol rhythm (e.g., flattened)	SCN dysfunction, impaired retinal input to SCN, direct effects of PD pathology on pineal gland or adrenal regulation, dopaminergic dysregulation.	Chen et al. (2024)
Core body temperature dysregulation	Blunted diurnal temperature rhythm, phase shifts	Hypothalamic dysfunction (including SCN), autonomic dysfunction common in PD.	Chen et al. (2024)
Clock gene expression changes	Altered expression/ rhythmicity of *BMAL1, PER1/2, CLOCK, CRY* in CNS and peripheral tissues	Direct impact of PD pathology (e.g., α-syn destabilizing *BMAL1* mRNA), neuroinflammation, oxidative stress affecting clock gene regulation, altered dopaminergic modulation of clock genes. Genetic polymorphisms in clock genes.	Chen et al. (2024)
Impact on PD pathogenesis	Exacerbation of neurodegeneration, oxidative stress, neuroinflammation, α-syn pathology	Impaired mitochondrial homeostasis, reduced antioxidant defense, pro-inflammatory state due to clock dysregulation, compromised BBB integrity, impaired proteostasis.	Chen et al. (2024)
Increased vulnerability to toxins	Enhanced neurotoxic effects of agents like MPTP	Weakened cellular defense mechanisms due to circadian disruption, impaired detoxification pathways.	Lauretti et al. (2017)

- **Changes in Clock Gene Expression:** Studies in PD patients and animal models have reported altered expression levels and rhythms of core clock genes (e.g., *BMAL1*, *PER1*, *PER2*, *CLOCK*, *CRY1*) in both central (e.g., SCN, substantia nigra, striatum) and peripheral tissues (e.g., blood cells, fibroblasts). Genetic polymorphisms in clock genes have also been associated with PD risk and symptom severity (Chen et al., 2024).

5.4.3 Bidirectional relationship between PD pathology and circadian dysfunction

The relationship between PD pathology and circadian dysfunction is increasingly viewed as bidirectional, forming a potential "vicious cycle" where each component can exacerbate the other (Asadpoordezaki et al., 2023).

5.4.3.1 Impact of PD pathology on circadian control systems

The neurodegenerative processes inherent to PD can directly impair the functionality of the circadian system:

- **Dopaminergic Degeneration:** Dopamine plays a modulatory role in circadian timing. Dopaminergic neurons project to the SCN, and dopamine signaling influences clock gene expression (e.g., *Per1*, *Per2*) in areas like the striatum and the retina's response to light (Asadpoordezaki et al., 2023). The profound loss of dopaminergic neurons in PD, therefore, disrupts these modulatory inputs to the circadian system. Animal models of PD (e.g., MPTP-induced) show that dopaminergic lesions lead to altered circadian rhythms of locomotor activity (Chen et al., 2024).
- **Alpha-Synucleinopathy:** Aggregated α-syn, the hallmark of PD, is not confined to the SNpc but also affects brain regions involved in circadian regulation, including the hypothalamus (where the SCN is located) and brainstem nuclei crucial for sleep-wake control. Furthermore, α-syn accumulation can directly interfere with clock gene function; for instance, it has been shown to destabilize *BMAL1* mRNA via miR-155, thereby disrupting core clock machinery (Chen et al., 2024). A continuum of circadian rhythm degradation is observed across α-synucleinopathies (Baser et al., 2025).
- **Neuroinflammation:** Chronic neuroinflammation in PD, driven by activated microglia and astrocytes, can release inflammatory mediators that disrupt SCN function and clock gene expression in various tissues (Chen et al., 2024).
- **SCN Pathology:** While not consistently reported, some studies suggest potential SCN neuronal loss or dysfunction in PD, which would directly impair the master clock's output. Hypothalamic volume loss has been observed in PD (Abbott et al., 2020).
- **Retinal Degeneration:** Degeneration of retinal ganglion cells, including ipRGCs that transmit light information to the SCN, can occur in PD, leading to impaired photic entrainment of the circadian clock (Abbott et al., 2020).

5.4.3.2 Contribution of circadian dysfunction to PD pathogenesis and symptoms

Conversely, primary or secondary circadian dysfunction can actively contribute to the development and progression of PD pathology and worsen symptoms:

- **Exacerbation of Neurodegeneration:** Disrupted circadian rhythms and clock gene dysregulation can impair fundamental cellular processes crucial for neuronal health, including:

- **Mitochondrial Homeostasis:** Clock genes regulate mitochondrial biogenesis, dynamics (fusion/fission), and mitophagy. Circadian disruption can lead to mitochondrial dysfunction, increased ROS production, and energy deficits, all implicated in PD neurodegeneration (Chen et al., 2024).
- **Oxidative Stress Response:** The expression of many antioxidant enzymes is under circadian control. Dysfunctional clocks can lead to impaired redox homeostasis and increased neuronal vulnerability to oxidative damage (Chen et al., 2024).
- **Proteostasis:** Autophagy and the ubiquitin-proteasome system, critical for clearing misfolded proteins like α-syn, exhibit circadian rhythmicity. Circadian disruption may impair these clearance mechanisms, promoting α-syn aggregation (Vallée et al., 2020).
- **Neuroinflammation:** Clock genes, particularly *BMAL1*, exert anti-inflammatory effects. Disruption of *BMAL1* or general circadian dysregulation can lead to a pro-inflammatory state, with increased microglial activation and cytokine production, thereby accelerating neurodegeneration (Chen et al., 2024).
- **Blood-Brain Barrier (BBB) Integrity:** The BBB's permeability is under circadian control. Disrupted rhythms can compromise BBB integrity, facilitating the entry of peripheral inflammatory factors and toxins into the brain (Chen et al., 2024).
- **Worsening of Motor and Non-Motor Symptoms:** Circadian misalignment can directly worsen PD symptoms. Sleep deprivation and fragmentation, common consequences of circadian disruption, are known to exacerbate motor deficits, cognitive impairment, fatigue, and mood disturbances in PD patients (Asadpoordezaki et al., 2023). The "wearing-off" phenomenon of levodopa may also have a circadian component, with drug absorption and efficacy varying across the day (Abbott et al., 2020).
- **Increased Disease Risk/Progression:** Chronic circadian disruption, such as that experienced by shift workers or due to societal factors ("social jet lag"), is increasingly considered an environmental risk factor that may lower the threshold for developing PD or accelerate its progression, especially in genetically susceptible individuals (Xu et al., 2024).

5.4.4 Interplay of environmental neurotoxins and circadian disruption in PD

The interaction between environmental neurotoxin exposure and circadian rhythm disruption represents a critical, yet less explored, facet of PD etiology. There is emerging evidence suggesting that these two factors can interact synergistically to promote neurodegeneration.

5.4.4.1 Neurotoxin-induced circadian disruption

Several environmental neurotoxins implicated in PD have been shown to disrupt circadian rhythms or clock gene expression in experimental models:

- **Pesticides:** Exposure to the pesticide rotenone in animal models of PD has been associated with altered expression of clock genes (e.g., phase shifts in *Bmal1* and *Per1*) in the SCN, reduced amplitude of locomotor and body temperature rhythms, and increased rhythm fragmentation (Asadpoordezaki et al., 2023). Co-exposure to lipopolysaccharide (LPS, an inflammagen) and rotenone in rats led to decreased expression of core clock genes (*Bmal1*, *Clock*, *Npas2*) and feedback genes (*Per1*, *Per2*), suggesting that inflammation potentiated by toxins can disrupt the clock (Li et al., 2019).

- **Heavy Metals:** Chronic lead exposure can cause alterations in SCN cells in developing rats. Cadmium has been shown to induce "chronotoxicity," disrupting circadian rhythms, partly via oxidative stress mechanisms. Copper overload may also adversely affect the circadian clock (Li et al., 2020).
- **General Pollutants/Endocrine Disruptors:** Some environmental pollutants and endocrine-disrupting chemicals (which can include certain pesticides) can dysregulate the endogenous circadian clock, potentially by interacting with xenobiotic response elements in the promoter regions of clock genes. Air pollution has also been linked to altered levels of circadian biomarkers like melatonin (Li et al., 2020).

These findings suggest that exposure to PD-relevant neurotoxins can directly impair the functioning of the circadian system, potentially contributing to the circadian abnormalities observed in PD patients.

5.4.4.2 Circadian disruption increasing vulnerability to neurotoxins

A disrupted circadian system may render the brain, particularly dopaminergic neurons, more susceptible to the damaging effects of environmental neurotoxins:

- Experimental studies have shown that pre-exposure to chronic circadian disruption (e.g., through altered light-dark cycles) significantly exacerbates MPTP-induced motor deficits, dopaminergic (TH-positive) cell loss in the SNpc, and neuroinflammation in mouse models of PD (Lauretti et al., 2017). This suggests that a compromised circadian system lowers the threshold for neurotoxin-induced parkinsonism.
- The circadian clock regulates cellular defense mechanisms, including antioxidant responses (e.g., glutathione levels) and xenobiotic metabolism (Li et al., 2020). Dysfunction of the clock could therefore impair the brain's ability to detoxify neurotoxins or protect against the oxidative stress they induce.

5.4.4.3 Shared pathophysiological mechanisms

Environmental neurotoxins and circadian dysfunction may converge on common downstream pathological pathways, thereby amplifying neurodegeneration in PD:

- **Oxidative Stress:** Both many neurotoxins (e.g., paraquat, rotenone, heavy metals) and circadian disruption (e.g., through mitochondrial dysregulation or impaired antioxidant gene expression) lead to increased oxidative stress. This convergence can create a particularly damaging environment for vulnerable neurons.
- **Neuroinflammation:** Neurotoxins can trigger microglial activation and inflammatory responses. Similarly, circadian disruption, particularly through *BMAL1* dysregulation, can lead to a pro-inflammatory state (Dias et al., 2013). The combined effect could lead to chronic, heightened neuroinflammation.
- **Impaired Proteostasis:** Both neurotoxic insults and circadian dysregulation can interfere with protein quality control mechanisms like the UPS and autophagy, leading to the accumulation of misfolded proteins such as α-syn.
- **Blood-Brain Barrier Disruption:** Neuroinflammation induced by either toxins or circadian disruption can compromise BBB integrity, creating a feed-forward loop of damage (Chen et al., 2024).

Understanding this three-way interaction between genetics, environmental neurotoxins, and circadian rhythm integrity is crucial for developing comprehensive preventative and therapeutic strategies for PD. The "vicious cycle" concept, where initial insults (be it toxin exposure or primary circadian dysfunction) trigger a cascade of pathological events that further weaken the system's resilience, is highly relevant here.

5.5 Pharmacological antagonists and therapeutic strategies

The growing understanding of the roles of environmental neurotoxins and circadian rhythm disruption in Parkinson's Disease (PD) pathogenesis has spurred research into pharmacological antagonists and therapeutic strategies aimed at mitigating these influences. These approaches range from targeting specific toxin-induced damage pathways to restoring circadian homeostasis, with the overarching goal of slowing disease progression and alleviating symptoms.

5.5.1 Counteracting environmental neurotoxin effects

Developing pharmacological interventions against environmental neurotoxins is challenging due to the diversity of toxins, their varied mechanisms, and the often long latency between exposure and disease onset. However, research has identified several potential avenues (Table 5.3).

5.5.1.1 Targeting pesticide/herbicide-induced neurotoxicity

Given the strong association between certain pesticides/herbicides and PD, strategies to counteract their specific toxic effects are of interest.

- **Rotenone:** As rotenone primarily acts by inhibiting mitochondrial Complex I and inducing oxidative stress and neuroinflammation, neuroprotective strategies focus on these mechanisms. The novel glucocorticoid receptor (GR) modulator, PT150, has shown promise in rotenone mouse models by reducing glial inflammation (microgliosis), diminishing dopaminergic neuron loss in the substantia nigra (SN), and decreasing the accumulation of neurotoxic misfolded α-synuclein (Latham et al., 2024). While PT150 did not prevent striatal terminal loss, its effect on SN neuronal survival highlights its potential. General neuroprotective agents targeting oxidative stress (e.g., antioxidants) and mitochondrial dysfunction (e.g., mitochondrial enhancers like Coenzyme Q10) are also theoretically relevant (Lin & Kang, 2005).
- **Paraquat (often with Maneb):** Paraquat induces oxidative stress via redox cycling. Caffeine, acting as an adenosine A2A receptor antagonist, has demonstrated neuroprotective effects against combined paraquat and maneb-induced dopaminergic neuron degeneration in mouse models, significantly reducing tyrosine hydroxylase (TH)-positive neuron loss (Kachroo et al., 2010). This suggests that A2A receptor antagonists could be a viable strategy.
- **Maneb:** The fungicide maneb, which contains manganese, induces PD-like neurotoxicity. Studies in mice have shown that inhibitors of asparagine endopeptidase (AEP) can attenuate the maneb-induced PD-like phenotype, suggesting AEP as a potential therapeutic target for maneb-induced toxicity (Liu et al., 2022).
- **Benomyl:** This fungicide inhibits aldehyde dehydrogenase (ALDH), leading to the accumulation of the toxic dopamine metabolite DOPAL (Fitzmaurice et al., 2013). While no specific antagonist for benomyl is highlighted, strategies to enhance ALDH activity or detoxify DOPAL could be beneficial.

Table 5.3 Investigational pharmacological antagonists for neurotoxin-induced effects relevant to Parkinson's disease.

Agent/Class	Target neurotoxin/ Mechanism	Proposed mechanism of action	Key preclinical/ Clinical findings	Developmental stage/Key snippets
Glucocorticoid receptor modulator (PT150)	Rotenone-induced neuroinflammation & neurodegeneration	Reduce glial activation, decrease α-syn accumulation, modulate astrocyte neuroprotective activity	Reduced DAn loss in SN, reduced microgliosis, modulated astrocyte reactivity in rotenone mouse model	Preclinical (Latham et al., 2024)
Adenosine A2A antagonist (caffeine)	Paraquat + Maneb-induced dopaminergic neurotoxicity	Blocks adenosine A2A receptors, potentially reducing excitotoxicity	Reduced TH + dopaminergic neuron loss in pesticide-exposed mice	Preclinical (for PD neuroprotection) (Kachroo et al., 2010)
Asparagine endopeptidase (AEP) inhibitor (compound #11)	Maneb-induced PD-like phenotype	Inhibits AEP activity	Attenuated PD-like motor impairment and neurochemical disturbances in maneb-exposed α-syn A53T transgenic mice	Preclinical (Liu et al., 2022)
N-Acetyl cysteine (NAC)	Organochlorine (Dieldrin)-induced oxidative stress	Antioxidant, restores glutathione levels	Blocked ROS generation and mitochondrial dysfunction, protected against dieldrin neurotoxicity in cell culture	Preclinical (Sharma et al., 2010)
Pomegranate juice	Carbon tetrachloride (CCl_4)-induced neurotoxicity	Antioxidant properties	Reversed CCl_4-induced increased AChE activity and cell death, suppressed oxidative stress markers in rat brain	Preclinical (Seidl & Potashkin, 2011)
Metal chelators (e.g., CaEDTA, PAS, PAS + CaEDTA)	Manganese (Mn) overload/ Manganism	Bind Mn ions, promoting their excretion and mobilizing from CNS	Improved clinical features of manganism, especially when combined (PAS + CaEDTA); increases urinary Mn excretion	Clinical use for Manganism (Evans & Masullo, 2023)
mGluR5 antagonist (MTEP)	MPTP-induced dopaminergic & noradrenergic neurodegeneration	Blocks mGluR5 receptors, modulating glutamate transmission	Significantly reduced MPTP toxicity toward DA and NA neurons in primate models	Preclinical (for PD neuroprotection) (Masilamoni et al., 2011)

- **Organochlorines (e.g., Dieldrin):** Dieldrin induces oxidative stress and mitochondrial dysfunction. The antioxidant N-acetyl cysteine (NAC) has been shown to block dieldrin-induced ROS generation and mitochondrial membrane potential decrease, protecting against its neurotoxicity in cell culture models (Sharma et al., 2010).

5.5.1.2 Addressing solvent-induced neurotoxicity

The neurotoxic mechanisms of solvents like TCE, PERC, and CCl_4 often involve oxidative stress and mitochondrial damage.

- **Trichlorethylene (TCE):** Currently, no specific pharmacological antagonists for TCE-induced neurotoxicity in the context of PD are well-established beyond general neuroprotective approaches targeting oxidative stress and mitochondrial health (Dorsey et al., 2023).
- **Perchlorethylene (PERC) and Carbon Tetrachloride (CCl_4):** For CCl_4-induced neurotoxicity, which involves significant oxidative stress, natural antioxidants like pomegranate juice have shown protective effects in animal models by reducing oxidative markers and apoptosis in brain tissue (Kalkan et al., 2024). Specific antagonists for PERC are not detailed in the provided materials (Goldman et al., 2012).

5.5.1.3 Mitigating heavy metal-induced neurotoxicity

Chelation therapy is the primary approach for heavy metal toxicity, aiming to remove the offending metal from the body.

- **Manganese (Mn):** For manganism, which shares features with PD, chelation therapy is employed. Traditional chelators like CaEDTA can increase Mn excretion but have limited efficacy on CNS symptoms due to poor BBB penetration. Newer strategies involve combination therapy, such as p-aminosalicylate (PAS) with CaEDTA. PAS is thought to penetrate the CNS and mobilize Mn from brain tissue, showing promise in improving clinical features of manganism, especially if initiated early (Aaseth & Nurchi, 2022). L-dopa has shown limited long-term benefit for manganism (Evans & Masullo, 2023).
- **Lead (Pb):** Lead toxicity also involves oxidative stress and interference with calcium signaling. While chelation is a general treatment for lead poisoning, specific chelating agents tailored for lead-induced neuroprotection in PD are not extensively detailed in the provided snippets, which focus more on iron chelation in PD (Seidl & Potashkin, 2011). General neuroprotective agents targeting oxidative stress and mitochondrial dysfunction may offer some benefit (Fahn & Sulzer, 2004).

5.5.1.4 General neuroprotective and anti-inflammatory strategies

Given that many environmental neurotoxins converge on common pathways like oxidative stress, mitochondrial dysfunction, and neuroinflammation, broad-spectrum neuroprotective and anti-inflammatory agents are relevant.

- **Metabotropic Glutamate Receptor 5 (mGluR5) Antagonists:** MTEP, an mGluR5 antagonist, showed significant neuroprotection against MPTP-induced dopaminergic and noradrenergic neuronal loss in primate models of PD, suggesting a role for glutamate modulation in mitigating toxin-induced damage (Masilamoni et al., 2011).

- **Antioxidants:** Agents like Coenzyme Q10, creatine, N-acetyl cysteine (NAC), and Vitamin E have been investigated for their potential to counteract oxidative stress in PD, with varying degrees of success in preclinical and clinical studies (Sharma et al., 2010).
- **Anti-inflammatory Agents:** Minocycline, an antibiotic with anti-inflammatory properties, has been explored for neuroprotection in PD (Seidl & Potashkin, 2011). Glucocorticoid receptor modulators like PT150 also act by reducing neuroinflammation (Latham et al., 2024).

The repurposing of existing drugs (e.g., caffeine, minocycline) and the investigation of natural compounds (e.g., pomegranate juice, ginsenosides offer potential avenues for accelerated drug development due to known safety profiles (Ma & Wang, 2024)). However, the translation from preclinical promise to clinical efficacy remains a significant hurdle for many neuroprotective agents.

5.5.2 Addressing circadian rhythm disruption in PD

Therapeutic strategies targeting circadian dysfunction in PD aim to restore rhythmicity, improve sleep, and potentially alleviate associated non-motor and even motor symptoms (Table 5.4).

5.5.2.1 Melatonin and melatonin receptor agonists

Melatonin, the primary hormone regulating sleep-wake cycles, and its agonists are logical candidates for treating circadian and sleep disturbances in PD.

- **Melatonin:** Supplementation with melatonin (e.g., 3 mg) has shown efficacy in improving subjective sleep quality (assessed by Pittsburgh Sleep Quality Index - PSQI), reducing daytime sleepiness (Epworth Sleepiness Scale - ESS), and improving polysomnography (PSG) parameters such as sleep latency and total sleep time in PD patients, as demonstrated in randomized controlled trials (Sugumaran et al., 2024). Furthermore, these improvements in sleep are often associated with benefits in overall non-motor symptoms (Non-Motor Symptoms Scale - NMSS) and quality of life (Parkinson's Disease Questionnaire - PDQ-39) (Sugumaran et al., 2024). Beyond its chronobiotic effects, melatonin possesses significant neuroprotective properties, including antioxidant (ROS scavenging, modulation of antioxidant enzymes), anti-inflammatory (cytokine inhibition, microglial modulation), anti-apoptotic, and anti-α-synuclein aggregation activities. It may also help prevent dopamine loss and restore circadian rhythm by influencing clock genes like *Bmal1* and *Per1* (Hu et al., 2023). The dual benefit of melatonin—addressing both circadian/sleep issues and potentially offering neuroprotection—makes it a particularly attractive agent.
- **Ramelteon:** This selective MT1/MT2 melatonin receptor agonist (typically 8 mg) has shown beneficial effects on RBD and general sleep disturbances in PD patients in open-label trials (Kashihara et al., 2016). While its efficacy for idiopathic RBD is less clear, it is generally well-tolerated, especially in elderly individuals, which is an advantage over agents like clonazepam (Esaki et al., 2016).
- **Agomelatine:** Agomelatine is unique as it combines MT1/MT2 receptor agonism with 5-HT2C serotonin receptor antagonism (Fornaro et al., 2010). This dual mechanism contributes to its efficacy in treating depression in PD patients. Importantly, studies have shown that agomelatine also improves sleep quality (assessed by SCOPA-Sleep and PSG, showing reduced PLMS and awakenings) and, surprisingly, has demonstrated benefits in motor symptoms (UPDRS scores) in

Table 5.4 Therapeutic interventions for circadian rhythm disruption in Parkinson's disease.

Intervention	Target circadian aspect/symptom	Mechanism of action	Key clinical findings in PD (examples)	References
Melatonin	Sleep quality, daytime sleepiness, RBD, NMS, QoL	MT1/MT2 receptor agonism, antioxidant, anti-inflammatory, anti-apoptotic, anti-α-syn aggregation, modulates *Bmal1*/*Per1* expression	Improved PSQI, ESS, NMSS, PDQ-39; improved sleep latency & TST (PSG) (3 mg RCT). Neuroprotective in preclinical models.	Sugumaran et al. (2024)
Ramelteon (MT1/MT2 agonist)	RBD, general sleep disturbances	Selective MT1/MT2 receptor agonism	Reduced severity of sleep disturbances, lowered RBD questionnaire scores in PD patients (8 mg open trial). Well-tolerated in elderly.	Kashihara et al. (2016)
Agomelatine (MT1/MT2 agonist, 5-HT2C antagonist)	Depression, sleep quality (nighttime sleep, daytime sleepiness, PLMS, awakenings), motor symptoms	MT1/MT2 agonism (resynchronizes circadian rhythms) + 5-HT2C antagonism (increases DA/NE in frontal cortex)	Significant decrease in HAM-D scores; improved SCOPA-sleep scores & PSG parameters (PLMS, awakenings); improved UPDRS motor scores.	Fornaro et al. (2010)
Bright light therapy (BLT)	Motor function, depression, sleep quality (PDSS), daytime sleepiness	Entrainment of SCN, regulation of melatonin-dopamine balance (light suppresses melatonin, may increase dopamine signaling), restoration of circadian rhythmicity	Meta-analysis shows improvements in motor function, depression, and PDSS scores. Mixed results for daytime sleepiness.	Rutten et al. (2012)
Novel clock gene modulators	Core clock function, downstream rhythmic processes	Direct modulation of clock gene/protein activity (e.g., stabilizing BMAL1, inhibiting CRY)	Primarily preclinical/bioinformatic research stage. *AK3, RTN3, LEPR* identified as	Videnovic and Willis (2016)

Continued

Table 5.4 Therapeutic interventions for circadian rhythm disruption in Parkinson's disease.—cont'd

Intervention	Target circadian aspect/symptom	Mechanism of action	Key clinical findings in PD (examples)	References
			potential biomarkers/ targets. No specific compounds in advanced PD trials yet.	
Chronotherapeutic medication timing	Optimize efficacy & reduce side effects of existing PD drugs (e.g., levodopa)	Aligning drug administration with endogenous rhythms of absorption, metabolism, and target sensitivity	Levodopa absorption slower at night. Potential to reduce "wearing-off" and improve symptom control by timed dosing.	Abbott et al. (2020)

PD patients (Avila et al., 2015). Its ability to resynchronize circadian rhythms is a key aspect of its therapeutic profile (Fornaro et al., 2010). Like melatonin, agomelatine's multifaceted benefits are highly valuable.

5.5.2.2 Bright light therapy (BLT)

BLT is a non-pharmacological intervention that uses exposure to high-intensity light to entrain and strengthen circadian rhythms.

- **Efficacy in PD:** Meta-analyses and reviews suggest that BLT can improve motor function, depression, and sleep quality (measured by PDSS) in PD patients (Rutten et al., 2012).
- **Mechanisms:** BLT is thought to work by restoring circadian rhythmicity, primarily by stimulating the retinohypothalamic tract and influencing SCN activity. This can lead to regulation of the melatonin-dopamine balance, as light suppresses melatonin production and can increase dopamine release (Rutten et al., 2012).
- **Administration Parameters:** Effective BLT typically involves exposure to 10,000 lux for about 30 min daily. The timing of BLT (morning vs. evening) is crucial and may need to be personalized based on the individual's chronotype and specific circadian disruption (e.g., phase advance often seen in PD might benefit from evening light, though morning light has also shown benefits for mood and sleep).Using a UV filter is recommended (Rutten et al., 2012).

5.5.2.3 Novel clock gene modulators

Directly targeting the molecular clockwork through pharmacological modulation of clock genes (*Per, Clock, Bmal1, Cry*) is an emerging research area with therapeutic potential for PD, but it is not yet an established therapy (Videnovic & Willis, 2016).

- Preclinical research and bioinformatic analyses are beginning to identify how clock gene dysregulation contributes to PD and to pinpoint potential targets. For instance, bioinformatic studies have identified genes like *AK3*, *RTN3*, and *LEPR* as potential circadian-related biomarkers or therapeutic targets in PD (Zhang et al., 2024).
- Currently, no specific clock gene modulator compounds are in advanced clinical trials for PD based on the available information, but this represents a significant future direction for drug development (Shkodina et al., 2022).

5.5.2.4 Chronotherapeutic approaches to PD management

Chronotherapy involves the timed administration of treatments to optimize efficacy and minimize adverse effects by aligning with the body's natural biological rhythms. This is a holistic approach that recognizes the importance of *when* a therapy is given, not just *what* is given.

- **Medication Timing:** The pharmacokinetics and pharmacodynamics of existing PD medications, such as levodopa, can be influenced by circadian rhythms. For example, levodopa absorption is reportedly slower at night (Abbott et al., 2020). Tailoring the timing of levodopa and other dopaminergic drug administration to an individual's circadian profile and symptom fluctuations could improve motor control and reduce "wearing-off" periods (Videnovic & Willis, 2016).
- **Integrated Strategies:** A comprehensive chronotherapeutic approach for PD would integrate pharmacological interventions (e.g., timed melatonin or agomelatine) with non-pharmacological strategies like BLT and timed physical exercise to synergistically restore circadian health and improve overall well-being (Fifel & Videnovic, 2019).

The development of such holistic and personalized chronotherapeutic strategies, which consider the individual's unique circadian profile and how it interacts with their PD symptoms and medication responses, is a key future direction.

5.5.3 Challenges and future directions in developing pharmacological antagonists

Despite promising preclinical findings for various agents targeting neurotoxin effects or circadian disruption, the translation to effective human therapies for PD faces significant challenges:

- **Translational Gap:** Many compounds that show neuroprotective effects in animal models fail to demonstrate efficacy in human clinical trials (Kachroo et al., 2010). This may be due to differences in species-specific metabolism, disease complexity in humans not fully recapitulated in models, and issues with trial design.
- **Complexity of Interactions:** PD pathogenesis involves intricate interactions between genetic predispositions, a wide array of potential environmental exposures occurring over decades, and endogenous factors like circadian rhythm status. Targeting a single neurotoxin or pathway may be insufficient (Dorsey & Bloem, 2024).
- **Lack of Biomarkers:** The absence of reliable biomarkers for early PD detection, specific toxin exposure, or individual circadian status hinders the ability to identify at-risk populations for preventative interventions or to stratify patients for targeted therapies.

- **Heterogeneity of PD:** PD is a heterogeneous disorder with varying clinical presentations and rates of progression. This variability, likely reflecting diverse underlying etiological contributions, makes it difficult to develop "one-size-fits-all" therapies.
- **Drug Delivery to the Brain:** Effectively delivering therapeutic agents across the BBB to target affected brain regions remains a challenge for many compounds.

Future directions in developing pharmacological antagonists and therapeutic strategies should focus on:

- **Improved Exposure Assessment:** Better characterization of the human "exposome" (the totality of environmental exposures over a lifetime) and its interaction with genetic susceptibility and circadian health.
- **Biomarker Development:** Identification and validation of robust biomarkers for early diagnosis, monitoring disease progression, and predicting therapeutic response.
- **Multi-Target Drug Development:** Designing agents that can address multiple pathological pathways simultaneously (e.g., compounds with combined antioxidant, anti-inflammatory, and chronobiotic properties, like melatonin or agomelatine, or iron chelators with additional neuroprotective actions (Geldenhuys & Van der Schyf, 2013)) may be more effective. The success of agents like melatonin and agomelatine, which offer dual benefits for circadian/sleep issues and core PD mechanisms, supports this approach.
- **Personalized Medicine:** Tailoring therapeutic interventions based on an individual's specific risk profile, including their genetic makeup, history of toxin exposure, and circadian characteristics (chronotype, degree of disruption).
- **Advanced Clinical Trial Designs:** Incorporating stratification based on biomarkers or risk factors, and focusing on clinically meaningful outcomes beyond motor scores.
- **Further Investigation of Clock Gene Modulators:** As understanding of the molecular clock's role in neurodegeneration deepens, direct pharmacological modulation of clock gene activity could emerge as a viable therapeutic strategy.

The development of effective pharmacological antagonists requires a multifaceted approach, combining strategies to mitigate specific neurotoxic insults with therapies aimed at restoring cellular and systemic homeostasis, including circadian rhythm integrity.

5.6 Conclusion and future perspectives

The evidence presented in this chapter underscores the significant and complex roles that environmental neurotoxins and circadian rhythm disruption play in the etiology and progression of Parkinson's Disease. A diverse array of environmental agents—ranging from pesticides like rotenone and paraquat, industrial solvents such as trichlorethylene, heavy metals including manganese and lead, to components of air pollution—have been implicated in PD pathogenesis. These toxins often converge on shared mechanistic pathways, primarily inducing oxidative stress, mitochondrial dysfunction, neuroinflammation, and promoting alpha-synucleinopathy, thereby contributing to the degeneration of dopaminergic neurons (Dorsey & Bloem, 2024). Concurrently, pervasive disruptions in the circadian system, manifesting as sleep-wake cycle disturbances, altered hormonal rhythms, and dysregulated clock gene expression, are not merely epiphenomena but appear to be intrinsically linked to PD pathology. This relationship is bidirectional: PD-related neurodegeneration can impair circadian control, while chronic circadian dysfunction can exacerbate neuroinflammatory processes, oxidative damage, and protein misfolding, potentially accelerating disease progression and increasing vulnerability to environmental insults (Chen et al., 2024).

The current pharmacological landscape for addressing these factors offers some promise, yet remains largely investigational. For specific neurotoxins, potential antagonists include chelating agents for heavy metals (e.g., PAS + CaEDTA for manganese), antioxidants (e.g., N-acetyl cysteine for dieldrin), anti-inflammatory agents (e.g., GR modulator PT150 for rotenone-induced effects), and compounds targeting specific enzymatic pathways (e.g., AEP inhibitors for maneb). For circadian rhythm disruption, melatonergic agents (melatonin, ramelteon, agomelatine) have shown efficacy in improving sleep and related non-motor symptoms in PD patients, with some agents like melatonin and agomelatine also possessing broader neuroprotective properties. Non-pharmacological interventions like Bright Light Therapy also show potential in resynchronizing circadian rhythms and alleviating some PD symptoms.

However, significant limitations persist. Many of these interventions are still in preclinical stages of development, and the translation of findings from animal models to human efficacy has proven challenging. The heterogeneity of PD, coupled with the diversity of potential environmental exposures and individual variations in genetic susceptibility and circadian makeup, makes a universal therapeutic approach elusive. The long latency between neurotoxin exposure and PD onset further complicates the design and implementation of preventative or early interventional strategies.

Future research must address these challenges through several key avenues:

- **Enhanced Characterization of Exposures and Interactions:** A deeper understanding of the human "exposome" and its complex interactions with individual genetic backgrounds and circadian status is crucial. This requires sophisticated epidemiological tools and longitudinal studies.
- **Biomarker Development:** There is an urgent need for reliable and accessible biomarkers that can identify individuals at high risk due to specific toxin exposures or profound circadian dysregulation, ideally before significant neurodegeneration occurs. Such biomarkers would also be invaluable for stratifying patients in clinical trials and monitoring therapeutic responses.
- **Novel Pharmacological Targets:** Continued exploration of molecular targets at the intersection of neurotoxic pathways and circadian regulatory mechanisms is warranted. This includes further investigation into direct clock gene modulators as a therapeutic strategy.
- **Robust Clinical Trials:** Well-designed, adequately powered clinical trials are essential to validate the efficacy of promising preclinical agents. These trials should consider combination therapies (e.g., a neuroprotective agent targeting toxin-induced damage combined with a chronobiotic agent to restore circadian health) and personalized medicine approaches. The potential for repurposing existing drugs with known safety profiles (e.g., caffeine, minocycline) and exploring natural compounds should continue to be investigated.
- **Preventative Strategies:** Given the strong evidence for environmental contributions and the role of circadian disruption as a potential risk factor, public health measures aimed at reducing exposure to known neurotoxicants (e.g., stricter regulations on pesticides and industrial emissions, remediation of contaminated sites) and promoting circadian health (e.g., public awareness about sleep hygiene and light exposure) are paramount. These preventative angles, while not pharmacological, are critical components of a comprehensive strategy to combat PD.

In conclusion, tackling Parkinson's Disease in the context of environmental neurotoxins and circadian rhythm disruption necessitates a multi-pronged approach. While the development of specific pharmacological antagonists and chronotherapeutic interventions holds significant promise, it must be complemented by robust public health initiatives aimed at prevention and a deeper commitment to personalized medicine that acknowledges the complex and individualized nature of this devastating disorder. Bridging the gap between promising preclinical research and clinically effective therapies remains a critical challenge, demanding innovative research methodologies and collaborative efforts across disciplines.

References

Aaseth, J. O., & Nurchi, V. M. (2022). Chelation combination—A strategy to mitigate the neurotoxicity of manganese, iron, and copper? *Biomolecules, 12*(11). https://doi.org/10.3390/biom12111713

Abbott, S. M., Malkani, R. G., & Zee, P. C. (2020). Circadian disruption and human health: A bidirectional relationship. *European Journal of Neuroscience, 51*(1), 567–583. https://doi.org/10.1111/ejn.14298

Armstrong, M. J., & Okun, M. S. (2020). Diagnosis and treatment of Parkinson disease: A review. *JAMA, 323*(6), 548–560. https://doi.org/10.1001/jama.2019.22360

Asadpoordezaki, Z., Coogan, A. N., & Henley, B. M. (2023). Chronobiology of Parkinson's disease: Past, present and future. *European Journal of Neuroscience, 57*(1), 178–200. https://doi.org/10.1111/ejn.15859

Atterling Brolin, K., Schaeffer, E., Kuri, A., Katharina Rumrich, I., Schuh, A. F. S., Darweesh, S. K. L., Kaasinen, V., Tolppanen, A.-M., Chahine, L. M., & Noyce, A. J. (2025). Environmental risk factors for Parkinson's disease: A critical review and policy implications. *Movement Disorders, 40*(2), 204–221. https://doi.org/10.1002/mds.30067

Avila, A., Cardona, X., Martin-Baranera, M., Leon, L., Caballol, N., Millet, P., & Bello, J. (2015). Agomelatine for depression in Parkinson disease: Additional effect on sleep and motor dysfunction. *Journal of Clinical Psychopharmacology, 35*(6), 719–723. https://doi.org/10.1097/JCP.0000000000000404

Ball, N., Teo, W.-P., Chandra, S., & Chapman, J. (2019). Parkinson's disease and the environment. *Frontiers in Neurology, 10*. https://doi.org/10.3389/fneur.2019.00218

Baser, K. H. C., Haskologlu, I. C., & Erdag, E. (2025). Molecular links between circadian rhythm disruption, melatonin, and neurodegenerative diseases: An updated review. *Molecules, 30*(9). https://doi.org/10.3390/molecules30091888

Bisbal, M., & Sanchez, M. (2019). Neurotoxicity of the pesticide rotenone on neuronal polarization: A mechanistic approach. *Neural Regeneration Research, 14*(5), 762–766. https://doi.org/10.4103/1673-5374.249847

Chen, Y.-C., Wang, W.-S., Lewis, S. J. G., & Wu, S.-L. (2024). Fighting against the clock: Circadian disruption and Parkinson's disease. *Journal of Movement Disorders, 17*(1), 1–14. https://doi.org/10.14802/jmd.23216

Coon, S., Stark, A., Peterson, E., Gloi, A., Kortsha, G., Pounds, J., Chettle, D., & Gorell, J. (2006). Whole-body lifetime occupational lead exposure and risk of Parkinson's disease. *Environmental Health Perspectives, 114*(12), 1872–1876. https://doi.org/10.1289/ehp.9102

Dias, V., Junn, E., & Mouradian, M. M. (2013). The role of oxidative stress in Parkinson's disease. *Journal of Parkinson's Disease, 3*(4), 461–491. https://doi.org/10.3233/JPD-130230

Domico, L. M., Zeevalk, G. D., Bernard, L. P., & Cooper, K. R. (2006). Acute neurotoxic effects of mancozeb and maneb in mesencephalic neuronal cultures are associated with mitochondrial dysfunction. *Neurotoxicology, 27*(5), 816–825.

Dorsey, E. R., & Bloem, B. R. (2024). Parkinson's disease is predominantly an environmental disease. *Journal of Parkinson's Disease, 14*(3), 451–465. https://doi.org/10.3233/JPD-230357

Dorsey, E. R., Zafar, M., Lettenberger, S. E., Pawlik, M. E., Kinel, D., Frissen, M., Schneider, R. B., Kieburtz, K., Tanner, C. M., De Miranda, B. R., Goldman, S. M., & Bloem, B. R. (2023). Trichloroethylene: An invisible cause of Parkinson's disease? *Journal of Parkinson's Disease, 13*(2), 203–218. https://doi.org/10.3233/JPD-225047

Esaki, Y., Kitajima, T., Koike, S., Fujishiro, H., Iwata, Y., Tsuchiya, A., Hirose, M., & Iwata, N. (2016). An open-labeled trial of Ramelteon in idiopathic rapid eye movement sleep behavior disorder. *Journal of Clinical Sleep Medicine, 12*(5), 689–693. https://doi.org/10.5664/jcsm.5796

Evans, G. R., & Masullo, L. N. (2023). *Manganese toxicity treasure Island (FL).* StatPearls Publishing.

Fahn, S., & Sulzer, D. (2004). Neurodegeneration and neuroprotection in Parkinson disease. *NeuroRx, 1*(1), 139–154.

Fifel, K., & Videnovic, A. (2019). Chronotherapies for Parkinson's disease. *Progress in Neurobiology, 174*, 16–27.

Fitzmaurice, A. G., Rhodes, S. L., Lulla, A., Murphy, N. P., Lam, H. A., O'Donnell, K. C., Barnhill, L., Casida, J. E., Cockburn, M., Sagasti, A., Stahl, M. C., Maidment, N. T., Ritz, B., & Bronstein, J. M. (2013). Aldehyde dehydrogenase inhibition as a pathogenic mechanism in Parkinson disease. *Proceedings of the National Academy of Sciences of the United States of America, 110*(2), 636–641. https://doi.org/10.1073/pnas.1220399110

Fornaro, M., Prestia, D., Colicchio, S., & Perugi, G. (2010). A systematic, updated review on the antidepressant agomelatine focusing on its melatonergic modulation. *Current Neuropharmacology, 8*(3), 287–304. https://doi.org/10.2174/157015910792246227

Geldenhuys, W. J., & Van der Schyf, C. J. (2013). Rationally designed multi-targeted agents against neurodegenerative diseases. *Current Medicinal Chemistry, 20*(13), 1662–1672.

Goldman, S. M., Quinlan, P. J., Ross, G. W., Marras, C., Meng, C., Bhudhikanok, G. S., Comyns, K., Korell, M., Chade, A. R., Kasten, M., Priestley, B., Chou, K. L., Fernandez, H. H., Cambi, F., Langston, J. W., & Tanner, C. M. (2012). Solvent exposures and Parkinson disease risk in twins. *Annals of Neurology, 71*(6), 776–784. https://doi.org/10.1002/ana.22629

Greenamyre, J. T., Cannon, J. R., Drolet, R., & Mastroberardino, P.-G. (2010). Lessons from the rotenone model of Parkinson's disease. *Trends in Pharmacological Sciences, 31*(4). https://doi.org/10.1016/j.tips.2009.12.006

Grotewold, N., & Albin, R. L. (2024). Update: Protective and risk factors for Parkinson disease. *Parkinsonism & Related Disorders, 125*, 107026.

Hu, X., Li, J., Wang, X., Liu, H., Wang, T., Lin, Z., & Xiong, N. (2023). Neuroprotective effect of melatonin on sleep disorders associated with Parkinson's disease. *Antioxidants, 12*(2), 396. https://doi.org/10.3390/antiox12020396

Kachroo, A., Irizarry, M. C., & Schwarzschild, M. A. (2010). Caffeine protects against combined paraquat and maneb-induced dopaminergic neuron degeneration. *Experimental Neurology, 223*(2), 657–661. https://doi.org/10.1016/j.expneurol.2010.02.007

Kalkan, Ö. F., Türk, A., Çitil, C., Uçkun, M., Özkaya, A., Yoloğlu, E., Özay, Y., Bülbül, S.Ç., Sahin, Z., & Kirbas, A. (2024). Pomegranate juice treatment reverses carbon tetrachloride (CCl4)-induced increased acetylcholinesterase activity and cell death via suppression of oxidative stress in rats. *Roczniki Panstwowego Zakladu Higieny, 75*(3), 293–302.

Kashihara, K., Nomura, T., Maeda, T., Tsuboi, Y., Mishima, T., Takigawa, H., & Nakashima, K. (2016). Beneficial effects of Ramelteon on rapid eye movement sleep behavior disorder associated with Parkinson's disease - Results of a multicenter open trial. *Internal Medicine, 55*(3), 231–236. https://doi.org/10.2169/internalmedicine.55.5464

Latham, A. S., Rocha, S. M., McDermott, C. P., Reigan, P., Slayden, R. A., & Tjalkens, R. B. (2024). Neuroprotective efficacy of the glucocorticoid receptor modulator PT150 in the rotenone mouse model of Parkinson's disease. *Neurotoxicology, 103*, 320–334.

Lauretti, E., Di Meco, A., Merali, S., & Praticò, D. (2017). Circadian rhythm dysfunction: A novel environmental risk factor for Parkinson's disease. *Molecular Psychiatry, 22*(2), 280–286. https://doi.org/10.1038/mp.2016.47

Li, H., Kilgallen, A. B., Münzel, T., Wolf, E., Lecour, S., Schulz, R., Daiber, A., & Van Laake, L. W. (2020). Influence of mental stress and environmental toxins on circadian clocks: Implications for redox regulation of the heart and cardioprotection. *British Journal of Pharmacology, 177*(23), 5393–5412. https://doi.org/10.1111/bph.14949

Li, H., Song, S., Wang, Y., Huang, C., Zhang, F., Liu, J., & Hong, J.-S. (2019). Low-grade inflammation aggravates rotenone neurotoxicity and disrupts circadian clock gene expression in rats. *Neurotoxicity Research, 35*(2), 421–431. https://doi.org/10.1007/s12640-018-9968-1

Lin, W., & Kang, U. J. (2005). Neuroprotective therapy in Parkinson's disease: Current status and new directions from experimental and genetic clues. *Journal of Clinical Neurology, 1*(2), 107–120. https://doi.org/10.3988/jcn.2005.1.2.107

Liu, C., Liu, Z., Fang, Y., Du, Z., Yan, Z., Yuan, X., Dai, L., Yu, T., Xiong, M., Tian, Y., Li, H., Li, F., Zhang, J., Meng, L., Wang, Z., Jiang, H., & Zhang, Z. (2022). Exposure to the environmentally toxic pesticide maneb induces Parkinson's disease-like neurotoxicity in mice: A combined proteomic and metabolomic analysis. *Chemosphere, 308*(Pt 2).

Lucchini, R., & Tieu, K. (2023). Manganese-induced parkinsonism: Evidence from epidemiological and experimental studies. *Biomolecules, 13*(8), 1190. https://doi.org/10.3390/biom13081190

Ma, X., & Wang, J. (2024). Research progress on the role of ginsenoside Rd in central nervous system diseases. *African Health Sciences, 24*(4), 325–331. https://doi.org/10.4314/ahs.v24i4.41

Magro, G., Laterza, V., Tosto, F., Torrente, A., & Neurotoxicity, M. (2025). A comprehensive review of pathophysiology and inherited and acquired disorders. *Journal of Xenobiotics, 15*(2), 54. https://doi.org/10.3390/jox15020054

Masilamoni, G. J., Bogenpohl, J. W., Alagille, D., Delevich, K., Tamagnan, G., Votaw, J. R., Wichmann, T., & Smith, Y. (2011). Metabotropic glutamate receptor 5 antagonist protects dopaminergic and noradrenergic neurons from degeneration in MPTP-treated monkeys. *Brain: Journal of Neurology, 134*(Pt 7), 2057–2073. https://doi.org/10.1093/brain/awr137

Ntetsika, T., Papathoma, P.-E., & Markaki, I. (2021). Novel targeted therapies for Parkinson's disease. *Molecular Medicine, 27*(1). https://doi.org/10.1186/s10020-021-00279-2

Rappold, P. M., Cui, M., Chesser, A. S., Tibbett, J., Grima, J. C., Duan, L., Sen, N., Javitch, J. A., & Kim, T. (2011). Paraquat neurotoxicity is mediated by the dopamine transporter and organic cation transporter-3. *Proceedings of the National Academy of Sciences of the United States of America, 108*(51), 20766–20771. https://doi.org/10.1073/pnas.1115141108

Rekatsina, M., Paladini, A., Piroli, A., Zis, P., Pergolizzi, J. V., & Varrassi, G. (2020). Pathophysiology and therapeutic perspectives of oxidative stress and neurodegenerative diseases: A narrative review. *Advances in Therapy, 37*(1), 113–139. https://doi.org/10.1007/s12325-019-01148-5

Richardson, J. R., Fitsanakis, V., Westerink, R. H. S., & Kanthasamy, A. G. (2019). Neurotoxicity of pesticides. *Acta Neuropathologica, 138*(3), 343–362. https://doi.org/10.1007/s00401-019-02033-9

Rutten, S., Vriend, C., van den Heuvel, O. A., Smit, J. H., Berendse, H. W., & van der Werf, Y. D. (2012). Bright light therapy in Parkinson's disease: An overview of the background and evidence. *Parkinson's Disease, 2012*. https://doi.org/10.1155/2012/767105

Sanders, T., Liu, Y., Buchner, V., & Tchounwou, P. B. (2009). Neurotoxic effects and biomarkers of lead exposure: A review. *Reviews on Environmental Health, 24*(1), 15–45. https://doi.org/10.1515/REVEH.2009.24.1.15

Seidl, S. E., & Potashkin, J. A. (2011). The promise of neuroprotective agents in Parkinson's disease. *Frontiers in Neurology, 2*. https://doi.org/10.3389/fneur.2011.00068

Sharma, H., Zhang, P., Barber, D. S., & Liu, B. (2010). Organochlorine pesticides dieldrin and lindane induce cooperative toxicity in dopaminergic neurons: Role of oxidative stress. *Neurotoxicology, 31*(2), 215–222. https://doi.org/10.1016/j.neuro.2009.12.007

Sherer, T. B., Betarbet, R., Testa, C. M., Seo, B. B., Richardson, J. R., Kim, J. H., Miller, G. W., Yagi, T., Matsuno-Yagi, A., & Timothy Greenamyre, J. (2003). Mechanism of toxicity in rotenone models of Parkinson's disease. *Journal of Neuroscience, 23*(34), 10756–10764.

Shkodina, A. D., Tan, S. C., Hasan, M. M., Abdelgawad, M., Chopra, H., Bilal, M., Ivanovych Boiko, D., Anatoliivna Tarianyk, K., & Alexiou, A. (2022). Roles of clock genes in the pathogenesis of Parkinson's disease. *Ageing Research Reviews, 74*, 101554.

Subramaniam, S. R., & Chesselet, M.-F. (2013). Mitochondrial dysfunction and oxidative stress in Parkinson's disease. *Progress in Neurobiology, 106–107*, 17–32.

Sugumaran, R., Sai Krishna, K. S., Saibaba, J., Narayan, S. K., Sandhiya, S., & Rajeswari, M. (2024). Melatonin on sleep in Parkinson's disease: A randomized double blind placebo controlled trial. *Sleep Medicine, 124*, 502–509.

Tanner, C. M., Kamel, F., Webster Ross, G., Hoppin, J. A., Goldman, S. M., Korell, M., Marras, C., Bhudhikanok, G. S., Kasten, M., Chade, A. R., Comyns, K., Richards, M. B., Meng, C., Priestley, B., Fernandez, H. H., Cambi, F., Umbach, D. M., Blair, A., Sandler, D. P., & Langston, J. W. (2011). Rotenone, paraquat, and Parkinson's disease. *Environmental Health Perspectives, 119*(6), 866–872. https://doi.org/10.1289/ehp.1002839

Tieu, K. (2011). A guide to neurotoxic animal models of Parkinson's disease. *Cold Spring Harbor Perspectives in Medicine, 1*(1), Article a009316. https://doi.org/10.1101/cshperspect.a009316

Vallée, A., Lecarpentier, Y., Guillevin, R., & Vallée, J.-N. (2020). Circadian rhythms, neuroinflammation and oxidative stress in the story of Parkinson's disease. *Cells, 9*(2), 314. https://doi.org/10.3390/cells9020314

Videnovic, A., & Willis, G. L. (2016). Circadian system - A novel diagnostic and therapeutic target in Parkinson's disease? *Movement Disorders, 31*(3), 260–269. https://doi.org/10.1002/mds.26509

Weed, D. L. (2021). Does paraquat cause Parkinson's disease? A review of reviews. *Neurotoxicology, 86*, 180–184.

Xie, C., Xia, X., Wang, K., Yan, J., Bai, L., Guo, L., Li, X., & Wu, S. (2025). Ambient air pollution and Parkinson's disease and Alzheimer's disease: An updated meta-analysis. *Toxics, 13*(2), 139. https://doi.org/10.3390/toxics13020139

Xu, K., Zhang, Y., Shi, Y., Zhang, Y., Zhang, C., Wang, T., Lv, P., Bai, Y., & Wang, S. (2024). Circadian rhythm disruption: A potential trigger in Parkinson's disease pathogenesis. *Frontiers in Cellular Neuroscience, 18*. https://doi.org/10.3389/fncel.2024.1464595

Zhang, J., Ma, X., Li, Z., Liu, H., Mei, T., Wen, Y., Wang, S., & Wang, L. (2024). Identification of key genes and diagnostic model associated with circadian rhythms and Parkinson's disease by bioinformatics analysis. *Frontiers in Aging Neuroscience, 16*. https://doi.org/10.3389/fnagi.2024.1458476

Zhou, Z. D., Yi, L. X., Wang, D. Q., Lim, T. M., & King Tan, E. (2023). Role of dopamine in the pathophysiology of Parkinson's disease. *Translational Neurodegeneration, 12*(1). https://doi.org/10.1186/s40035-023-00378-6

CHAPTER

6

Oral bacteriome dysbiosis and mechanisms in cognitive impairment among older people and Parkinson's disease: A systematic review

Nur Sabrina Ameerah Mohd Nazri[1], Mohd Shaiful Ehsan Shalihin[2], Sulhi Abidin[3], Hairul Aini Hamzah[4], Edre Mohamad Aidid[5] and Ramli Musa[6]

[1]*Kulliyyah of Medicine, International Islamic Univeristy of Malaysia, Kuantan, Pahang, Malaysia;* [2]*Department of Family Medicine, Kulliyyah of Medicine, International Islamic University of Malaysia, Kuantan, Pahang, Malaysia;* [3]*Department of Prosthodontics, Kulliyyah of Dentistry, International Islamic University of Malaysia, Kuantan, Pahang, Malaysia;* [4]*Department of Basic Medical Sciences, Kulliyyah of Medicine, International Islamic University of Malaysia, Kuantan, Pahang, Malaysia;* [5]*Department of Community Medicine, Kulliyyah of Medicine, International Islamic University of Malaysia, Kuantan, Pahang, Malaysia;* [6]*Department of Psychiatry, Kulliyyah of Medicine, International Islamic University of Malaysia, Kuantan, Pahang, Malaysia*

We conducted a systematic search of the PubMed and Scopus databases for studies published between January 2014 and June 2024. Eligible studies included human participants aged 60 and above and reported data on oral bacteria and cognitive outcomes. Data extraction followed a standardized protocol, and study quality was assessed using the Newcastle–Ottawa Scale, Cochrane Risk of Bias Tool, and CASP Case Report Checklist.

Twenty studies, including case reports, cross-sectional, case-control, cohort studies, and clinical trials, were reviewed. Pathogenic bacteria like Porphyromonas gingivalis, Streptococcus mutans, Fusobacterium nucleatum, Treponema denticola, and Tannerella forsythia were often linked to a decline in cognitive function. *Porphyromonas gingivalis, Streptococcus mutans, Fusobacterium nucleatum, Treponema denticola*, and *Tannerella forsythia* were often connected to a decrease in thinking ability. Proposed mechanisms included systemic inflammation, neuroinflammation, blood-brain barrier disruption, and microbial dysbiosis. Additionally, biomarkers such as oral acidity and antibody titers against periodontal pathogens showed potential for early detection. Some studies also suggested a possible role of oral microbiota alterations in Parkinson's disease-related cognitive impairment, though further research is needed to confirm these associations.

Findings suggest that oral bacteria play a crucial role in cognitive impairment through inflammatory and neurodegenerative pathways. While evidence continues to grow, knowledge gaps remain regarding the full spectrum of bacterial species and mechanisms involved. Future research should prioritize standardized methodologies and longitudinal studies to establish causal relationships and assess the impact of oral health interventions in mitigating cognitive decline.

Pharmacological Foundations of Parkinson's Disease. https://doi.org/10.1016/B978-0-443-27702-3.00007-8

6.1 Introduction

Cognitive impairment is a growing global health concern, particularly among the elderly population. Mild cognitive impairment (MCI) is often seen as a transitional stage between normal aging and more severe conditions such as dementia, including Alzheimer's disease (AD). While aging is the most significant risk factor for cognitive decline, other modifiable risk factors have gained attention in recent years (Anand & Schoo, 2024). Among these, oral health has emerged as an area of interest due to its potential systemic effects on overall health, including cognitive function.

The proportion of the population that is elderly has increased dramatically during the last few decades. According to the United Nations estimates, 1 in 6 people of our population will be older adults who are 65 years of age or older by 2050, approximately 1.5 billion in total ("World population ageing 2020 highlights: Living arrangements of older persons," 2020). The positive consequences of healthy aging extend to the elderly as well as to their families and communities as it improves the quality of life for older adults, strengthens family ties, and lowers the strain on society's resources. However, the issue of dental caries in the elderly has drawn more attention as the population ages. While oral bacteria generally preserve homeostasis, a dysbiosis of oral microbes can result in oral diseases such as periodontitis and dental caries, as well as systemic chronic inflammation (Plachokova et al., 2021).

Researchers have implicated oral bacteria, particularly those associated with periodontal disease, in systemic inflammation, a condition known to contribute to cognitive impairment. Specific bacteria, such as *Porphyromonas gingivalis, Treponema denticola, Fusobacterium nucleatum,* and *Tannerella forsythia* elicit the release of cytokines that have been found in higher concentrations in individuals with cognitive disorders, as well as their virulence factors might potentially contributing to neuroinflammation and blood-brain barrier disruption (Visentin et al., 2023). Neurofibrillary tangles and amyloid plaques build up due to overall inflammation, making it harder for the nervous system to remove abnormal cells and proteins, which is linked to the development of several long-term diseases like heart disease, diabetes, and lung infections. Emerging evidence suggests that systemic inflammation caused by oral bacteria could also contribute to the development or progression of cognitive impairment (Lu et al., 2019).

Despite growing evidence linking oral bacteria to cognitive impairment, there remains a significant gap in the study regarding the specific types of bacteria involved and the detailed mechanisms by which they may contribute to cognitive impairment. Some studies have found strong associations between specific bacterial taxa and cognitive outcomes, while others have yielded more inconclusive results. This gap underscores the need for a systematic review to synthesize the current knowledge on the types of oral bacteria associated with cognitive impairment and the biological pathways through which they exert their effects. Therefore, a systematic review aims to address the following questions:

1. What types of oral bacteria are associated with cognitive impairment in elderly populations?
2. What are the proposed mechanisms through which these bacteria influence cognitive function?
3. Are there any links between oral bacteria and cognitive impairment in Parkinson's disease, and what potential mechanisms might contribute to neurodegeneration?

6.2 Materials and methods

6.2.1 Study design

This systematic review was performed in accordance with the Preferred Reporting Items for Systematic Reviews and Meta-Analyses (PRISMA 2020) guidelines (Page et al., 2021). A statement of ethics was not required.

In this review, we aim to summarize the evidence on the association between oral bacteria and cognitive impairment, with a specific focus on identifying bacterial types and their mechanisms of influence. We structure our research question using the PICO framework (Population, Intervention/Exposure, Comparator, and Outcome) as follows: In elderly populations aged 60 years and above (P), what types of oral bacteria and mechanisms involved (I) are associated with cognitive impairment (O) compared to cognitively healthy elderly individuals (C)?

6.2.2 Search strategy

A systematic literature search of PubMed and Scopus was performed for studies published from January 2014–June 2024 and included papers from all countries. The databases were searched for eligible records using search terms about "oral bacteria", "geriatric", and "cognitive impairment" "bacteria types" and "mechanisms". These search terms are "oral bacteria" "bacteria colony" "microorganism" "geriatric" "older people" "elderly" "cognitive impairment" "cognitive deterioration" "cognitive decline" "dementia" "bacteria types" "bacteria species" "mechanisms" "process" "pathogenesis" "association". Keywords were combined using the Boolean operators "OR" and "AND". The search was conducted with English language restrictions and was limited to human studies.

6.2.3 Selection criteria

All studies (including full paper, cross-sectional, case-control, cohort, case report, case series, commentary studies, and randomized controlled trials studies) providing quantitative measures of the association between oral bacteria and cognitive impairment among geriatric (age 60 and above) were included in our review without regards to the region or country where the study was conducted. Studies needed to focus on the association between oral bacteria and cognitive impairment and report on the bacteria types and mechanisms involved. We did not adopt any pre-specified restriction criteria for the assessment of dementia or cognitive impairment in our study inclusion process. We excluded studies that did not involve human participants, reviews, meta-analysis articles, presentation papers, and abstract proceedings, or those lacking relevant data on oral bacteria or cognitive outcomes. This selection process aimed to capture high-quality evidence directly relevant to our research questions.

6.2.4 Data extraction and synthesis

Data extraction and synthesis for this systematic review involved a structured approach to collect and analyze relevant information from the included studies. Data extraction was conducted using a standardized form to capture key details, including study characteristics, population characteristics, types of oral bacteria studied, bacteria sample types, bacterial identification methods, mechanisms or pathogenesis of influence, as well as the outcomes and findings. Two independent reviewers performed the extraction to ensure accuracy, resolving discrepancies through discussion or a third reviewer if necessary. For synthesis, we conducted a narrative summary of the findings from the included studies, highlighting patterns and inconsistencies in the data. This comprehensive approach allowed us to integrate and interpret the evidence effectively, providing insights into the relationship between oral bacteria and cognitive decline.

6.2.5 Quality assessment

The quality assessment of the studies included in this systematic review was conducted using a variety of tools tailored to the different study designs as showed in Table 6.1. For case-control and cohort studies, we employed the Newcastle–Ottawa Scale (NOS) to evaluate the selection of participants, comparability of groups, and outcome assessment. Cross-sectional studies were assessed using a modified version of the NOS, focusing on sample selection, control for confounders, and outcome measurement. Each category has specific criteria, and studies are scored based on whether they meet the recommended criteria. For selection, higher scores are given for representative samples and clear case definitions. Meanwhile, for comparability, studies are rated on how well they control for confounders, and for outcome assessment, points are awarded based on the adequacy of outcome measurement and follow-up. The total score ranges from 0 to 9, with higher scores indicating better study quality. Generally, studies scoring 7–9 are considered high quality, 4–6 are moderate, and 0–3 are low quality.

Additionally, clinical trial studies were evaluated with the Cochrane Risk of Bias Tool, which checks for random sequence generation, blinding, and outcome assessment to determine the quality of the study. A study is rated low risk for sequence generation if random methods are used, and high risk if non-random methods are employed. It is rated low risk for blinding if both participants and outcome assessors are blinded, and high risk if there is no blinding. For outcome assessment, a low-risk rating requires the blinding of assessors and reliable measurement methods, while high-risk applies if assessors are not blinded or methods are biased. The study's overall risk of bias increases if any domain receives a high risk rating. Meanwhile, reviewers used the CASP (Critical Appraisal Skills Program) Case Report Checklist to evaluate the case report, ensuring that the study has a clear aim, provides a thorough case description, and includes appropriate ethics considerations. Each study was independently assessed by two reviewers, and any disagreements were resolved through discussion or consultation with a third reviewer. This rigorous approach ensured a comprehensive evaluation of the methodological quality across all study types included in the review.

6.3 Results

The electronic searches initially identified a total of 120 records. We retained 108 studies after excluding duplicates. Of these, 83 abstracts did not meet the inclusion criteria, leaving 25 abstracts for further investigation. We obtained full-text articles for all 25 studies and thoroughly evaluated them. We included 20 studies that met the full inclusion criteria in this review. With regards to the classification of the studies according to study design, we obtained one case report, nine cross-sectional studies, two clinical trials, seven case-control studies, and two cohort studies. Fig. 6.1 illustrates the flowchart of the study selection process.

Table 6.1 Quality assessment of studies using Newcastle–Ottawa Scale (NOS), cochrane risk of bias tool and CASP case report checklist.

References	Study design	Newcastle–Ottawa Scale (NOS)	Cochrane risk of bias tool	CASP case report checklist	Overall quality rating
Cobo et al. (2018)	Case report study	–	–	Clear aim: Yes Case description: Yes Ethics consideration: Yes	High
Merchant et al. (2023)	Cross-sectional study	Selection: 4 Comparability: 2 Outcome: 2	–	–	High
Bathini et al. (2020)	Cross-sectional study	Selection: 4 Comparability: 1 Outcome: 3	–	–	High
Chung and Chan (2023)	Case-control study	Selection: 3 Comparability: 2 Outcome: 2	–	–	Moderate
Troci et al. (2024)	Cross-sectional study	Selection: 3 Comparability: 1 Outcome: 2	–	–	Moderate
Leblhuber et al. (2020)	Cross-sectional study	Selection: 3 Comparability: 1 Outcome: 2	–	–	Moderate
Arıkan et al. (2023)	Cross-sectional study	Selection: 3 Comparability: 2 Outcome: 3	–	–	High
Vanhatalo et al. (2021)	Clinical trial	–	Random sequence generation: Low Blinding: Low Outcome assessment: Low	–	High
Hosoki et al. (2020)	Cohort study	Selection: 3 Comparability: 1 Outcome: 2	–	–	Moderate
Watanabe et al. (2016)	Cross-sectional study	Selection: 4 Comparability: 1 Outcome: 3	–	–	High

Continued

Table 6.1 Quality assessment of studies using Newcastle–Ottawa Scale (NOS), cochrane risk of bias tool and CASP case report checklist.—cont'd

References	Study design	Newcastle–Ottawa Scale (NOS)	Cochrane risk of bias tool	CASP case report checklist	Overall quality rating
Panzarella et al. (2022)	Case-control study	Selection: 3 Comparability: 2 Outcome: 3	–	–	High
Da et al. (2023)	Case-control study	Selection: 4 Comparability: 1 Outcome: 3	–	–	High
Li et al. (2024)	Case-control study	Selection: 3 Comparability: 1 Outcome: 2	–	–	Moderate
Wu et al. (2021)	Case-control study	Selection: 4 Comparability: 1 Outcome: 2	–	–	Moderate
Qiu et al. (2024)	Cross-sectional study	Selection: 4 Comparability: 1 Outcome: 3	–	–	High
Noble et al. (2014)	Cohort study	Selection: 3 Comparability: 2 Outcome: 2	–	–	Moderate
Fogelholm et al. (2023)	Cross-sectional study	Selection: 3 Comparability: 1 Outcome: 2	–	–	Moderate
Holmer et al. (2021)	Case-control study	Selection: 4 Comparability: 1 Outcome: 3	–	–	High
Yang et al. (2021)	Cross-sectional study	Selection: 4 Comparability: 1 Outcome: 3	–	–	High
Tadjoedin et al. (2022)	Case-control study	Selection: 3 Comparability: 1 Outcome: 2	–	–	Moderate

Data from 20 studies on the oral bacteria focusing on the bacteria types and mechanisms involved in the elderly subjects ($\geq$60 years of age) with cognitive impairment that were diagnosed and confirmed based on histopathologic analysis were extracted and qualitatively synthesized in two tables. Table 6.2 displays data on study characteristics which provides an overview of the key features of the included studies, including the authorship, study design, population details, sample size, methods used for bacterial analysis, and primary findings related to the association between oral bacteria and cognitive impairment.

Part of your document could not be imported as it contained an unsupported element. For more information about unsupported elements, please visit the Support Center.

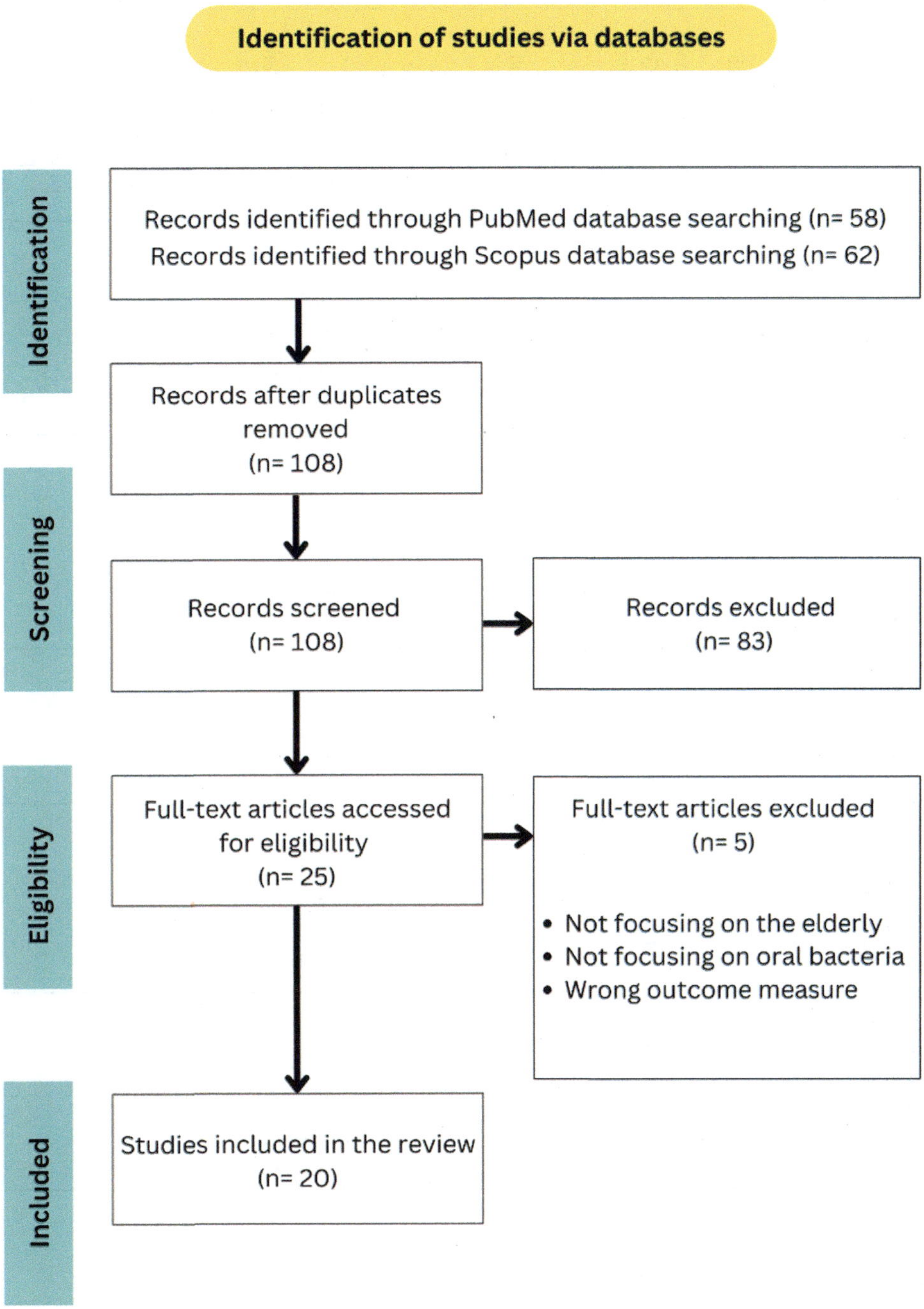

FIGURE 6.1

PRISMA flow diagram.

Table 6.2 Summary of study characteristics on oral bacteria and cognitive impairment.

Author (Year)	Study design	Population	Sample size (n)	Cognitive outcome measured	Methodology	Key findings
Cobo et al. (2018)	Case report	Older adult (88)	1	Cognitive impairment	(1) Aerobic and anaerobic culture (2) MALDI-TOF MS (3) 16S rRNA sequencing (4) E-test method	- *Prevotella dentalis* was identified as the sole causative agent of the pleural effusion through culture and molecular methods.
Merchant et al. (2023)	Cross- sectional	Older adults (60+)	5162	Cognitive impairment and AD	(1) Analysis of IgG antibody titers against 19 periodontal bacteria. (2) Checkerboard immunoblotting	- Groups of IgG antibodies against periodontal microorganisms, specifically the Orange-Red and Yellow-Orange clusters, were associated with lower cognitive scores in older adults.
Bathini et al. (2020)	Cross- sectional study	Older adults (60+)	78	MCI and AD	(1) 16S rRNA sequencing (2) Bead- based immunoassay	- The salivary microbiome analysis revealed stage-dependent changes in oral bacteria, with a decline in periodontal pathogens like *Filifactor villosus* and an enrichment of opportunistic oral bacteria like Leptotrichia wadei in the MCI group.

Chung and Chan (2023)	Case-control study	Older adults (50–80)	196	MCI and non-MCI	(1) SILL-Ha® saliva test system to assess oral health. (2) CatBoost (classification prediction for cognitive decline)	- Significant differences in oral diadochokinesis (ODK) rate ($P = .003$) and acidity from SILL-Ha ($P = .04$) between cognitive decline and normal groups were identified. - The prediction model using these digital oral health biomarkers had high accuracy, with an AUC of 0.86 and 0.99 for the sensitivity analysis.
Troci et al. (2024)	Cross- sectional study	Older adults (60+)	151	MCI and non-MCI	(1) 16S rRNA sequencing	- These findings suggest stage-dependent alterations in the oral microbiota that may contribute to the pathogenesis of Alzheimer's disease through facilitated intestinal and systemic inflammation leading to neuroinflammation and neurodegeneration.
Leblhuber et al. (2020)	Cross- sectional study	Older adults (60+)	20	Cognitive impairment and AD	(1) RNA-based analysis: specifically utilizing the	- The presence of the periodontal pathogen Porphyromonas

Continued

Table 6.2 Summary of study characteristics on oral bacteria and cognitive impairment.—cont'd

Author (Year)	Study design	Population	Sample size (n)	Cognitive outcome measured	Methodology	Key findings
					PerioPOC® system (Genspeed Biotech, Henry Schein Dental, Vienna, Austria) to detect the presence of periodontal pathogens in saliva alveolar fluid.	gingivalis was associated with lower Mini-Mental State Examination (MMSE) scores, indicating a potential link between this pathogen and neuroinflammation and the dementia process.
Arıkan et al. (2023)	Cross- sectional study	Older adults (60+)	115	Cognitive impairment	(1) 16S rRNA Sequencing	- The study identified specific bacterial genera and protein groups that were associated with different stages of cognitive impairment in Parkinson's disease.
Vanhatalo et al. (2021)	Clinical Trial	Older adults (70–80)	30	Cognitive impairment	(1) 16 S rRNA Sequencing	- Several significant correlations were found between oral bacteria modules and indices of cognitive and physiological function, representing promising avenues for developing

						biomarkers and therapies for cognitive and cardiovascular impairment in older age.
Hosoki et al. (2020)	Cohort study	Older adults (60+)	111	Cognitive impairment	(1) Anaerobic culture (2) Polymerase Chain Reaction (PCR)	- Patients with cnm-positive *S. mutans* had a significantly higher incidence of new cerebral microbleeds (CMB), especially in deep brain regions, compared to patients without cnm-positive *S. mutans*.
Watanabe et al. (2016)	Cross- sectional study	Older adults (65+)	279	Cognitive impairment	(1) Polymerase Chain Reaction (PCR)	- Cnm-positive *Streptococcus mutans*, especially those expressing collagen binding activity, are associated with a higher risk of cerebral microbleeds, particularly deep cerebral microbleeds.
Panzarella et al. (2022)	Case-control study	Older adults (70+)	60	MCI and AD	(1) RT-PCR Analysis (2) Oral health-related quality of life (OHR-QoL)	- The Alzheimer's disease group had a significantly higher load of the periodontal bacteria *Fusobacterium*

Continued

Table 6.2 Summary of study characteristics on oral bacteria and cognitive impairment.—cont'd

Author (Year)	Study design	Population	Sample size (n)	Cognitive outcome measured	Methodology	Key findings
						nucleatum compared to controls, while the amnestic mild cognitive impairment group had a higher load of Treponema denticola compared to Alzheimer's disease.
Da et al. (2023)	Case-control study	Older adults (60+)	157	MCI and non-MCI	(1) 16S rDNA gene sequencing	- The oral microbiome of older adults with MCI showed significant differences in alpha diversity (sequencing depth and richness) and beta diversity (community structure) compared to cognitively normal older adults.
Li et al. (2024)	Case-control study	Older adults (60+)	50	MCI and dementia	(1) 16S rRNA sequencing. (2) Quantitative real-time PCR (qPCR)	- Certain bacterial genera, including *Prevotella, Lactobacillus, Megasphaera, Atopobium*, and *Howardella*, were more abundant in

						the PD-MCI group and negatively correlated with cognitive scores. - The Kgp genotype of *P. gingivalis* was more prevalent in the PD-MCI group and associated with lower cognitive scores.
Wu et al. (2021)	Case-control study	Older adults (60+)	35	Cognitive impairment and AD	(1) 16S rDNA sequencing using PacBio SMRT platform	- Patients with Alzheimer's disease had significantly more missing teeth, higher dental plaque weight, and lower overall oral microbiome diversity compared to healthy controls. -The PacBio SMRT sequencing platform could detect oral microbiome changes that may serve as biomarkers to identify patients with Alzheimer's disease.
Qiu et al. (2024)	Cross- sectional study	Older adults (60+)	96	MCI and AD	(1) 16S rRNA Sequencing:	- The study found that periodontal microbial dysbiosis and metabolic disorders may be involved in the etiology and progression of AD.

Continued

Table 6.2 Summary of study characteristics on oral bacteria and cognitive impairment.—cont'd

Author (Year)	Study design	Population	Sample size (n)	Cognitive outcome measured	Methodology	Key findings
Noble et al. (2014)	Cohort study	Older adults (65+)	219	Cognitive impairment and AD	(1) Checkerboard immunoblotting	- High serum IgG antibody levels to the periodontal bacteria *Actinomyces naeslundii* were associated with an increased risk of incident Alzheimer's disease.
Fogelholm et al. (2023)	Cross-sectional study	Older adults (50–80)	376	Cognitive impairment	(1) 16S rRNA gene sequencing	- Cognitive decline was associated with substantial changes in the composition of the subgingival microbiome, with increased abundance of the Lachnospiraceae [XIV] family being a key finding.
Holmer et al. (2021)	Case-control study	Older adults (60+)	195	MCI and non-MCI, AD, SCD	(1) 16S rRNA gene sequencing	- The subgingival microbiota of individuals with cognitive dysfunction exhibited higher microbial richness and evenness compared to cognitively healthy controls.

Yang et al. (2021)	Cross- sectional study	Older adults (60+)	68	MCI and non-MCI	(1) 16S rRNA gene sequencing	- The overall composition and diversity of the oral microbiome did not differ between the MCI and control groups. -The study suggests that pursuing the relationship between oral health, the microbiome, and inflammation could provide opportunities for new diagnostic tools and illuminate mechanisms for the prevention and mitigation of Alzheimer's disease.
Tadjoedin et al. (2022)	Case-control study	Older adults (60+)	28	MCI and non-MCI	(1) 16S rRNA gene sequencing	- The subgingival microbiome was distinct between cognitively impaired and cognitively normal elderly subjects with periodontitis.

This systematic review synthesized findings from 20 studies (Table 6.2) that examined the association between oral health, periodontal microbiota, and cognitive decline in older adults. The studies included various designs such as case reports, cross-sectional studies, case-control studies, cohort studies, and clinical trials. Participants were older adults aged 60 years and above, with sample sizes ranging from a single individual to over 5000. The cognitive outcomes assessed included MCI, AD, and other forms of dementia. The studies employed advanced molecular techniques to investigate the role of oral bacteria in cognitive decline. The most commonly used methods were 16S rRNA sequencing, quantitative polymerase chain reaction (qPCR), and immunoassays. These methods enabled detailed profiling of the oral microbiome and its potential impact on cognitive health. Cognitive impairment was assessed using various standardized tools, including the Mini-Mental State Examination (MMSE) and diagnostic criteria for MCI and AD.

A consistent finding across studies was the significant association between oral microbiome alterations and cognitive status. Several studies reported stage-dependent shifts in bacterial genera. Pathogenic bacteria, such as *Porphyromonas gingivalis* and *Fusobacterium nucleatum*, were found to increase in abundance among cognitively impaired individuals, while beneficial bacteria like *Filifactor villosus* decreased. Diversity measures also revealed marked differences; cognitively impaired individuals displayed distinct microbial richness and evenness compared to healthy controls. Subgingival microbiota composition, in particular, showed significant variation between groups. Plus, specific bacterial species and their associated biomarkers were frequently linked to cognitive outcomes. For instance, individuals with cnm-positive *Streptococcus mutans* had an increased likelihood of cerebral microbleeds, particularly in deep brain regions. Similarly, high IgG antibody levels against periodontal bacteria, such as *Actinomyces naeslundii*, were associated with an elevated risk of AD.

These findings underscore the role of particular pathogens in the progression of cognitive decline. Meanwhile, several studies explored the potential of oral health biomarkers as diagnostic tools for cognitive impairment. For instance, digital biomarkers, such as oral acidity and oral diadochokinesis rates, were significantly different between cognitively impaired and healthy groups. Predictive models leveraging these markers demonstrated high accuracy, with area under the curve (AUC) values ranging from 0.86 to 0.99 suggesting that oral health assessments could serve as non-invasive methods for early detection of cognitive decline.

6.4 Discussion

6.4.1 The role of oral bacteria species in cognitive impairment

Due to growing evidence, oral bacteria have been identified as key contributors to periodontal diseases such as gingivitis and periodontitis, which have also been linked to cognitive impairment. classifies list of oral bacteria species based on their bacterial classes, while also outlining their characteristics and roles in oral health and disease. In subsequent sections, particular focus is given to the bacteria most frequently associated with cognitive decline among older people.

6.4.2 Porphyromonas gingivalis

Among the bacterial species implicated in cognitive decline, *Porphyromonas gingivalis* was proven to be the most frequent bacteria found in the oral cavity (Leblhuber et al., 2020; Merchant et al., 2023;

Panzarella et al., 2022; Troci et al., 2024). This gram-negative anaerobe, a key pathogen in chronic periodontitis, produces virulence factors such as lipopolysaccharides (LPS) and gingipains (proteolytic enzymes) that can enter the systemic circulation and cross the blood-brain barrier (Da et al., 2023; Noble et al., 2014; Tadjoedin et al., 2022). Once in the brain, these factors stimulate neuroinflammation, induce amyloid-beta production, and contribute to tau protein hyperphosphorylation which is the factor contributing to AD. Studies have consistently linked elevated levels of antibodies against *P. gingivalis* with lower cognitive scores and increased risk of dementia (Da et al., 2023; Leblhuber et al., 2020; Merchant et al., 2023; Noble et al., 2014; Panzarella et al., 2022; Tadjoedin et al., 2022; Troci et al., 2024).

6.4.3 Streptococcus mutans

Streptococcus mutans, a gram-positive bacteria particularly strains expressing the *cnm* gene (Hosoki et al., 2020; Noble et al., 2014; Watanabe et al., 2016; Wu et al., 2021). These strains produce collagen-binding proteins that allow the bacteria to adhere to vascular endothelial cells, leading to endothelial damage and increased expression of MMP-9, which can degrade the extracellular matrix and cause cerebral microbleeds. These microbleeds have been identified as a risk factor for both vascular dementia and AD. Studies suggest that individuals harboring *cnm*-positive *S. mutans* have a significantly higher risk of cognitive decline, underscoring the importance of targeting this bacterium in prevention strategies (Hosoki et al., 2020; Noble et al., 2014; Watanabe et al., 2016; Wu et al., 2021).

6.4.4 Fusobacterium nucleatum

According to recent studies, Merchant et al. (2023) and Panzarella et al. (2022), elderly patients with AD had poorer dental health, with lower DMFT scores indicating more missing, decayed, and filled teeth which had significantly higher load of the periodontal bacteria *Fusobacterium nucleatum* (Merchant et al., 2023; Panzarella et al., 2022). Two main ways these periodontal bacteria might be linked to memory problems are by causing more inflammation in the body from the gum infection, which can impact the brain, and by directly reaching the central nervous system, possibly leading to brain cell damage. *F. nucleatum* acts as a "bridge bacterium" in biofilms, facilitating the attachment of other pathogens. The combined presence of multiple pathogens in systemic circulation can enhance inflammation and immune activation, indirectly affecting brain function.

6.4.5 Treponema denticola and Tannerella forsythia

Members of the "red complex" bacteria, including *Treponema denticola* and *Tannerella forsythia*, are strongly associated with periodontal disease and cognitive impairment. These bacteria are capable of invading host tissues, evading immune responses, and promoting chronic systemic inflammation (Da et al., 2023; Leblhuber et al., 2020; Panzarella et al., 2022; Tadjoedin et al., 2022). *Treponema denticola* in the saliva was found to be associated with lower levels of neopterin and kynurenine, respectively, suggesting they may suppress adaptive immunity and downregulate the inflammatory response. Plus, the presence of these bacteria in oral dysbiosis is linked to lower cognitive scores and increased risk of neurodegeneration, highlighting their potential role in disease progression (Da et al., 2023; Leblhuber et al., 2020; Panzarella et al., 2022; Tadjoedin et al., 2022).

6.4.6 Opportunistic and commensal bacteria

In addition to classical periodontal pathogens, opportunistic bacteria such as *Leptotrichia wadei, Veillonella spp.,* and *Lactobacillus spp* (Arıkan et al., 2023; Bathini et al., 2020; Da et al., 2023). have been detected in higher abundance in individuals with MCI or Parkinson's disease with cognitive impairment. Conversely, beneficial bacteria like *Neisseria spp.* and *Gemella haemolysans* are often reduced in these populations, suggesting that a shift in the balance between pathogenic and commensal species may drive disease progression (Arıkan et al., 2023; Bathini et al., 2020; Da et al., 2023).

6.5 Mechanisms linking oral bacteria to cognitive impairment

6.5.1 Systemic inflammation and neuroinflammation

Oral pathogens are at the forefront of the connection between periodontal disease and neurodegenerative conditions such as AD and MCI. Certain bacteria species, including *Porphyromonas gingivalis, Treponema denticola,* and *Prevotella* species, produce virulence factors that harm host tissues. For instance, *Prevotella dentalis*, a Gram-negative anaerobic rod, is typically associated with oral infections. Study highlights the clinical manifestation of the infection, including the presence of pleural effusion, the patient's underlying chronic respiratory disease, and the development of cognitive impairment in the patient (Cobo et al., 2018). Besides, oral bacteria such as *P. gingivalis* and *F. nucleatum* release LPS and other inflammatory mediators that enter the bloodstream, triggering systemic inflammation. This process activates immune cells, including microglia and astrocytes in the central nervous system, leading to chronic neuroinflammation. This state of inflammation contributes to neuronal damage, synaptic dysfunction, and the aggregation of amyloid-beta and tau proteins, ultimately accelerating cognitive decline (Chung & Chan, 2023; Wu et al., 2021).

6.5.2 Chronic inflammation

Chronic inflammation driven by periodontal disease has a systemic impact on cognitive function. The release of pro-inflammatory cytokines such as tumor necrosis factor-alpha (TNF-α) and interleukin-6 (IL-6) into circulation creates a pro-inflammatory milieu that affects the central nervous system (CNS) (Merchant et al., 2023). Periodontal microorganisms can induce an inflammatory response, and chronic inflammation has been linked to cognitive decline and neurodegenerative diseases. Bacteria species such as *Aggregatibacter actinomycetemcomitans* and *Tannerella forsythia* have been implicated in these processes. *Aggregatibacter actinomycetemcomitans,* for example, triggers an exaggerated immune response, promoting amyloid beta secretion in hippocampal cells which can result in the formation of AD (Leblhuber et al., 2020).

6.5.3 Direct neurotoxicity

Neurotoxic effects arise from bacterial byproducts such as lipopolysaccharides (LPS), a major component of Gram-negative bacteria like *Prevotella intermedia*. LPS induces microglial activation in the brain, promoting neuroinflammation and the production of reactive oxygen species (ROS), which damage neuronal structures (Da et al., 2023; Panzarella et al., 2022). Additionally, a study by Chung et al. stated that the involvement of *Streptococcus mutans*, particularly *cnm*-positive strains with collagen-binding capabilities, has been linked to vascular injury and deep cerebral microbleeds, further contributing to cognitive impairment (Chung & Chan, 2023). Certain oral bacteria have been detected in the brains of individuals with AD. The study by Troci et al. (2024) mentioned that some oral bacteria produce neurotoxic compounds that can directly affect neuronal health and function (Troci et al., 2024). For example, *P. gingivalis* and *T. denticola* are believed to reach the brain via systemic circulation or through cranial nerves such as the trigeminal or olfactory nerves. Once in the brain, these bacteria exacerbate neurodegeneration through the release of proteolytic enzymes and inflammatory mediators (Noble et al., 2014; Tadjoedin et al., 2022).

6.5.4 Blood-brain barrier disruption

Certain oral bacteria, such as *Porphyromonas gingivalis*, have been suggested to cross the blood-brain barrier (BBB), a protective membrane that prevents harmful substances from entering the brain. Inflammation may compromise the integrity of the blood-brain barrier, allowing inflammatory mediators and bacteria to enter the central nervous system (CNS) (Troci et al., 2024). Pathogens present may affect the blood-brain barrier permeability, influencing local immune responses and amyloid clearance in the brain. Plus, the mechanisms leading to cerebral microbleeds (CMB), such as endothelial injury and blood-brain barrier disruption, may impair cerebral blood flow and function, impacting cognitive abilities. The increased incidence of CMB is associated with cognitive decline and dementia (Hosoki et al., 2020).

6.5.5 Immune dysregulation

Furthermore, immune dysregulation is caused by oral pathogens that compromise adaptive immunity. These pathogens can inhibit the function of regulatory T cells, leading to an imbalance between pro-inflammatory and anti-inflammatory responses. For example, bacteria species such as *Treponema denticola* and *Tannerella forsythia* may alter the host immune response, affecting immune biomarkers which are neopterin and kynurenine levels. This dysregulation exacerbates systemic inflammation and increases the risk of cognitive decline, particularly in elderly individuals with existing periodontal disease (Leblhuber et al., 2020).

6.5.6 Microbial dysbiosis

Microbial dysbiosis, an imbalance in the oral microbiota can lead to the overgrowth of pathogenic bacteria, which may induce inflammation and contribute to cognitive decline. The study by Arıkan et al. (2023) and Holmer et al. (2021) mentioned that alterations in the composition of the oral microbiota, particularly the decrease in beneficial bacteria such as *Neisseria* and *Rothia* the increase in *Lactobacillus*, *Streptococcus*, *Prevotella,* and *Fusobacterium* which affect the cognitive function. These changes have been linked to systemic inflammation and neurodegeneration. For example, patients with AD have shown altered salivary microbiota, with increased levels of *Lactobacillus* and *Streptococcus*, which are associated with cognitive decline. Conversely, dietary interventions, such as the consumption of nitrate-rich foods, promote the growth of beneficial bacteria like *Rothia* and *Neisseria*, which produce nitric oxide known as a molecule crucial for vascular health and cognitive function.

6.5.7 Neurodegenerative process

Periodontal pathogens directly contribute to neurodegeneration by influencing amyloid and tau pathology in the brain. Oral bacteria may influence the accumulation of amyloid-β (Aβ) plaques and tau tangles, which are significant features of AD pathology (Troci et al., 2024). Studies by Panzarella et al. (2022) and Leblhuber et al. (2020), suggest that MCI is linked to early neurodegenerative processes, potentially leading to the development of AD. MCI may involve the accumulation of amyloid-beta plaques and tau tangles in the brain, which are characteristic of neurodegenerative diseases. *Porphyromonas gingivalis* has been shown to exacerbate amyloid beta accumulation, *while Treponema denticola* and *Tannerella forsythia* produce enzymes that degrade neuronal proteins, accelerating neurodegenerative processes (Leblhuber et al., 2020).

6.5.8 Vascular and functional changes in oral health

Bacteria such as *cnm*-positive S. mutans directly affect vascular health by damaging the endothelium and promoting the formation of cerebral microbleeds. Watanabe et al. (2016) stated that this mechanism involves the ability of the *cnm*-positive strain of *Streptococcus mutans* to bind to collagen, a component of dentin and the vascular endothelium (Watanabe et al., 2016). This binding activity is associated with an increased risk of deep cerebral microbleeds (CMBs) and cognitive impairment. Periodontal pathogens can also contribute to atherogenesis, reducing cerebral blood flow and impairing cognitive function. This vascular component highlights the multifactorial nature of oral bacteria's impact on brain health (Fogelholm et al., 2023; Hosoki et al., 2020).

6.5.9 The link between Parkinson's disease and cognitive impairment

6.5.9.1 Cognitive impairment in Parkinson's disease

Cognitive impairment (CI) is a prevalent and progressive non-motor symptom of Parkinson's disease (PD), affecting a significant proportion of patients as the disease advances. Studies indicate that nearly half of PD patients develop dementia within 10 years of diagnosis, with a substantial proportion of PD-MCI cases progressing to Parkinson's disease dementia (PDD) over time (Arıkan et al., 2023; Li et al., 2024). The high conversion rate from PD-MCI to PDD suggests an urgent need for early detection and intervention to delay or prevent cognitive decline in PD patients.

6.5.9.2 Pathological mechanisms of cognitive decline

The underlying mechanisms contributing to cognitive decline in PD are complex and multifactorial, involving neuroinflammatory responses, α-synuclein deposition, and Alzheimer's disease-like pathologies, including amyloid-β accumulation and tau tangles (Li et al., 2024). These pathological changes lead to neuronal dysfunction, affecting key cognitive domains such as memory, executive function, and attention. In addition, vascular abnormalities and oxidative stress further contribute to neurodegeneration, worsening cognitive impairment in PD patients. Identifying patients at risk of cognitive deterioration is crucial for early intervention, as timely diagnosis and targeted therapeutic strategies may help slow the progression of cognitive decline in PD patients.

6.5.10 Oral microbiome and Parkinson's disease

6.5.10.1 Microbiome dysbiosis in Parkinson's disease

A growing body of evidence suggests that alterations in the oral microbiome contribute to the pathogenesis of PD and its associated cognitive impairment. PD patients exhibit significant dysbiosis in their oral microbiota, characterized by an increased abundance of specific bacterial genera, such as *Lactobacillus, Megasphaera*, and *Prevotella,* while beneficial bacteria like *Neisseria* show a marked decline (Arıkan et al., 2023; Li et al., 2024). This imbalance may have widespread implications, influencing systemic inflammation, gut-brain axis dysfunction, and neurodegenerative processes. Changes in the oral microbiome may also be linked to impaired immune responses, further promoting bacterial colonization and infection, which may contribute to disease progression.

6.5.10.2 Oral health and cognitive function

Oral health deterioration, including reduced saliva secretion and dysphagia, has been strongly correlated with worsening cognitive status in PD patients. Saliva plays a crucial role in maintaining oral microbiota homeostasis, and reduced secretion can exacerbate microbial imbalances, increasing the risk of periodontal disease and systemic inflammation. The presence of specific bacterial and protein markers in saliva suggests that monitoring and modulating the oral microbiome could play a crucial role in mitigating disease progression and preserving cognitive function (Arıkan et al., 2023). Further research is needed to determine whether oral health interventions, such as improved hygiene practices or probiotic treatments, can have a protective effect on cognitive function in PD patients.

6.5.11 Potential mechanisms linking oral bacteria, Parkinson's disease, and cognitive impairment

6.5.11.1 Neuroinflammation and systemic effects

Neuroinflammation is a key mechanism connecting oral microbiota alterations to cognitive impairment in PD. Chronic oral infections, particularly those involving *Porphyromonas gingivalis* (*P. gingivalis*), can trigger systemic inflammation, elevating pro-inflammatory cytokine levels in the brain and accelerating neurodegeneration (Li et al., 2024). The immune response to these infections may exacerbate neuronal damage, leading to further cognitive deterioration. Variations in the lysine-gingipain (Kgp) genotype of *P. gingivalis* have been significantly associated with cognitive decline in PD patients, indicating that bacterial virulence factors contribute to disease pathology. These findings suggest that targeting specific bacterial strains or virulence factors may be a potential therapeutic avenue to reduce neuroinflammation and slow cognitive decline in PD patients.

6.5.11.2 Bacterial translocation and blood-brain barrier dysfunction

Bacterial translocation and reduced bactericidal permeability-increasing protein (BPI) levels may lead to increased endotoxin exposure and blood-brain barrier (BBB) disruption, further exacerbating cognitive decline (Arıkan et al., 2023). The weakening of the BBB allows harmful bacterial metabolites and inflammatory molecules to enter the brain, intensifying neuroinflammatory responses and promoting neuronal loss. The role of bacterial translocation highlights the importance of maintaining both oral and gut microbiome balance to prevent further neurodegeneration. Future research should focus on how interventions aimed at preserving BBB integrity might mitigate PD-associated cognitive impairment.

6.5.11.3 Metabolic disruptions and cognitive decline

The metabolic influence of oral bacteria is another important aspect, as microbial metabolites, such as reduced pyruvate phosphate dikinase (PPDK) levels, may impair energy metabolism and contribute to neurodegenerative processes (Arıkan et al., 2023). Impaired metabolic pathways can affect mitochondrial function, reduce cellular energy production, and increase oxidative stress, all of which contribute to the progressive cognitive decline observed in PD patients. These findings suggest that dietary modifications, probiotics, or metabolic-targeting drugs could be potential strategies for mitigating the impact of oral dysbiosis on cognitive function in PD.

6.6 Conclusion

This systematic review underscores the significant association between oral bacteriome dysbiosis and cognitive impairment among older adults, including those with mild cognitive impairment (MCI), Alzheimer's disease (AD), and Parkinson's disease (PD). Pathogenic bacteria such as *Porphyromonas gingivalis, Fusobacterium nucleatum, Treponema denticola,* and *Streptococcus mutans* contribute to neuroinflammation, systemic inflammation, blood-brain barrier disruption, and microbial dysbiosis, all of which are implicated in cognitive decline. In Parkinson's disease, alterations in the oral microbiome, particularly an increased abundance of *Lactobacillus* and *Prevotella* species and a decline in *Neisseria,* have been linked to both motor and cognitive dysfunction. Additionally, bacterial virulence factors such as the lysine-gingipain (Kgp) genotype of *P. gingivalis* may play a role in neurodegeneration in PD-related cognitive impairment.

Emerging biomarkers, including oral acidity levels, antibody titers against periodontal bacteria, and specific microbial profiles, show promise for early detection of cognitive impairment. However, despite growing evidence, key knowledge gaps remain regarding the causal mechanisms linking oral bacteria to neurodegenerative diseases. Future research should focus on standardized methodologies, longitudinal studies, and intervention-based trials to establish causation and explore whether improving oral health could help in slowing down the progression of cognitive decline. Given the increasing aging population and the burden of dementia-related disorders, integrating oral health management into cognitive and neurodegenerative disease prevention strategies may offer a valuable approach for early intervention and improved health outcomes.

Acknowledgments

This study is funded by a research grant from the Ministry of Higher Education (MOHE) – Fundamental Research Grant Scheme (FRGS); FRGS21-211-0820 FRGS/1/2021/SKK05/UIAM/03/1.

Ethical statement

We would like to acknowledge our Kulliyyah of Medicine, International Islamic University of Malaysia (IIUM) and Research Management Center IIUM for full support of this research. This research is sponsored by grant from the Ministry of Higher Education of Malaysia (MOHE) – Fundamental Research Grant Scheme (FRGS); FRGS/1/2021/SKK05/UIAM/03/1. The authors also thank the research management center (IIUM) for facilitating the grant management (FRGS21-211-0820).

Conflict of interest

The authors declare no conflict of interest.

References

Anand, S., & Schoo, C. (2024). In *Mild cognitive impairment.*

Arıkan, M., Demir, T. K., Yıldız, Z., Nalbantoğlu, Ö. U., Korkmaz, N. D., Yılmaz, N. H., Sen, A., Özcan, M., Muth, T., Hanoğlu, L., & Yıldırım, S. (2023). Metaproteogenomic analysis of saliva samples from Parkinson's disease patients with cognitive impairment. *NPJ Biofilms and Microbiomes, 9*(1). https://doi.org/10.1038/s41522-023-00452-x

Bathini, P., Foucras, S., Dupanloup, I., Imeri, H., Perna, A., Berruex, J. L., Doucey, M. A., Annoni, J. M., & Auber Alberi, L. (2020). Classifying dementia progression using microbial profiling of saliva. *Alzheimer's and Dementia: Diagnosis, Assessment and Disease Monitoring, 12*(1). https://doi.org/10.1002/dad2.12000

Chung, P.-C., & Chan, T.-C. (2023). Digital oral health biomarkers for early detection of cognitive decline. *BMC Public Health, 23*(1), 16897. https://doi.org/10.1186/s12889-023-16897-w

Cobo, F., Calatrava, E., Rodríguez-Granger, J., Sampedro, A., Aliaga-Martínez, L., & Navarro-Marí, J. M. (2018). A rare case of pleural effusion due to Prevotella dentalis. *Anaerobe, 54*, 144–145. https://doi.org/10.1016/j.anaerobe.2018.09.004

Da, D., Zhao, Q., Zhang, H., Wu, W., Zeng, X., Liang, X., Jiang, Y., Xiao, Z., Yu, J., Ding, S., Zheng, L., Zhang, Y., Xu, X., & Ding, D. (2023). Oral microbiome in older adults with mild cognitive impairment. *Journal of Oral Microbiology, 15*(1). https://doi.org/10.1080/20002297.2023.2173544

Fogelholm, N., Leskelä, J., Manzoor, M., Jacob, H., Paju, S., Hiltunen, K., Roitto, H.-M., Kt Saarela, R., Pitkälä, K., Eriksdotter, M., Buhlin, K., Pussinen, P. J., & Mäntylä, P. (2023). Subgingival microbiome at different levels of cognition. *Journal of Oral Microbiology, 15*(1). https://doi.org/10.1080/20002297.2023.2178765

Holmer, J., Aho, V., Eriksdotter, M., Paulin, L., Pietiäinen, M., Auvinen, P., Schultzberg, M., Pussinen, P. J., & Buhlin, K. (2021). Subgingival microbiota in a population with and without cognitive dysfunction. *Journal of Oral Microbiology, 13*(1). https://doi.org/10.1080/20002297.2020.1854552

Hosoki, S., Saito, S., Tonomura, S., Ishiyama, H., Yoshimoto, T., Ikeda, S., Ikenouchi, H., Yamamoto, Y., Hattori, Y., Miwa, K., Friedland, R. P., Carare, R. O., Jin, N., Suzuki, N., Koga, M., Toyoda, K., Nomura, R., Nakano, K., Takegami, M., & Ihara, M. (2020). Oral carriage of Streptococcus mutans harboring the cnm gene relates to an increased incidence of cerebral microbleeds. *Stroke, 51*(12), 3632–3639. https://doi.org/10.1161/strokeaha.120.029607

Leblhuber, F., Huemer, J., Steiner, K., Gostner, J. M., & Fuchs, D. (2020). Knock-on effect of periodontitis to the pathogenesis of Alzheimer's disease? *Wiener Klinische Wochenschrift, 132*(17–18), 493–498. https://doi.org/10.1007/s00508-020-01638-5

Li, D., Ren, T., Li, H., Huang, M., Chen, J., He, Q., et al. (2024). Oral microbiota and *Porphyromonas gingivalis Kgp* genotypes altered in Parkinson's disease with mild cognitive impairment. *Molecular Neurobiology, 61.* https://doi.org/10.1007/s12035-024-04119-2

Lu, M., Xuan, S., & Wang, Z. (2019). Oral microbiota: A new view of body health. *Food Science and Human Wellness, 8*(1), 8–15. https://doi.org/10.1016/j.fshw.2018.12.001

Merchant, A. T., Yi, F., Vidanapathirana, N. P., Lohman, M., Zhang, J., Newman-Norlund, R. D., & Fridriksson, J. (2023). Antibodies against periodontal microorganisms and cognition in older adults. *JDR Clinical & Translational Research, 8*(2), 148–157. https://doi.org/10.1177/23800844211072784

Noble, J. M., Scarmeas, N., Celenti, R. S., Elkind, M. S. V., Wright, C. B., Schupf, N., & Papapanou, P. N. (2014). Serum IgG antibody levels to periodontal microbiota are associated with incident alzheimer disease. *PLoS One, 9*(12). https://doi.org/10.1371/journal.pone.0114959

Page, M. J., McKenzie, J. E., Bossuyt, P. M., Boutron, I., Hoffmann, T. C., Mulrow, C. D., et al. (2021). The PRISMA 2020 statement: An updated guideline for reporting systematic reviews. *Journal of Clinical Epidemiology, 134*, 178–189.

Panzarella, V., Mauceri, R., Baschi, R., Maniscalco, L., Campisi, G., & Monastero, R. (2022). Oral health status in subjects with amnestic mild cognitive impairment and Alzheimer's disease: Data from the Zabút Aging Project. *Journal of Alzheimer's Disease, 87*(1), 173–183. https://doi.org/10.3233/jad-200385

Plachokova, A. S., Andreu-Sánchez, S., Noz, M. P., Fu, J., & Riksen, N. P. (2021). Oral microbiome in relation to periodontitis severity and systemic inflammation. *International Journal of Molecular Sciences, 22*(11). https://doi.org/10.3390/ijms22115876

Qiu, C., Zhou, W., Shen, H., Wang, J., Tang, R., Wang, T., Xie, X., Hong, B., Ren, R., Wang, G., & Song, Z. (2024). Profiles of subgingival microbiomes and gingival crevicular metabolic signatures in patients with amnestic mild cognitive impairment and Alzheimer's disease. *Alzheimer's Research & Therapy, 16*(1). https://doi.org/10.1186/s13195-024-01402-1

Tadjoedin, F. M., Masulili, S. L. C., Rizal, M. I., Kusdhany, L. S., Turana, Y., Ismail, R. I., & Bachtiar, B. M. (2022). The red and orange complex subgingival microbiome of cognitive impairment and cognitively normal elderly with periodontitis. *Geriatrics, 7*(1). https://doi.org/10.3390/geriatrics7010012

Troci, A., Philippen, S., Rausch, P., Rave, J., Weyland, G., Niemann, K., Jessen, K., Schmill, L.-P., Aludin, S., Franke, A., Berg, D., Bang, C., Bartsch, T., & Dupont, C. (2024). Disease- and stage-specific alterations of the oral and fecal microbiota in Alzheimer's disease. *PNAS Nexus, 3*(1). https://doi.org/10.1093/pnasnexus/pgad427

Vanhatalo, A., L'Heureux, J. E., Kelly, J., Blackwell, J. R., Wylie, L. J., Fulford, J., Winyard, P. G., Williams, D. W., van der Giezen, M., & Jones, A. M. (2021). Network analysis of nitrate-sensitive oral microbiome reveals interactions with cognitive function and cardiovascular health across dietary interventions. *Redox Biology, 41*. https://doi.org/10.1016/j.redox.2021.101933

Visentin, D., Gobin, I., & Maglica, Ž. (2023). Periodontal pathogens and their links to neuroinflammation and neurodegeneration. *Microorganisms, 11*(7), 1832. https://doi.org/10.3390/microorganisms11071832

Watanabe, I., Kuriyama, N., Miyatani, F., Nomura, R., Naka, S., Nakano, K., Ohi, T., Kato, Y., Ozaki, E., Iwasaki, M., Yamashita, Y., Ihara, M., Miyamoto, T., & Nakagawa, M. (2016). Oral Cnm-positive Streptococcus mutans expressing collagen binding activity is a risk factor for cerebral microbleeds and cognitive impairment. *Scientific Reports, 6*(1). https://doi.org/10.1038/srep38561

World population ageing 2020 highlights: Living arrangements of older persons. (2020). United Nations.

Wu, Y. F., Lee, W. F., Salamanca, E., Yao, W. L., Su, J. N., Wang, S. Y., Hu, C. J., & Chang, W. J. (2021). Oral microbiota changes in elderly patients, an indicator of Alzheimer's disease. *International Journal of Environmental Research and Public Health, 18*(8). https://doi.org/10.3390/ijerph18084211

Yang, I., Arthur, R. A., Zhao, L., Clark, J., Hu, Y., Corwin, E. J., & Lah, J. (2021). The oral microbiome and inflammation in mild cognitive impairment. *Experimental Gerontology, 147*. https://doi.org/10.1016/j.exger.2021.111273

CHAPTER

Pharmacokinetics and pharmacodynamics in Parkinson's disease

7

Kholoud Mohamed Ibrahim, Ganna Ameen, Esraa M. Sakr, Basant Osama and Yomna Mostafa
Biophysics Department, Faculty of Science, Cairo University, Cairo, Egypt

7.1 Introduction

Parkinson disease (PD) is defined as a progressive neurodegenerative disease that is characterized by the loss of dopaminergic neurons in the substantia nigra, followed by motor and nonmotor symptoms affecting the quality of life of patients. The treatment of choice for PD primarily involves pharmacotherapy intended to restore, improve, or modify dopamine concentrations and neurotransmission to treat symptoms. To utilize this knowledge effectively for achieving optimized efficacy with minimal side effects, one needs a thorough knowledge of the pharmacokinetics (Pk) and pharmacodynamics (Pd) of the antiparkinsonian drugs (Isaacson et al., 2023; Woitalla et al., 2023).

Pk of a drug refers to its absorption, distribution, metabolism, and excretion (ADME) into or out of the body, which are important determinants of drug concentrations at the site of action. In PD, various physiological changes can influence drug Pk, such as the permeability of the blood-brain barrier and hepatic metabolism. Such changes give variability to therapeutic responses. One of the important ways of treatment is that levodopa undergoes almost complete first-pass metabolism and hence is administered with dopa decarboxylase inhibitors to enhance its bioavailability, thus prolonging its therapeutic effects. Other dopaminergic agents such as dopamine agonists (DAs), MAO-B inhibitors, and COMT inhibitors present different pharmacokinetic profiles with implications for their clinical utility. Subsequently, novel drug delivery systems are being evaluated for controlled-release formulations and continuous infusion therapies to optimize pharmacokinetic consistency while minimizing the peaks and troughs in drug levels (Gharat et al., 2024; Lewitt, 2015).

Pharmacodynamics, on the other hand, examines the biochemical and physiological effects of drugs and their mechanisms of action. In PD, the primary pharmacodynamic target is the dopaminergic system, where therapies aim to restore dopaminergic neurotransmission or modulate related pathways. The therapeutic response to levodopa and other drugs is often complicated by motor fluctuations, such as wearing-off phenomena and dyskinesias, which are closely linked to drug-receptor interactions and adaptive neuroplastic changes over time. Understanding receptor binding, downstream signaling pathways, and compensatory mechanisms is crucial for refining treatment strategies and developing novel therapeutics with improved efficacy and tolerability. Moreover, pharmacodynamic research is increasingly focusing on nondopaminergic systems, including glutamatergic, cholinergic, and

Pharmacological Foundations of Parkinson's Disease. https://doi.org/10.1016/B978-0-443-27702-3.00014-5

adenosinergic pathways, to develop adjunctive treatments that target motor and nonmotor symptoms more effectively (Gharat et al., 2024; Lewitt, 2015).

In this chapter, we provide detailed information on the Pk and Pd of drugs that are key to the treatment of PD. The chapter discusses problems of factors affecting drug disposition, interpatient variation, and therapy optimization issues in a progressive neurodegenerative disorder. New pharmacological approaches, such as novel delivery systems and continuous-drug infusions, will be examined for their importance in Pk and pharmacodynamics. In this effort, the chapter will combine the principles with clinical observations to explain drug effects in PD for the ultimate objective of improved individualized treatment strategies for patients with this incapacitating disorder. It will also underscore the relevance of personalized medicine systems, therapeutic drug monitoring, and patient-centered approaches toward the long-term management of the disease and enhancement of the quality of life.

7.2 Levodopa

7.2.1 L-DOPA

Following the hydroxylation of tyrosine, L-DOPA (L-3,4-dihydroxyphenylalanine), a precursor of dopamine (dihydroxy-3,4-phenyl-ethylamine), was introduced in the late 1960s. The discovery of L-dopa, the precursor of dopamine that crosses the blood-brain barrier, was revolutionary. It has significantly improved the lives of several people worldwide by effectively treating motor symptoms. The L-DOPA response is increasingly used as a diagnostic standard (Demailly et al., 2024; Müller, 2020).

Dopamine-decarboxylase (aromatic L-amino acid decarboxylase) later converts L-DOPA into dopamine. Dopamine β-hydroxylase can further convert dopamine into noradrenaline within adrenergic and noradrenergic neurons. Lastly, a variety of enzymatic and nonenzymatic processes catabolize dopamine, most notably the sequential activity of two enzymes: catecholamine O-methyl transferase (COMT) and monoamine oxidases A and B. Antiparkinsonian medications, such as entacapone and tolcapone for COMT inhibitors, target both enzymes in conjunction with L-DOPA to increase its effects by about 30% (Demailly et al., 2024).

Because the gut's peripheral aromatic L-amino acid decarboxylase (AADC) significantly metabolizes oral levodopa into dopamine, it has a 30% bioavailability (Xu et al., 2023; di Biase et al., 2023). By increasing levodopa's bioavailability by up to three times, concurrent administration of AADC peripheral inhibitors (AADCI) lowers the necessary therapeutic dose. Levodopa interferes with the neutral amino acid transport pathway in the blood–brain barrier and intestinal mucosa. High-protein meals raise the plasmatic concentrations of neutral amino acids, which decreases levodopa absorption and its therapeutic effect. To maximize levodopa's therapeutic efficacy, the delivery schedule should be adjusted to coincide with mealtimes (di Biase et al., 2023; Leta et al., 2023).

A serine-rich diet may even increase the bioavailability by 22% when compared to the administration of ante-cibum, according to mathematical simulations that also show that not all amino acids compete with levodopa absorption. Research on how pharmacokinetic and pharmacodynamic factors change as an illness progresses has been extensive (di Biase et al., 2023).

7.2.2 Pharmacokinetics

One of the most important Pk properties for L-DOPA is its short plasma half lifetime. It has a brief half-life of 30–90 min. Levodopa plasma concentrations fluctuate throughout the day because of this rapid metabolism. After levodopa is administered orally in plasma, its peripheral rise and fall is converted into pulsatile dopamine levels in the brain by the blood-brain barrier and its presynaptic dopa decarboxylase-mediated conversion to dopamine (Müller et al., 2024).

The short half-life maintains steady control over motor symptoms, so patients must take doses extremely often (every two to 3 hours) throughout the day. The neurons in the substantia nigra must retain L-DOPA when it is intermittently consumed. This storage capacity decreases as the disease progresses because fewer of these neurons are present. Patients are forced to reduce the time between doses as a result of this trend, which increases Pk inconsistencies and causes motor irregularities. Dopaminergic neurons are abnormally activated on a big scale and intermittently because of the short half-life and higher dosage frequency (Demailly et al., 2024).

Another challenge for Pk of oral Levodopa is the variable intragastric bioavailability. As some conditions worsen, dysphagia—a condition marked by trouble swallowing liquids, solid meals, or saliva—becomes more common. The main cause of it is bradykinesia. Drug retention in the esophagus or the epiglottic vallecula has been documented in a number of clinical cases (Demailly et al., 2024; Safarpour et al., 2022).). The peak plasma concentration of L-DOPA may decrease because of this retention. Nonetheless, studies have proved that a more typical Pk profile for oral L-DOPA can be achieved by successfully addressing dysphagia, particularly through speech therapy (Demailly et al., 2024).

Sometimes due to neuronal death the decrease in dopamine storage may cause problems with pharmacokinetics. As PD advances, the gradual death of dopamine neurons significantly impacts the Pk of L-DOPA. Imaging studies have shown that with disease progression, there is a heightened release of dopamine in the brain following an L-DOPA dose, potentially explaining L-DOPA-induced dyskinesias. This can be attributed to multiple factors: the diminished capacity for vesicular dopamine storage, a decrease in dopamine reuptake sites due to vanishing DATs, and the unintended utilization of L-DOPA by nondopaminergic cells. Continuous dopaminergic administration may reduce the impact of this problem on treatment Pk (Demailly et al., 2024).

7.2.3 Pharmacodynamics

Numerous dopamine receptors and transduction systems spread throughout diverse parts of the central nervous system result in distinct actions with varying time courses, making the Pd of L-dopa complicated. As a result, "the" reaction to L-dopa in Pd is the culmination of numerous dopamine-induced alterations in neuronal activity. Despite the wide range of responses, the short-duration antiparkinsonian response is the most common Pd therapy used to treat Parkinsonism. The concentrations of plasma L-dopa and, most likely, striatal synaptic dopamine are approximately paralleled by the short-duration response. The motor fluctuations or, in extreme situations, the "on-off phenomenon" is caused by this short-duration motor response (Fabbri et al., 2023; Nutt, 2008).

7.2.4 Factors affecting

Each drug sometimes has factors affecting its Pk and Pd, however, gender is the most affecting factor for LD. Regretfully, long-term use of LD causes problems, primarily dyskinesias and motor/nonmotor swings. It appears that women are more likely to experience certain LD-related issues. However, few prospective studies have looked at gender-related determinants of dyskinesias and motor/nonmotor variations. The effectiveness of medicine is influenced by variations in LD pharmacokinetics, among other parameters that concur with a very complex scenario (Conti et al., 2022). As the most relevant clinically practical finding, women might require a 25% reduced weight-normalized LD dose compared with men to achieve the same LD bioavailability, contributing to minimize the development of LD induced dyskinesias in the long term (Conti et al., 2022).

7.3 Dopamine agonists

DAs are a crucial part of the therapy in PD since they substitute for dopamine deficiency in the basal ganglia. DAs are split into two subsets ergoline agonists (ergot-like derivatives, e.g., bromocriptine, cabergoline, lisuride, and pergolide) and non-ergoline-derived agonists (e.g., pramipexole, ropinirole, rotigotine, and apomorphine) (Isaacson et al., 2023).

7.3.1 Ergoline derivatives

Ergoline derivatives like bromocriptine, pergolide, lisuride, and cabergoline are ergot alkaloid-derived and act primarily on dopamine receptors. Their Pk and Pd profile in the management of PD will be discussed.

7.3.1.1 Bromocriptine

Bromocriptine is also administered as adjunct therapy alongside levodopa, lowering the dose of levodopa needed as well as increasing motor fluctuations toward the end of a dosing interval. In de novo patients with a new diagnosis, bromocriptine monotherapy has been shown to delay the treatment with levodopa and prevent motor complications. It is normally administered three times a day (Ozery & Wadhwa, 2024). Bromocriptine is a D2 dopamine receptor agonist that selectively activates D2 receptors while acting as a partial antagonist at D1 receptors. It is tissue-selective in its action. In PD, bromocriptine causes activation of striatal D2 receptors in order to facilitate movement and relief from bradykinesia due to degeneration of dopaminergic neurons in the nigrostriatal pathway. Similarly, its stimulation of D2 receptors in the anterior pituitary suppresses prolactin release, which controls hyperprolactinemia, particularly in pituitary prolactinoma.

7.3.1.1.1 Pk of bromocriptine

After oral administration, the peak plasma concentration of bromocriptine is reached in about 2.5 h, and its elimination half-life is about 4.85 h. Its systemic absorption is not affected by food intake in a clinically significant way, but bromocriptine should be taken with food to avoid nausea and vomiting that may occur if taken under fasting conditions. Bromocriptine is bound to plasma proteins, usually between 90% and 96%, and primarily binds to serum albumin. Bromocriptine undergoes extensive liver first-pass metabolism mainly by CYP3A4 enzymes. Due to its high CYP3A affinity, other drugs blocking or competing with CYP3A4 can reduce the clearance of bromocriptine and consequently elevate plasma levels. Bromocriptine is also a CYP3A4 inhibitor. Bromocriptine is eliminated mainly through bile, whereas only 2%–6% of it is removed through urine (Kvernmo et al., 2006).

7.3.1.2 Pergolide

Pergolide is a synthetic ergot-derived DA with a major activity at D2-type dopamine receptors but also with agonist action at D1-type receptors. Pergolide also has high affinity for serotonin receptors 5-HT2A (Ki = 8.3 nmol/L) and 5-HT2B (Ki = 7.1 nmol/L), with reported agonist action at 5-HT2B. A randomized, controlled trial assessed the use of pergolide compared to levodopa for motor complication prevention in early PD. This trial differed from previous trials by prohibiting levodopa rescue treatment and recruiting individuals with mild severity (Hoehn-Yahr stage 1–1.5). A total of 294 participants were allocated at random to receive either pergolide (3.23 mg/day) or levodopa (504 mg/day). The treated patients had significantly more dyskinesia after 3 years ($P < .001$), but their wearing-off effect and motor fluctuation were no different from their controls. A further 6-month double-blind, placebo-controlled trial investigated pergolide as an adjunct to levodopa in advanced PD (Hoehn-Yahr grade 2–4). Patients (n = 376) were randomized to pergolide (2.94 mg/day) + levodopa (671 mg/day) or placebo + levodopa (894 mg/day). Pergolide reduced levodopa requirements significantly ($P < .001$) but improved total Pd scores ($P < .001$), though prevalence and severity of dyskinesia were not different between groups. While pergolide showed clinical usefulness, its high affinity for serotonin 5-HT2A and 5-HT2B receptors precipitated valvular heart disease (VHD) risk. Studies indicate that there is a dose-dependent relationship, although valvulopathic fibrotic cases have been observed even on low doses (Kvernmo et al., 2006; Oertel et al., 2006).

7.3.1.2.1 Pk of pergolide

Pergolide has linear Pk up to a dose of 3 mg/day, only slightly more than half its therapeutic window for PD treatment. Pergolide is metabolized primarily by the CYP3A4 enzyme, and thus coadministration with CYP3A4 inhibitors would lead to increased plasma levels of pergolide, similar to that with bromocriptine and cabergoline. Co-administration with CYP3A4 Ind.ucers, on the other hand, could lead to subtherapeutic concentrations of pergolide and thus possibly undermine its effectiveness. Additionally, pergolide is a potent CYP2D6 inhibitor ($IC_{50} = 0.08$ μmol/L), just like paroxetine ($K_i = 0.15$ μmol/L) and quinidine ($K_i = 0.03$ μmol/L). Due to its inhibition of CYP2D6, pergolide has the potential to interact with other substrates of CYP2D6 like tricyclic antidepressants and antiarrhythmics and alter their metabolism and plasma concentration. Understanding such metabolic pathways is critical for controlling potential drug interactions, providing therapeutic effects, and evading unfavorable effects in patients taking pergolide (Kvernmo et al., 2006).

7.3.1.3 Lisuride

Lisuride is a PD drug that possesses a chemical structure similar to dopaminergic ergoline. It has also recently been found in some studies to bind with the histamine H1 receptor (Cacabelos, 2017; Kumar et al., 2023). Unlike pergolide, lisuride does not bind to 5HT2B receptors, meaning it is unlikely to contribute to valvular heart disease (Reichmann et al., 2006).

7.3.1.3.1 Pk of lisuride

Lisuride is rapidly absorbed from the gastrointestinal tract. When given orally, it is extensively metabolized by the liver during the first pass, with very marked interindividual variation due to differences in cytochrome P450 enzyme activity, particularly CYP2D6. Lisuride thus must be slowly and gradually titrated according to patient tolerance and therapeutic response. The clearance value of lisuride has been found to be approximately 0.80 ± 0.25 L/min in healthy volunteers. In patients with

PD, the calculated clearance values using the area under the curve (AUC) analysis were 0.39–7.13 L/min with a mean of 1.95 ± 1.99 L/min (Burns & Calne, 1981; Burns et al., 1984; Horowski, 2022, pp. 3199–3241). The drug also undergoes moderate enterohepatic circulation (Horowski, 2022, pp. 3199–3241).

Lisuride undergoes metabolism in different ways, including oxidative des-alkylation, hydroxylation, mono-oxygenation, and oxidation. None of the metabolites are responsible for more than 10% of the high-pressure liquid chromatography (HPLC) spectrum, and none of them would be expected to influence lisuride's pharmacological effect greatly. The medication is eliminated largely through urine and to a limited extent through feces, as with other ergoline derivatives (Horowski, 2022, pp. 3199–3241).

The systemic availability of lisuride is very inconstant between different individuals but more or less consistent within individuals. It has an average bioavailability of 10%–20%, however, ranging between 5% and 50% in a few individuals. The degree of the first-pass effect and thus the bioavailability of lisuride are variably dependent upon liver blood flow and the extent of activity of the liver microsomal enzymes, particularly CYP2D6. It must be noted that a clinical trial has reported a 100% increase in lisuride clearance after 2–4 weeks of continuous treatment (Burns et al., 1984; Horowski, 2022, pp. 3199–3241).

7.3.1.4 Cabergoline

Cabergoline (1-[(6-allylergolin-8β-yl) carbonyl]-1-[3-(dimethylamino) propyl]-3-ethyl-urea) is a novel dopamine D2 receptor agonist utilized for managing PD. It possesses distinct pharmacological characteristics, including an extended plasma half-life of approximately 68 h, enabling once-daily dosing. Multiple clinical studies have demonstrated that cabergoline is generally well tolerated (Pastor & Tolosa, 2003).

Cabergoline is used for PD treatment (except in the United States) and reproductive medicine. In addition to its strong D2 receptor agonist activity, it also has a significant affinity for D1 receptors and 5-HT2A (Ki = 6.2 nmol/L) and 5-HT2B (Ki = 1.2 nmol/L) serotonin receptors. A meta-analysis found that cabergoline increases the risk of dyskinesia compared to bromocriptine (OR = 1.57; $P = .03$), possibly due to its D1 receptor activity. Another meta-analysis reviewed three large, randomized, double-blind clinical trials:

Study 1: 412 patients took either cabergoline (0.25 mg/day to 4 mg/day) or L-dopa (100–600 mg/day) for 5 years.

Study 2: 301 patients received either pramipexole (1.5–4.5 mg/day) or L-dopa (300–600 mg/day) for 2 years.

Study 3: 268 patients were given either ropinirole (0.75 mg/day to 24 mg/day) or L-dopa (50–1200 mg/day) for 5 years.

Rescue L-dopa was allowed in all three studies. The meta-analysis revealed that cabergoline was less effective at reducing dyskinesia risk compared to L-dopa (OR = 0(0.38; $P < .008$), while pramipexole (OR = 0(0.25; $P < .001$) and ropinirole (OR = 0(0.31; $P < .001$) were more effective in lowering dyskinesia incidence. These findings suggest that cabergoline might have D1 agonist properties, but due to variations in the definitions of dyskinesia among the studies, the results should be interpreted with caution (Kvernmo et al., 2006; Nakatsuka et al., 2006).

7.3.1.4.1 Pk of cabergoline

Cabergoline has a long elimination half-life ranging from 63 to 110 h, meaning it takes over 3 weeks to reach steady-state levels after dose titration. While no studies have specifically determined its inhibition constant (K_i) for CYP3A4, it is believed that cabergoline, like other ergot-derived DAs may interact with this enzyme.

Cabergoline is primarily metabolized by CYP3A4, similar to bromocriptine and pergolide. Coadministration with CYP3A4 inhibitors can significantly increase cabergoline plasma levels. For example, when taken with itraconazole (a strong CYP3A4 inhibitor), cabergoline levels increased by 300%. Likewise, when combined with clarithromycin, cabergoline's maximum concentration (C_{max}) increased 2.6-fold in healthy volunteers and 1.7-fold in PD patients. Additionally, grapefruit juice was found to raise cabergoline concentrations by 1.7 times in PD patients. Conversely, CYP3A4 inducers may lower cabergoline levels, reducing its therapeutic efficacy. Cabergoline exhibits linear Pk only up to doses of 1.5 mg/day, which is below the recommended therapeutic range for PD. Due to the risk of elevated plasma levels, coadministration with certain antibiotics, such as clarithromycin, is generally not advised (Kvernmo et al., 2006; Nakatsuka et al., 2006).

7.3.2 Nonergoline dopamine agonist

Nonergoline derivatives like **pramipexole**, **ropinirole**, and **rotigotine** primarily refer to DAs that are not derived from the ergot alkaloid family. These drugs are extensively used in the treatment of PD both as monotherapy and add-on therapy to levodopa. They work by stimulating dopamine receptors in the brain, providing symptomatic relief for PD.

Nonergoline DAs may be administered in various ways. Pramipexole and ropinirole are taken orally and are available in both immediate-release (IR) and extended-release (ER) formulations. Rotigotine is delivered transdermally through a patch formulation, while apomorphine is given subcutaneously via injection (Cánovas et al., 2014).

Extended-release oral formulations were developed to achieve more stable plasma drug concentrations, helping to reduce motor fluctuations which are partially derived from oscillations in plasma drug concentrations. DA called rotigotine was recently developed for the same purpose. It is the first nonergoline DA delivered through the skin (transdermally) and has a similar effectiveness and safety profile compared to other drugs in its class (Cánovas et al., 2014).

Although the new DAs can cause serious side effects, such as impulse control disorders (ICD), they have clearly improved the quality of life for PD patients. They have also considerably widened the range of treatment strategies available to neurologists (Cánovas et al., 2014).

7.3.2.1 Pk and Pd of non-ergoline dopamine agonist

7.3.2.1.1 Pramipexol

Pramipexole's chemical name is (S)-2-amino-4,5,6,7-tetrahydro-6-(propylamino) benzothiazole (Cánovas et al., 2014).

Pharmacokinetics:

Absorption:

Immediate-release (IR) formulation of pramipexole is rapidly absorbed from the gastrointestinal tract, reaching a maximum concentration in plasma within 1–2 h after oral administration, or later if administered with food. It has a high bioavailability around 90% (Cánovas et al., 2014).

Extended-release (ER) formulation of Pramipexole is designed as a matrix tablet containing carbomer, which promotes slow and constant release of the drug by diffusion and erosion. The drug reaches its maximum concentration in plasma within approximately 6 h after administration, with minimal fluctuations in drug plasma levels compared to those reached in patients taking the IR formulation three times per day. Plasma concentrations stabilize after 5 days of treatment (Cánovas et al., 2014).

Distribution: Pramipexole exhibits linear pharmacokinetics, characterized by low protein-binding (<20%), which allows most of the drug to remain free and pharmacologically active. It has a large volume of distribution of approximately 400 L, indicating extensive distribution throughout the body. The drug is widely distributed in the body, including the brain, where it exerts its therapeutic effects (Cánovas et al., 2014).

Metabolism and elimination: The agent undergoes minimal metabolism within the body and is predominantly eliminated through renal excretion, accounting for approximately 90% of its clearance. The renal clearance rate is about 400 mL/min, indicating efficient removal of the drug from the bloodstream by the kidneys (Hametner et al., 2012).

Most of the administered dose (around 80%) is eliminated unchanged in the urine through active tubular secretion (Cánovas et al., 2014). The elimination half-life (t½) varies with age, ranging from 8 h in younger individuals to 12 h in the elderly (Hametner et al., 2012).

Pramipexole should not be used in patients with advanced renal failure, and adjustments are necessary for patients with mild to moderate renal insufficiency. No significant drug interactions have been reported, except for potential decrease in urinary excretion of pramipexole among patients treated concurrently with cimetidine and amantadine (Cánovas et al., 2014).

Pharmacodynamics:

Pramipexole acts as full intrinsic DAs. The aminobenzothiazole compound exhibits strong selectivity for the D2 receptor family and, intragroup, has higher affinity for D3 receptor subtype compared to the D2 and D4 dopamine receptors. The agent shows lack affinity for the D1 and D5 dopamine receptors and only minimal affinity for the D2 and D4 receptors subtype (Constantinescu, 2008; Hametner et al., 2012).

Pramipexole simultaneously activates the direct striatopallidal pathway through D3 receptor stimulation and inhibits the indirect striatopallidal pathway via D2 receptor activation. This dual action helps alleviate PD symptoms by mimicking dopamine's effects within the striatum (Constantinescu, 2008).

Since the D3 receptors are most predominance in the limbic system, pramipexole may have an impact on psychiatric symptoms in PD. Additionally, pramipexole has lower affinity for 5-HT2A, 5-HT2B, and D1 receptors, partly explaining its positive effects in reducing the risk of cardiac valvulopathy and dyskinesias (Constantinescu, 2008).

7.3.2.2 Ropinirole

Ropinirole is a compound classified as an indole derivative whose chemical name is 4-[2-(dipropylamino) ethyl]-1,3-dihydroindol-2-one. This potent DA interacts with both peripheral and central receptors, demonstrating the highest affinity for the D3 subtype (Cánovas et al., 2014).

Pharmacokinetics:

Absorption:

The immediate-release formulation is rapidly absorbed, reaching its maximum concentration within 1–2 h and later if taken with food. Its bioavailability is approximately 50% (Cánovas et al., 2014).

The extended-release (ER) formulation utilizes a matrix core with a double-layer coating, consisting of an impermeable layer and a semi-permeable layer. When exposed to intestinal fluids, the tablet becomes gelatinous, which permits slow and uniform release and absorption of the drug over 24 h, irrespective of food intake. Comparative studies indicate that the ER formulation achieves more stable ropinirole plasma concentrations, with fewer oscillations compared to similar doses of immediate-release (IR) formulations, which are administered 3 times per day. The bioavailability of extended-release (ER) formulations remains approximately 50%, demonstrating linear pharmacokinetics, with the maximum concentration being reached after a delay of 6–10 h (Cánovas et al., 2014).

Distribution: The drug is highly lipophilic, allowing it to penetrate cell membranes and cross the blood-brain barrier. It has a large volume of distribution (6.7 L/kg), indicating extensive movement from the bloodstream into body tissues, including fat and organs. The plasma protein binding is relatively low (10%–39%), which is not clinically relevant (Cánovas et al., 2014).

Metabolism and elimination: Ropinirole is metabolized in the liver by cytochrome P450 enzymes before being eliminated through the urine, with approximately 10% of the drug remaining active at elimination. The clearance of ropinirole is estimated to be about 15% lower in individuals older than 65 years (Cánovas et al., 2014).

Pharmacodynamics:

Ropinirole is a potent DA that has a high affinity for postsynaptic dopamine receptors located in the central and peripheral nervous systems, exhibiting its maximum affinity for the D3 subtype (Cánovas et al., 2014).

Ropinirole demonstrates a preferential binding affinity for D2-like receptors (D2, D3, and D4) receptors. Among these, it has the highest affinity for the D3 receptors, which are predominantly found in the limbic areas of the brain and may contribute to some of the neuropsychiatric effects. Although the D2 receptor in the striatum has a slightly lower affinity compared to D3, it significantly contributes to the motor symptom relief seen in PD (Shill & Stacy, 2009).

Ropinirole exhibits negligible affinity for α2 adrenoreceptors in the periphery and 5HT-1 receptors. Additionally, it shows no affinity for D1-like receptors, benzodiazepine, or GABA receptors (Shill & Stacy, 2009).

Dopamine receptors (D2) are G-protein-coupled inhibitory neurons predominantly located in the striatonigral, mesolimbic, and tuberoinfundibular systems. These receptors inhibit adenylyl cyclase and calcium channels while activating potassium channels. This mechanism increases the duration of the "on" time while reducing the "off" time associated with disease progression, making ropinirole an attractive choice for management both early and advanced stages of PD (Rewane et al., 2024).

7.3.2.3 Rotigotine

Rotigotine's chemical name is (6S)-6-[propyl(2-thiophen-2-ylethyl) amino]-5,6,7,8 tetrahydronaphthalen-1-ol. It has a high affinity for D3 receptors, and it has an agonist effect on 5HT1A serotonin receptors and an antagonist effect on α_{2B} and α_{2C} adrenergic receptors (Cánovas et al., 2014).

Pharmacokinetics:

Absorption:

This compound has a low molecular weight, and it is highly lipid-soluble, allowing it to efficiently diffuse through the stratum corneum of the skin. It is delivered via a silicone adhesive matrix with an aluminized polyester film coating. The drug release from the patch is constant and proportional to the patch's surface area (Cánovas et al., 2014).

Although oral bioavailability is less than 1%, Rotigotine demonstrates effective transdermal absorption, averaging 46.1% ± 10.6% of the total patch content, despite individual variations. As a result, the patches contain a higher amount of the drug to achieve the desired dosage: the 2 mg patch contains 4.5 mg, the 4 mg patch contains 9 mg, the 6 mg patch contains 13.5 mg, and the 8 mg patch contains 18 mg. Additionally, two new patch formats are recently added which deliver 1 and 3 mg and nonabsorbed content remains in the patch (Cánovas et al., 2014).

Distribution: Rotigotine exhibits a high protein binding rate, with over 90% of the drug bound to plasma proteins, leaving only a small fraction unbound and pharmacologically active. Despite this, no significant drug interactions have been identified (not even for drugs metabolized by cytochrome P450). Additionally, there are no reports of plasma concentration changes in cases of hypoalbuminaemia or administration of other plasma protein-bound drugs (Cánovas et al., 2014).

When the patch is changed daily, plasma concentrations remain stable without significant fluctuations, regardless of patch placement. Plasma concentrations stabilize within 2–3 days of initiating treatment. However, unchanging the patch for more than 24 h may result unstable concentrations and undesirable fluctuations (Cánovas et al., 2014).

Metabolism and elimination: Rotigotine is primarily metabolized in the liver through cytochrome P450 enzymes and glucuronidation. Its metabolites are excreted in urine (<1% eliminated actively), and hemodialysis does not affect its plasma concentrations (Cánovas et al., 2014).

Pharmacodynamics:

Rotigotine acts as a dopamine receptor agonist, primarily targeting D1, D2, and D3 receptors in the brain, which play a crucial role in motor coordination. This activity makes rotigotine particularly effective in managing symptoms of PD. Recent studies confirmed the high affinity binding of rotigotine on D3 and D2 receptors but also showed a similarly high affinity toward the D1 receptor. Unlike many other DAs that primarily stimulate D2 and D3 receptors, rotigotine also activates D1 receptors, making it more similar to dopamine or apomorphine compared to other DAs (Elshoff et al., 2015).

Additionally, rotigotine exhibits in vitro activity not only at dopamine receptors (D1 to D5) but also at select adrenergic and serotonergic receptor sites. It acts as an antagonist at α_{2B} adrenergic receptors and an agonist at 5-HT1A receptors, which may further enhance its therapeutic effects in vivo. Importantly, rotigotine does not interact with 5-HT2B receptors.

Overall, the ability of rotigotine to stimulate D1–D3 receptors within the caudate putamen regions of the brain is likely to underlie its effectiveness in treating PD (Elshoff et al., 2015).

Animal studies have explored both presynaptic and postsynaptic activity of rotigotine. Presynaptic activity is observed by hypomotility (reduced movement) after taking low doses of the agonist, as well as reduction in γ-butyrolactone stimulated dopamine synthesis and extracellular dopamine level. Postsynaptic activity of rotigotine has been demonstrated in rats through two experimental models: reserpine reversal and stereotypy induction. Moreover, evidence of its postsynaptic activity on dopamine receptors is supported by observations of controversies turning and increased locomotors activity in models treated with 6-hydroxydopamine (rats) and MPTP (monkeys), confirming its postsynaptic activity on dopamine receptors (Elshoff et al., 2015).

7.3.3 Aporphines

7.3.3.1 Apomorphine

Progressive loss of dopaminergic neurons in the pars compacta of the substantia nigra causes striatal dopamine deficit; neuropathological hallmarks are intracellular inclusions comprising aggregates of alpha-synuclein. PD was the first neurodegenerative illness for which highly effective therapies became available. Matched only by apomorphine in its effect size on motor symptoms, oral levodopa remains the gold standard of symptomatic treatment by replacing dopamine. The oldest dopaminergic medication for PD is apomorphine, which still is the only one with effectiveness roughly equal to that of levodopa. From a structural standpoint, it is a morphine opioid derivative. At D1 and D2 receptors, it has short-acting agonist action; at low doses, it acts on presynaptic auto receptors to reduce dopamine turnover. Though, many patients experience difficult motor problems like motor fluctuations and dyskinesia as the disease advances, the long-term response to levodopa is preserved. Apomorphine's present function in treating PD is to control levodopa-related motor problems—as either continuous subcutaneous mini-pump delivery or intermittent subcutaneous pen injections (Carbone et al., 2019).

7.3.3.1.1 History

Though its first use almost certainly goes back to ancient civilizations, apomorphine is a recognized DA for the treatment of advanced PD, with intriguing parallels between cultures as far apart as those of the Mayas and the ancient Egyptians. The iconography of these two civilizations reveals many hints supporting the central significance of Nymphaea plants (water lilies) in magical-religious ceremonies. Today, we are aware that some aporphines, including apomorphine, can be found in the roots and bulbs of water lilies. The plants were most likely employed as an emetic in purifying rituals and as an aphrodisiac and hallucinogenic for the upper castes. Interestingly, the effects sought and experienced by these ancient civilizations are the very same that were clinically evaluated thousands of years later, after the discovery of synthetic apomorphine. Credit for finding apomorphine goes to Matthiessen and Wright's research, which in 1868 synthetized apomorphine hydrochloride by heating morphine with concentrated hydrochloric acid. To emphasize its source and its difference from the mother compound, morphine, the compound was called apomorphia. Although apomorphine began to draw attention in human and veterinary medicine only after Matthiessen and Wright's studies, it is reasonable to say that Arppe was likely the first to synthesize the molecule in 1845 by heating morphine with an excess of sulfuric acid, thus naming it sulfomorphide. Apomorphine was used in various animal and human studies in the years after its discovery, demonstrating a spectrum of effects that led to its application in various medical domains. The studies done by Gee, Hare, Pierce, Siebert, and Harnack in people and animals helped to connect apomorphine's effects to central nervous system activity. Most especially, people and dogs with oral and parenteral doses almost always showed an emetic reaction. An unwanted effect of today's use of apomorphine, emesis became the main indication for the medication for several decades and led to its use in removing foreign objects from the esophagus or in treating poisoning. In cases of drug, alcohol, and smoking dependence, this emetic reaction was also employed to cause negative conditioning by giving the drug with unwanted stimulus. In cases of drug, alcohol, and smoking dependence, the drug was given with the unwanted stimulus to cause negative conditioning using this emetic reaction (Carbone et al., 2019).

Pharmacokinetic: Poorly absorbed, oral apomorphine has a bioavailability of under 4%. Moreover, oral doses must be 10 to 20 times the parenteral dose to generate comparable therapeutic response. With the simultaneous use of vitamin C, sublingual apomorphine's relative bioavailability drops to 6%. Though significant interindividual differences are seen, the area under the curve (AUC) is higher after sublingual administration of apomorphine 30 mg than after 3 mg subcutaneously. The medication is quite lipophilic. Studies on plasma concentration-effect after rising doses of given apomorphine have shown a therapeutic window between 28 and 56 nmol/L. A two-compartment model describes the vanishing of drug. Apart from glucuronidation and sulfate conjugation, which each contribute 10% of metabolic transformation, (auto)oxidation is the primary metabolic path. There have been no active metabolites found. Apomorphine's total body clearance surpasses the liver blood flow, indicating extrahepatic clearance. The urine excretes only 4% unaltered (Carbone et al., 2019). **Pharmacodynamic features:** Derived from acidification of morphine, apomorphine is an aporphine alkaloid. Molecularly, it is $C_{17}H_{17}NO_2$. The lipophilicity and the affinity to dopaminergic receptors are caused by its structure, which is made up of a tetracycline aporphine ring. Specifically, the ortho-catechol group gives structural resemblance to dopamine. Apomorphine, like many antipsychotic medications, has piperidine moiety. Though it differs somewhat from other oral DAs used in PD, apomorphine is frequently characterized as a DA. Apomorphine is a strong dopamine receptor agonist with a wide range on all D1-and D2-like receptors (D1, D2S, D2L, D3, D4, and D5), thanks to its catechol moiety. By contrast, the oral DAs ropinirole and pramipexole mostly bind to D2 and D3 receptors with little affinity for D1 receptors. Thus, the way apomorphine works is more similar to that of dopamine or its precursor levodopa. Apomorphine also has antagonist effects on serotonergic 5HT2A, 5HT2B, and 5HT2C and adrenergic alpha2A, alpha2B, and alpha2C receptors and agonist effects at serotonergic 5HT1A receptors. Unlike its mother compound, morphine, apomorphine shows no affinity for opioid receptors. Almost total first-pass hepatic metabolism, in which the molecule is metabolized following various pathways including sulfation, glucuronidation, and catechol O-methylation, causes apomorphine to have extremely low oral bioavailability (<4%). Clinical trials have thus used various parenteral administration routes. Currently, apomorphine is given by subcutaneous injections or infusions as a licensed treatment for PD. The drug absorption (bioavailability 100%), volume of distribution, plasma clearance, and half-lives (t\u00bd) of subcutaneous injections or infusions are comparable to those of intravenous infusion. The latter, though, is not appropriate for chronic use since apomorphine may crystallize in the catheter and cause thrombi formation. The subcutaneous absorption of the drug can be influenced by several factors: injection site (abdominal injection appears to have the best outcomes), skin condition (vascularization, skin temperature, body fat), volume and depth of injection (a larger volume increases the area of subcutaneous absorption and affects the time to peak concentration [tmax]), and the presence of subcutaneous nodules that may impede absorption both mechanically and through inflammation-related modification of the blood flow. Peak blood concentration (Cmax) is about 10 min after subcutaneous injection; maximum cerebrospinal fluid concentration is reached after 30 min. Apomorphine is very lipophilic; hence, it has a significant volume of distribution and, unlike levodopa, can freely cross the blood-brain barrier. It also appears to be more concentrated in the brain, with a brain-to-blood ratio of 8:1. Apomorphine has a t\u00bd of about 33 min due to its fairly quick metabolism and clearance. All things considered, a range of factors—including regional fat, blood flow and differences in metabolic enzymatic profiles—causes great interindividual variability in tmax, Cmax, and area under the plasma concentration–time curve (AUC). Conversely, intraindividual variation is low. In clinical practice, this means that beginning apomorphine treatment calls for personal titration. In patients with PD, a clinical response often starts within 7–10 min following the subcutaneous injection and lasts for approximately

45–60 min after one dose, so intermittent subcutaneous injections of apomorphine are a very appropriate rescue treatment for those undergoing "on/off" fluctuations during chronic levodopa therapy (Carbone et al., 2019).

Parkinsonian patients with motor fluctuations respond with a latency to effect of 5–20 and 30 min, respectively, following subcutaneous and sublingual administration of apomorphine. The stage of the disease inversely affects the duration of the antiparkinsonian action (0.5 h in advanced PD compared to nearly 1 h in early PD) and its efficacy half-life following a single subcutaneous dose. This might verify that most postsynaptic elements are engaged. A single dose given sublingually offers a longer duration of action (128 min). Longer duration of action (0.6–2.5 h) is provided by chronic administration. Clinical studies have shown apomorphine to be effective. Over 16 months, Frankel et al. investigated 57 individuals. Patients on bolus apomorphine (2.2 mg per injection, five injections daily) or continuous infusion, augmented with bolus doses as required, showed about 5-hour reductions in "off" periods in their research. Twelve patients kept up the study for more than 2 years. During the study, just 7% of their patients experienced psychiatric responses. The writers suggested apomorphine for patients with disabling "off" times unresponsive to oral treatment. Other research has demonstrated that apomorphine's positive effects last up to 5 years. Generally, apomorphine appears to be as effective as lisuride but with lower chances of neuropsychiatric responses. Nausea and vomiting—up to 73% of patients—are the main side effects of apomorphine, which domperidone pretreatment can help to reduce. Long-term use causes neuropsychiatric negative effects, but the frequency is lower than with other DAs. Patients with severe neuropsychiatric reactions to other antiparkinsonian medications have used the drug. Compared to placebo, long-term use of apomorphine can lead to a notable rise (by 67%) in the mean daily length of dyskinesia. Though careful skin care can help to some extent, continuous subcutaneous infusion can lead to local damage including subcutaneous nodules. Careful skin care can help prevent continuous subcutaneous infusion's local damage, such subcutaneous nodules (Deleu et al., 2002).

Managing levodopa-related motor problems has three main strategies: the use of 'on demand' drugs meant to quickly abort OFF episodes, continuous drug delivery (e.g., infusion), and the addition of oral adjuncts. Apomorphine, a short-acting dopamine (D)1 and D2 receptor agonist, is the only drug shown to reduce motor symptoms with an efficacy equal to that of levodopa; it has a quicker onset of action than levodopa but a shorter effect duration. Approved for use in the United States are two kinds of "on demand" apomorphine therapy: the subcutaneous (SC) formulation and the sublingual (SL) formulation; the SL formulation is no longer commercially supported in the US. For SC administration, the advised apomorphine dose is 2–6 mg: for SL administration, 10–30 mg. The two bioavailabilities on demand formulations are quite different. Similar absorption, distribution volume, plasma clearance, and half-life properties to intravenous infusion make the SC formulation 100% bioavailable. SC absorption, on the other hand, can be affected by many elements including skin condition at the injection site, injection depth, and volume. By nonexclusive absorption via the SL or buccal routes, when part of it is being swallowed and absorbed in the stomach, the SL apomorphine, on the other hand, has only 17%–18% bioavailability. These variations in Pk traits can cause variations in the time course of the effect intensity between different formulations. Previously developed were the models characterizing Pk of SC and SL apomorphine formulations as well as the Pk/Pd model of apomorphine. Using a Pk/Pd modeling technique, the goal of this study was to evaluate the SC and SL formulations of apomorphine for the management of motor fluctuations in PD (Nasser et al., 2024).

7.3.3.1.2 Pk model for SC apomorphine

The Pk time course of apomorphine after SC administration was best described by a one-compartment model with first order absorption and elimination processes (Fig. 7.1) The model was defined by two differential equations:

A and *C* are the amounts of drug in the depot and central compartments, *ka* and *kel* are the first-order absorption and elimination rate constants, *V/F* is the volume of distribution, *F* is the

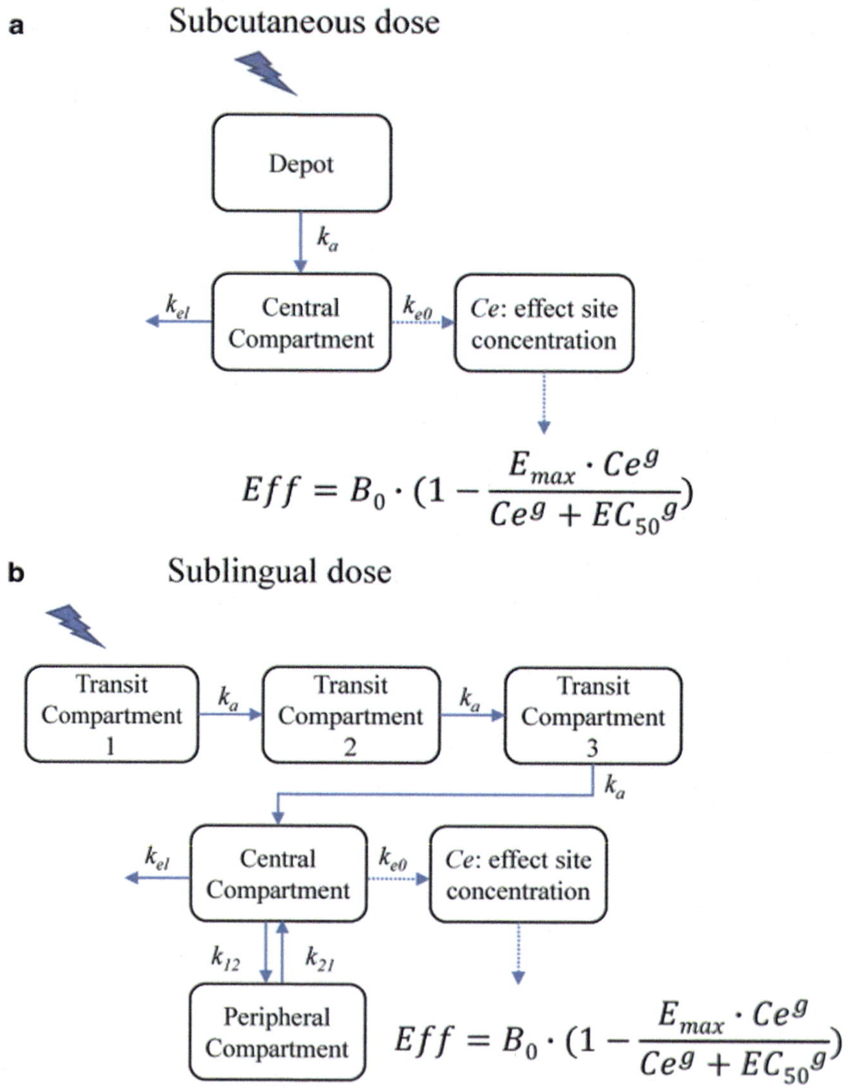

FIGURE 7.1

Schematic of the apomorphine Pk model fol.

bioavailability (assumed equal to one), and *Cp* is the drug concentration in the central compartment (Nasser et al., 2024), lowering subcutaneous administration. Abbreviations: *B0*, baseline motor score; *Ce*, drug concentration at the site of action; *EC50*, drug concentration that causes 50% of the maximum effect; *Emax*, maximum inhibitory effect; *g*, Hill's sigmoid coeffcient; *ka*, first-order absorption constant; *ke0*, first-order plasma-effect site equilibration rate constant; *kel*, elimination constant; Pk, pharmacokinetics. **b** Schematic of the apomorphine Pk model following sublingual administration. Abbreviations: *B0*,baseline motor score; *Ce*, drug concentration at the site of action; *EC50*, drug concentration that causes 50% of the maximum effect; *Emax*, maximum inhibitory effect; *g*, Hill's sigmoid coeffcient; *k12* and *k21*, first-order transfer rate constants between the central and peripheral compartments; *ka*, first-order absorption constant; *ke0*, first-order plasma-effect site equilibration rate constant; *kel*, elimination constant; Pk (Nasser et al., 2024).

7.3.3.1.3 Pk model for SL apomorphine

The Pk time course of apomorphine after SL administration was best described by a two-compartment model with a delayed absorption process, which was described by a transit compartments model, a first-order distribution from/to a peripheral compartment, and a first-order elimination rate constant (Fig. 7.1b). The model was defined by five differential equations:

T1, *T2*, and *T3* are the amount of drug in the transit compartments, *C* and *P* are the amount of drug in the central and peripheral compartments, *ka* and *kel* are the first-order absorption and elimination rate constants, and *k12* and *k21* are the first-order transfer rate constants between the central and peripheral compartments,

V/F is the volume of distribution, *F* is the bioavailability, and *Cp* is the drug concentration in the central compartment (Nasser et al., 2024).

30 mg, 40 mg, and 50 mg SL administration. The recommended dose for SC administration is 2–6 mg and 10 mg to 30 mg for SL administration. Abbreviations: min, minute; SC, subcutaneous; SL, sublingual (Nasser et al., 2024).

7.4 Anticholinergic drugs

Motor incoordination is caused by reduced dopaminergic signaling in comparison to increased cholinergic signaling. Parkinsonism is typified by bradykinesia, akathisia (inability to sit still), rigidity, resting tremors, and an unstable posture. Atypical parkinsonism, secondary parkinsonism, and parkinsonism are all considered parkinsonian disorders. As of right now, the only way to treat parkinsonism is to reinforce the dopaminergic pathway, for example, by giving levodopa, a precursor to dopamine (DA). Another option is to use central anticholinergic medications to block the cholinergic pathway. In the early stages of the disease, anticholinergic antiparkinsonian medications are used as monotherapy, which postpones the need for levodopa (Abdelmissih et al., 2025). DA and acetylcholine levels are balanced in healthy individuals without PD, but PD patients release less DA than is necessary. The imbalance is caused by an increase in acetylcholine as a result of that decrease. Patients are administered anticholinergics to help them regain equilibrium (El-Shorbagi et al., 2020). A class of drugs known as anticholinergic drugs work by preventing the neurotransmitter acetylcholine (ACh) from acting in the central and autonomic nervous systems (Marzoughi et al., 2021). Consequently, the neuronal activity will be reduced, and the DA-acetylcholine balance will be restored. Nicotinic (Nn;

Nm) and muscarinic (M1, M2, and M3) receptors are both impacted by acetylcholine. Skeletal muscle contractions and cognitive function are both impacted by nicotinic receptor actions. Acetylcholine attaches itself to the muscarinic receptor's arm. Ionic bonds, two hydrogen bond acceptors, and van der Waals interactions are the three potential interactions that lead to binding (El-Shorbagi et al., 2020). This can have a wide range of both positive and negative effects. Anticholinergic properties are present in between one-third and half of the most often prescribed medications for elderly patients Therefore, it is essential to comprehend the clinical significance of long-term use of these drugs on the development and course of neurodegenerative diseases. The word "anticholinergic" implies that these medications have a wide range of effects (Marzoughi et al., 2021). Prior to the commercialization of levodopa, anticholinergic medications were mainly prescribed for parkinsonism and were the first pharmaceutical agents used to treat PD. Anticholinergics have been used to treat dystonia, PD, and parkinsonism brought on by neuroleptics. Although the exact mechanism is unknown, it has been thought that blocking muscarinic acetylcholine receptors resolves the imbalance between dopamine and acetylcholine in the brain (Kawabata & Katsuno, 2022, pp. 3333–3340). Procyclidine, benztropine, biperiden, orphenadrine, trihexyphenidyl (benzhexol), and other centrally acting antimuscarinic medications still have a role in the treatment of early PD. These substances are structurally similar to atropine. Using high-resolution positron emission tomography (PET) scans and [N-methyl-11C] benztropine, the regional distribution of muscarinic M1 and M2 receptors in the living human brain has been investigated in both young and elderly adult male volunteers. Muscarinic cholinergic receptor binding decreases with age in the corpus striatum, frontal, parietal, temporal, and occipital cortices. Numerous studies have demonstrated that many of these compounds act as strong inhibitors of the presynaptic carrier-mediated dopamine transport mechanism, in which each dopamine molecule entering the nerve terminal via the carrier is accompanied by two or more sodium ions and one chloride ion. This is even though the mechanism of action of this class of agents is most likely related to blocking the muscarinic receptors in the striatum. Two or more sodium ions and one chloride ions accompany the molecule as it enters the nerve terminal through the carrier (Deleu et al., 2002).

7.4.1 Trihexyphenidyl

7.4.1.1 Its synthesis

Acetophenone, paraformaldehyde, and piperidine are the three compounds used in the initial aminomethylation synthesis of 2-(1-piperdino) propiophenone. Trihexyphenidyl is the product of this reaction with cyclohexyl magnesium bromide (El-Shorbagi et al., 2020).

7.4.1.2 Pk properties

Its total oral daily dose is 5–15 mg, its daily time is three to four, its peak plasma concentration (C_{max}) is 7 μg/L for 10 mg dose, t_{max} which is time to C_{max} is 1.3 h, its oral bioavailability is 100b%, its clearance is 25.8 (430) L/h (mL/min), its $t_1/_2\beta$ which is elimination half-life is 33 h (Deleu et al., 2002).

b = Tablet versus elixir.

7.4.1.3 Pd properties

According to preliminary research, 76% of patients experienced an average 24% reduction in parkinsonian symptoms when taking trihexyphenidyl. Takahashi et al. assessed cognitive function and motor disability in de novo PD patients in a PET scan study both before and after they took trihexyphenidyl 6 mg daily for 5–11 weeks. All PD patients showed improvement on the motor disability scale at the conclusion of the treatment period, and there was no discernible change in their cognitive function. According to PET results, trihexyphenidyl inhibits the cortical cholinergic system at this point in the disease without impairing cognitive function. In a double-blind, randomized study, Guthrie et al. assessed the central (memory, sedation) and peripheral (salivation, ratio of RR interval on electrocardiogram) muscarinic function in 14 healthy volunteers who were given trihexyphenidyl, biperiden, and a placebo. Biperiden and trihexyphenidyl continuously raised the RR ratio while decreasing saliva production. Biperiden or trihexyphenidyl also had an impact on delayed recall and selective reminding tasks. Biperiden had a more sedative effect than trihexyphenidyl or a placebo, but otherwise there were no differences between the two medications (Deleu et al., 2002). Trihexyphenidyl is used to treat and manage PD symptoms. Weakness, dizziness, dry mouth, and unsettling behavior are some of the adverse effects. In effector cells, trihexyphenidyl is similar to atropine. Additionally, it blocks acetylcholine at specific synaptic locations in the brain. Other drugs are administered in addition to the trihexyphenidyl when the body does not react to the medication. trihexyphenidyl works by blocking cholinergic activity in the central nervous system, which causes the disease's symptoms. It also raises DA (El-Shorbagi et al., 2020). THP considerably reduced overall motor symptoms in the current study (29%), but this improvement was much smaller than the response to LD (61%). When tremors, bradykinesia, and rigidity were evaluated separately, tremors exhibited the best response (54%), followed by rigidity (29%), and bradykinesia (22%). The tremor sub-score of the UPDRS-III improved by more than 50% after treatment with THP and LD (53.8% vs. 67.1%, $P = .057$). In terms of tremor control, LD outperformed THP by a small margin, but the difference was not statistically significant. According to subgroup analysis, patients who responded to THP or LD with the same or better tremor response (measured by percentage improvement) had a noticeably lower baseline tremor severity than those who responded better to LD. This suggests that THP may provide modest improvement that is more beneficial for patients with less severe tremors. When measured by electromyography, one of the earliest studies to evaluate the anticholinergic effect revealed a 40% improvement in THP compared to a placebo in tremor amplitude. However, there was no difference in performance on the pegboard test (Sahoo et al., 2020). Trihexyphenidyl is used clinically, but side effects such as dry mouth, blurred vision, bradycardia, nausea, vomiting, urinary retention, constipation, and erythema are also becoming more frequently reported. However, another uncommon side effect of trihexyphenidyl is a high fever (Zhao et al., 2020).

7.4.2 Benztropine

One medication that helps lessen PD symptoms is benztropine. Verify dosages based on patient needs. Benztropine may cause addiction; therefore, patients must stick with the doctor's prescription. Benztropine has a number of adverse effects, including dry mouth, nausea, constipation, and dizziness, just like any other medication. The mechanism of action of benztropine works by blocking the relative excess of the acetylcholine in the striatum. The equilibrium between acetylcholine and DA will be restored as a result (El-Shorbagi et al., 2020).

7.4.2.1 Its synthesis

Diphenylmethane and bromine are combined to create benztropine. Benztropine is created when the intermediate combines with tropine and undergoes a work-up (El-Shorbagi et al., 2020).

7.4.2.2 Pharmacokinetic properties

There are not many pharmacokinetic studies on benztropine, we only know that its total oral daily dose is 2–16 mg, its daily time is two to four, its peak plasma concentration (C_{max}) is 2.5 μg/L for 1.5 mg dose, t_{max} which is time to C_{max} is 7 h, its oral bioavailability is low. Benztropine is absorbed more slowly than the other centrally acting antimuscarinic drugs. Rat urine and bile have been found to contain four glucuronide conjugates and eight phase I metabolites following oral benztropine administration. Benztropine undergoes N-oxidation, N-dealkylation, and ring hydroxylation, just like the majority of other centrally acting antimuscarinic medications (Deleu et al., 2002).

7.4.2.3 Pharmacodynamic aspects

Benztropine is said to start working 1–2 h and a few minutes after oral and intramuscular administration, respectively. The action lasts for 24 h in studies involving both administration routes. Compared to the majority of other antimuscarinic medications, the drug has a stronger sedative effect. For this medication, there are no pharmacodynamic studies available (Deleu et al., 2002).

7.4.3 Biperiden

Biperiden lessens PD side effects, such as movements brought on by other drugs. It functions by assisting in the correction of the chemical imbalance. By blocking the muscarinic cholinergic receptor, it reduces the action of acetylcholine and corrects the excitatory system's imbalance. It is categorized as an acetylcholine competitive antagonist (El-Shorbagi et al., 2020).

7.4.3.1 Its synthesis

Beginning with 2-(1-piperidino) propiophenone, the synthetic steps produce biperiden through a reaction with the Grignard reagent made from 5-chloro-2-norbornene (El-Shorbagi et al., 2020).

7.4.3.2 Pharmacokinetic properties

Compared to the immediate-release tablet, the slow-release formulation of biperiden exhibits significantly slower absorption; a first peak is observed roughly 4.5 h after ingestion. After 10–12 h, a peak of roughly 1.0 μg/L is reached in all recipients. At 24 h, the slow-release formulation's plasma concentrations are approximately 0.5 μg/L, which is roughly twice as high as the immediate-release formulation's. Less than 1% of the drug is eliminated unaltered in the urine after being metabolized by the liver. Biperiden's removal from the plasma is biexponential. The aliphatic tertiary amine moiety undergoes N-oxidation and N-dealkylation during the metabolism of biperiden (Deleu et al., 2002).

7.4.3.3 Pharmacodynamic aspects

Biperiden's muscarinic receptor occupancy in the frontal cortex was 10%–45% 3 hours after the drug's oral administration of 4 mg, according to a recent PET scan study conducted on healthy volunteers. Furthermore, there was a strong curvilinear correlation between the occupancy and the biperiden plasma concentration. The slow-release formulation had less of an impact on near-point accommodation, pupil size, and salivary secretion than the immediate-release tablet, or no effect at all. These symptoms started to show up two to 7 hours after taking the tablet and peaked 5 hours later. According to one study, biperiden helped PD patients with their tremors but was unable to suppress their sebum production. Patients with PD often exhibit an increase in their sebum excretion rate. According to some authors, the parasympathetic nervous system is hyperactive, which is why antimuscarinic medications may help it. This was not proven in this study, though, as an acute single-dose comparison of intravenous biperiden 5 mg and subcutaneous apomorphine showed that both medications were successful in lowering tremor, but that biperiden had no effect on rigidity or akinesia in contrast to apomorphine (Deleu et al., 2002).

7.5 Dopamine releasers

7.5.1 Amantadine

Amantadine was initially marketed as an antiviral medication. Interestingly, Schwab discovered that a woman taking 200 mg daily for antiviral prophylaxis had improved parkinsonian motor symptoms. Since then, a number of studies have verified amantadine's weakness to moderate antiparkinsonian effectiveness. There is ongoing debate regarding a potential neuroprotective potential to slow the degenerative process in PD due to antiglutamatergic properties. However, amantadine's use in treating levodopa-induced motor fluctuations and dyskinesia in PD has garnered the majority of clinical attention in recent years (Kuhn & Müller, 2022).

7.5.1.1 Synthesis of amantadine

Amantadine's synthesis. In acidic media, the tricyclic ring serves as the starting material and reacts with bromine to produce acetonitrile. Alkaline hydrolysis of the carbamide intermediate yields the final compound, which is then separated as a hydrochloride salt (El-Shorbagi et al., 2020).

7.5.1.2 Pk and Pd

The 50% effective amantadine plasma concentration (EC50), needed to significantly reduce dyskinesia in a variety of species, including mice and nonhuman primates, is *1400 ng/mL (or * 9 lM), according to a pharmacokinetic (Pk)/pharmacodynamic analysis conducted in animal models. This EC50 is in line with amantadine's known half maximal inhibitory concentration (IC50), which is 12 lM, for inhibiting the NMDA receptor in striatal neurons. An immediate-release (IR) form of amantadine alleviated dyskinesia in a few small clinical trials. Nonetheless, there was ongoing discussion regarding amantadine IR's long-term effects. Amantadine IR treatment was found to have an average benefit of 4.9 months on dyskinesia, while placebo administration showed an average benefit of 1.3 months. After receiving amantadine IR treatment for an average of 3.4 years, PD patients who switched to a placebo saw a worsening of their dyskinesia within a median of 7 days. When taking amantadine IR doses ranging from 81 to 161 mg daily, the majority of PD patients exhibit no issues. Higher dosages that might have more antidyskinetic effects are not as well tolerated. Despite amantadine IR's comparatively long half-life (*17 h), clinicians typically administer this medication in divided doses. As a result, they attempt to delay the onset of adverse effects. An extended-release amantadine formulation (GOCOVRITM; Adamas Pharma, LLC, Emeryville, CA, USA) is the novel aspect of the ADS5102 preparation. Throughout the day, this formulation produces greater plasma drug concentrations (roughly 1500 ng/mL). Conventionally applied amantadine infrared cannot produce these plasma concentrations (Müller et al., 2019). Research on both humans and animals shows that amantadine has a good concentration-effect relationship when it comes to lowering dyskinesia. Higher amantadine concentrations were obtained in PD patients (* 1500 ng/mL) in study 3, which approximated the EC50 for the reduction in dyskinesia observed in rodents and nonhuman primates (* 1400 ng/mL), even though scaling the dose of ADS-5102 to the recommended dose of 274 mg in healthy volunteers indicated that the Cmax,ss would be approximately 1000 ng/mL. Given that most PD patients are diagnosed at 60 years of age or older, and because elderly people frequently have diminished renal function (Hauser et al., 2019).

7.5.1.3 Side effects

One of Amantadine's main advantages is its low frequency of adverse effects. Pedal edema and liver reticularis are frequent. Livedo reticularis, a reddish-purple reticular mottling that is typically restricted to the leg skin, is usually asymptomatic and does not always necessitate stopping the medication. Persistent pedal edema rarely becomes incapacitating, and stopping the medication is not always required. However, more clinical research is required for significant secondary causes like vein thrombosis or cardiac or renal failure. Mental side effects like confusion, visual hallucinations, and insomnia are much less common but more problematic. These side effects go away quickly when the medication is stopped. Generally speaking, people who already have cognitive dysfunction are more likely to experience cognitive side effects. Therefore, it is essential to avoid use even in patients with mild cognitive impairment and to use it sparingly in the elderly. Additionally, treating patients with impaired kidney function may carry a high risk of toxicity due to amantadine's predominant renal excretion. Amantadine's mild anticholinergic effects are most likely the cause of dry mouth and blurred vision (Kuhn & Müller, 2022).

7.6 Catechol-O-methyltransferase inhibitors

A novel therapeutic choice in the management of PD sufferers is catechol-O-methyltransferase (COMT) inhibitors. By inhibiting the enzyme COMT, they slightly extend the effect of levodopa treatment, therefore increasing dopamine levels in the brain by letting more levodopa reach it. Representatives of COMT are part of the nitrocatechols class of medications; two of them, entacapone and tolcapone, are only used with levodopa. Somewhat like carbidopa and benserazide, their action inhibits the enzyme converting levodopa into a compound unable to cross the blood-brain barrier. Side effects are mostly those ascribed to a boosted levodopa effect, including a higher likelihood of involuntary movements (dyskinesias). Their use has also another drawback: the possibility of significant liver (Vardanyan & Hruby, 2016, pp. 1–846).

AADC = aromatic amino acid decarboxylase; MAOB = monoamine oxidase B; 3-MT = 3-methoxytyramine

DOP-AC = 3,4-dihydroxyphenylacetic acid.

COMT converts levodopa to 3-O-methyl-DOPA (3-OMD). While the peripheral component is essential for the CNS bioavailability of levodopa, COMT is found in all peripheral tissues and in the CNS. Peripheral COMT not only lowers levodopa levels but also its product 3-OMD competes with levodopa for blood-brain barrier transport and CNS dopamine absorption, therefore impairing motor function. Consequently, COMT inhibiting works not only by raising levodopa levels carried into the CNS but also by means of a continuous decrease of its rival 3-OMD, an effect that is enhanced in the presence of dopamine decarboxylase inhibitors (DDCI) (Bonifacio et al., 2012). Approved three COMT inhibitors are opicapone, entacapone, and tolcapone. O-methylation is the most obvious pathway of levodopa catabolism when a PDI blocks decarboxylation of levodopa, causing large quantities of 3-OMD to build up. Though, given that no link has been shown between the short-term changes or buildup in circulating 3-OMD levels and motor performance, it seems improbable that the buildup of plasma 3-OMD plays a major role in the development of motor fluctuations in PD. Since no link has been shown between the short-term changes or buildup in circulating 3-OMD levels and motor performance, it seems improbable that the buildup of plasma 3-OMD plays a major role in the pathogenesis of motor fluctuations in PD.20 Moreover, the frequency of levodopa in the CSF does not correspond with the fractional rise in CSF 3-OMD levels, which implies that the rate of production of 3-OMD from levodopa in the periphery more influences the availability of levodopa to the brain than competition for entrance into the brain at the blood-brain barrier. Therefore, the systemic pool of 3-OMD could possibly act as a significant sink for exogenously delivered levodopa, and COMT inhibitors could positively affect levodopa Pk in plasma, skeletal muscle, and brain. In liver, kidney, small intestine, and red blood cells, COMT inhibitors (entacapone and tolcapone) cause strong, selective, reversible, and dose-dependent suppression of soluble COMT (Deleu et al., 2002).

7.6.1 Entacapone

While tolcapone also affects O-methylation in brain, entacapone is a peripherally acting COMT inhibitor. COMT inhibition in primary mesencephalic cultures from rats has been shown in vitro to reduce levodopa toxicity on dopaminergic neurons; this is unrelated to 3-OMD or S-adenosyl-L-methionine. Two hundred forty-three patients with motor fluctuations, COMT inhibitors greatly extend the antiparkinsonian response following single-dose and during long-term levodopa treatment. Long-term studies still to come will verify the effectiveness and safety of COMT inhibitors as adjuvants in the management of PD (Deleu et al., 2002). A selective COMT inhibitor, entacapone stops levodopa from degrading in peripheral tissues, therefore improving its effects by prolonging the half-life by up to 75% and raising the maximum plasma concentration. More levodopa thus reaches the CNS over a longer period, therefore guaranteeing a more consistent availability of dopamine. Notably, it has little effect on the metabolism of other catecholamines, including norepinephrine and epinephrine (Muranova & Shanina, 2023).

7.6.1.1 Pharmacokinetic properties

After oral administration of a single dose, entacapone [the (E)-isomer] is quickly absorbed. Oral entacapone's distribution half-life is around 0.3 h. Older patients show higher Cmax and tmax values. Entacapone does not reach notable concentrations in the brain since it does not cross the blood-brain barrier. Moreover, at therapeutic doses, regular use of entacapone does not cause plasma build-up. Entacapone Pks are not much affected by the combination of levodopa/PDI with entacapone. Patients with liver damage should lower their dose. Though it has a catechol structure, entacapone is not a COMT substrate. In plasma and red blood cells, entacapone quickly isomerizes to the (Z)-isomer, the only phase I metabolite discovered in human plasma. Though present in low amounts and lacking clinical COMT inhibitory effect, the (Z)-isomer has a comparable plasma-time profile to its parent compound. Entacapone and its (Z)-isomer's glucuronide conjugates are the main metabolites and account for roughly 70% and 25%, respectively, of the urinary metabolites. Biliary excretion seems to remove a significant portion of an entacapone dose. Over 8 hours, less than 10 percent of it is excreted unchanged in the urine. In healthy volunteers, two best phases describe the elimination of entacapone after oral administration of therapeutic doses: the β phase and γ phase, which correspond to 90% and 10% of elimination, respectively (Deleu et al., 2002).

Absorption: Entacapone is rapidly absorbed through the intestinal mucosa and reaches peak concentration (Cmax) in the plasma within 0.5–0.7 h.

Distribution: Entacapone exhibits a high plasma protein binding capacity, with 98% of the active substance bound to albumin.

Metabolism: Entacapone has an average half-life of 1 h, and the liver predominantly metabolizes the medication through glucuronidation before its elimination via the biliary tract.

Elimination: Only 0.2% of nonmetabolized substance is excreted in the urine (Muranova & Shanina, 2023).

7.6.1.2 Effect on levodopa Pk and metabolism

Entacapone's COMT-inhibiting effects significantly influence levodopa's peripheral absorption and elimination. Combined use of entacapone and levodopa/PDI in healthy volunteers and parkinsonian patients greatly changes the AUC and t1/2β of levodopa relative to levodopa/PDI alone but has no impact on its Cmax or tmax. Less fluctuating levels of levodopa follow from this, therefore causing less peak dose toxicity in the shape of hallucinations and dyskinesia. Both after acute (29%–65% rise) and chronic (21% increase) administration of entacapone, entacapone raises the AUC of levodopa in a dose-dependent way. Dose-finding studies suggest that in parkinsonian patients with wearing-off phenomenon, a single 200 mg dose of entacapone is linked with best pharmacokinetic effects on levodopa. In patients with PD, long-term entacapone therapy raises mean plasma levodopa levels (+22%), interdose trough levels (+29%), and interdose peak levels (+13%) despite a 27% levodopa-sparing effect. During either acute or long-term administration of entacapone, a corresponding drop in the AUC of 3-OMD and HVA of up to 45%–60% and 21%, respectively, is seen. In patients with PD, the acute or long-term co-administration of entacapone 200 mg with controlled-release levodopa/PDI raises the AUC of levodopa against the controlled-release preparation alone by 36% and 33%, respectively. When entacapone is administered with controlled-release levodopa/PDI, repeated doses of entacapone (600–800 mg/day for 10 days) significantly raise the Cmax of levodopa and extend its tmax to a more degree than when the drug is given with immediate release levodopa/PDI. A population pharmacodynamic model of the dose-response study indicated that entacapone had no effect on the concentration-effect curve of levodopa, implying that entacapone operates only at the peripheral level (Deleu et al., 2002).

7.6.1.3 Pharmacodynamics

7.6.1.3.1 Advanced PD with motor fluctuations

Entacapone has been used to extend the duration of levodopa action in patients wearing off motor fluctuations since it can lengthen the elimination half-life of levodopa. Panel of several randomized, placebo controlled trials has revealed 1–2 h more on time per day (and less off-time) as well as a drop in the levodopa dose in PD patients with motor fluctuations on levodopa (with a dopa-decarboxylase inhibitor). In one study, this impact was more noticeable in people with less on-time and appeared to be most helpful toward the day's end. entacapone's effectiveness has been demonstrated with either conventional or controlled-release levodopa in combination. Off-time was decreased even in patients already on a DA (or other antiparkinsonian medication) in addition to levodopa; no changes in the pharmacokinetic and pharmacodynamic characteristics of subcutaneous apomorphine with entacapone have been observed. Therefore, when given with DAs, entacapone appears safe and successful. There have been no published direct comparisons of entacapone and an active comparator. One study, though, looked at rasagiline—an irreversible selective monoamine-oxidase-B inhibitor—and entacapone against placebo. Though no direct comparisons between the medications were done, the decrease of off-time and enhancement of unified PD rating scale (UPDRS) scores were comparable for both drugs. While entacapone only affects the peripheral metabolism of levodopa, rasagiline works by blocking the central breakdown of dopamine; these two drugs extend the action of levodopa by means of separate mechanisms (Fig. 7.4). Adding entacapone mostly causes dyskinesias, especially in people with prior dyskinesias and those on high doses of levodopa. Increased bioavailability of levodopa causes this side effect, which can be controlled by a 10%–30% reduction in the levodopa dose; with dose control of levodopa, dyskinesias either improve or return to baseline. Adding entacapone has other side effects including nausea, dizziness, sleepiness, stomach discomfort, diarrhea, and urine discoloration. Though innocuous, urine discoloration might cause concern and shame for patients. Typically 2–12 weeks after start, diarrhea affects about 6%–10% of patients, while this side-effect can be significant and limit the dose given, it seldom is as explosive as claimed with tolcapone. Though high concentrations of liver enzymes are seen sometimes and a report of three cases of hepatic dysfunction during entacapone treatment has been published. These anomalies could not clearly be linked to entacapone and, unlike with tolcapone, regular monitoring of liver function is not required. With mean reductions in unified PD rating scale (UPDRS) motor scores between 2.7 and 6.5 and activities of daily living scores between 0.5 and 1.7, several studies have revealed modest but significant reductions in disease severity in entacapone patients. HRQOL (measured with disease-specific [PDQ-39] and generic [SF 36] scales) also significantly improved in entacapone-treated patients in several studies, implying that the increase of clinical score reflects better subjective health experience. Other short-term studies, meanwhile, showed no change in HRQOL in entacapone-treated patients with fluctuations despite strong efficacy as assessed on motor performance, global function, and activities of daily living. Thirty-two. The lack of improvement in HRQOL scores could indicate a lack of sensitivity of such scales, especially to changes in intermittent events like on-off oscillations. On the other hand, the lack of improvement might be attributed to the failure of motor improvements in short-term studies to influence patients' general well-being. A cost effectiveness study in PD patients with motor fluctuations on levodopa treatment indicated that entacapone is cost effective in patients with wearing-off fluctuations, assessed as increases in quality-adjusted life years and years without progression to more than 25% off-time. Results from randomized controlled trials can be duplicated in more routine clinical practice, according to several open-label trials—some lasting three years—which have shown improvements on global impression scores, UPDRS motor scores and activities of daily living scores, off time, and HRQOL scores in patients with wearing-off fluctuations treated with entacapone. Results from open-label trials should be interpreted with caution, though, as there is no control for possible placebo effects, which may be significant, at least if follow-up was brief (Schrag, 2005) (Fig. 7.5).

7.6.1.3.2 Advanced PD without motor fluctuations

Entacapone's effectiveness in patients with stable treated PD—i.e., without motor fluctuations (with or without dyskinesias)—has also been evaluated. Two of these studies found that adding entacapone to carbidopa and levodopa modestly improved motor and daily living activity scores and let a lowering of levodopa dose (panel); the average drop in motor and daily living activity scores on the UPDRS was

2.3 and 0.6 in one study and 2.5 and 1.0 in the other. Twenty-three, 24. Entacapone did not enhance UPDRS motor or activities of daily living scores in a third double-blind, placebo-controlled, multicenter trial of 750 patients without motor fluctuations taking levodopa and carbidopa with or without other dopaminergic treatments. Still, many disease-specific and generic HRQOL measures, as well as investigator and subject Clinical Global Assessment scores, revealed notable improvement. The group of patients who got entacapone showed improvements in HRQOL measures of mobility, daily living activities, physical function, vitality, and distress scores. Furthermore, levodopa "rescue" was less frequent in the entacapone group than in the placebo group, implying that the UPDRS might not be sensitive to certain areas of improvement early in disease, possibly due to floor effects and skewness. Moreover, long-term dopaminergic action could help nonmotor aspects of PD like depression, sleep, or autonomic dysfunction without changing UPDRS motor scores. Overall evaluation of their own health by patients, such the HRQOL scales, could offer a better evaluation of these features of PD. On the other hand, motor benefit prolongation in the entacapone group at peak dose might not have been noticed given the motor assessment, therefore enhancing quality of life ratings. The discrepancy between HRQOL and clinical rating scales in stable and fluctuating patients confirms that, regardless of their origin, HRQOL and clinical rating scales offer valuable, albeit often different, information on the impact of drug treatment on PD. Clinical measures are probably used in trials of possibly neuroprotective medications. On the other hand, in trials of symptomatic treatment it could be argued that patient rated scores—which are probably to include motor and nonmotor effects and side-effects—might be the most relevant outcome measures. Future studies will probably include HRQOL measurements in addition to clinical rating scales; the findings of those completed so far underline the need of tailoring the selection of scales to the particular research (Schrag, 2005).

7.6.2 Tolcapone

Unlike entacapone, tolcapone's lipophilic composition allows it to cross the blood-brain barrier and inhibit COMT in the periphery as well as the central nervous system. After showing considerable decrease of OFF time in randomized placebo-controlled trials, tolcapone became the first COMT inhibitor approved for PD with motor fluctuations in 1997. Daily OFF time decreased significantly compared to placebo (100 mg vs. placebo:8.5% points of daily OFF time; 200 mg vs. placebo:5.6% points, corresponding to roughly −0.85 and −0.56 h of absolute OFF time reduction, respectively). Marketing was suspended in 1998 following four instances of liver damage, three of which were fatal. Hepatic toxicity could come from (Regensburger et al., 2023).

A single dose's oral administration causes tolcapone to be quickly absorbed. Tolcapone's great bioavailability and low metabolic rate relative to entacapone help to explain why the former can be taken three times daily, during which tolcapone shows dose-proportional Pk for doses up to 200 mg. 19 studies on population Pk show that a two-compartment open model with first-order absorption most accurately describes the Pk of tolcapone. Two-hundred doses of 400 mg and above have been linked to tolcapone accumulation, perhaps as a consequence of reduced or saturated metabolic clearance.201. Changes in protein binding—hypoalbuminemia state, liver failure, drug interactions—cause unbound tolcapone to rise, which could possibly cause negative dopaminergic effects. Quantified in CSF, tolcapone appears to be concentrated enough to roughly 75% COMT activity suppression. First-pass metabolism is low for tolcapone. Before excretion, it is nearly totally metabolized in the liver; 60% of it is eliminated by the kidney. Cirrhosis patients have lower clearance and distribution volume than healthy people; thus, it is advised to cut the dose in those with liver damage. The main metabolite of tolcapone is an inactive glucuronide conjugate. An inactive glucuronide conjugate is the main metabolite of tolcapone. Being a COMT substrate, tolcapone produces 3-omethyltolcapone. Though rather low, plasma levels of this metabolite only show with supratherapeutic doses.19. With a t1/2β of about 32 h, this metabolite does not add to the inhibitory action of the parent compound. Produced by CYP3A4 and CYP2A6, another metabolite is the carboxylic acid compound. In the urine, only tiny doses (0.5%) remain unchanged; renal clearance is 0.02 L/h. Of the dose, only 0.5% remains unchanged in the urine (renal clearance 0.02 L/h) (Deleu et al., 2002).

7.6.2.1 Effect on levodopa Pk and metabolism

Like entacapone, concomitant use of tolcapone and levodopa/PDI causes a dose-dependent rise in AUC of levodopa without notable alteration in the pharmacokinetic characteristics of levodopa absorption (Cmax and tmax). Among advanced PD patients, a single 200 mg dose of tolcapone shows the best pharmacokinetic effects on immediate-release levodopa. Tolcapone lowers the Cmax and AUC of 3-OMD by 80% and 70%, respectively, with all levodopa/carbidopa combinations. Plasma 3-OMD levels drop sixfold with repeated doses of tolcapone (200 mg three times daily). Clinical trials show that tolcapone 200 or 400 mg raises the AUC of levodopa by 32%–81% relative to placebo. Levodopa clearance is lowered by 38% after tolcapone 200 mg, and its t1/2β rises by 32%–78%. Thus, a decrease in levodopa dose should be recommended during simultaneous use of tolcapone and levodopa/PDI. The simultaneous use of tolcapone, compared to levodopa/carbidopa treatment alone, causes notable increases in levodopa and dopamine levels and a drop in 3-OMD concentration in CSF. Interestingly, the clinical effects of tolcapone were more closely related to the drop in 3-OMD concentration than to the rise in CSF dopamine and levodopa levels. Interestingly, the decrease in 3-OMD concentration rather than the rise in dopamine and levodopa levels in the CSF seemed to closely correlate with the clinical effects of tolcapone (Deleu et al., 2002).

7.6.2.2 Pharmacodynamics

Usually, tolcapone is given in oral daily doses of 100 mg or 200 mg tid. The Pk of the 100 and 200 mg doses reveal comparable Pk either alone or in combination with levodopa plus a DDCI. In healthy volunteer studies, tolcapone exhibits linear Pk across the 50–400 mg dose range. In healthy volunteers, tolcapone's Pk mirror those in PD sufferers. Tolcapone is quickly absorbed after oral administration; first pass metabolism gives it 60% bioavailability. Peak plasma concentration is attained in 30 minutes to 2 hours. Highly plasma protein bound (over 99.9%), tolcapone has limited distribution. Cite 13. With only 0.5% of the drug excreted unchanged, tolcapone undergoes significant metabolism mostly via glucuronidation to inactive 3-O\u03b2, D-glucuronic acid conjugate. With an elimination half-life of 1.6–3.4 h, the tolcapone is removed rather fast. Dose-dependent is the area under the tolcapone plasma-concentration time curve; its Pk stays constant in the presence of food, after single versus repeated doses, or as a function of age. Repeated dosing shows no evidence of pharmacodynamic tolerance. Long-term use of tolcapone results in little accumulation of the methylated metabolite. With a fast to maximum inhibition of under 2 h, tolcapone reversibly lowers S-COMT activity in erythrocytes in a dose-dependent fashion. Maximum COMT inhibition after oral doses of 100 mg or 200 mg is 72% and 80% respectively; it returns to baseline roughly 18 h after the 200 mg dose. Without affecting Cmax or Tmax, COMT inhibition with tolcapone causes dose-dependent rises in the plasma half-life of levodopa as well as its area under the curve (AUC). Administration of tolcapone, according to Factor et al. increased the half-life of levodopa by 80%. Studies conducted on healthy volunteers as well as PD patients have revealed that tolcapone in 100 or 200 mg doses raises the bioavailability of levodopa by up to 2.1-fold. Therefore, levodopa levels are more constant (less fluctuating), which should lower the onset of dyskinesias. In fact, tolcapone tid has been shown in clinical studies in PD to increase the advantage of levodopa. Tolcapone has also been shown to reduce the increased homocysteine levels linked with levodopa/DDCI therapy in PD patients, which could help to lower long-term degenerative changes and dementia connected with hyperhomocysteinemia. Since its first arrival on the market in 1997/1998, tolcapone's safety and tolerability have generated much debate and discussion based on increased liver transaminases and hepatotoxicity in a small number of initial patients and postmarketing studies. Several writers have noted that some were kept on tolcapone despite liver function tests indicating differently and that these patients were not handled per protocol. Still, these results caused a black box warning in the United States, tolcapone's withdrawal in Europe and Canada, and a black box warning in the US. The warning called for strict liver enzyme monitoring, patient informed consent before treatment, and doctors using tolcapone only after considering or trying other drugs. Significantly, the alert said that tolcapone treatment should be stopped if liver enzymes even once during the course of treatment exceeded the upper limits of normal. Over the following seven years and 40,000 more tolcapone patient years, no further cases of fatal hepatotoxicity have been connected to the therapy. Given this, a rethinking of tolcapone brought it back to Europe and the FDA's monitoring policies were reviewed. Indeed, more recent research has indicated that tolcapone could have a larger safety window than once thought. A Valeant Pharmaceuticals International review of tolcapone global safety (data on file), for instance, revealed that only 0.04% of patients over the last 7 years experienced severe hepatocellular damage; most of those with liver toxicity showed raised liver transaminases but no clinical signs or symptoms. Olanow's review of 1535 PD patients revealed that half of those who stayed on tolcapone showed ALT/AST normalization within 1–3 months compared to 2–3 weeks for those who stopped the medication. These results imply that nonresponses could be found early in the progression of any liver abnormalities and could be switched to a different drug as warranted. In another study, 677 patients who had never taken levodopa were randomly assigned to either placebo add-on therapy or tolcapone add-on therapy to standard doses of levodopa. Twenty-point 2% and twenty-seven-point 5% of patients in the placebo and active treatment groups, respectively, experienced liver function elevations at the upper limit of normal (ULN); increases more than three times the ULN occurred in 1.2% and 1.7% of patients. There was no significant hepatoxicity. Though the mechanism of tolcapone-induced hepatotoxicity is unknown, it could have something to do with mitochondrial respiration abnormalities in hepatocytes caused by uncoupling of oxidative phosphorylation. In patients taking other medications with adrenergic receptor-mediated toxicity, increased catecholamine levels may also be linked to tolcapone-induced hepatotoxicity. Current advice is to conduct liver function tests before beginning tolcapone and to refrain from using it in those with signs of liver disease or who have had two aminotransferase levels over the ULN. During the first year of treatment, aminotransferase should be checked every 2 weeks; for the following 6 months, every 4 weeks; and then every 8 weeks after that. Tolcapone might also cause dopaminergic adverse effects connected to the higher levodopa availability, including most especially dyskinesia but also nausea, dizziness, orthostatic hypotension, vomiting, anorexia, sleep disturbances, somnolence, and hallucinations. Usually, lowering the levodopa dose will help to offset these negative effects. Tolcapone can also cause major headaches, stomach discomfort, urine discoloration, and significant diarrhea (Truong, 2009).

7.7 Selegiline

MAO inhibitors inhibit MAO B, which metabolizes brain dopamine. When added to carbidopa-levodopa, these medications can increase the risk of hallucinations. These medications include selegiline and rasagiline (Fig. 7.2) (Vardanyan & Hruby, 2016, pp. 1–846) (Fig. 7.3)

7.7.1 Selegiline rasagiline

Approved by the U.S. Food and Drug Administration (FDA), monoamine oxidase (MAO) inhibitor selegiline is an adjunct treatment for adults with major depressive disorder and PD. Catabolizing neurotransmitters including norepinephrine, serotonin, and dopamine, the MAO enzymes preventing the reuptake of these neurotransmitters in the central nervous system by blocking these enzymes will increase biologically active monoamine levels at the synaptic cleft. Selegiline is also used off-label to control early PD and treat attention-deficit hyperactivity disorder. This exercise summarizes selegiline's indications, mechanism of action, routes of administration, notable side effects, contraindications, and monitoring. This knowledge also improves the ability of members of the healthcare team to properly direct patient therapy and manage indicated conditions as part of an interprofessional team (Truong, 2009). Selegiline functions as an irreversible MAO inhibitor (MAOI). Catabolizing neurotransmitters including norepinephrine, serotonin, and dopamine, the MAO enzymes blocking these enzymes from working will prevent the reuptake of these neurotransmitters in the CNS, so increasing the levels of biologically active monoamines at the synaptic cleft. Selegiline shows selective inhibition of B-type monoamine oxidase (MAO-B) at lower doses. PD is brought on by the loss of dopamine-containing neurons in the midbrain's substantia nigra, which depletes dopamine in the striatum. The treatment of PD thus seeks for particular MAO-B inhibition since MAO-B is mostly responsible for metabolizing dopamine. By contrast, using selegiline to treat MDD in adults calls for selective MAO-B inhibition rather than the preferred result. Selegiline's efficient mechanism of action in treating MDD is ascribed to its inhibition of both the isoenzymes, MAO-A and MAO-B. The monoamine theory of depression holds that the pathophysiological foundation of depression is a drop in serotonin, norepinephrine, and dopamine levels in the central nervous system. Nonselective inhibition of both MAO subtypes is preferred since the aimed result for treating MDD is raising the levels of all three of these monoamine neurotransmitters. Like many psychotropic drugs, selegiline's whole

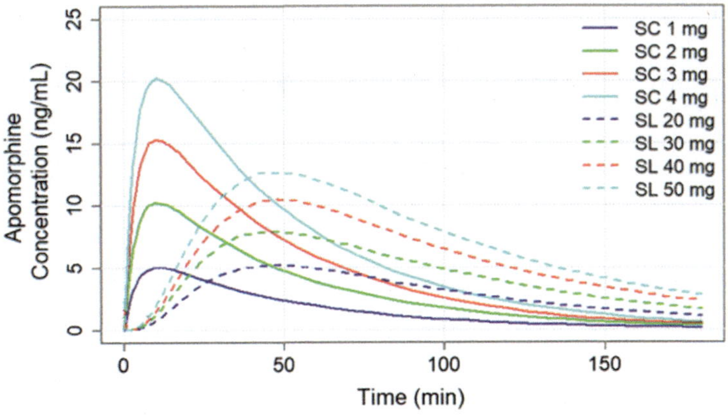

FIGURE 7.2

Mean apomorphine concentration–time profles for the 1 mg, 2 mg, 3 mg, and 4 mg SC administration and 20 mg.

FIGURE 7.3

Structure of entacapone and tolcapone.

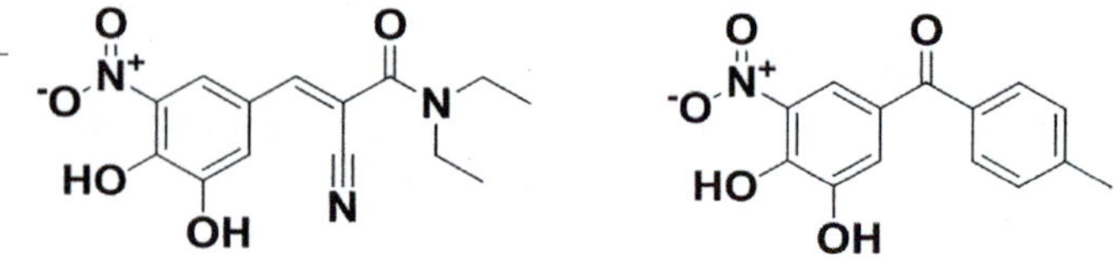

Entacapone 10.5.1 **Tolcapone 10.5.2**

mechanism of action is not fully known. Though the above-mentioned mechanisms are generally accepted, selegiline's clinical effectiveness might also be influenced by other suggested ones. A theory holds that by increasing the release of monoamine neurotransmitters, selegiline's metabolites, including amphetamine, might influence its mechanism of action. Moreover, by encouraging the synthesis of neurotrophins like brain-derived neurotrophic factor, nerve growth factor, and glial cell line-derived neurotrophic factor, selegiline may also have neuroprotective properties possibly delaying the course of PD. These neurotrophins are absolutely essential for protecting neurons from the inflammatory process. Selegiline's induction and activation of several antiapoptosis and antioxidative stress factors could help to maintain healthy brain tissue (Moore & Saadabadi, 2018).

7.7.2 Pharmacokinetics

Absorption: Selegiline undergoes extensive first-pass metabolism in the liver and gastrointestinal tract. As a result, the oral formulation has low bioavailability (4%).

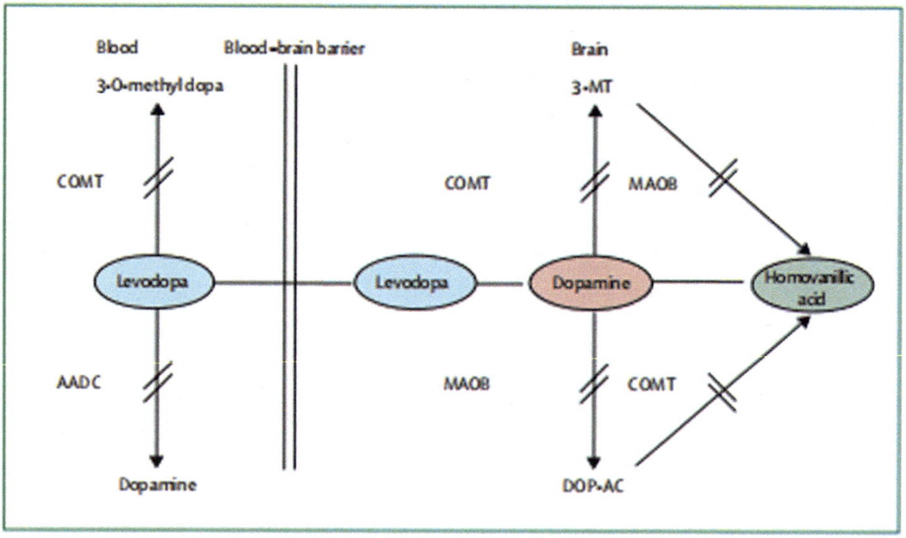

Figure: Breakdown of levodopa
AADC=aromatic amino acid decarboxylase; MAOB=monoamine oxidase B; 3-MT=3-methoxytyramine; DOP-AC=3,4-dihydroxyphenylacetic acid

FIGURE 7.4

Breakdown of levodopa (Schrag, 2005).

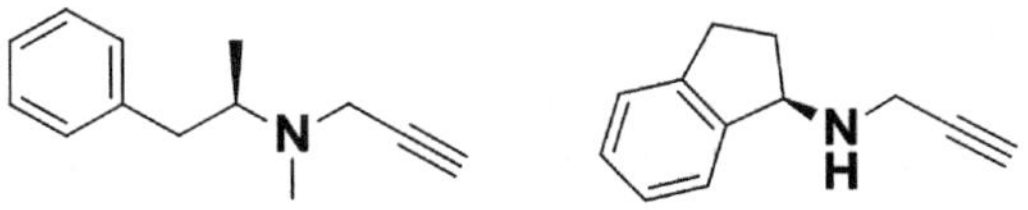

Selegiline 10.4.1 Rasagiline 10.4.2

FIGURE 7.5

Structure of selegiline and rasagiline (Vardanyan & Hruby, 2016, pp. 1–846).

Distribution: The peak plasma levels of metabolites are approximately 4–20 times higher than the maximum plasma concentration of selegiline. However, the concentrations of amphetamine and methamphetamine do not induce stimulatory effects. Selegiline exhibits high plasma protein binding, specifically with macroglobulin and albumin.

Metabolism: Selegiline undergoes metabolism to produce *N*-desmethylselegiline, *L*-amphetamine, and *L*-methamphetamine. Notably, *N*-desmethylselegiline possesses MAO-B inhibitory activity. Excretion: The mean elimination half-life of selegiline is 2 h. However, under steady-state concentration, the elimination of half-life extends to 10 h.

Selegiline use may lead to the following adverse effects in patients using the medication.

- Selegiline may lead to a hypertensive crisis, a severe elevation of blood pressure, if the patient consumes the medication alongside food, drink, or supplements rich in tyramine.
- Other dangerous adverse effects of selegiline include sudden sleep episodes, orthostatic hypotension, arrhythmias, mental status alteration, hallucinations, extrapyramidal symptoms, dyskinesia, and serotonin syndrome.
- The common adverse events associated with selegiline use include xerostomia and constipation, which are primarily attributed to the drug's anticholinergic effects. Other commonly reported adverse reactions experienced by patients include headaches, dizziness, insomnia, and nausea.
- Abrupt cessation of selegiline is not recommended due to the potential risk of antidepressant and antiparkinsonian discontinuation syndromes.
- Selegiline may also lead to transient elevation of the enzymes aspartate aminotransferase and alanine transaminase in 40% of patients. However, these enzyme elevations are typically mild and do not require therapy cessation.
- Selegiline is not an FDA-approved medication for bipolar depression, as it has the potential to precipitate a manic episode.
- The transdermal use of selegiline commonly causes skin irritation at the application site, whereas the drug's ODT form can irritate the buccal mucosa (Moore & Saadabadi, 2018).

7.7.3 Pharmacodynamics

While it extends the effectiveness of levodopa, selegiline's symptomatic benefits on motor symptoms in PD patients are modest. Periods off decrease. Selegiline's main effects were seen under chronic levodopa use. They increase dopamine bioavailability in the synaptic cleft and lower dopamine metabolism. Selegiline might increase dopamine release from nerve cells and stop dopamine removal in the synaptic cleft. Selegiline blocks the free radical generation caused by the dopamine metabolism via MAO and inhibits the oxidative metabolism of dopamine. The discovery of selegiline was the finding that this substance could extend life expectancy in PD patients treated with levodopa. Mostly 7.5 mg, in 5 mg tablets up to 10 mg, selegiline is given once or twice daily (Riederer & Müller, 2022, pp. 3149–3157).

7.7.4 Selegiline in long-term trials

These studies mostly used clinical measures in studies with PD patients. They focused on

1. halting or slowing of the emergence or worsening of disability in everyday activities,
2. diminishing the decline with the help of rating scales, which aim on distinctive disease features,
3. alteration of the speed of disease progression,
4. avoidance of reaching specific clinical milestones associated with disease progression, such as time to administer levodopa, interval to onset of motor complications, and
5. improving long-term outcomes for patients or slowing disease progression by impacting underlying disease processes (Riederer & Müller, 2022, pp. 3149–3157).

Several clinical trials aimed to demonstrate these benefits on disease progression. The design of these trials predominantly investigated a possible protective effect of additional monoamine oxidase-B inhibition on disease progression in association with concomitant levodopa intake in monotherapy, initially or in the further course over at least 1 year even in an open-label fashion (see Table 2 for summary) (Riederer & Müller, 2022, pp. 3149–3157).

Table 1Plasma levels and Pk of selegiline and its metabolites (Riederer & Müller, 2022, pp. 3149–3157).

Statistically significant difference compared with Day 1, $^{*}P < .05$; $^{**}P < .001$.

a - All data are given as mean values SD for 12 subjects

b - tmax is given as median (range).

c n = 3

Table 2:Synopsis of essential selegiline studies (Riederer & Müller, 2022, pp. 3149–3157).

Innovative approaches:

As PD is one of the fastest growing neurodegenerative disorders, research is increasing in this area. In this part the chapter will discuss the future perspectives and new approaches in Pd and Pk for drugs used in PD including different models and insightful techniques.

Integrative model of PD treatment:

In 2021, Véronneau-Veilleux and colleagues created an integrative model for PD that predicts levodopa plasma concentration, its associated dopamine concentration in the brain, and the response performance of a motor task for various disease stages. It also assesses how motor function changes in response to levodopa treatment as the disease advances.

The most recent pathophysiological and pharmacological understanding forms the basis of the current model. Numerous physiological markers were assessed in both humans and animals. A group of six patients' tapping frequency data, which was recorded 12 times across 200 min, was previously used to fit the parameters of the neurocomputational model of basal ganglia (Véronneau-Veilleux et al., 2021).

The key underlying mechanisms were represented by combining three models. A two-compartment pharmacokinetic model of levodopa was first modified and linked to a third compartment of the drug's brain concentration. Then, by include the three primary components—release, DAT-recapture, and removal—dopamine kinetics in the striatum were modeled. Lastly, the three neurotransmission pathways and the effects of dopamine on these pathways as well as on cholinergic interneurons were represented using a neurocomputational model of the basal ganglia. After that, these models were linked by changing the units or scaling (Véronneau-Veilleux et al., 2021). In conclusion, by illustrating its key mechanisms, the integrative model created here was able to replicate the behavior of levodopa's effect, particularly the fact that the medication's therapeutic effect begins to resemble plasma concentration as the disease worsens (Pedrosa De Menezes et al., 2024). Developing the best medication regimens and comprehending key mechanisms behind PD are made possible by this quantitative systems approach (Véronneau-Veilleux et al., 2021).

Targeting α-Synuclein for PD:

Vodobatinib, another name for K0706, is a third-generation c-Abl tyrosine kinase inhibitor that has been demonstrated to trigger autophagy. Clinical research on vodobatinib's antileukemic effects in patients with chronic myeloid leukemia is presently underway (Baggett et al., 2024; Mosley et al., 2024, pp. 943–973).

Trial in phase one. In both healthy volunteers and PD patients, vodobatinib's safety, plasma pharmacokinetics, and CSF penetration were assessed in an open-label, multiple-dose research phase 1 trial (NCT03445338, NCT02970019). To evaluate safety and plasma and cerebrospinal fluid (CSF) Pk, PD patients and healthy human volunteers were given different oral dosages of vodobatinib once daily for seven and 14 days, respectively. These investigations revealed a better potential for c-Abl inhibition in the brain by demonstrating greater potency in vitro than nilotinib and achieving higher CSF concentrations in both healthy and PD patients. A positive CSF Pk profile indicates the drug's potential for neuroprotection in PD patients, and it was safe and well tolerated at all dosages (Baggett et al., 2024).

$$\frac{dA}{dt} = -k_a * A$$

$$\frac{dC}{dt} = k_a * A - k_{el} * C$$

$$C_p = \frac{C}{V/F}$$

$$\frac{dT_1}{dt} = -k_a * T_1$$

$$\frac{dT_2}{dt} = -k_a * (T_1 - T_2)$$

$$\frac{dT_3}{dt} = -k_a * (T_2 - T_3)$$

$$\frac{dC}{dt} = k_a * T_3 - k_{el} * C - k_{12} * C + k_{21} * P$$

$$\frac{dP}{dt} = k_{12} * C - k_{21} * P$$

$$Cp = \frac{C}{V/F}$$

Parameter	Day 1	Day 4	Day 8
Selegiline			
AUC_{τ} (ng/mL · h)[a]	1.0 ± 0.9	2.2 ± 2.4[b]	2.7 ± 1.8[b]
C_{max} (ng/mL)[a]	0.8 ± 2.8	1.4 ± 1.6[a]	1.6 ± 1.3[a]
t_{max} (h)	0.75 (0.5–1.5)	0.5 (0.25–1.0)	0.5 (0.25–1.0)
$t_{1/2}$ (h)[a]	1.5 ± 0.6[c]	2.6 ± 2.7	3.5 ± 2.7
$R_{ac/obs}$	–	2.2	2.7
$R_{ac/est}$	(1.0)[c]	1.0	1.0
Desmethylselegiline			
AUC_{τ} (ng/ml · h)[a]	31.3 ± 7.5	40.7 ± 11.6[b]	45.7 ± 13.8[b]
C_{max} (ng/mL)[a]	17.2 ± 6.7	19.0 ± 5.8	17.9 ± 5.8
t_{max} (h)	1.0 (0.5–1.5)	0.5 (0.5–2.0)[b]	0.75 (0.5–1.5)
$t_{1/2}$ (h)[a]	3.4 ± 3.0	3.6 ± 1.7	5.3 ± 3.0[a]
$R_{ac/obs}$	–	1.3	1.5
$R_{ac/est}$	1.0	1.0	1.0
L-Methamphetamine			
AUC_{τ} (ng/ml · h)[a]	161 ± 38	274 ± 84[b]	278 ± 92[b]
C_{max} (ng/mL)[a]	13.8 ± 3.3	20.3 ± 5.2	20.5 ± 5.3[b]
t_{max} (h)	1.5 (1.0–4.0)	1.0 (1.0–8.0)	1.5 (1.0–3.0)
$t_{1/2}$ (h)[a]	11.3 ± 2.7	12.2 ± 6.0	12.3 ± 3.6
$R_{ac/obs}$	–	1.7	1.7
$R_{ac/est}$	1.5	1.3	1.3
L-Amphetamine			
AUC_{τ} (ng/ml · h)[a]	49.5 ± 6.8	91.5 ± 19.2[b]	95.8 ± 19.9[b]
C_{max} (ng/mL)[a]	3.3 ± 0.4	5.9 ± 1.9[a]	6.2 ± 1.6[b]
t_{max} (h)	2.0 (1.0–8.0)	1.5 (1.0–8.0)	1.0 (1.0–8.0)
$t_{1/2}$ (h)[a]	15.8 ± 4.6	13.1 ± 4.2	13.1 ± 4.2
$R_{ac/obs}$	–	1.8	1.9
$R_{ac/est}$	1.3	1.3	1.4

Name	Participants	Comparison	Outcome
DATATOP	800 previously untreated PD patients	Four arms: 1. Selegiline plus placebo 2. Tocopherol plus placebo 3. Selegiline plus tocopherol 4. Placebo	Selegiline delayed the need for additional levodopa No beneficial effect of tocopherol
SIN-DEP-PAR	101 mild to moderate PD patients	Two arms 1. Selegiline 2. Placebo Supplemental dosing of levodopa/ carbidopa and/or bromocriptine	After 2-month lasting washout of bromocriptine and/or levodopa/carbidopa, patients on selegiline had less deterioration compared to placebo-treated study participants
Swedish Parkinson Study Group trial	157 previously untreated PD patients	Two arms 1. Selegiline 2. Placebo	Selegiline reduced disease symptoms and delayed the need for levodopa/carbidopa
Norwegian-Danish Study	163 early PD patients	Two arms 1. Selegiline plus levodopa/carbidopa 2. Placebo plus levodopa/carbidopa	Selegiline-treated PD patients performed better and needed less additional levodopa/ carbidopa
SELEDO trial	116 prior optimum levodopa/carbidopa titrated PD patients	Two arms 1. Selegiline 2. Placebo	Time to 150% dosage of initial levodopa/carbidopa dose was shorter with placebo More patients on placebo reached this endpoint after 5 years compared with selegiline Dosage increment of levodopa/ carbidopa was distinct less in selegiline-treated patients

References

Abdelmissih, S., Rashed, L. A., Negm, M. S. I., Walaa, M. S., Mahmoud, H. M., & Emorsy, S. (2025). Dabigatran combined with benztropine ameliorates cobalt chloride-induced parkinsonism in rats, restores protease-activated receptor 1 (PAR1), and mitigates oxidative stress. *Cureus*. https://doi.org/10.7759/cureus.80486

Baggett, D., Olson, A., & Parmar, M. S. (2024). Novel approaches targeting α-synuclein for Parkinson's disease\uff00\uff00cgress and future directions for the disease-modifying therapies. *Brain Disorders, 16*. https://doi.org/10.1016/j.dscb.2024.100163. https://www.sciencedirect.com/science/journal/26664593

Burns, R. S., & Calne, D. B. (1981). Treatment of parkinsonism with artificial dopaminomimetics: Pharmacokinetic considerations. *Apomorphine and Other Dopaminomimetics, 2*, 93–106.

Burns, R. S., Gopinathan, G., Huempel, M., Dorow, R., & Calne, D. B. (1984). Disposition of oral lisuride in Parkinson's disease. *Clinical Pharmacology & Therapeutics, 35*(4), 548–556.

Cacabelos, R. (2017). Parkinson's disease: From pathogenesis to pharmacogenomics. *International Journal of Molecular Sciences, 18*(3), 551. https://doi.org/10.3390/ijms18030551

Cánovas, A. A., Piudo, R. L., Ruiz-Espiga, P. G., Burguera, J. A., Arillo, V. C., Castro, A., & Castrillo, J. M. (2014). Dopaminergic agonists in Parkinson's disease. *Neurologia, 29*(4), 230–241.

Carbone, F., Djamshidian, A., Seppi, K., & Werner, P. (2019). Apomorphine for parkinson's disease: Efficacy and safety of current and new formulations. *CNS Drugs, 33*(9), 905–918. https://doi.org/10.1007/s40263-019-00661-z

Constantinescu, R. (2008). Update on the use of pramipexole in the treatment of Parkinson's disease. *Neuropsychiatric Disease and Treatment, 4*(2), 337–352. https://doi.org/10.2147/ndt.s2325

Conti, V., Izzo, V., Russillo, M. C., Picillo, M., Amboni, M., Scaglione, C. L. M., Nicoletti, A., Cani, I., Cicero, C. E., De Bellis, E., Charlier, B., Giudice, V., Somma, G., Corbi, G., Barone, P., Filippelli, A., & Pellecchia, M. T. (2022). Gender differences in levodopa pharmacokinetics in levodopa-naïve patients with parkinson's disease. *Frontiers of Medicine, 9*. https://doi.org/10.3389/fmed.2022.909936

Deleu, D., Northway, M. G., & Hanssens, Y. (2002). Clinical pharmacokinetic and pharmacodynamic properties of drugs used in the treatment of Parkinson's disease. *Clinical Pharmacokinetics, 41*, 261–309.

Demailly, A., Moreau, C., & Devos, D. (2024). Effectiveness of continuous dopaminergic therapies in parkinson's disease: A review of L-DOPA Pharmacokinetics/pharmacodynamics. *Journal of Parkinson's Disease, 14*(5), 925–939. https://doi.org/10.3233/jpd-230372

di Biase, L., Pecoraro, P. M., Carbone, S. P., Caminiti, M. L., & Di Lazzaro, V. (2023). Levodopa-induced dyskinesias in Parkinson's disease: An overview on pathophysiology, clinical manifestations, therapy management strategies and future directions. *Journal of Clinical Medicine, 12*(13). https://doi.org/10.3390/jcm12134427. https://www.mdpi.com/journal/jcm

El-Shorbagi, A. N., Chaudhary, S., Alshemali, K. A., Alabdulrazzaq, R. F., & Alqahtani, F. Y. (2020). A comprehensive review on management of Parkinson's disease, inclusive of drug discovery and pharmacological approaches. *Journal of Applied Pharmaceutical Science, 10*(10), 130–150. https://doi.org/10.7324/JAPS.2020.1010015

Elshoff, J. P., Cawello, W., Andreas, J. O., Mathy, F. X., & Braun, M. (2015). An update on pharmacological, pharmacokinetic properties and drug-drug interactions of rotigotine transdermal system in Parkinson's disease and restless legs syndrome. *Drugs, 75*(5), 487–501. https://doi.org/10.1007/s40265-015-0377-y

Fabbri, M., Barbosa, R., & Rascol, O. (2023). Off-time treatment options for Parkinson's disease. *Neurology and Therapy, 12*(2), 391–424. https://doi.org/10.1007/s40120-022-00435-8

Gharat, S. A., Momin, M. M., & Khan, T. (2024). *Pharmacokinetics and pharmacodynamics of novel drug delivery systems: From basic concepts to applications: A machine-generated literature overview.* Singapore: Springer Nature. https://doi.org/10.1007/978-981-99-7858-8

Hametner, E. M., Seppi, K., & Poewe, W. (2012). Role and clinical utility of pramipexole extended release in the treatment of early Parkinson's disease. *Clinical Interventions in Aging, 7*, 83–88. https://doi.org/10.2147/CIA.S11829Austria

Hauser, R. A., Pahwa, R., Wargin, W. A., Souza-Prien, C. J., McClure, N., Johnson, R., Nguyen, J. T., Patni, R., & Went, G. T. (2019). Pharmacokinetics of ADS-5102 (amantadine) extended release capsules administered once daily at bedtime for the treatment of dyskinesia. *Clinical Pharmacokinetics, 58*(1), 77–88. https://doi.org/10.1007/s40262-018-0663-4

Horowski, R. (2022). *Lisuride: An 8-Alpha-ergoline with ergot antagonistic properties Neuro-Psychopharmacotherapy.* Germany: Springer International Publishing. https://doi.org/10.1007/978-3-030-62059-2_287. https://link.springer.com/book/10.1007/978-3-030-62059-2

Isaacson, S. H., Hauser, R. A., Pahwa, R., Gray, D., & Duvvuri, S. (2023). Dopamine agonists in Parkinson's disease: Impact of D1-like or D2-like dopamine receptor subtype selectivity and avenues for future treatment. *Clinical Parkinsonism and Related Disorders, 9*. https://doi.org/10.1016/j.prdoa.2023.100212. https://www.journals.elsevier.com/clinical-parkinsonism-and-related-disorders

Kawabata, K., & Katsuno, M. (2022). *Trihexyphenidyl, biperiden, and other anticholinergics in the treatment of Parkinson's disease NeuroPsychopharmacotherapy* (pp. 3333–3340). Japan: Springer International Publishing. https://doi.org/10.1007/978-3-030-62059-2_221. https://link.springer.com/book/10.1007/978-3-030-62059-2

Kuhn, W., & Müller, T. (2022). *Amantadine for treating Parkinson's disease NeuroPsychopharmacotherapy.* Germany: Springer International Publishing. https://doi.org/10.1007/978-3-030-62059-2_220, 3327–3332 https://link.springer.com/book/10.1007/978-3-030-62059-2.

Kumar, S., Gupta, S. K., & Pahwa, R. (2023). Designing lisuride intranasal nanocarrier system for reduction of oxidative damage with enhanced dopamine level in brain for parkinsonism. *Journal of Psychiatric Research, 165*, 205–218. https://doi.org/10.1016/j.jpsychires.2023.07.030

Kvernmo, T., Härtter, S., & Burger, E. (2006). A review of the receptor-binding and pharmacokinetic properties of dopamine agonists. *Clinical Therapeutics, 28*(8), 1065–1078. https://doi.org/10.1016/j.clinthera.2006.08.004

Leta, V., Klingelhoefer, L., Longardner, K., Campagnolo, M., Levent, H.Ç., Aureli, F., Metta, V., Bhidayasiri, R., Chung-Faye, G., Falup-Pecurariu, C., Stocchi, F., Jenner, P., Warnecke, T., & Ray Chaudhuri, K. (2023). Gastrointestinal barriers to levodopa transport and absorption in Parkinson's disease. *European Journal of Neurology, 30*(5), 1465–1480. https://doi.org/10.1111/ene.15734. http://onlinelibrary.wiley.com/journal/10.1111/(ISSN)1468-1331

Lewitt, P. A. (2015). Levodopa therapy for Parkinson's disease: Pharmacokinetics and pharmacodynamics. *Movement Disorders, 30*(1), 64–72. https://doi.org/10.1002/mds.26082

Marzoughi, S., Banerjee, A., Jutzeler, C. R., Prado, M. A. M., Rosner, J., Cragg, J. J., & Cashman, N. (2021). Tardive neurotoxicity of anticholinergic drugs: A review. *Journal of Neurochemistry, 158*(6), 1334–1344. https://doi.org/10.1111/jnc.15244. http://onlinelibrary.wiley.com/journal/10.1111/(ISSN)1471-4159

Moore J.J., SaadabadiA., (2018). Selegiline.

Mosley, R. L., Saleh, M., & Olson, K. E. (2024). *Immunotherapy for neurodegenerative movement disorders* (pp. 943–973). Springer Science and Business Media LLC. https://doi.org/10.1007/978-3-031-68237-7_52

Müller, T. (2020). Pharmacokinetics and pharmacodynamics of levodopa/carbidopa cotherapies for Parkinson's disease. *Expert Opinion on Drug Metabolism and Toxicology, 16*(5), 403–414. https://doi.org/10.1080/17425255.2020.1750596

Müller, T., Gerlach, M., Hefner, G., Hiemke, C., Jost, W. H., & Riederer, P. (2024). Therapeutic drug monitoring in Parkinson's disease. *Journal of Neural Transmission, 131*(10), 1247–1262. https://doi.org/10.1007/s00702-024-02828-5

Müller, T., Kuhn, W., & Möhr, J. D. (2019). Evaluating ADS5102 (amantadine) for the treatment of Parkinson's disease patients with dyskinesia. *Expert Opinion on Pharmacotherapy, 20*(10), 1181–1187. https://doi.org/10.1080/14656566.2019.1612365

Muranova, A., & Shanina, E. (2023). *Levodopa/carbidopa/entacapone combination therapy StatPearls*. StatPearls Publishing.

Nakatsuka, A., Nagai, M., Yabe, H., Nishikawa, N., Nomura, T., Moritoyo, H., Moritoyo, T., & Nomoto, M. (2006). Effect of clarithromycin on the pharmacokinetics of cabergoline in healthy controls and in patients with Parkinson's disease. *Journal of Pharmacological Sciences, 100*(1), 59–64. https://doi.org/10.1254/jphs.fp0050711

Nasser, A., Gomeni, R., Ceresoli-Borroni, G., Xie, L., Busse, G. D., Melyan, Z., & Rubin, J. (2024). Model-based comparison of subcutaneous versus sublingual apomorphine administration in the treatment of motor fluctuations in Parkinson's disease. *Journal of Pharmacokinetics and Pharmacodynamics, 51*(4), 385–393. https://doi.org/10.1007/s10928-024-09914-x

Nutt, J. G. (2008). Pharmacokinetics and pharmacodynamics of levodopa. *Movement Disorders, 23*(3), Article S580. https://doi.org/10.1002/mds.22037

Oertel, W. H., Wolters, E., Sampaio, C., Gimenez-Roldan, S., Bergamasco, B., Dujardin, M., Grosset, D. G., Arnold, G., Leenders, K. L., Hundemer, H. P., Lledó, A., Wood, A., Frewer, P., & Schwarz, J. (2006). Pergolide versus levodopa monotherapy in early Parkinson's disease patients: The PELMOPET study. *Movement Disorders, 21*(3), 343–353. https://doi.org/10.1002/mds.20724

Ozery, M., & Wadhwa, R. (2024). Bromocriptine. In *StatPearls*. StatPearls Publishing. Retrieved on.

Pastor, P., & Tolosa, E. (2003). Cabergolina en el tratamiento de la enfermedad de parkinson. *Neurologia, 18*(4), 202–209.

Pedrosa De Menezes, A. L., Bloem, B. R., Beckers, M., Piat, C., Benarroch, E. E., & Savica, R. (2024). Molecular variability in levodopa absorption and clinical implications for the management of Parkinson's disease. *Journal of Parkinson's Disease, 14*(7), 1353–1368. https://doi.org/10.3233/JPD-240036

Regensburger, M., Ip, C. W., Kohl, Z., Schrader, C., Urban, P. P., Kassubek, J., & Jost, W. H. (2023). Clinical benefit of MAO-B and COMT inhibition in Parkinson's disease: Practical considerations. *Journal of Neural Transmission, 130*(6), 847–861. https://doi.org/10.1007/s00702-023-02623-8

Reichmann, H., Bilsing, A., Ehret, R., Greulich, W., Schulz, J. B., Schwartz, A., & Rascol, O. (2006). Ergoline and non-ergoline derivatives in the treatment of Parkinson's disease. *Journal of Neurology*. https://doi.org/10.1007/s00415-006-4009-z

Rewane, A., Patel, P., & Nagalli, S. (2024). Ropinirole. In *StatPearls*. StatPearls Publishing.

Riederer, P., & Müller, T. (2022). *Selegiline for treating Parkinson's disease neuropsychopharmacotherapy* (p. 3149). Germany: Springer International Publishing. https://doi.org/10.1007/978-3-030-62059-2_237. https://link.springer.com/book/10.1007/978-3-030-62059-2

Safarpour, D., Sharzehi, K., & Pfeiffer, R. F. (2022). Gastrointestinal dysfunction in Parkinson's disease. *Drugs, 82*(2), 169–197. https://doi.org/10.1007/s40265-021-01664-1

Sahoo, L. K., Holla, V. V., Batra, D., Prasad, S., Bhattacharya, A., Kamble, N., Yadav, R., & Pal, P. K. (2020). Comparison of effectiveness of trihexyphenidyl and levodopa on motor symptoms in Parkinson's disease. *Journal of Neural Transmission, 127*(12), 1599–1606. https://doi.org/10.1007/s00702-020-02257-0

Schrag, A. (2005). Entacapone in the treatment of Parkinson's disease. *The Lancet Neurology, 4*(6), 366–370. https://doi.org/10.1016/s1474-4422(05)70098-3

Shill, H. A., & Stacy, M. (2009). Update on ropinirole in the treatment of Parkinson's disease. *Neuropsychiatric Disease and Treatment, 5*(1), 33–36.

Truong D.D. (2009). Tolcapone: Review of its pharmacology and use as adjunctive therapy in patients with Parkinson's disease. Clinical Interventions in Aging, 109–113.

Vardanyan, R., & Hruby, V. (2016). *Synthesis of best-seller drugs synthesis of best-seller drugs* (p. 1). United States: Elsevier. https://doi.org/10.1016/C2012-0-07004-4. https://www.sciencedirect.com/book/9780124114920

Véronneau-Veilleux, F., Robaey, P., Ursino, M., & Nekka, F. (2021). An integrative model of Parkinson's disease treatment including levodopa pharmacokinetics, dopamine kinetics, basal ganglia neurotransmission and motor action throughout disease progression. *Journal of Pharmacokinetics and Pharmacodynamics, 48*(1), 133–148. https://doi.org/10.1007/s10928-020-09723-y

Woitalla, D., Buhmann, C., Hilker-Roggendorf, R., Höglinger, G., Koschel, J., Müller, T., & Weise, D. (2023). Role of dopamine agonists in Parkinson's disease therapy. *Springer, Germany Journal of Neural Transmission, 130*(6), 863–873. https://doi.org/10.1007/s00702-023-02647-0

Xu, K., Sheng, S., & Zhang, F. (2023). Relationship between gut bacteria and levodopa metabolism. *Current Neuropharmacology, 21*(7), 1536–1547. https://doi.org/10.2174/1570159x21666221019115716

Zhao, J., Xu, G., Feng, C., Chen, Y., Kang, Y., Liu, F., & Ma, W. (2020). Trihexyphenidyl induced malignant hyperthermia in a patient with Parkinson's disease complicated with pneumonia. *Medicine, 99*(20), Article e20129. https://doi.org/10.1097/md.0000000000020129

SECTION

Established pharmacotherapies

II

CHAPTER

8 Dopaminergic treatments for Parkinson's disease: Seeing the unseen

Maha Awan
Sulaiman Al Rajhi University, Al Bukayriyah, Saudi Arabia

8.1 Introduction: The central role of dopamine in Parkinson's disease

8.1.1 The dopaminergic deficit in PD pathophysiology

Parkinson's disease (PD) is pathologically defined by the progressive and relentless loss of dopaminergic neurons originating in the substantia nigra pars compacta (SNc) and projecting to the striatum. This neurodegeneration results in a profound decrease in dopamine (DA) content within the striatum, disrupting the delicate balance of basal ganglia circuitry responsible for motor control (Zhou et al., 2023). The consequent dopamine deficiency directly underlies the emergence of the cardinal motor symptoms of PD: bradykinesia (slowness of movement), muscular rigidity, resting tremor, and, in later stages, postural instability (Muranova and Shanina, 2023).

However, the pathophysiology extends beyond simple neuronal attrition. Accumulating evidence suggests that functional deficits within the dopaminergic system may precede widespread cell death. Research indicates that dysregulation of axonal dopamine release can occur before significant neurodegeneration is evident (Cramb et al., 2023). This early dysfunction involves impairments in various presynaptic processes, including dopamine synthesis, vesicular loading via the vesicular monoamine transporter 2 (VMAT2), synaptic vesicle trafficking and docking (involving the SNARE complex), exocytosis, and dopamine reuptake via the dopamine transporter (DAT), as well as disruptions caused by protein aggregation. These findings imply that impaired dopamine release itself, resulting from diverse genetic and molecular disturbances associated with PD, could be considered an early pathophysiological hallmark (Cramb et al., 2023).

Furthermore, dopamine itself presents a biological paradox. While essential for neurotransmission, it is an inherently unstable molecule. Its metabolism and autooxidation can generate potentially toxic byproducts, including reactive oxygen species (ROS), electrophilic dopamine quinones (such as dopamine-o-quinone (DOQ) and its cyclized form, aminochrome (AM)), and 3,4-dihydroxyphenylacetaldehyde (DOPAL) (Zhou et al., 2023). These reactive species can damage cellular components, including proteins and lipids, contributing to oxidative stress and neuronal vulnerability. Key enzymes involved in dopamine metabolism, monoamine oxidase (MAO) and catechol-O-methyltransferase (COMT), participate in pathways that can either detoxify dopamine metabolites (e.g., forming 3-methoxytyramine (3-MT), homovanillic acid (HVA), or 3,4-

Pharmacological Foundations of Parkinson's Disease. https://doi.org/10.1016/B978-0-443-27702-3.00028-5

dihydroxyphenylacetic acid (DOPAC)) or generate reactive intermediates like DOPAL (via MAO). Genetic factors, such as mutations in LRRK2 or PINK1, can further perturb dopamine homeostasis and increase neuronal susceptibility by influencing dopamine synthesis and the production of these toxic by-products (Zhou et al., 2023). This dual nature of dopamine – being both the deficient neurotransmitter requiring replacement and a potential endogenous contributor to neurodegeneration – poses a significant challenge for therapeutic strategies. Increasing dopamine levels is crucial for symptomatic relief, yet the very molecule being replaced carries inherent chemical risks that might exacerbate the underlying pathology if not carefully managed (Tables 8.1–8.6).

8.1.2 Rationale for dopaminergic replacement therapy (DRT)

Given the central role of dopamine deficiency in PD motor symptoms, the primary therapeutic strategy aims to restore dopaminergic neurotransmission within the basal ganglia. Dopaminergic replacement therapy (DRT) encompasses various pharmacological approaches designed to enhance dopamine levels or stimulate dopamine receptors, thereby compensating for the endogenous deficit (Muranova and Shanina, 2023). The goal is to alleviate motor symptoms and improve the patient's functional capacity and quality of life. It is crucial to recognize, however, that current DRT strategies are purely symptomatic; they do not alter the underlying neurodegenerative process or prevent disease progression (Armstrong and Okun, 2020).

8.1.3 Chapter scope: Seeing the unseen

This chapter provides a comprehensive overview of dopaminergic treatments for PD, extending beyond the readily apparent motor benefits – "the seen" – to explore the often less visible, yet critically important, aspects of therapy – "the unseen." These encompass:

- The intricate relationship between drug pharmacokinetics and pharmacodynamics and the resulting variability in individual patient responses.
- The significant, yet often complex, impact of DRT on the wide spectrum of non-motor symptoms (NMS) that frequently cause substantial disability (Schaeffer and Berg, 2017).
- The inevitable emergence of treatment-related complications over the long term, including motor fluctuations, dyskinesias, and challenging non-motor side effects like impulse control disorders.
- The influence of individual genetic makeup (pharmacogenomics) on treatment efficacy and the risk of adverse events (Corvol and Poewe, 2017).
- The continuous evolution of therapeutic strategies, including advanced drug delivery systems and novel pharmacological agents, aimed at overcoming the limitations of current treatments.

By examining these "unseen" dimensions, this chapter aims to equip readers with a deeper understanding of the nuances involved in optimizing dopaminergic therapy for the multifaceted challenge of Parkinson's disease.

8.2 Levodopa: The gold standard and its challenges

8.2.1 Mechanism of action and pharmacology

Levodopa (L-DOPA), the metabolic precursor of dopamine, remains the cornerstone of PD pharmacotherapy. Unlike dopamine itself, levodopa can cross the blood-brain barrier (BBB) via the large

Table 8.1 Overview of dopaminergic drug classes in Parkinson's disease therapy.

Drug class	Primary mechanism	Key agents	Primary clinical use	Major advantages	Major disadvantages/ Key side effects
Levodopa	Dopamine precursor; converted to dopamine in CNS	Levodopa/ Carbidopa, levodopa/ Benserazide	Most effective for motor symptoms (all stages); gold standard	Highest motor symptom efficacy	Motor fluctuations, dyskinesias with longterm use; nausea, orthostatic hypotension
Dopamine agonists (DAs)	Direct stimulation of postsynaptic dopamine receptors (mainly D2/ D3)	Pramipexole, ropinirole, rotigotine, apomorphine	Early PD monotherapy (younger patients); adjunct in advanced PD for fluctuations	Lower risk of motor complications versus levodopa; various formulations	Less motor efficacy than levodopa; higher risk of ICDs, somnolence, hallucinations, edema, orthostatic hypotension
MAO-B inhibitors	Inhibit MAO-B enzyme, reducing dopamine breakdown in CNS	Selegiline, rasagiline, safinamide	Mild monotherapy (early PD); adjunct in advanced PD for fluctuations	Modest motor benefit; May improve some NMS; generally well-tolerated	Potential for dyskinesia worsening (adjunct); insomnia (selegiline); serotonin syndrome risk (rare)
COMT inhibitors	Inhibit peripheral COMT enzyme, reducing levodopa breakdown, increasing bioavailability	Entacapone, tolcapone, opicapone	Adjunct to levodopa in advanced PD for wearing-off fluctuations	Reduce "off" time; extend levodopa effect; opicapone may improve NMS	Dyskinesia worsening; diarrhea; urine discoloration; hepatotoxicity risk (tolcapone only)

CNS: Central Nervous System; ICDs: Impulse Control Disorders; MAO-B: Monoamine Oxidase type B; COMT: Catechol-O-Methyltransferase; NMS: Nonmotor Symptoms.

neutral amino acid (LNAA) transport system. Once in the central nervous system (CNS), it is decarboxylated by the enzyme aromatic L-amino acid decarboxylase (AADC) to dopamine, directly replenishing the depleted neurotransmitter stores within the remaining nigrostriatal terminals and other cells capable of this conversion. This restoration of striatal dopamine levels effectively alleviates the cardinal motor symptoms of PD (Muranova and Shanina, 2023).

Table 8.2 Levodopa formulations for Parkinson's disease.

Formulation type	Brand examples (US)	Key PK characteristics	Primary clinical use case	Key advantages	Key disadvantages/ Considerations
Immediate release (IR) tablet/Capsule	Sinemet, Parcopa (dissolvable)	Rapid onset (~30 min), short duration (~2–4 h), high peak-trough fluctuation	Standard initial therapy, dose titration	Reliable efficacy, flexible dosing	Short duration leads to wearingoff ; requires frequent dosing; contributes to pulsatile stimulation (Contin and Martinelli, 2010)
Controlled release (CR)/ Sustained release (SR) tablet	Sinemet CR	Slower absorption, delayed onset, lower Çmax, longer duration (variable)	Attempt to reduce fluctuations, overnight coverage[1]	Reduced dosing frequency potentially	Erratic/ unpredictable absorption; delayed onset ("dose failure"); lower bioavailability than IR; May worsen peakdose dyskinesia if peaks still occur (Contin and Martinelli, 2010)
Extended release (ER) capsule (IR/ER beads)	Rytary, numient (EU)	Faster onset than CR, longer duration than IR (~4–5 h), smoother profile than IR	Management of fluctuations, reduced dosing frequency	Combines faster onset with longer duration; more predictable than CR (Livingston and Monroe-Duprey, 2024)	Cannot be crushed/ chewed; higher cost; dose conversion from IR is complex
Oral disintegrating tablet (ODT)	Parcopa	Rapid disintegration in mouth, absorption still primarily intestinal, PK similar to IR	Ease of administration (dysphagia), potentially faster onset (minor)	Convenient for swallowing difficulties (Livingston and Monroe-Duprey, 2024)	Similar duration/ fluctuation issues as IR tablets

Table 8.2 Levodopa formulations for Parkinson's disease.—cont'd

Formulation type	Brand examples (US)	Key PK characteristics	Primary clinical use case	Key advantages	Key disadvantages/ Considerations
Levodopa/ Carbidopa intestinal gel (LCIG)	Duopa (US), Duodopa (EU)	Continuous jejunal infusion via PEG-J tube, stable plasma levels	Advanced PD with severe motor fluctuations/ dyskinesia refractory to oral therapy	Provides continuous dopaminergic stimulation (CDS); reduces "off" time and dyskinesia; improves NMS (Batzu and Qamar, 2023)	Invasive (surgery, pump maintenance); tube/pump complications; high cost (Livingston and Monroe-Duprey, 2024)
Inhaled levodopa Powder	Inbrija	Rapid pulmonary absorption, fast onset (~10–30 min)	On-demand ("rescue") treatment for "off" episodes	Rapid relief of "off" symptoms (Livingston and Monroe-Duprey, 2024)	Treats only individual "off" episodes, not underlying fluctuations; Cough, respiratory irritation, sputum discoloration (Jimenez-Shahed, 2016)
Subcutaneous (SC) infusion (investigational)	Foslevodopa/ Foscarbidopa	Continuous SC infusion of levodopa prodrugs, aims for stable plasma levels	Potential alternative to LCIG for CDS in advanced PD with fluctuations	Less invasive than LCIG; provides CDS; potential NMS benefits (sleep) (Batzu and Qamar, 2023)	Injection site reactions; pump management; still under investigation (Batzu and Qamar, 2023)

PK: Pharmacokinetics; Cmax: Maximum concentration; EU: European Union; PEG-J: Percutaneous Endoscopic Gastrostomy with Jejunal tube; NMS: Nonmotor Symptoms; CDS: Continuous Dopaminergic Stimulation.

However, AADC is also abundant in peripheral tissues. If administered alone, levodopa undergoes extensive peripheral decarboxylation, leading to high circulating levels of dopamine, which causes significant side effects (primarily nausea and vomiting) and drastically limits the amount of levodopa reaching the brain (estimated at only ~1%). To overcome this, levodopa is almost universally coadminsitered with a peripheral AADC inhibitor, such as carbidopa or benserazide. These inhibitors do not cross the BBB significantly but effectively block peripheral levodopa metabolism. This combination dramatically increases the CNS bioavailability of levodopa (up to ~10%), allows for a

Table 8.3 Commonly used nonergoline dopamine agonists.

Agent	Receptor profile	Available formulations	Typical use case	Key efficacy points	Major adverse effects
Pramipexole	D3 > D2 agonist	Oral IR, oral ER	Early monotherapy; adjunct for fluctuations; potential antidepressant effect?	Good motor benefit; reduces "off" time; delays motor complications (early use)	ICDs, somnolence/ Sleep attacks, hallucinations, nausea, orthostatic hypotension, edema
Ropinirole	D3 > D2 agonist	Oral IR, oral ER	Early monotherapy; adjunct for fluctuations	Good motor benefit; reduces "off" time; delays motor complications (early use)	ICDs, somnolence/ Sleep attacks, hallucinations, nausea, orthostatic hypotension
Rotigotine	D3 > D2 agonist (also 5-HT, α-adrenergic)	Transdermal patch	Early monotherapy; adjunct for fluctuations; continuous delivery	Good motor benefit; reduces "off" time; improves sleep/NMS; stable levels	ICDs, somnolence, nausea, orthostatic hypotension; application site reactions (common)
Apomorphine	Potent D1/D2 agonist	SC intermittent injection, SC continuous infusion (CSAI)	Rapid rescue for "off" episodes (injection); severe fluctuations (infusion)	Potent, rapid motor improvement; reduces "off" time (infusion); improves NMS (infusion)	Nausea (often requires antiemetic cotreatment), orthostatic hypotension, injection site nodules (infusion), somnolence, hallucinations

IR: Immediate Release; ER: Extended Release; SC: Subcutaneous; ICDs: Impulse Control Disorders; NMS: Nonmotor Symptoms; 5-HT: Serotonin.

significant reduction in the required levodopa dose (by approximately 75%–80%), extends its effective half-life, and markedly reduces peripheral side effects (Muranova and Shanina, 2023).

8.2.2 Pharmacokinetics: The basis of fluctuation

The pharmacokinetic (PK) profile of levodopa presents inherent challenges that significantly influence its long-term use. Levodopa is rapidly absorbed primarily from the proximal small intestine, utilizing

Table 8.4 MAO-B and COMT inhibitors used in Parkinson's disease.

Agent	Class	Specific mechanism notes	Primary use	Key efficacy	Key safety/ Tolerability issues
Selegiline	MAO-BI	Irreversible; metabolites include amphetamines	Early monotherapy (mild); adjunct for fluctuations	Modest motor benefit; reduces "off" time	Insomnia, confusion, orthostatic hypotension; Dyskinesia worsening (adjunct); low tyramine risk at PD doses; serotonin syndrome risk
Rasagiline	MAO-BI	Irreversible; nonamphetamine metabolite (aminoindan)	Early monotherapy; adjunct for fluctuations	Modest motor benefit; reduces "off" time; potential NMS benefit (pain, fatigue?)	Generally well-tolerated; dyskinesia worsening (adjunct); low tyramine risk at PD doses; serotonin syndrome risk
Safinamide	MAO-BI	Reversible; also inhibits glutamate release	Adjunct for fluctuations	Reduces "off" time; potential NMS benefit (pain, fatigue, sleep?)	Dyskinesia worsening (adjunct); slightly higher TAEs versus placebo in meta-analysis; low tyramine risk; serotonin syndrome risk
Entacapone	COMT-I	Peripheral; short-acting (requires dosing with each levodopa dose)	Adjunct for wearing-off	Reduces "off" time; extends levodopa effect	Dyskinesia worsening, nausea, diarrhea, urine discoloration; No hepatotoxicity risk
Tolcapone	COMT-I	Peripheral and central; longer acting than entacapone	Adjunct for wearingoff (when others fail)	Potent reduction in "off" time; extends levodopa effect	**Hepatotoxicity risk (requires strict monitoring)**; dyskinesia worsening, nausea, severe diarrhea

Continued

Table 8.4 MAO-B and COMT inhibitors used in Parkinson's disease.—cont'd

Agent	Class	Specific mechanism notes	Primary use	Key efficacy	Key safety/ Tolerability issues
Opicapone	COMT-I	Peripheral; long acting (once-daily dosing)	Adjunct for wearingoff	Reduces "off" time; extends levodopa effect; improves/ stabilizes NMS	Dyskinesia worsening, nausea, dry mouth, urine discoloration; No hepatotoxicity risk

TAEs: Treatment-Associated Adverse Events.

the same saturable LNAA transporter responsible for its BBB passage. This shared transport mechanism means that dietary proteins, composed of LNAAs, can compete with levodopa for both intestinal absorption and entry into the brain. Consequently, high-protein meals can reduce and delay levodopa absorption, leading to inconsistent clinical responses. Standardizing levodopa dosing relative to meal times and managing dietary protein intake are therefore important strategies to enhance the reproducibility of its effects (Contin and Martinelli, 2010).

Even when coadministered with an AADC inhibitor, levodopa possesses a very short plasma half-life, typically around 60–90 min (Muranova and Shanina, 2023). This rapid clearance results in significant oscillations in plasma drug concentrations following standard oral dosing regimens (Contin and Martinelli, 2010). Early in the disease, the brain's remaining dopaminergic neurons can buffer these fluctuations by storing dopamine synthesized from levodopa and releasing it more physiologically. However, as neurodegeneration progresses, this buffering capacity diminishes, and the clinical response becomes increasingly dependent on the fluctuating plasma levodopa levels. This pharmacokinetic limitation is a fundamental driver of the motor complications that emerge with long-term therapy. The inherent variability in absorption and the short half-life conspire to create a non-physiological, pulsatile stimulation of postsynaptic dopamine receptors, contrasting sharply with the tonic stimulation provided by intact nigrostriatal neurons.

8.2.3 Clinical efficacy: Unmatched motor symptom control

Despite its pharmacokinetic challenges and long-term complications, the combination of levodopa and a peripheral AADC inhibitor remains the most potent pharmacological treatment available for the motor symptoms of PD (Pandey and Srivanitchapoom, 2013). Its introduction revolutionized PD management, dramatically improving motor function, activities of daily living, and quality of life. Levodopa typically provides significant improvement in bradykinesia and rigidity, with a more variable effect on tremor and postural instability (Lee and Koh, 2015).

The robust efficacy of levodopa is quantifiable through objective measures. Dopaminergic challenge tests, involving the administration of a standardized dose of levodopa followed by motor

Table 8.5 Summary of dopaminergic therapy effects on key nonmotor symptoms.

NMS domain	Effect of levodopa (IR/ Oral)	Effect of levodopa (CDS - LCIG)	Effect of DAs (non-ergot)	Effect of MAO-BIs	Effect of COMT-Is (entacapone/ Opicapone)
Depression/ Anxiety	+/–	+	+	+/–	0/+
Psychosis/ Hallucinations	–	- (Potential risk)	–	- (Potential risk)	- (Potential risk via L-dopa)
Impulse control disorders (ICDs)	- (Lower risk than DAs)	? (may allow DA reduction)	–	0/?	0
Sleep: Insomnia	- (Can disrupt sleep)	+	+/–	+/–	+
Sleep: EDS	–	0/-	–	+/–	0/+
Sleep: RLS/ PLM	+	+	++	?	?
Sleep: RBD	0	?	0	+/–	?
Autonomic: Orthostatic hypotension (OH)	–	?	–	+/–	0
Autonomic: Constipation	–	+/–	–	?	+/0
Pain (fluctuation-related)	+ (during "on" time)	+	+	+	+/+
Fatigue	+/–	+	+/–	+	+/+
Olfaction	0	0	0	0	0
Cognition (global)	0	0/+?	0/- (psychosis risk)	0	0/+?

Symbol Key: ++ Strongly beneficial; + Beneficial; +/– Mixed/Variable/Potential benefit; 0 Neutral/Unclear/No significant effect; - Detrimental/Worsening; – Strongly detrimental; — Very high risk.

assessment using scales like the Unified Parkinson's Disease Rating Scale Part III (UPDRS-III), consistently demonstrate significant motor improvement in PD patients. Meta-analyses indicate an average UPDRS-III improvement rate of approximately 41.5% following an acute levodopa challenge in established PD patients. However, this responsiveness is not uniform and exhibits considerable heterogeneity. Patients newly diagnosed de novo typically show a lower improvement rate (around 25.9%) compared to those already on treatment (around 42.4%), likely reflecting differences in disease stage and potentially compensatory mechanisms. Furthermore, responsiveness is dose-dependent, with higher doses (e.g., 200–250 mg) eliciting greater improvement than lower doses (e.g., 100 mg), and positively correlates with baseline motor severity (Kou et al., 2025).

Table 8.6 Selected pharmacogenomic associations in dopaminergic therapy for Parkinson's disease.

Gene	SNP/Variant	Associated Drug (s)	Potential clinical association	Strength of evidence/ Consistency
COMT	rs4680 (Val158Met)	Levodopa, entacapone	LL genotype: Lower L-dopa dose, ↑LID risk?, ↑Sleepiness (Liu et al., 2023); influences acute entacapone response (Corvol and Poewe, 2017)	Replicated associations, some conflicting
	rs165815	Levodopa	C Allele: ↑Visual hallucination risk (Liu et al., 2023)	Preliminary/Needs replication
DRD2	rs1800497 (TaqIA)	Levodopa, DAs	Associated with L-dopa dose; ↑LID risk (14/15 genotype); ↓Peak dose dyskinesia (13/14 alleles); C allele: ↑Delayed hallucinations (Liu et al., 2023)	Conflicting/ Inconsistent
DRD3	rs6280 (Ser9Gly)	Levodopa, DAs	C Genotype: ↑Visual hallucination risk (Liu et al., 2023); associated with ICD risk; possibly influences pramipexole response (Corvol and Poewe, 2017)	Some replication, needs more validation
SLC6A3 (DAT)	VNTR, rs28363170, rs393795	Levodopa	Associated with LID risk/timing; hallucination/ psychosis risk; dose requirement (9R allele) (Liu et al., 2023); motor response? (Corvol and Poewe, 2017)	Some replication, complex associations
MAO-A	rs1799836	Levodopa	A allele/AA genotype: ↑LID risk (Liu et al., 2023)	Preliminary/Needs replication
BDNF	rs6265 (Val66Met)	Levodopa	Met allele: ↑LID risk? (Liu et al., 2023)	Conflicting

Table 8.6 Selected pharmacogenomic associations in dopaminergic therapy for Parkinson's disease.—cont'd

Gene	SNP/Variant	Associated Drug (s)	Potential clinical association	Strength of evidence/ Consistency
HOMER1	rs4704560	Levodopa	G allele: ↓LID risk (Liu et al., 2023)	Preliminary/Needs replication
AADC	Promoter deletion	Levodopa	Lower motor response to acute challenge (Corvol and Poewe, 2017)	Single study/Needs replication
UGT1A	Various polymorphisms	Tolcapone, entacapone	Associated with COMT-I induced liver toxicity/ adverse reactions (Corvol and Poewe, 2017)	Preliminary

LID: Levodopa Induced Dyskinesia; ICD: Impulse Control Disorder; VNTR: Variable Number Tandem Repeat.

8.2.4 Formulations: Striving for stability

Recognizing the limitations imposed by levodopa's short half-life and the desire to achieve more stable plasma concentrations and clinical effects, various formulations have been developed (Livingston and Monroe-Duprey, 2024). These aim to improve convenience, manage fluctuations, or provide rapid relief from "off" periods (Fig. 8.1).

8.2.5 Long-term complications: The waning honeymoon

While highly effective initially, the benefits of levodopa therapy often diminish over time, accompanied by the emergence of debilitating treatment-related complications, primarily motor fluctuations and dyskinesias (Pandey and Srivanitchapoom, 2013).

- **Motor Fluctuations ("Wearing-off"):** Early in PD, the response to a single levodopa dose typically lasts longer than predicted by its short plasma half-life, a phenomenon known as the "long-duration response" (LDR) (Chaudhuri et al., 2013). This is attributed to the buffering capacity of surviving nigrostriatal neurons. As the disease progresses and neuronal loss continues, this buffering capacity is lost, and the duration of benefit from each dose shortens, increasingly mirroring the drug's rapid elimination. This results in the "short-duration response" (SDR), where parkinsonian symptoms re-emerge predictably before the next scheduled dose – the "wearing-off" phenomenon (Contin and Martinelli, 2010). Motor fluctuations develop in approximately 10% of patients per year of levodopa treatment, with prevalence reaching very high levels (up to 80%–100%) after 5–10 years (Antonini et al., 2008).
- **Dyskinesias (LID):** Levodopa-induced dyskinesias are involuntary movements that arise as a consequence of chronic, pulsatile levodopa administration interacting with the progressively

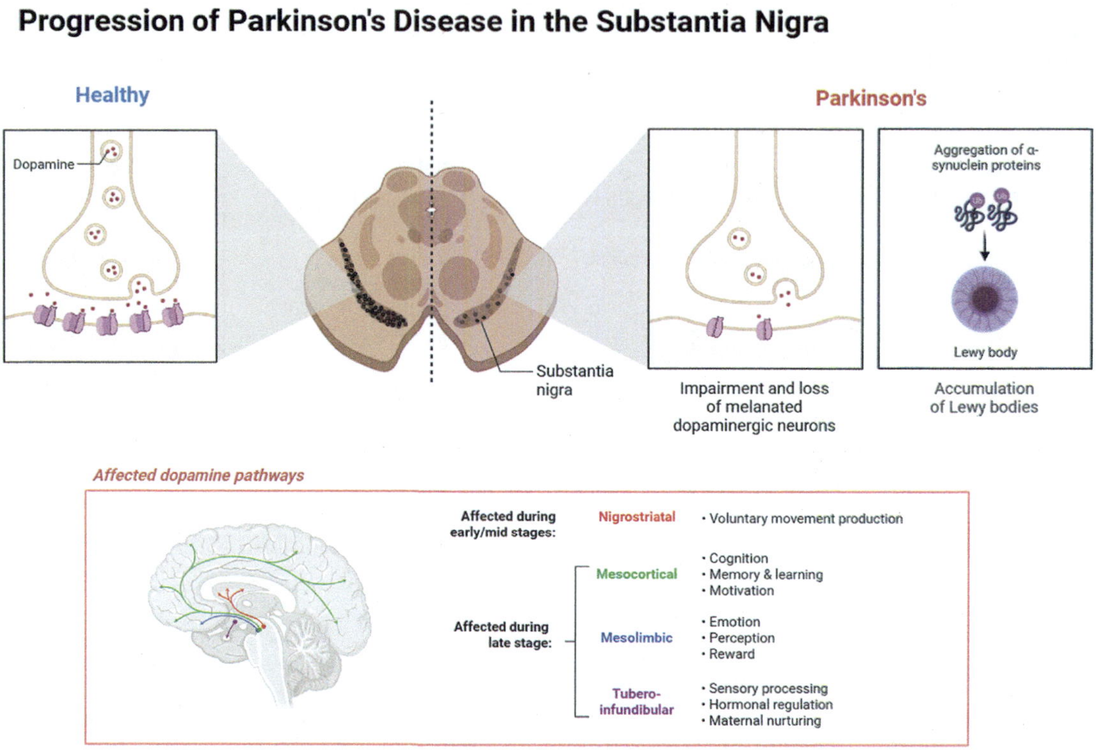

FIGURE 8.1

Progression of Parkinson's disease in the Substantia Nigra.

Created with BioRender.com

denervated and sensitized postsynaptic dopamine receptors. LID can manifest as chorea (rapid, dance-like movements), dystonia (sustained muscle contractions causing abnormal postures), ballism (large-amplitude flinging movements), myoclonus (brief muscle jerks), or a combination thereof. They commonly affect the limbs, trunk, and orofacial region (Pandey and Srivanitchapoom, 2013).

- *Types of LID*: Accurate phenotyping of LID is crucial for management as different types relate differently to levodopa levels.
  Peak-dose dyskinesia is the most frequent type, occurring when plasma levodopa concentrations are highest. It is typically choreiform but can include other movement types. Management often involves reducing individual levodopa doses, fractionating the total daily dose into smaller, more frequent administrations, or adding amantadine (Pandey and Srivanitchapoom, 2013).
  Off-period dyskinesia, often presenting as painful dystonia (especially in the foot or leg, commonly in the early morning), occurs when levodopa levels are low. Management strategies aim to extend dopaminergic coverage, such as adding a long-acting DA, MAO-BI, or COMT-I, or using long-acting levodopa formulations at bedtime (Pandey and Srivanitchapoom, 2013).

Diphasic dyskinesia occurs as levodopa levels are rising and falling, often manifesting as dystonia in the lower limbs. It can be challenging to manage, sometimes requiring a reduction in levodopa dose alongside an increase in DA dose, or consideration of advanced therapies like LCIG. Rarer forms like respiratory, abdominal ("belly dancer's"), or ocular dyskinesias have also been described, typically coinciding with peak levodopa effect (Pandey and Srivanitchapoom, 2013).

- *Pathophysiology of LID*: The mechanisms are complex and involve multiple neurotransmitter systems and adaptive changes within the basal ganglia circuitry. Key factors include:
- *Pulsatile Dopamine Receptor Stimulation*: Non-physiological fluctuations in dopamine levels from standard levodopa formulations lead to abnormal downstream signaling (Thanvi and Lo, 2004).
- *Postsynaptic Supersensitivity*: Dopamine receptors, particularly D1 receptors located on direct pathway neurons, become hypersensitive.
- *Altered Basal Ganglia Output*: An imbalance occurs, with overactivity of the pro-kinetic direct pathway and underactivity of the inhibitory indirect pathway, leading to excessive, involuntary movements.
- *Neurotransmitter Dysregulation*: Changes involve not only dopamine but also glutamate (via NMDA receptors, explaining amantadine's efficacy), serotonin (5-HT1A receptors modulate dopamine release), GABA, adenosine (A2A receptors), and endocannabinoids.
- *Abnormal Synaptic Plasticity*: Chronic intermittent stimulation induces maladaptive changes in synaptic strength and connectivity within the cortico-basal ganglia loops.
- *Management of LID*: Strategies focus on smoothing levodopa delivery and modulating neurotransmitter systems involved. This includes optimizing levodopa dosing (fractionation, smaller doses), adding adjunct therapies (DAs, MAO-BIs, COMT-Is to reduce "off" time and potentially allow levodopa dose reduction), utilizing amantadine, considering atypical antipsychotics with caution, and, in refractory cases, advanced therapies like LCIG, continuous subcutaneous apomorphine infusion (CSAI), or deep brain stimulation (DBS) (Pandey and Srivanitchapoom, 2013).

The inherent pharmacokinetic limitations of levodopa, particularly its short half-life and variable absorption, are thus central to the development of long-term motor complications (Contin and Martinelli, 2010). The shift from a stable LDR to a fluctuating SDR is a direct consequence of disease progression interacting with these PK properties (Chaudhuri et al., 2013). This pulsatile stimulation is widely considered the primary driver of the maladaptive neuroplastic changes underpinning both wearing-off and dyskinesia (Thanvi and Lo, 2004). This understanding provides a strong rationale for therapeutic strategies aimed at achieving more continuous dopaminergic stimulation (CDS), such as utilizing advanced formulations or adjunct therapies that prolong levodopa's action (Antonini et al., 2008). Furthermore, the distinct pathophysiological basis and timing relative to levodopa dosing for different types of dyskinesia necessitate careful clinical assessment. Effective management requires tailoring interventions to the specific LID phenotype, rather than applying a uniform approach (Pandey and Srivanitchapoom, 2013).

8.3 Dopamine agonists: Direct receptor stimulation

8.3.1 Classification and receptor pharmacology

Dopamine agonists (DAs) constitute a major class of antiparkinsonian drugs that exert their therapeutic effect by directly stimulating postsynaptic dopamine receptors within the basal ganglia, thereby mimicking the action of endogenous dopamine (Borovac, 2016). Unlike levodopa, they do not require enzymatic conversion and bypass the degenerating presynaptic nigrostriatal neurons.

DAs are broadly classified into two groups based on their chemical structure:

- **Ergot Derivatives:** These were the first DAs developed (e.g., bromocriptine, pergolide, cabergoline, lisuride). However, their use has become significantly restricted or withdrawn in many regions due to the risk of inducing fibrotic reactions, including cardiac valvulopathy (heart valve thickening and regurgitation), pulmonary fibrosis, and retroperitoneal fibrosis. Consequently, regulatory agencies and clinical guidelines strongly advise against their use as first-line agents, reserving them only for specific situations where non-ergot options are ineffective or not tolerated, and requiring careful monitoring (e.g., serial echocardiograms) (Borovac, 2016).
- **Non-Ergot Derivatives:** This newer generation includes pramipexole, ropinirole, rotigotine, and apomorphine. They lack the ergoline structure and are not associated with the risk of fibrosis, making them the preferred DAs in current clinical practice (Dopamine Agonist Market Size, Share & Trends Analysis Report By Drug (Non-ergot Dopamine Agonists, Ergot Alkaloids), By Route Of Administration (Oral, Injectable), By Application, By Distribution Channel, By Region, And Segment Forecasts, 2025 - 2030, 2024).

Dopamine receptors belong to the G protein-coupled receptor superfamily and are divided into two main families: D1-like (D1, D5) and D2-like (D2, D3, D4). Most clinically used non-ergot DAs exhibit preferential affinity for the D2-like receptors, particularly the D2 and D3 subtypes, with lower affinity for D1 receptors (Borovac, 2016). Pramipexole and ropinirole have notable D3 affinity, while rotigotine also interacts with serotonin and alpha-adrenergic receptors. Apomorphine is distinct in being a potent agonist at both D1 and D2 receptors. The specific receptor binding profiles may contribute to differences in efficacy and side effects. For instance, D2 receptor stimulation is strongly linked to motor improvement but also psychosis, while D3 receptor stimulation, particularly in the limbic system, has been implicated in the development of impulse control disorders and potentially mood effects (Borovac, 2016).

8.3.2 Pharmacokinetics and formulations

Pharmacokinetic properties can vary among different DAs. They are available in various formulations designed to optimize delivery and improve patient convenience:

- **Oral Immediate Release (IR):** Pramipexole and ropinirole are available as IR tablets, typically requiring multiple daily doses.
- **Oral Extended Release (ER/PR):** Both pramipexole and ropinirole are also available in ER formulations that allow for once-daily dosing. These formulations utilize different technologies to provide slower drug absorption and more stable plasma concentrations over 24 h compared to IR versions. This smoother PK profile may contribute to more consistent symptom control and potentially better tolerability, with some evidence suggesting ER ropinirole is better tolerated than IR (*Dopaminergic agonists in Parkinson's disease*, no date).
- **Transdermal Patch:** Rotigotine is formulated as a transdermal patch applied once daily. This delivery system provides continuous drug absorption through the skin, resulting in stable plasma levels over a 24-hour period (Borovac, 2016).

- **Subcutaneous (SC) Administration:** Apomorphine, due to poor oral bioavailability and extensive first-pass metabolism, is administered subcutaneously. It is available as an intermittent injection pen for rapid relief ("rescue") of unpredictable "off" episodes and as a continuous subcutaneous apomorphine infusion (CSAI) via a portable pump for patients with severe motor fluctuations refractory to other therapies.

8.3.3 Clinical efficacy

DAs play a significant role in both early and advanced stages of PD management.

- **Early PD:** DAs (pramipexole, ropinirole, rotigotine) are established as effective monotherapy options, particularly for younger patients (generally <60–70 years) (Borovac, 2016). Clinical guidelines often recommend considering DAs as an initial treatment strategy in this population (Recommendations | Parkinson's disease in adults | Guidance | NICE, 2017). Large clinical trials have demonstrated that initiating treatment with a DA, compared to levodopa, significantly delays the onset of motor complications, specifically dyskinesia and motor fluctuations, over several years (Borovac, 2016). However, this benefit comes at the cost of generally less potent control of motor symptoms compared to levodopa (Hitzeman and Rafii, 2009). The Brazilian Academy of Neurology guidelines assign Level A evidence for pramipexole and rotigotine as monotherapy in early PD (Saba et al., 2022).
- **Advanced PD:** In patients experiencing motor fluctuations and dyskinesias on levodopa therapy, adding a DA is a standard strategy (Borovac, 2016). As adjunct therapy, DAs effectively reduce total daily "off" time, improve motor function during both "on" and "off" periods (as measured by UPDRS scores), and often allow for a reduction in the total daily levodopa dose, which may help mitigate LID (Borovac, 2016). Level A evidence supports the use of pramipexole and rotigotine for managing motor fluctuations in advanced PD (Hitzeman and Rafii, 2009). Apomorphine, administered via intermittent injection or continuous infusion, provides potent and rapid motor improvement, demonstrating significant UPDRS-III score reductions (~40.1%) in challenge tests and effectively managing refractory "off" periods (Borovac, 2016).

DAs appear to interact with levodopa in a synergistic manner. Studies using intravenous levodopa infusions have shown that coadministration of a DA (pramipexole) potentiates the motor response to levodopa, increasing the peak effect (finger tapping speed, walking speed) and duration of response beyond what would be expected from a simple additive effect. However, this augmentation of motor benefit is often accompanied by an increase in the severity of levodopa-induced dyskinesia (Brodsky et al., 2010).

8.3.4 Key adverse effects: The trade-offs

While offering advantages in terms of delaying motor complications, DAs have a distinct adverse effect profile compared to levodopa. Overall, they are associated with a higher incidence of non-motor side effects, leading to higher rates of treatment withdrawal in clinical trials (Hitzeman and Rafii, 2009).

- **Common Side Effects:** Frequently encountered adverse effects include nausea, vomiting, orthostatic hypotension (dizziness upon standing), peripheral edema (swelling, particularly in the legs), constipation, somnolence (daytime sleepiness), and hallucinations. Application site reactions (redness, itching) are common with the rotigotine patch (Borovac, 2016).

- **Serious Adverse Effects:** Certain adverse effects associated with DAs require careful monitoring and management due to their potential severity and impact on quality of life:
- **Impulse Control Disorders (ICDs):** This is arguably the most concerning class-specific adverse effect of DAs. ICDs represent a failure to resist urges or impulses that are harmful, manifesting as pathological gambling, compulsive sexual behavior (hypersexuality), compulsive shopping, binge eating, or related behaviors like punding (stereotyped, repetitive activities) and dopamine dysregulation syndrome (compulsive medication use) (Park and Stacy, 2011). The prevalence in DA-treated patients is significant, estimated between 14% and 30%, potentially reaching nearly 50% cumulative incidence over 5 years. The risk is substantially higher with DAs than with levodopa monotherapy (Carbone and Djamshidian, 2024). Key risk factors include DA use itself (potentially dose- and duration-dependent), younger age, male gender (for gambling/hypersexuality), personal or family history of addictive behaviors or substance abuse, smoking, and preexisting depression or anxiety (Recommendations | Parkinson's disease in adults | Guidance | NICE, 2017). The underlying mechanism is thought to involve dopaminergic overstimulation of the mesolimbic reward pathway, particularly the ventral striatum, which is relatively spared from neurodegeneration in PD and rich in D3 receptors. Management is challenging and necessitates patient/family education, screening (e.g., using the QUIP-RS questionnaire), and primarily involves reducing or discontinuing the DA, often requiring a switch to levodopa. Advanced therapies like apomorphine infusion or DBS may be considered in refractory cases, alongside behavioral therapies (Carbone and Djamshidian, 2024).
- **Excessive Daytime Sleepiness (EDS) and Sleep Attacks:** DAs are well-known to cause somnolence and, more alarmingly, sudden, irresistible episodes of sleep ("sleep attacks") that can occur without warning, posing significant risks, particularly when driving or operating machinery. Patients must be warned about this risk. The likelihood appears higher with DAs compared to levodopa (Park and Stacy, 2011).
- **Psychosis and Hallucinations:** The risk of developing hallucinations (typically visual) and delusions is generally higher with DAs than with levodopa. Management involves reducing antiparkinsonian medications (starting with anticholinergics, amantadine, then DAs before levodopa) and potentially using atypical antipsychotics like quetiapine or clozapine.
- **Dopamine Agonist Withdrawal Syndrome (DAWS):** Abrupt discontinuation or rapid tapering of DAs can trigger a severe withdrawal syndrome characterized by anxiety, panic attacks, depression, apathy, fatigue, pain, orthostatic hypotension, and drug craving. Therefore, gradual tapering over weeks to months is essential when stopping DA therapy (*Dopaminergic agonists in Parkinson's disease*, no date).

The clinical use of DAs exemplifies a critical therapeutic dilemma in PD management. While they offer a valuable strategy to delay or mitigate levodopa-induced motor complications, particularly beneficial for younger patients, this advantage must be weighed against the substantially increased risk of neuropsychiatric adverse effects, especially ICDs and somnolence (Hitzeman and Rafii, 2009). The direct stimulation of D2/D3 receptors, while potentially providing smoother dopaminergic tone compared to pulsatile levodopa, appears to preferentially impact non-motor circuits involved in reward, behavior, and wakefulness (Borovac, 2016). This highlights an "unseen" cost associated with this class of drugs, demanding vigilant patient monitoring, education, and a willingness to adjust therapy if problematic behaviors emerge. The decision to initiate DA therapy requires a careful discussion of these risks and benefits, tailored to the individual patient's profile and priorities.

Furthermore, the development of ER oral formulations and transdermal delivery systems reflects the persistent drive toward achieving more continuous dopaminergic stimulation, a principle shared with advanced levodopa strategies. By providing more stable plasma concentrations, these formulations aim to optimize efficacy in managing fluctuations and potentially improve tolerability compared to IR DAs(*Dopaminergic agonists in Parkinson's disease*, no date). While not eliminating the inherent risks of the drug class (e.g., ICDs), these advanced DA formulations offer alternative approaches within the CDS paradigm, expanding the therapeutic armamentarium for managing PD throughout its course.

8.4 Modulating levodopa metabolism: MAO-B and COMT inhibitors

Beyond direct dopamine replacement or receptor stimulation, two major classes of drugs enhance dopaminergic neurotransmission indirectly by inhibiting key enzymes responsible for dopamine or levodopa metabolism: Monoamine Oxidase type B (MAO-B) inhibitors and Catechol-O-Methyltransferase (COMT) inhibitors. These agents are primarily used as adjuncts to levodopa, particularly in patients experiencing motor fluctuations.

8.4.1 MAO-B inhibitors (Selegiline, rasagiline, safinamide)

- **Mechanism of Action:** MAO-B is one of the two main isoenzymes of monoamine oxidase and is predominantly found in the brain, where it plays a significant role in the oxidative deamination of dopamine. MAO-B inhibitors selectively block the activity of this enzyme, thereby reducing the breakdown of dopamine in the synaptic cleft and prolonging the action of both endogenously produced dopamine (in early PD) and dopamine derived from exogenous levodopa. Selegiline and rasagiline are irreversible inhibitors, forming a covalent bond with the enzyme, while safinamide is a reversible inhibitor. A key advantage of selective MAO-B inhibitors, when used at recommended therapeutic doses, is that they largely spare the MAO-A isoenzyme, which is primarily responsible for metabolizing dietary amines like tyramine in the gut and liver. This selectivity avoids the significant risk of hypertensive crisis ("cheese effect") associated with older, non-selective MAO inhibitors when patients consume tyramine-rich foods (Riederer and Laux, 2011). Safinamide possesses additional non-dopaminergic mechanisms, notably the inhibition of voltage-gated sodium channels and modulation of stimulated glutamate release, which may contribute to its clinical effects, including potential benefits beyond motor control (Pandey and Srivanitchapoom, 2013). Rasagiline is metabolized to aminoindan, which is non-amphétaminique and may contribute to its favorable side effect profile compared to selegiline, whose metabolites include L-amphetamine and L-methamphetamine (Riederer and Laux, 2011).
- **Clinical Efficacy:**
- *Motor Symptoms*: MAO-B inhibitors provide mild symptomatic improvement when used as monotherapy in early PD. Rasagiline has demonstrated Level A evidence for efficacy as monotherapy, while selegiline has Level B evidence (Saba et al., 2022). Their primary role,

however, is as adjunct therapy to levodopa in patients experiencing motor fluctuations (Recommendations | Parkinson's disease in adults | Guidance | NICE, 2017). Selegiline, rasagiline, and safinamide have all shown Level A evidence for reducing total daily "off" time and improving motor function in fluctuating patients (Saba et al., 2022).

- *Non-Motor Symptoms (NMS)*: The impact of MAO-BIs on NMS is an area of active investigation, but current evidence is often mixed or derived from secondary analyses. Some studies suggest potential benefits for depression, with positive signals reported for selegiline, rasagiline, and safinamide in certain patient subgroups or trial settings. Evidence for sleep disturbances is inconsistent; rasagiline might improve sleep maintenance, and safinamide showed potential benefit for REM sleep behavior disorder (RBD) in one open-label study, while selegiline's stimulant metabolites can cause insomnia. MAO-BIs, particularly rasagiline and safinamide, may improve pain, especially fluctuation-related pain in more advanced PD (Tsuboi et al., 2022). There is emerging evidence suggesting potential benefits for fatigue, possibly linked to selegiline's metabolites, rasagiline's effect on motor/non-motor symptoms, or safinamide's dual mechanism (Galli et al., 2025). However, MAO-BIs are generally considered unlikely to improve global cognition or olfactory dysfunction (Tsuboi et al., 2022). Effects on overall quality of life (QoL) have been inconsistent across studies and often not clinically meaningful. Data regarding effects on autonomic dysfunction, apathy, and impulse control disorders (ICDs) remain limited and inconclusive (Tsuboi et al., 2022).
- **Safety Profile:** MAO-BIs are generally well-tolerated. Common side effects can include nausea, dizziness, dry mouth, and orthostatic hypotension. Insomnia is more frequently reported with selegiline due to its amphetamine metabolites (Riederer and Laux, 2011). When added to levodopa, MAO-BIs can potentiate dopaminergic effects, potentially leading to or worsening dyskinesias, confusion, or hallucinations, which may necessitate a reduction in levodopa dosage (Muranova and Shanina, 2023). While the risk of hypertensive crisis with tyramine is minimal at selective MAO-B inhibiting doses, caution is still advised with very high tyramine intake. There is a theoretical risk of serotonin syndrome when MAO-BIs are combined with certain serotonergic medications (e.g., SSRIs, SNRIs, tricyclics, meperidine), although the clinical risk appears lower than with non-selective MAOIs; careful coadministration and monitoring are recommended (Riederer and Laux, 2011). Safinamide was associated with a slightly higher incidence of treatment-associated adverse events compared to placebo in meta-analyses, but was still deemed effective in improving QoL (Liu et al., 2025).

8.4.2 COMT inhibitors (Entacapone, tolcapone, opicapone)

- **Mechanism of Action:** COMT is another major enzyme involved in dopamine and levodopa metabolism. Peripherally, COMT converts levodopa to 3-O-methyldopa (3-OMD). 3-OMD serves no therapeutic purpose and competes with levodopa for transport across the intestinal wall and the BBB via the LNAA transporter. COMT inhibitors block this peripheral conversion, thereby reducing 3-OMD formation and increasing the fraction of administered levodopa that reaches the brain. This results in a prolonged plasma elimination half-life and increased (Saba et al., 2022) area under the concentration-time curve (AUC) for levodopa, leading to more sustained dopamine levels in the CNS without significantly increasing peak concentrations

(Cmax). Entacapone acts only peripherally due to its short half-life and limited BBB penetration. Tolcapone inhibits both peripheral and central COMT, potentially offering additional benefit by reducing dopamine breakdown within the brain, but its use is limited by hepatotoxicity concerns (Antonini et al., 2008). Opicapone is a newer, third-generation, peripherally selective COMT inhibitor with a longer duration of action, allowing for convenient once-daily dosing (Santos García et al., 2022).

- **Clinical Efficacy:**
- *Motor Symptoms*: COMT inhibitors are indicated solely as adjunct therapy to levodopa/AADC inhibitor combinations in PD patients experiencing end-of-dose "wearing-off" motor fluctuations. They effectively increase levodopa bioavailability, prolong its clinical effect, reduce total daily "off" time, and may allow for a reduction in the total daily levodopa dose (Antonini et al., 2008). Level A evidence supports the use of COMT inhibitors for managing motor fluctuations (Saba et al., 2022). Clinical trial data suggest tolcapone may be more potent than entacapone in reducing "off" time and improving motor scores, likely due to its dual central/peripheral action and higher potency. Opicapone (50 mg once daily) has demonstrated superiority over placebo in reducing "off" time without increasing troublesome dyskinesia in phase III trials (Santos García et al., 2022).
- *Non-Motor Symptoms (NMS)*: While primarily targeting motor fluctuations, evidence is emerging for the potential benefits of COMT inhibitors on NMS, particularly with the newer agent, opicapone. An open-label study (OPEN-PD) found that opicapone significantly improved the global NMS burden (total NMSS score) over 6 months, with notable improvements in the **sleep/fatigue**, **mood/apathy**, and **gastrointestinal** domains, accompanied by enhanced QoL (Santos García et al., 2022). Furthermore, a retrospective comparative study suggested that opicapone **stabilized NMS burden and sleep dysfunction** (PDSS scores) over 1 year, whereas patients initiated on entacapone experienced a worsening in these measures (Leta et al., 2023). This suggests the more sustained COMT inhibition provided by once-daily opicapone might translate into better control of non-motor fluctuations compared to shorter-acting entacapone. Data on tolcapone's NMS effects are limited, though its central action raises theoretical possibilities for mood or cognitive benefits (Antonini et al., 2008). Entacapone has also been suggested to improve aspects of sleep and NMS in some studies (Leta et al., 2023).
- **Safety Profile:** Since COMT inhibitors enhance levodopa's effects, many common side effects are dopaminergic in nature and result from increased central dopamine stimulation. These include the onset or worsening of **dyskinesias** (often requiring a reduction in levodopa dosage), nausea, vomiting, hallucinations, and orthostatic hypotension (Antonini et al., 2008). **Diarrhea** is a common non-dopaminergic side effect associated with COMT inhibition, sometimes severe, and reported more frequently with tolcapone (Antonini et al., 2008). Benign **urine discoloration** (brownish-orange or reddish) is expected with entacapone and opicapone due to drug metabolites (Muranova and Shanina, 2023). The most significant safety concern relates to **tolcapone**, which carries a black box warning due to the risk of potentially fatal **hepatotoxicity** (liver failure). Strict monitoring of liver function tests (transaminases) is mandatory during tolcapone treatment (Antonini et al., 2008). Entacapone and opicapone have not been associated with significant hepatotoxicity and do not require routine liver monitoring (Santos García et al., 2022).

MAO-B and COMT inhibitors represent indirect strategies to augment dopaminergic signaling, primarily by modulating the metabolism of dopamine or its precursor, levodopa. Unlike the direct supply of precursor (levodopa) or direct receptor agonism (DAs), these inhibitors work by preserving existing dopaminergic molecules. Their main clinical utility lies in extending and smoothing the effect of levodopa, making them valuable adjuncts for managing motor fluctuations (Saba et al., 2022). Their efficacy is thus dependent on the coadministration of levodopa (for COMT inhibitors) or the presence of levodopa-derived or residual endogenous dopamine (for MAO-B inhibitors). Safinamide stands out within the MAO-BI class due to its additional non-dopaminergic actions targeting glutamate release, potentially offering broader therapeutic effects (Pandey and Srivanitchapoom, 2013).

While developed primarily to address the "seen" problem of motor wearing-off, there is growing appreciation for the potential impact of these inhibitors on the "unseen" NMS. Stabilizing dopamine levels may indirectly alleviate non-motor fluctuations, and specific agents like safinamide (via glutamate modulation) or opicapone (potentially via more consistent COMT inhibition) show promise for improving domains like sleep, mood, fatigue, and pain (Santos García et al., 2022). However, the evidence remains inconsistent for many NMS, and clinically meaningful improvements in overall QoL are not always observed (Tsuboi et al., 2022). This underscores the need for further research specifically targeting NMS outcomes with these agents. The contrasting 1-year NMS outcomes between opicapone and entacapone suggest that the *duration* and *consistency* of COMT inhibition might be important factors influencing benefits beyond motor control, favoring longer-acting agents (Leta et al., 2023).

8.5 Seeing the unseen: Dopaminergic therapy and non-motor symptoms

8.5.1 The burden of non-motor symptoms (NMS)

While Parkinson's disease is defined by its motor features, it is increasingly recognized as a complex, multi-system disorder characterized by a wide array of non-motor symptoms (NMS) (Lee and Koh, 2015). These NMS are highly prevalent throughout the disease course, often appearing years before the onset of motor signs (prodromal NMS), and significantly contribute to disability and reduced quality of life, frequently exceeding the impact of the motor symptoms themselves (Schaeffer and Berg, 2017).

The spectrum of NMS is broad and encompasses multiple domains (Schaeffer and Berg, 2017):

- **Neuropsychiatric:** Depression, anxiety, apathy, psychosis (hallucinations, delusions), impulse control disorders (ICDs), cognitive impairment (ranging from mild deficits to dementia).
- **Sleep Dysfunction:** Insomnia (difficulty initiating or maintaining sleep), excessive daytime sleepiness (EDS), restless legs syndrome (RLS), REM sleep behavior disorder (RBD - acting out dreams), sleep fragmentation, nocturnal akinesia.
- **Autonomic Dysfunction:** Orthostatic hypotension (OH), constipation, urinary urgency/frequency/nocturia, erectile dysfunction, excessive sweating (hyperhidrosis) or reduced sweating (anhidrosis), dysphagia, sialorrhea (drooling).
- **Sensory Symptoms:** Pain (musculoskeletal, dystonic, central/neuropathic, radicular), olfactory dysfunction (hyposmia/anosmia), visual disturbances (blurred vision, diplopia, dry eyes), paresthesias (numbness, tingling).

- **Fatigue:** Overwhelming sense of tiredness not solely related to exertion or sleepiness.

Several NMS, including RBD, constipation, depression, and hyposmia, are now recognized as potential prodromal markers, often preceding the classical motor diagnosis by years or even decades (Armstrong and Okun, 2020). The underlying pathophysiology of NMS is heterogeneous; some arise directly from the dopaminergic denervation affecting non-motor basal ganglia loops or other dopaminergic pathways (e.g., mesolimbic, mesocortical), while many others result from the degeneration of non-dopaminergic neuronal systems (e.g., serotonergic, noradrenergic, cholinergic, peptidergic) throughout the brainstem, cortex, and peripheral nervous system (Lee and Koh, 2015). Furthermore, some NMS can be induced or exacerbated by dopaminergic therapies themselves (Park and Stacy, 2011).

Systematic assessment of NMS is crucial for comprehensive PD care. Validated tools like the Non-Motor Symptoms Questionnaire (NMSQ) for screening and the Non-Motor Symptoms Scale (NMSS) for quantifying severity across different domains are widely used in clinical practice and research (Santos García et al., 2022). Quality of life measures, such as the Parkinson's Disease Questionnaire (PDQ-39), also capture the impact of both motor and non-motor features (Liu et al., 2025).

8.5.2 Differential effects of dopaminergic drugs on NMS

The response of NMS to standard dopaminergic therapies is highly variable and often unpredictable, reflecting the diverse underlying pathologies (Schaeffer and Berg, 2017). A specific DRT may improve one NMS while worsening another or having no effect on a third.

- **Levodopa:** Its effects on NMS are complex. Symptoms clearly linked to dopamine levels or fluctuations, such as off-period anxiety, panic attacks, fluctuation-related pain, and some sleep disorders like RLS and periodic limb movements (PLM), may improve with optimized levodopa therapy. Depression and apathy might also show some response (Lee and Koh, 2015). However, levodopa can induce or worsen nausea, orthostatic hypotension, psychosis (hallucinations), and excessive daytime sleepiness (Park and Stacy, 2011). Its impact on core cognitive deficits or olfactory loss is generally minimal (Lee and Koh, 2015). Continuous delivery via LCIG appears to offer broader NMS benefits compared to oral levodopa, particularly for sleep disturbances, fatigue, and potentially mood/anxiety, likely due to the stabilization of dopamine levels (Batzu and Qamar, 2023).
- **Dopamine Agonists (DAs):** There is growing evidence supporting the use of DAs for certain NMS, particularly **depression and anxiety**, where they may exert intrinsic beneficial effects (Schaeffer and Berg, 2017). They are also effective treatments for **RLS** (Batzu and Qamar, 2023). However, DAs are strongly associated with inducing or worsening several NMS, including **psychosis, ICDs, EDS/sleep attacks, nausea, orthostatic hypotension, and peripheral edema** (Park and Stacy, 2011). Continuous delivery via the rotigotine patch has shown benefits for nocturnal sleep disturbances and overall sleep quality, and CSAI has demonstrated improvements in sleep and global NMS scores (Batzu and Qamar, 2023).
- **MAO-B Inhibitors:** As discussed previously, evidence for NMS benefits is emerging but inconsistent (Tsuboi et al., 2022). Potential improvements in **depression, fatigue, and pain** have been reported in some studies, but effects on QoL are often not significant (Liu et al., 2025). Their

impact on sleep is variable, and they are unlikely to improve cognition or olfaction (Tsuboi et al., 2022).

- **COMT Inhibitors:** Primarily used to manage motor fluctuations, their NMS effects are less studied, though recent data for **opicapone** suggest benefits for **global NMS burden, sleep/fatigue, mood/apathy, and GI symptoms**, potentially offering better NMS stabilization than entacapone (Santos García et al., 2022). They can worsen dopaminergic side effects like dyskinesia and nausea, and cause diarrhea (Antonini et al., 2008).

8.5.3 Managing non-motor fluctuations

Just as motor symptoms can fluctuate in relation to levodopa dosing ("wearing-off"), many NMS can also exhibit cyclical patterns, worsening during "off" periods and improving during "on" periods. These **non-motor fluctuations** can involve anxiety, panic attacks, depression, pain, fatigue, cognitive slowing ("mental fog"), sweating, akathisia (inner restlessness), and urinary urgency (Antonini et al., 2008). They are common in patients with motor fluctuations and can be equally or even more disabling (Chaudhuri et al., 2013). Recognizing these fluctuations is crucial, as they often respond to adjustments aimed at providing more continuous dopaminergic stimulation (CDS) (Schaeffer and Berg, 2017). Strategies include optimizing levodopa timing and formulation (e.g., using ER capsules), adding adjunct inhibitors (MAO-BIs, COMT-Is) or DAs, or employing continuous delivery systems like LCIG, CSAI, or transdermal rotigotine (Batzu and Qamar, 2023). Studies investigating LCIG and CSAI have indeed shown improvements across various NMS domains, supporting the concept that stabilizing dopamine levels can mitigate both motor and non-motor fluctuations (Chaudhuri et al., 2013).

The complex relationship between dopaminergic therapy and NMS underscores the limitations of viewing PD solely through a dopaminergic lens (Schaeffer and Berg, 2017). While motor symptoms are the primary target of DRT, the variable, often limited, or even detrimental effects on NMS highlight the involvement of widespread non-dopaminergic pathology in PD (Lee and Koh, 2015). Many NMS require targeted treatments beyond DRT, such as antidepressants, cognitive enhancers, or specific agents for autonomic dysfunction (Armstrong and Okun, 2020). Furthermore, the fact that DRT itself can induce significant NMS like psychosis and ICDs (Park and Stacy, 2011) emphasizes the need for careful therapeutic balancing. Effectively managing PD necessitates "seeing" and addressing this NMS burden, tailoring treatment not just to motor needs but to the patient's overall symptom profile and minimizing therapy-induced NMS.

The observation that strategies providing more continuous dopaminergic stimulation (CDS) often lead to improvements in NMS, particularly sleep quality and non-motor fluctuations (Batzu and Qamar, 2023), suggests that the benefits of stabilizing dopamine levels extend beyond motor control circuits. Dopamine plays modulatory roles in brain regions governing mood, arousal, motivation, and autonomic function. It is plausible that the non-physiological peaks and troughs associated with standard oral levodopa disrupt these non-motor functions, contributing to cyclical NMS. By providing a smoother, more tonic dopaminergic signal, CDS approaches may help stabilize these systems, leading to broader symptom improvement and enhanced QoL (Chaudhuri et al., 2013). This reinforces the rationale for developing and utilizing advanced delivery systems and adjunct therapies that promote more physiological dopamine receptor stimulation.

References indicate sources supporting the assessment. CDS: Continuous Dopaminergic Stimulation; LCIG: Levodopa-Carbidopa Intestinal Gel; DAs: Dopamine Agonists; MAO-BIs: MAO-B

Inhibitors; COMT-Is: COMT Inhibitors; EDS: Excessive Daytime Sleepiness; RLS/PLM: Restless Legs Syndrome/Periodic Limb Movements; RBD: REM Sleep Behavior Disorder.

8.6 Individualizing therapy: Pharmacogenomics and patient factors

8.6.1 The need for personalized medicine

Parkinson's disease manifests with remarkable heterogeneity. Patients differ significantly in their age of onset, rate of progression, specific constellation of motor and non-motor symptoms, response to dopaminergic therapies, and propensity to develop treatment-related complications (Corvol and Poewe, 2017). Pharmacokinetic and pharmacodynamic variability for antiparkinsonian drugs is substantial, estimated at 60%–90% (Liu et al., 2023). This high degree of inter-individual variation underscores the critical need for a personalized approach to treatment, moving beyond standardized protocols to tailor therapy based on the unique characteristics and needs of each patient.

8.6.2 Pharmacogenomics: Unveiling genetic influences

Pharmacogenomics investigates how variations in an individual's genetic makeup influence their response to medications (Corvol and Poewe, 2017). In PD, research has focused on identifying genetic polymorphisms that might predict efficacy, optimal dosage, or the risk of adverse reactions to DRT, with the ultimate goal of enabling precision medicine (Liu et al., 2023). Genes encoding drug metabolizing enzymes, transporters, dopamine receptors, and other related targets have been investigated.

While numerous associations have been reported, it is crucial to note that findings are often inconsistent across studies, may be specific to certain ethnic populations, and require further replication and validation before they can be implemented in routine clinical practice (Liu et al., 2023).

Currently, there are no established, evidence-based clinical guidelines recommending pharmacogenetic testing to guide DRT decisions in PD (Corvol and Poewe, 2017). Nonetheless, the existing research provides valuable insights into the biological basis of treatment variability. Key findings include:

These genetic findings offer intriguing clues about why patients respond differently, but they represent only one facet of a complex interplay. The modest effect sizes of individual polymorphisms and the inconsistencies across studies highlight that genetics alone cannot currently dictate therapeutic choices (Corvol and Poewe, 2017). Personalized medicine in PD remains largely driven by clinical judgment integrating multiple patient factors. Pharmacogenomics holds promise for the future, likely as part of multi-factorial algorithms that combine genetic data with clinical and pharmacological information to predict treatment outcomes more accurately (Corvol and Poewe, 2017). The "unseen" genetic contribution is undoubtedly relevant but requires further deciphering before it can be routinely applied.

8.6.3 Integrating clinical factors

In current practice, treatment individualization relies heavily on considering various clinical factors:

- **Age:** As previously mentioned, age significantly influences the initial choice between levodopa and DAs. Younger patients (<60–70 years) might start with a DA to delay motor complications, accepting the higher risk of neuropsychiatric side effects, while older patients often begin with levodopa due to its superior tolerability profile regarding psychosis, somnolence, and orthostatic hypotension (Borovac, 2016).

- **Disease Stage and Severity:** Treatment intensity and complexity typically increase with disease progression. Monotherapy may suffice initially, but combination therapies become necessary to manage motor fluctuations and dyskinesia in later stages (Saba et al., 2022). Motor severity also influences the magnitude of response observed in dopaminergic challenge tests (Kou et al., 2025).
- **Symptom Profile:** The specific pattern of motor and non-motor symptoms guides treatment selection. For instance, patients with significant tremor might benefit from specific agents, while those with prominent NMS like depression, cognitive impairment, or autonomic dysfunction require targeted management, which may influence the choice or tolerability of DRT (Armstrong and Okun, 2020). The presence of risk factors for ICDs warrants caution with DAs (Recommendations | Parkinson's disease in adults | Guidance | NICE, 2017).
- **Patient Preferences and Lifestyle:** Individual tolerance for side effects, desired level of symptom control, complexity of the medication regimen, cost considerations, and personal preferences regarding formulations (e.g., tablets vs. patches vs. infusions) are all important factors in shared decision-making.

8.6.4 Role of dopaminergic challenge tests

Acute pharmacological challenge tests, typically using oral levodopa or subcutaneous apomorphine, can be employed to objectively assess dopaminergic responsiveness. A significant improvement in motor scores (e.g., UPDRS-III) following the challenge supports a diagnosis of PD, particularly in differentiating it from atypical parkinsonian syndromes (APS) which generally show a much poorer response. These tests demonstrate moderate diagnostic accuracy, with apomorphine challenges potentially offering slightly better sensitivity and specificity than levodopa challenges in distinguishing PD from APS (Kou et al., 2025).

However, these tests provide only a snapshot of the *current* dopaminergic responsiveness and have limitations. As noted, the magnitude of response varies considerably based on disease stage, baseline severity, and treatment history, with significant overlap observed between de novo PD and some early-stage APS (Kou et al., 2025). Therefore, while useful adjuncts in the diagnostic workup, challenge tests do not reliably predict the long-term course of the disease or the future development of treatment complications. They confirm the presence of a dopaminergic deficit responsive to therapy but do not fully capture the complexity of the underlying pathology or future therapeutic needs.

8.7 Future directions: Novel dopaminergic strategies

The quest to improve PD management continues, with ongoing research focused on developing novel dopaminergic strategies that offer enhanced efficacy, better tolerability, improved convenience, and potentially disease-modifying effects. Key areas of development include optimizing drug delivery, identifying novel drug targets, and exploring biological therapies like gene therapy.

8.7.1 Optimizing delivery: The quest for continuous stimulation

Recognizing that the pulsatile stimulation provided by standard oral levodopa contributes significantly to long-term motor complications (Thanvi and Lo, 2004), a major focus is on developing methods to achieve more continuous dopaminergic stimulation (CDS). The goal is to mimic the physiological tonic release of dopamine more closely, thereby reducing fluctuations and dyskinesias, and potentially improving NMS (Batzu and Qamar, 2023).

- **Subcutaneous Infusion Pumps:** These offer a less invasive alternative to LCIG for providing CDS.
- *Apomorphine (CSAI)*: Already established in clinical practice for advanced PD with refractory fluctuations (Batzu and Qamar, 2023).
- *Foslevodopa/Foscarbidopa*: These are soluble prodrugs of levodopa and carbidopa designed for continuous subcutaneous infusion. Late-stage clinical trials have shown efficacy in reducing "off" time and improving "on" time without troublesome dyskinesia, as well as potential benefits for sleep (Batzu and Qamar, 2023). This approach aims to provide levodopa-based CDS without requiring intestinal surgery.
- **Novel Oral Formulations:** Research continues into developing oral levodopa formulations with improved pharmacokinetic profiles, potentially offering longer duration of action and reduced peak-trough variability beyond current ER technologies (Livingston and Monroe-Duprey, 2024).
- **Inhaled Levodopa:** While not providing CDS, inhaled levodopa (Inbrija) represents an advance in rapid, on-demand treatment for "off" episodes, addressing an unmet need for quick symptom relief (Livingston and Monroe-Duprey, 2024).

8.7.2 Novel drug targets and pipeline agents

Efforts are underway to develop dopaminergic agents with novel mechanisms or improved therapeutic profiles:

- **Agents with Dual Actions:** Safinamide, combining MAO-B inhibition with glutamate modulation, exemplifies a move toward multi-target therapy (Pandey and Srivanitchapoom, 2013).
- **Optimized Existing Classes:** Opicapone offers a long-acting, once-daily COMT inhibitor with potential NMS benefits, improving upon older agents in the class (Ntetsika et al., 2021; Santos García et al., 2022).
- **Novel Receptor Subtype Agonists:** Tavapadon, an investigational D1/D5 partial agonist, represents a departure from traditional D2/D3-preferring DAs. By targeting different dopamine receptor subtypes, it may offer a distinct efficacy and side effect profile. Positive Phase 3 results in early PD showed significant motor improvement. Other pipeline DAs like IRL1117 (D1/D2 agonist) are also in development (Dopamine Agonist Market Size, Share & Trends Analysis Report By Drug (Non-ergot Dopamine Agonists, Ergot Alkaloids), By Route Of Administration (Oral, Injectable), By Application, By Distribution Channel, By Region, And Segment Forecasts, 2025 - 2030, 2024).
- **Disease-Modifying Therapies Targeting Core Pathology:** A significant portion of the 2024 pipeline has shifted beyond symptomatic treatment to focus on potentially disease-modifying therapies (DMTs). These agents target the underlying biological processes of PD, primarily the aggregation of alpha-synuclein (alpha-syn) and pathways implicated by genetic discoveries (McFarthing et al., 2024).
- **Alpha-Synuclein Immunotherapies:** Multiple strategies aim to clear pathological alpha-syn aggregates. Prasinezumab, a monoclonal antibody developed by Prothena and Roche, targets

aggregated alpha-syn to promote its clearance. In 2024, the Phase 2b PADOVA study reported positive results, showing that prasinezumab significantly slowed motor progression on specific measures in patients with rapidly progressing disease (McFarthing et al., 2024). Other antibody-based approaches and active vaccines remain in various stages of clinical development.

- **LRRK2 Kinase Inhibition:** Targeting mutations in the Leucine-Rich Repeat Kinase 2 (*LRRK2*) gene, a major genetic risk factor for PD, is a leading strategy for precision medicine. BIIB094 (DNL151), a LRRK2 inhibitor from Biogen and Denali, is currently in Phase 3 trials (LUMA and LIGHTHOUSE studies). The goal is to normalize LRRK2 kinase activity, which is thought to play a role in lysosomal function and neuroinflammation, thereby slowing disease progression in both *LRRK2* mutation carriers and potentially idiopathic PD patients (McFarthing et al., 2024).
- **GBA1 Pathway Modulators:** Mutations in the *GBA1* gene, which encodes the lysosomal enzyme glucocerebrosidase, are the most common genetic risk factor for PD. Strategies to enhance GBA activity are being actively pursued. Ambroxol, a repurposed mucolytic agent that acts as a GBA chaperone, has shown promise in earlier-phase studies and is being investigated in the large Phase 3 ASPro-PD trial. The aim is to improve lysosomal function and reduce alpha-syn accumulation (McFarthing et al., 2024).

8.7.3 Gene therapy: Modifying the system

Gene therapy offers a potentially transformative approach by aiming to genetically modify cells within the brain to restore function or provide long-term therapeutic benefit (Ntetsika et al., 2021). Strategies relevant to the dopaminergic system include:

- **Enhancing Dopamine Synthesis:** Using viral vectors (typically AAV or lentivirus) to deliver genes encoding key dopamine synthesis enzymes (AADC, TH, GCH1) directly into the striatum. The goal is to enable local, continuous production of dopamine from exogenous levodopa (AAV-AADC) or even from endogenous tyrosine (using the enzyme triad). Clinical trials (Phase I/II) have demonstrated feasibility, safety, and sustained motor improvements with approaches like AAV2-AADC and LV-GCH1-TH-AADC (ProSavin and its successor OXB-102) (Ntetsika et al., 2021).
- **Neuroprotection/Neurorestoration:** Delivering genes encoding neurotrophic factors (e.g., GDNF, neurturin) via viral vectors to protect surviving dopaminergic neurons or promote their recovery. Results from clinical trials have been mixed, with challenges in delivery and demonstrating clear efficacy over placebo (Ntetsika et al., 2021).
- **Genetic Neuromodulation:** Modifying the activity of specific basal ganglia circuits, for example, by delivering the gene for glutamate decarboxylase (GAD) to the subthalamic nucleus (STN) to increase local GABAergic inhibition and improve motor control. Phase I/II trials showed safety and motor benefits (Ntetsika et al., 2021).

These gene therapy approaches, particularly those aimed at restoring dopamine synthesis, align conceptually with the goal of achieving continuous, localized dopaminergic stimulation within the striatum (Ntetsika et al., 2021).

The diverse array of future strategies, encompassing advanced drug delivery technologies, novel pharmacological targets, and biological therapies like gene therapy, reflects a clear convergence on the principle of providing more stable, continuous, and potentially more physiological dopaminergic stimulation (Ntetsika et al., 2021). Decades of clinical experience have underscored the limitations and detrimental long-term consequences of pulsatile dopaminergic stimulation inherent in standard oral levodopa therapy (Thanvi and Lo, 2004). Whether through sophisticated pumps delivering levodopa prodrugs subcutaneously (Batzu and Qamar, 2023), next-generation oral formulations (Livingston and Monroe-Duprey, 2024), or gene therapies enabling endogenous dopamine production within the target brain region (Ntetsika et al., 2021), the overarching goal is to smooth out dopamine levels, thereby mitigating motor complications and potentially improving non-motor fluctuations.

Furthermore, the development pipeline indicates a move beyond simple dopamine replacement toward more nuanced approaches (Dopamine Agonist Market Size, Share & Trends Analysis Report By Drug (Non-ergot Dopamine Agonists, Ergot Alkaloids), By Route Of Administration (Oral, Injectable), By Application, By Distribution Channel, By Region, And Segment Forecasts, 2025 - 2030, 2024). Targeting specific dopamine receptor subtypes (Dopamine Agonist Market Size, Share & Trends Analysis Report By Drug (Non-ergot Dopamine Agonists, Ergot Alkaloids), By Route Of Administration (Oral, Injectable), By Application, By Distribution Channel, By Region, And Segment Forecasts, 2025 - 2030, 2024), combining dopaminergic actions with modulation of other neurotransmitter systems (Galli et al., 2025), and utilizing gene therapy to precisely modify cellular function within specific circuits (Ntetsika et al., 2021) all represent efforts to address the multifaceted pathophysiology of PD more effectively. These strategies aim to tackle the "unseen" complexities of the disease and its treatment, offering hope for improved long-term outcomes.

8.8 Conclusion: Optimizing dopaminergic therapy in PD

8.8.1 Synthesizing key principles

Dopaminergic replacement therapy remains the symptomatic bedrock for managing Parkinson's disease. Levodopa, particularly when combined with a peripheral AADC inhibitor, provides unparalleled efficacy in alleviating motor symptoms, establishing it as the gold standard against which other therapies are measured. However, its long-term use is invariably complicated by motor fluctuations and dyskinesias, driven largely by its unfavorable pharmacokinetic profile and the progressive nature of the underlying neurodegeneration. Adjunct therapies, including dopamine agonists, MAO-B inhibitors, and COMT inhibitors, play crucial roles in optimizing levodopa therapy, managing these complications, and providing alternative strategies, especially in early disease. Critically, effective management extends beyond the visible motor symptoms ("the seen") to encompass the broad spectrum of non-motor symptoms ("the unseen"), which profoundly impact patient quality of life and require careful consideration during treatment selection and adjustment.

8.8.2 Balancing efficacy and complications

Optimizing dopaminergic therapy involves navigating inherent trade-offs. Levodopa offers maximal motor benefit but carries the highest risk of long-term motor complications. Dopamine agonists can help avoid motor problems for a while, but they can also cause serious mental health issues like trouble controlling impulses, feeling very sleepy, and experiencing hallucinations. MAO-B and COMT inhibitors help smooth levodopa's effects but provide only modest direct symptomatic benefit and can potentiate dopaminergic side effects. Strategies aimed at providing more continuous dopaminergic stimulation – through advanced formulations, delivery systems, or adjunct combinations – represent a key paradigm for mitigating fluctuations and potentially improving both motor and non-motor outcomes, though they come with their own challenges related to invasiveness, side effects, or complexity.

8.8.3 The imperative of a personalized, patient-centered approach (Precision medicine)

Given the profound clinical and biological heterogeneity of Parkinson's Disease (PD), a "one-size-fits-all" approach is inadequate. This reality underscores the imperative for a precision medicine framework, which aims to tailor treatment to the individual's unique characteristics. Optimal dopaminergic therapy necessitates meticulous individualization that integrates not only traditional clinical factors but also emerging biological data. Treatment decisions must incorporate patient age, disease phenotype (e.g., tremor-dominant vs. akinetic-rigid), the specific profile of motor and non-motor symptoms (NMS), and cognitive status.

Furthermore, insights from biomarkers are becoming increasingly crucial for subtyping the disease and predicting its course. For instance, genetic screening for pathogenic variants in genes like *Glucocerebrosidase* (*GBA*) can identify patients at risk for a more rapid disease course and associated cognitive decline, which may influence long-term treatment strategies and eligibility for targeted clinical trials. Similarly, the field of pharmacogenomics holds significant promise for refining predictions of therapeutic response and adverse events. Variants in the *Catechol-O-methyltransferase* (*COMT*) gene, for example, can influence the efficacy and side effect profile of levodopa, helping to guide the selection of COMT inhibitors.

Beyond genetics, molecular imaging (e.g., Dopamine Transporter Scan) and fluid biomarkers, such as cerebrospinal fluid alpha-synuclein seed amplification assays (α-syn SAAs), are providing objective measures of underlying pathophysiology that can aid in diagnosis and stratification. While many of these tools are still transitioning into routine clinical practice, their growing use highlights the shift toward a more biologically-informed approach.

Truly "seeing the unseen" in PD management means leveraging these advancing tools to uncover the hidden biological drivers of the disease, alongside the subtle onset of treatment complications and the unique personal context of each individual. By integrating these precision medicine principles with careful clinical monitoring, assessment of lifestyle factors, and—crucially—the patient's own preferences and treatment goals, clinicians can create a truly comprehensive and patient-centered strategy. Only through such an approach can we hope to maximize the benefits of dopaminergic therapy while minimizing its risks, ultimately improving long-term function and quality of life for those living with Parkinson's disease.

References

Antonini, A., Abbruzzese, G., Barone, P., Bonuccelli, U., Lopiano, L., Onofrj, M., Zappia, M., & Quattrone, A. (2008). COMT inhibition with tolcapone in the treatment algorithm of patients with Parkinson's disease (PD): Relevance for motor and non-motor features. *Neuropsychiatric Disease and Treatment, 4*(1), 1–9.

Armstrong, M. J., & Okun, M. S. (2020). Diagnosis and treatment of Parkinson disease: A review. *JAMA, 323*(6), 548–560. https://doi.org/10.1001/jama.2019.22360

Batzu, L., & Qamar, M. A. (2023). *Where are we? Continuous dopaminergic stimulation for Parkinson's disease continuous dopaminergic stimulation and nonmotor symptoms of Parkinson's.*

Borovac, J. A. (2016). Side effects of a dopamine agonist therapy for Parkinson's disease: A mini-review of clinical pharmacology. *Yale Journal of Biology & Medicine, 89*(1), 37–47.

Brodsky, M. A., Park, B. S., & Nutt, J. G. (2010). Effects of a dopamine agonist on the pharmacodynamics of levodopa in Parkinson disease. *Archives of Neurology, 67*(1), 27–32. https://doi.org/10.1001/archneurol.2009.287

Carbone, F., & Djamshidian, A. (2024). Impulse control disorders in Parkinson's disease: An overview of risk factors, pathogenesis and pharmacological management. *CNS Drugs, 38*(6), 443–457. https://doi.org/10.1007/s40263-024-01087-y

Chaudhuri, K. R., Rizos, A., & Sethi, K. D. (2013). Motor and nonmotor complications in Parkinson's disease: An argument for continuous drug delivery? *Journal of Neural Transmission, 120*(9), 1305–1320. https://doi.org/10.1007/s00702-013-0981-5

Contin, M., & Martinelli, P. (2010). Pharmacokinetics of levodopa. *Journal of Neurology, 257*(Suppl. 2). https://doi.org/10.1007/s00415-010-5728-8

Corvol, J.-C., & Poewe, W. (2017). Pharmacogenetics of Parkinson's disease in clinical practice. *Movement Disorders Clinical Practice, 4*(2), 173–180. https://doi.org/10.1002/mdc3.12444

Cramb, K. M. L., Beccano-Kelly, D., Cragg, S. J., & Wade-Martins, R. (2023). Impaired dopamine release in Parkinson's disease. *Brain: A Journal of Neurology, 146*(8), 3117–3132. https://doi.org/10.1093/brain/awad064

Dopamine Agonist Market Size, Share and trends analysis report by drug (Non-ergot dopamine agonists, ergot alkaloids), 2025 *By route of administration (oral, injectable), by application, by distribution channel, by region, and segment forecasts, 2025 - 2030* https://www.grandviewresearch.com/industry-analysis/dopamine-agonist-market-report.

Galli, S., Pacilio, P., Bianchini, E., Alborghetti, M., De Carolis, L., Lombardo, P., Garramone, F., Salvetti, M., & Rinaldi, D. (2025). The role of MAO-B inhibitors in fatigue in Parkinson's disease: A narrative review. *Journal of Clinical Medicine, 14*(8), 2598. https://doi.org/10.3390/jcm14082598, 2077-0383.

Hitzeman, N., & Rafii, F. (2009). Dopamine agonists for early Parkinson disease. *American Family Physician, 80* (1), 28–30.

Jimenez-Shahed, J. (2016). A review of current and novel levodopa formulations for the treatment of Parkinson's disease. *Therapeutic Delivery,* 2041-5990. *7*(3), 179–191. https://doi.org/10.4155/tde.15.96

Kou, W., Cai, H., Cui, Y., Zhu, J., Li, S., Yang, C., Chen, H., & Feng, T. (2025). Dopaminergic responsiveness and dopaminergic challenge tests of Parkinson's disease: A systematic review and meta-analysis. *Journal of Neurology, 272*(2). https://doi.org/10.1007/s00415-025-12894-8

Lee, H. M., & Koh, S.-B. (2015). Many faces of parkinson's disease: Non-motor symptoms of Parkinson's disease. *Journal of Movement Disorders, 8*(2), 92–97. https://doi.org/10.14802/jmd.15003

Leta, V., van Wamelen, D. J., Aureli, F., Metta, V., Trivedi, D., Cortelli, P., Rodriguez-Blazquez, C., Rizos, A., & Chaudhuri, K. R. (2023). The real-life effect of catechol-O-methyltransferase inhibition on non-motor symptoms in levodopa-treated Parkinson's disease: Opicapone versus entacapone. *Journal of Neural Transmission, 130*(7), 925–930. https://doi.org/10.1007/s00702-023-02603-y

Liu, J.-S., Chen, Y., Shi, D.-D., Zhang, B.-R., & Pu, J.-L. (2023). Pharmacogenomics-a new frontier for individualized treatment of Parkinson's disease. *Current Neuropharmacology, 21*(3), 536–546. https://doi.org/10.2174/1570159X21666221229154830

Liu, X., Su, J., Zhang, J., Li, Z., Huang, K., Lin, D., & Tao, E. (2025). Effects of MAO-B inhibitors in life quality of Parkinson's disease patients: A systematic review and meta-analysis. *Behavioural Brain Research, 480.*

Livingston, C., & Monroe-Duprey, L. (2024). A review of levodopa formulations for the treatment of Parkinson's disease available in the United States. *Journal of Pharmacy Practice, 37*(2), 485–494. https://doi.org/10.1177/08971900221151194

McFarthing, K., Buff, S., Rafaloff, G., Pitzer, K., Fiske, B., Navangul, A., Beissert, K., Pilcicka, A., Fuest, R., Wyse, R. K., & Stott, S. R. (2024). Parkinson's disease drug therapies in the clinical trial pipeline: 2024 update. *Journal of Parkinson's Disease, 14*(5), 899–912. https://doi.org/10.3233/JPD-240272

Muranova, A., & Shanina, E. (2023). *Levodopa, Carbidopa, Treasure Island (FL)*. StatPearls Publishing.

Ntetsika, T., Papathoma, P.-E., & Markaki, I. (2021). Novel targeted therapies for Parkinson's disease. *Molecular Medicine, 27*(1). https://doi.org/10.1186/s10020-021-00279-2

Pandey, S., & Srivanitchapoom, P. (2013). Levodopa-induced dyskinesia: Clinical features, pathophysiology, and medical management. *Annals of Indian Academy of Neurology, 20*(3), 190–198. https://doi.org/10.4103/aian.AIAN_239_17

Park, A., & Stacy, M. (2011). Dopamine-induced nonmotor symptoms of Parkinson's disease. *Parkinson's Disease, 2011*. https://doi.org/10.4061/2011/485063

Recommendations. (2017). *Parkinson's disease in adults | guidance | NICE*, 2025 5 13 https://www.nice.org.uk/guidance/ng71/chapter/recommendations.

Riederer, P., & Laux, G. (2011). MAO-Inhibitors in Parkinson's disease. *Experimental Neurobiology, 20*(1), 1–17. https://doi.org/10.5607/en.2011.20.1.1

Saba, R. A., Palma Maia, D., Eduardo Costa Cardoso, F., Borges, V., Andrade, L. A. F., Ferraz, H. B., Reis Barbosa, E., Rieder, C. R.de M., Silva, D. J.da, Chien, H. F., Capato, T., Rosso, A. L., Lima, C. F. S., Bezerra, J. M. F., Nicaretta, D., Povoas Barsottini, O. G., Godeiro-Júnior, C., Barcelos, L. B., Cury, R. G., … Colletta, M. V. Della (2022). Guidelines for parkinson's disease treatment: Consensus from the movement disorders scientific department of the Brazilian academy of neurology - Motor symptoms. *Arquivos de neuro-psiquiatria, 80*(3), 316–329. https://doi.org/10.1590/0004-282X-ANP-2021-0219

Santos García, D., Fernández Pajarín, G., Oropesa-Ruiz, J. M., Escamilla Sevilla, F., Rahim López, R. R. A., & Muñoz Enríquez, J. G. (2022). Opicapone improves global non-motor symptoms burden in Parkinson's disease: An open-label prospective study, 20763425 *Brain Sciences, 12*(3). https://doi.org/10.3390/brainsci12030383

Schaeffer, E., & Berg, D. (2017). Dopaminergic therapies for non-motor symptoms in parkinson's disease. *CNS Drugs, 31*(7), 551–570. https://doi.org/10.1007/s40263-017-0450-z

Thanvi, B. R., & Lo, T. C. N. (2004). Long term motor complications of levodopa: Clinical features, mechanisms, and management strategies. *Postgraduate Medical Journal, 80*(946), 452–458.

Tsuboi, T., Satake, Y., Hiraga, K., Yokoi, K., Hattori, M., Suzuki, M., Hara, K., Ramirez-Zamora, A., Okun, M. S., & Katsuno, M. (2022). Effects of MAO-B inhibitors on non-motor symptoms and quality of life in Parkinson's disease: A systematic review. *Npj Parkinson's Disease, 8*(1). https://doi.org/10.1038/s41531-022-00339-2, 2373-8057.

Zhou, Z. D., Yi, L. X., Wang, D. Q., Lim, T. M., & King Tan, E. (2023). Role of dopamine in the pathophysiology of Parkinson's disease. *Translational Neurodegeneration, 12*(1). https://doi.org/10.1186/s40035-023-00378-6

CHAPTER

9

Catechol-o-methyl-transferase (COMT) inhibitors: Present problems and relevance of the new ones

Yusuf Olalekan Ahmed[1], Ebele Joan Ajagun[2], Abraham Olufemi Asuku[2] and Peace Ayo Olaoluwa[3]

[1]*Department of Clinical Pharmacology and Therapeutics, Faculty of Basic Clinical Sciences, Federal University of Health Sciences Azare, Azare, Bauchi, Nigeria;* [2]*Bioresources Development Centre, National Biotechnology Research and Development Agency, Ogbomoso, Oyo, Nigeria;* [3]*Department of Physiology, Faculty of Basic Medical Sciences, University of Ilorin, Ilorin, Kwara, Nigeria*

9.1 Introduction

Parkinson's disease (PD) is the second most prevalent neurodegenerative disorder, affecting both motor functions and nonmotor functions (Asuku, Ayinla, Olajide, Oyerinde, et al., 2024; Khan et al., 2021). It majorly affects the elderly and significantly impacts their quality of life. PD affects well over six million individuals globally, accounting for 1% of the elderly (Söderbom, 2020). The cause of the disease is linked to the nigrostriatal pathway, where damage occurs in a part of the brain called the substantia nigra, leading to the buildup of insoluble α-synuclein (α-Syn) Lewis bodies. The disease's etiopathology is influenced by several factors, including age, environmental pollutants, chronic neuroinflammation, and genetics (Asuku et al., 2022; Bogers et al., 2023). The loss of dopamine is key to how PD develops, as shown by the connection between low dopamine in the substantia nigra and how long the disorder lasts. As a result, drugs that increase dopamine levels continue to be the mainstay for the treatment of PD.

PD is associated with complicated problems in the body that include oxidative stress, issues with mitochondria, problems with the endosomal-lysosomal system, stress in the endoplasmic reticulum, abnormal protein behavior, activation of the immune response, and neuroinflammation (Obeso et al., 2022). After the discovery of mutations in α-Syn (SNCA) and parkin (PRKN) genes, more than 20 gene mutations have been connected to PD risk, but mutations in *SNCA, VPS35, LRRK2, PINK1, PRKN, DJ1*, and *GBA1* have been undoubtedly connected with Mendelian forms of PD (Obeso et al., 2022; Periñán et al., 2022). Advancing age is the primary determinant of the manifestation of PD, but other "modifiers" such as environmental factors also influence the expression of the mutant genes associated with PD (Ben-Shlomo et al., 2024; Periñán et al., 2022).

This disease has diverse clinical presentation and progression; therefore hypothesis-driven subtype classification has been employed in clinical research and treatment of PD (Deng et al., 2024). The

Pharmacological Foundations of Parkinson's Disease. https://doi.org/10.1016/B978-0-443-27702-3.00017-0

classification of PD subtypes is according to criteria, such as prominent symptoms. Classic PD shows reduced movement, including shaking when at rest, slow movements, stiffness, and trouble with balance, which happen because of a lack of dopamine in the substantia nigra (Asuku, Ayinla, Olajide, Ajagun, et al., 2024). Recently, patients have been reported to have nonmotor symptoms (NMS) such as depression, decline in cognition, insomnia, urinary dysfunction, blood pressure dysregulation, and sensory symptoms (Daniels et al., 2024). However, the increase in NMS is primarily attributable to PD pharmacotherapy, which has turned PD into a chronic disease. The motor subtype is the most common in the clinical setting, in which COMT inhibitors play a major role in reducing the symptoms. Akinetic-rigid (AR) and tremor predominant (TD) are the main subtypes of classic PD (Eisinger et al., 2017). In this chapter, we will introduce the current limitations and future perspective on the use of COMT inhibitors in PD.

9.2 Overview of pharmacotherapy strategies for PD

Pharmacotherapy is the use of drugs in the management of disease conditions; in the case of PD, it provides relief from symptoms and ameliorates the quality of life of PD (DeMaagd & Philip, 2015). Restoring depleted dopamine in the midbrain remains the focus of PD treatment. But the effectiveness of this option is for the short term because its effect reduces as the disease progresses, and this has become a main limitation in the use of drugs to treat PD. Up to-date, the wearing off of these medications, especially levodopa, has been a focus of drug development for this condition (Ajagun et al., 2024). The strategy for drug treatment of PD is to maintain a balance between clinical efficacy and adverse effects because this condition is incurable; thus patients will be on the medications for the long term. The mainstay of PD drug treatment is optimal control of motor symptoms and NMS; this requires frequent dose adjustment and correct combinations or treatment options.

There is no drug to stop the progression of PD, but there are drugs that target proteins involved in the pathogenesis of the disease, particularly dopamine receptors (Cheong et al., 2019). Alternatively, PD treatment also employs drugs that enhance the activity of the dopaminergic system or inhibit the enzymatic breakdown of dopamine to boost its concentration. Because of the complex nature of PD, single-target pharmacotherapies are no longer effective. Thus multitarget strategies are now considered to treat PD, particularly as the disease continues to the advanced stages (Cheong et al., 2019). Furthermore, some of the current drugs used as single targets have been found to act in more than one pathophysiology pathway of PD (Rai et al., 2021). Notably, biperiden is a muscarinic receptor blocker that effectively alleviates motor symptoms and may also improve cognitive impairment associated with PD (Zaccara & Schmidt, 2016). Another example is a dopamine receptor blocker known as talipexole that has demonstrated neuroprotection against neuronal cell apoptosis (Ma et al., 2016).

The current drug therapies for PD are focused on increasing dopamine signaling in the central nervous system, such as the administration of levodopa, a dopamine precursor that can penetrate the blood–brain barrier (Lee et al., 2024). DOPA decarboxylase converts levodopa to dopamine in the CNS; this enzyme is found in the periphery and *substantia nigra pars compacta* (Siddiqi et al., 2016). Thus DOPA decarboxylase can convert levodopa to dopamine outside the CNS to cause side effects such as nausea, vomiting, arrhythmia, and postural hypotension (Muleiro Alvarez et al., 2024). Thus carbidopa, a DOPA decarboxylase inhibitor, is combined with levodopa to reduce these adverse effects (Masood & Jimenez-Shahed, 2023). Although this strategy does not eliminate adverse effects associated with prolonged use of levodopa, such as worsening of function at the end of the dose, dyskinesia, and the treated patients' on/off phenomenon (Cheong et al., 2019).

Inhibition of enzymes involved in dopamine metabolism can also be utilized as another strategy to treat PD. They primarily aim to extend the half-life of dopamine in the central nervous system. Catechol-o-methyltransferase (COMT) and monoamine oxidase-B (MAO-B) are the major enzymes (Fig. 9.1) responsible for the breakdown of dopamine into 3-methoxytyramine and 3,4-dihydroxyphenyacetic, respectively (Regensburger et al., 2023). Thus agents that can inhibit these enzymes are useful in PD management. Selective MAO-B inhibitors (MAO-Is), such as selegiline, rasagiline, and safinamide, prevent the catabolism of dopamine by MAO-B and are currently used either as monotherapy or in conjunction with levodopa to reduce the motor symptoms of PD (Tan et al., 2022). The focus of this chapter is COMT inhibitors; thus other pharmacotherapy options will not be considered. However, it is generally agreed that an optimized PD drug treatment that involves multitarget strategies should be supplemented by other forms of treatment, such as physiotherapy.

9.3 Role of COMT enzymes in PD

Tyrosine hydrolase catalyzes the rate-limiting step in catecholamine synthesis; it converts tyrosine, an amino acid, to L-DOPA that is further converted into dopamine (Fig. 9.1). COMT enzymes are coded by the *COMT* gene; its distinctive transcription led to two isoforms that have similar catalytic mechanisms but different substrate affinity and cellular localization (Moskovitz et al., 2015). Chromosome 22q11.21 is the site of the human COMT gene; two isoforms of COMT, the membrane-bound form (MB-COMT) and cytosolic soluble form (S-COMT), have been reported (Xiao et al., 2017).

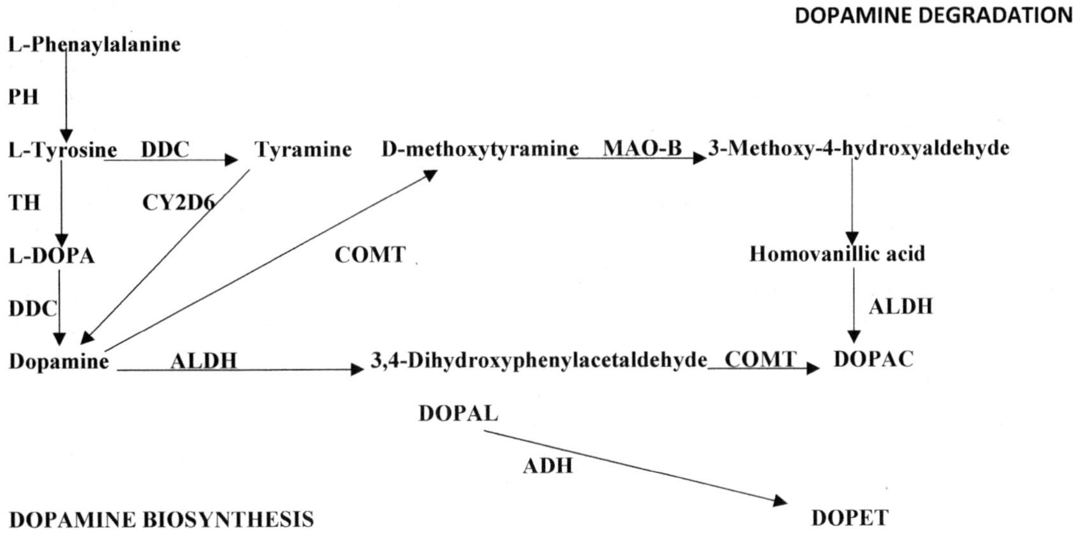

FIGURE 9.1

Highlights dopamine biosynthesis and the role of COMT in its degradation.

COMT variations linked to high, medium, and low enzyme activity may affect the risk of PD and its treatment. The *rs4680* single nucleotide polymorphisms that occur due to the substitution of A with G in the fourth exon of the COMT gene lead to the substitution of valine 158 with a methionine (Val158-Met), with consequent low COMT enzyme activity (Bonetti et al., 2020). The protein present in the L allele is thermolabile, predisposing individuals with this variant to PD and variations in therapeutic response to levodopa (Hao et al., 2014). There are other single nucleotide polymorphisms that affect PD treatment and its susceptibility; therefore COMT enzymes have both therapeutic and pathogenesis role in PD. Thus it is important to individualize patient care based on their genotypic variations and other factors.

COMT enzyme catalyzes the O-methylation reaction of catechol substrate (Fig. 9.1), this reaction requires magnesium ions as a cofactor, which results in loss of pharmacological activity of the catechol substrate (Männistö et al., 2024). The inhibition of COMT activity reduces levodopa breakdown, thus maintaining the plasma level and providing a more stable clinical response (Müller, 2010). Levodopa is the gold standard in PD pharmacotherapy, but prolonged use of this drug results in complications such as wearing off and dyskinesias (Hao et al., 2014). However, levodopa has a short half-life (1 h), leading to fluctuations in its blood concentration. This leads to the "wearing-off" phenomenon seen in the advanced stage of PD (Murakami et al., 2023). So, blocking COMT activity helps to lessen the ups and downs seen at the end of a dose in levodopa treatment (Ferreira et al., 2022). Additionally, stopping COMT activity increases the creation of more breakdown products of levodopa, such as trihydroxyphenylacetate and dihydroxyphenylpyruvate acetate. Thus the GIT pH milieu is altered to improve the gastrointestinal conditions, leading to an enhanced duodenal absorption rate of levodopa (Müller, 2015).

Dopamine is synthesized by tyrosine and phenylalanine through a major pathway involving a series of reactions catalyzed by PH, TH, and DDC. A minor pathway is also involved in the synthesis of dopamine, utilizing tyramine to synthesize dopamine, a reaction catalyzed by CYP2D6. Dopamine is inactivated through reactions catalyzed by COMT, MAO, ALDH, and ADH. *PH phenylalanine hydroxylase, TH tyrosine hydroxylase, DDC DOPA decarboxylase, COMT catechol-O-methyltransferase, MAO- monoamine oxidase-B, ALDH aldehyde dehydrogenase, ADH alcohol dehydrogenase, DOPAC 3,4-dihydroxylphenylacetic acid, DOPET 3,4-dihydroxyphenylethanol.*

9.4 COMT inhibitors

COMT inhibitors are drugs used to treat PD and extend the effectiveness of levodopa therapy by inhibiting dopamine metabolism in the periphery and brain (Lees et al., 2023). This class of drugs is classified based on their mechanism of action and chemical structure; examples include entacapone (ENT) and opicapone (OPC), recommended as first-line COMT inhibitors, and the second-line drug is tolcapone (TOL), which requires regular liver function tests to monitor the liver. It can also be classified as a first-generation and second-generation COMT inhibitor. The COMT inhibitors first produced are known as "first-generation" inhibitors; they inhibit COMT activity to extend the functional activity of catecholamines (Bindra et al., 2024). They are quercetin, caffeic acid, rutin, and 2-hydroxy estrogens. Second-generation COMT inhibitors were later discovered with a better pharmacokinetic profile than the first-generation COMT inhibitors. Examples of the second generation are nitecapone, entacapone, tolcapone, and nebicapone, while opicapone belongs to the third generation of COMT inhibitors, having an improved toxicity and inhibitory profile.

There is a compensatory pathway for the metabolism of levodopa that follows the inhibition of dopa decarboxylase. Such a pathway involved COMT, leading to an increased plasma level of 3-O-*methyldopa* (3-OMD). Higher levels of 3-OMD can make levodopa treatment less effective because this substance competes with the transporter that helps move levodopa through the intestines. However, the peripheral metabolism of levodopa is prolonged by COMT inhibitors such as ENT; thus levodopa clearance is decreased, and its bioavailability is increased (Männistö et al., 2024).

9.5 Current and future pharmacotherapies of COMT inhibitors

The main goal of COMT inhibitor therapy is to ameliorate the problems with levodopa therapy. Levodopa/carbidopa combination was designed to overcome the short half-life of levodopa; this approach improved motor activity, especially during the daytime (Murakami et al., 2023). Even though this combined drug can still be broken down in the body, adding COMT inhibitors can help extend how long levodopa/carbidopa works and increase its availability in the brain. The benefits of this triple drug combination include reducing "off" time and prolonging "on" time in patients with fluctuating motor symptoms (Greenwood et al., 2021).

ENT and TOL are two of the recently approved COMT inhibitors used as adjuncts for levodopa/carbidopa therapy to ameliorate the "wearing-off" effect and "on" time. These drugs are different in their adverse effects and pharmacokinetic profile. TOL is capable of inhibiting both the peripheral and central COMT activity; therefore it has a longer half-life than ENT, which only inhibits peripheral COMT activity. Unlike ENT, only TOL can cross the blood–brain barrier because of its lipophilicity (Regensburger et al., 2023). Both drugs cause hypotension, confusion, vomiting, and nausea, but only TOL causes fulminant hepatic failure. OPC is a third-generation COMT inhibitor that was approved by the Food and Drug Administration (FDA) in 2020 as adjunctive treatment of patients with "off" episodes (Lewitt et al., 2023). It has high COMT inhibition affinity and reduced toxicity. It does not pass through the blood–brain barrier and only inhibits peripheral COMT enzyme activity (Bicker et al., 2016). COMT inhibition and half-life by OPC are dose-dependent; the inhibition of COMT and its half-life is higher at high doses (Lewitt et al., 2023).

The current drug treatment for PD has not met the need for clinical therapy for this disease. To date, there is no available pharmacotherapeutic approach that restores or repairs the underlying pathology of PD. The current COMT inhibition clinical strategies are largely symptomatic, focusing on optimizing dopamine deficiency and associated motor activity deficit. Although there is an increased insight into the pathology of PD, its pharmacotherapy approaches remain unchanged from the symptom's alleviation strategy. The current COMT inhibitors, with the exception of TOL, are strictly peripheral; therefore the future direction for pharmacotherapy involving COMT inhibitors is to develop more effective drugs that have synergistic effects (Cruz-Vicente, Gonçalves, Barroca-Ferreira, et al., 2022; Cruz-Vicente, Gonçalves, Ferreira, et al., 2022). Thus the new advanced techniques, including computational, biomolecular, and structural techniques, and the determination of more than 100 3D COMT crystal structures provide information about interactions between protein active sites and many substrates/inhibitors (Cruz-Vicente, Gonçalves, Barroca-Ferreira, et al., 2022; Cruz-Vicente, Gonçalves, Ferreira, et al., 2022). This advancement in computational algorithms and information on COMT structures is now regarded as the future in the discovery of more effective and safe COMT inhibitors (Ferreira et al., 2015). The available in silico tools have now changed researchers' focus on plant-based COMT inhibitors, for instance, garcinol, a natural product with in vitro similar effects to TOL, was studied using in silico tools, and it was found to have identical protein interactions with TOL (Deb et al., 2019). Another future research perspective is in the development of dual MAO-B and COMT inhibitors that may enhance the pharmacokinetic profile of levodopa and attenuate the side effects connected with levodopa-only therapy (Cruz-Vicente, Gonçalves, Barroca-Ferreira, et al., 2022; Cruz-Vicente, Gonçalves, Ferreira, et al., 2022).

9.6 Conclusion

Currently available COMT inhibitors are associated with several side effects, and the complexity of PD often worsens despite treatment with COMT inhibitors and levodopa; this limits the usefulness of the standard pharmacotherapy approach against PD. However, there are significant promising reports on the development of better pharmacokinetic and pharmacodynamic profiles of COMT inhibitors. Although these new promising COMT inhibitors are plant-derived bioactive phytochemicals, there are still existing knowledge gaps in terms of their pharmacokinetics and pharmacodynamics. Thus the direction of research on COMT inhibitors pharmacotherapy is to develop compounds that can cross the blood–brain barrier, are safe and affordable, and alternative to the standard COMT inhibitors.

References

Ajagun, E. J., Asuku, A. O., Ayinla, M. T., Abdulsalam, T. A., Ajibare, A. J., Olajide, T. S., Hamza, Y. O., & Ganiyu, K. O. (2024). Pharmacotherapy of parkinson's disease and their limitations. In W. Mohamed (Ed.), *Zebrafish as a model for parkinson's disease*. Taylor and Francis. https://doi.org/10.1201/9781003402893-17. CRC.

Asuku, A. O., Adeyemo, M. B., Adeyemo, R. O., Agoro, S. A., Odugbesan, O. A., & Ayoola, S. A. (2022). Applications of stem cell therapy in neurodegenerative diseases. *European Journal of Biotechnology and Bioscience, 10* (2), 17–24.

Asuku, A. O., Ayinla, M. T., Olajide, T. S., Ajagun, E. J., Ganiyu, K. O., Hamza, Y. O., Ajibare, A. J., & Abdulsalam, T. A. (2024). Diagnosis and biomarkers of parkinson's disease. In W. Mohamed (Ed.), *Zebrafish as a model for parkinson's disease*. Taylor and Francis. https://doi.org/10.1201/9781003402893-15. CRC.

Asuku, A. O., Ayinla, M. T., Olajide, T. S., Oyerinde, T. O., Yusuf, J. A., Bayo-Olugbami, A. A., & Fajemidagba, G. A. (2024). Coffee and Parkinon's disease. In N. Moradikor, & I. Chatterjee (Eds.), *Progress in Brain Research, 289: Neuroscience of Coffee*. Elsevier. https://doi.org/10.1016/bs.pbr.2024.06.001

Ben-Shlomo, Y., Darweesh, S., Llibre-Guerra, J., Marras, C., San Luciano, M., & Tanner, C. (2024). The epidemiology of Parkinson's disease. *The Lancet, 403*(10423), 283–292. https://doi.org/10.1016/S0140-6736(23)01419-8

Bicker, J., Alves, G., Fortuna, A., Soares-Da-Silva, P., & Falcão, A. (2016). A new PAMPA model using an in-house brain lipid extract for screening the blood–brain barrier permeability of drug candidates. *International Journal of Pharmaceutics, 501*(1–2), 102–111. https://doi.org/10.1016/J.IJPHARM.2016.01.074

Bindra, S., Datta, A., Yasin, H. K. A., Thomas, R. R., Verma, S., Patel, A., Parambi, D. G. T., Mali, S. N., Rangarajan, T. M., & Mathew, B. (2024). Recent progress in synthetic and natural Catechol-O-methyltransferase inhibitors for neurological disorders. *ACS Omega*. https://doi.org/10.1021/acsomega.4c06190

Bogers, J. S., Bloem, B. R., & Den Heijer, J. M. (2023). The etiology of parkinson's disease: New perspectives from gene-environment interactions. *Journal of Parkinson's Disease, 13*(8), 1281–1288. https://doi.org/10.3233/JPD-230250

Bonetti, L., Sedghi, N. A., Bruzzone, S. E. P., Haumann, N. T., Paunio, T., Kantojärvi, K., Kliuchko, M., Vuust, P., & Brattico, E. (2020). Association between COMT gene Val^{158}Met heterozygote polymorphism and enhanced brain predicting processes. *bioRxiv*. https://doi.org/10.1101/2020.09.26.314732

Cheong, S. L., Federico, S., Spalluto, G., Klotz, K. N., & Pastorin, G. (2019). The current status of pharmacotherapy for the treatment of Parkinson's disease: Transition from single-target to multitarget therapy. *Drug Discovery Today, 24*(9), 1769–1783. https://doi.org/10.1016/j.drudis.2019.05.003

Cruz-Vicente, P., Gonçalves, A. M., Barroca-Ferreira, J., Silvestre, S. M., Romão, M. J., Queiroz, J. A., Gallardo, E., & Passarinha, L. A. (2022). Unveiling the biopathway for the design of novel COMT inhibitors. *Drug Discovery Today, 27*(10), Article 103328. https://doi.org/10.1016/J.DRUDIS.2022.07.013

Cruz-Vicente, P., Gonçalves, A. M., Ferreira, O., Queiroz, J. A., Silvestre, S., Passarinha, L. A., & Gallardo, E. (2022). Discovery of small molecules as membrane-bound Catechol-O-methyltransferase inhibitors with interest in parkinson's disease: Pharmacophore modeling, molecular docking and in vitro experimental validation studies. *Pharmaceuticals, 15*(1). https://doi.org/10.3390/ph15010051

Daniels, C., Rodríguez-Antigüedad, J., Jentschke, E., Kulisevsky, J., & Volkmann, J. (2024). Cognitive disorders in advanced Parkinson's disease: Challenges in the diagnosis of delirium. *Neurological Research and Practice, 6*(1). https://doi.org/10.1186/s42466-024-00309-4

Deb, S., Phukan, B. C., Mazumder, M. K., Dutta, A., Paul, R., Bhattacharya, P., Sandhir, R., & Borah, A. (2019). Garcinol, a multifaceted sword for the treatment of Parkinson's disease. *Neurochemistry International, 128*, 50–57. https://doi.org/10.1016/J.NEUINT.2019.04.004

DeMaagd, G., & Philip, A. (2015). Parkinson's disease and its management: Part 2: Introduction to the pharmacotherapy of Parkinson's disease, with a focus on the use of dopaminergic agents. *P and T, 40*(9), 590–600.

Deng, X., Mehta, A., Xiao, B., Ray Chaudhuri, K., Tan, E. K., & Tan, L. C. (2024). Parkinson's disease subtypes: Approaches and clinical implications. *Parkinsonism & Related Disorders, 130*(November 2024), Article 107208. https://doi.org/10.1016/j.parkreldis.2024.107208

Eisinger, R. S., Hess, C. W., Martinez-Ramirez, D., Almeida, L., Foote, K. D., Okun, M. S., & Gunduz, A. (2017). Motor subtype changes in early Parkinson's disease. *Parkinsonism & Related Disorders, 43*, 67–72. https://doi.org/10.1016/j.parkreldis.2017.07.018

Ferreira, L. G., Dos Santos, R. N., Oliva, G., & Andricopulo, A. D. (2015). Molecular docking and structure-based drug design strategies. *Molecules, 20*(7). https://doi.org/10.3390/molecules200713384

Ferreira, J. J., Poewe, W., Rascol, O., Stocchi, F., Antonini, A., Moreira, J., Pereira, A., Rocha, J. F., & Soares-da-Silva, P. (2022). Opicapone as an Add-on to levodopa in patients with parkinson's disease without motor fluctuations: Rationale and design of the phase III, double-blind, randomised, placebo-controlled EPSILON trial. *Neurology and Therapy, 11*(3), 1409–1425. https://doi.org/10.1007/s40120-022-00371-7

Greenwood, J., Pham, H., & Rey, J. (2021). Opicapone: A third generation COMT inhibitor. *Clinical Parkinsonism and Related Disorders, 4*, Article 100083. https://doi.org/10.1016/j.prdoa.2020.100083

Hao, H., Shao, M., An, J., Chen, C., Feng, X., Xie, S., Gu, Z., Chan, P., Xu, Y., Feng, T., Liang, Z., Bao, H., Liu, Y., Guan, X., Ye, Q., Chen, H., Shen, X., Chen, Q., Gu, P., … Xuan, C. (2014). Association of Catechol-O-Methyltransferase and monoamine oxidase B gene polymorphisms with motor complications in parkinson's disease in a Chinese population. *Parkinsonism & Related Disorders, 20*(10), 1041–1045. https://doi.org/10.1016/j.parkreldis.2014.06.021

Khan, S. T., Ahmed, S., Gul, S., Khan, A., & Al-Harrasi, A. (2021). Search for safer and potent natural inhibitors of Parkinson's disease. In *Neurochemistry international, 149*Pergamon, Article 105135. https://doi.org/10.1016/j.neuint.2021.105135

Lee, H., Elkamhawy, A., Rakhalskaya, P., Lu, Q., Nada, H., Quan, G., & Lee, K. (2024). Small molecules in parkinson's disease therapy: From dopamine pathways to new emerging targets. *Pharmaceuticals, 17*(12). https://doi.org/10.3390/ph17121688

Lees, A., Tolosa, E., Stocchi, F., Ferreira, J. J., Rascol, O., Antonini, A., & Poewe, W. (2023). Optimizing levodopa therapy, when and how? Perspectives on the importance of delivery and the potential for an early combination approach. *Expert Review of Neurotherapeutics, 23*(1), 15–24. https://doi.org/10.1080/14737175.2023.2176220

Lewitt, P., Liang, G. S., Olanow, C. W., Kieburtz, K. D., Jimenez, R., Olson, K., Klepitskaya, O., & Loewen, G. (2023). Opicapone pharmacokinetics and effects on Catechol- O -Methyltransferase activity and levodopa pharmacokinetics in patients with parkinson disease receiving carbidopa/levodopa. *Clinical Neuropharmacology, 46*(2), 43–50. https://doi.org/10.1097/WNF.0000000000000538

Ma, J., Wang, Z., Liu, C., Shen, H., Chen, Z., Yin, J., Zuo, G., Duan, X., Li, H., & Chen, G. (2016). Pramipexole-Induced Hypothermia Reduces Early Brain Injury via PI3K/AKT/GSK3β pathway in Subarachnoid Hemorrhage rats OPEN. https://doi.org/10.1038/srep23817.

Männistö, P. T., Keränen, T., Reinikainen, K. J., Hanttu, A., & Pollesello, P. (2024). The catechol O-Methyltransferase inhibitor entacapone in the treatment of parkinson's disease: Personal reflections on a first-in-class drug development programme 40 years on. *Neurology and Therapy, 13*(4), 1039–1054. https://doi.org/10.1007/s40120-024-00629-2

Masood, N., & Jimenez-Shahed, J. (2023). Effective management of "OFF" episodes in parkinson's disease: Emerging treatment strategies and unmet clinical needs. *Neuropsychiatric Disease and Treatment, 19*, 247–266. https://doi.org/10.2147/NDT.S273121

Moskovitz, J., Walss-Bass, C., Cruz, D. A., Thompson, P. M., Hairston, J., & Bortolato, M. (2015). The enzymatic activities of brain catechol-O-methyltransferase (COMT) and methionine sulphoxide reductase are correlated in a COMT Val/Met allele-dependent fashion. *Neuropathology and Applied Neurobiology, 41*(7), 941–951. https://doi.org/10.1111/nan.12219

Muleiro Alvarez, M., Cano-Herrera, G., Osorio Martínez, M. F., Vega Gonzales-Portillo, J., Monroy, G. R., Murguiondo Pérez, R., Torres-Ríos, J. A., van Tienhoven, X. A., Garibaldi Bernot, E. M., Esparza Salazar, F., & Ibarra, A. (2024). A comprehensive approach to parkinson's disease: Addressing its molecular, clinical, and therapeutic aspects. *International Journal of Molecular Sciences, 25*(13). https://doi.org/10.3390/ijms25137183

Müller, T. (2010). The impact of COMT-Inhibition on gastrointestinal levodopa absorption in patients with parkinson's disease. *Clinical Medicine Insights: Therapeutics, 2*. https://doi.org/10.4137/cmt.s1169. CMT.S1169.

Müller, T. (2015). Catechol-O-methyltransferase inhibitors in Parkinson's disease. *Drugs, 75*(2), 157–174. https://doi.org/10.1007/s40265-014-0343-0

Murakami, H., Shiraishi, T., Umehara, T., Omoto, S., & Iguchi, Y. (2023). Recent advances in drug therapy for parkinson's disease. *Internal Medicine, 62*(1), 33–42. https://doi.org/10.2169/internalmedicine.8940-21

Obeso, J. A., Monje, M. H. G., & Matarazzo, M. (2022). Major advances in Parkinson's disease over the past two decades and future research directions. *The Lancet Neurology, 21*(12), 1076–1079. https://doi.org/10.1016/S1474-4422(22)00448-3

Periñán, M. T., Brolin, K., Bandres-Ciga, S., Blauwendraat, C., Klein, C., Gan-Or, Z., Singleton, A., Gomez-Garre, P., Swanberg, M., Mir, P., & Noyce, A. (2022). Effect modification between genes and environment and parkinson's disease risk. *Annals of Neurology, 92*(5), 715–724. https://doi.org/10.1002/ana.26467

Rai, S. N., Singh, P., Varshney, R., Chaturvedi, V. K., Vamanu, E., Singh, M. P., & Singh, B. K. (2021). Promising drug targets and associated therapeutic interventions in Parkinson's disease. *Neural Regeneration Research, 16*(9), 1730–1739. https://doi.org/10.4103/1673-5374.306066

Regensburger, M., Ip, C. W., Kohl, Z., Schrader, C., Urban, P. P., Kassubek, J., & Jost, W. H. (2023). Clinical benefit of MAO-B and COMT inhibition in Parkinson's disease: Practical considerations. *Journal of Neural Transmission, 130*(6), 847–861. https://doi.org/10.1007/s00702-023-02623-8

Siddiqi, S. H., Abraham, N. K., Geiger, C. L., Karimi, M., Perlmutter, J. S., & Black, K. J. (2016). The human experience with intravenous levodopa. *Frontiers in Pharmacology, 6*(JAN). https://doi.org/10.3389/fphar.2015.00307

Söderbom, G. (2020). Status and future directions of clinical trials in Parkinson's disease. *International Review of Neurobiology, 154*, 153–188. https://doi.org/10.1016/bs.irn.2020.02.009

Tan, Y. Y., Jenner, P., & Chen, S. Di (2022). Monoamine Oxidase-B inhibitors for the treatment of parkinson's disease: Past, present, and future. *Journal of Parkinson's Disease, 12*(2), 477–493. https://doi.org/10.3233/JPD-212976

Xiao, Q., Qian, Y., Liu, J., Xu, S., & Yang, X. (2017). Roles of functional catechol-O-methyltransferase genotypes in Chinese patients with Parkinson's disease. *Translational Neurodegeneration, 6*(1), 1–11. https://doi.org/10.1186/s40035-017-0081-9

Zaccara, G., & Schmidt, D. (2016). Do traditional anti-seizure drugs have a future? A review of potential anti-seizure drugs in clinical development. *Pharmacological Research, 104*, 38–48. https://doi.org/10.1016/j.phrs.2015.12.011

Further reading

Ramesh, S., & Arachchige, A. S. P. M. (2023). Depletion of dopamine in Parkinson's disease and relevant therapeutic options: A review of the literature. *AIMS Neuroscience, 10*(3), 200–231. https://doi.org/10.3934/NEUROSCIENCE.2023017

Zhou, Z. D., Yi, L. X., Wang, D. Q., Lim, T. M., & Tan, E. K. (2023). Role of dopamine in the pathophysiology of Parkinson's disease. *Translational Neurodegeneration, 12*(1), 1–15. https://doi.org/10.1186/s40035-023-00378-6

CHAPTER

Non-dopaminergic therapies for Parkinson's disease

10

Abraham Olufemi Asuku[1], Peace Ayo Olaoluwa[2], Ebele Joan Ajagun[1] and Yusuf Olalekan Ahmed[3]

[1]*Bioresources Development Centre, National Biotechnology Research and Development Agency, Ogbomoso, Oyo, Nigeria;* [2]*Department of Physiology, Faculty of Basic Medical Sciences, University of Ilorin, Ilorin, Kwara, Nigeria;* [3]*Department of Clinical Pharmacology and Therapeutics, Faculty of Basic Clinical Sciences, Federal University of Health Sciences Azare, Azare, Bauchi, Nigeria*

10.1 Introduction

Parkinson's disease (PD) is a neurological disorder that results in progressive mobility problems. Stiffness, tremor, motor and balance problems are some of the symptoms that result from the weakening, loss, and death of nerve cells (neurons) in certain parts of the brain (Ajagun et al., 2024; Asuku, Adeyemo, Adeyemo, Agoro, & Odugbesan, 2022). PD patients may have difficulty walking, talking, or performing other daily activities when their symptoms worsen (National Institute of Neurological Disorders and Stroke, 2024).

PD involves many areas of the brain; however, the most common symptoms are brought on by the death of neurons in the substantia nigra (SN), which is a region toward the bottom of the brain (Asuku, Adeyemo, Adeyemo, Agoro, Odugbesan, et al., 2022). The neurons in this region produce dopamine. Dopamine is a chemical messenger that sends impulses that result in voluntary and smooth motion. When the symptoms begin to appear, the majority of PD patients have lost at least 60 to 80% of their dopamine-producing neurons in the substantia nigra (National Institute of Neurological Disorders and Stroke, 2024).

Norepinephrine, a neurotransmitter, is the main chemical messenger of the nervous system responsible for regulating many of the body natural functions, including heart rate and blood pressure. Most of the non-motor symptoms of PD, including fatigue and fluctuations in blood pressure, are due to the loss of norepinephrine (National Institute of Neurological Disorders and Stroke, 2024). Lewy bodies and alpha-synuclein, are present in the brain cells of patients with PD (Asuku, Ayinla, Olajide, Ajagun, et al., 2024). Scientists have not yet identified the origin of Lewy bodies and how they lead to the disease. Some research claims that PD patients may have a defective protein waste elimination system in their cells, causing toxic protein accumulation and cell death. Other research has revealed findings indicating that protein aggregates that form in PD patients' brain cells are involved in inducing neuronal death (National Institute of Neurological Disorders and Stroke, 2024).

New studies using animal models have uncovered more about how PD works, showing that the ND system is also affected and might cause various PD symptoms (Villalba et al., 2015). Within the basal

Pharmacological Foundations of Parkinson's Disease. https://doi.org/10.1016/B978-0-443-27702-3.00002-9

ganglia and its targets, the ND system includes different neurotransmitters and neuromodulatory systems like glutamatergic, adrenergic, adenosine, serotonergic, histaminic, opioid, and cholinergic systems (Stayte & Vissel, 2014). In the basal ganglia and its targets, the ND system is made up of various neurotransmitters and neuromodulatory systems, including glutamatergic, adrenergic, adenosine, serotonergic, histaminic, opioid, and cholinergic systems (Stayte & Vissel, 2014). Even though dopaminergic medication is currently the best treatment for both movement and non-movement symptoms, it can lead to side effects like levodopa-induced dyskinesia (LID) and changes in movement. Furthermore, dopaminergic medication may trigger or exacerbate non-motor symptoms, which is usually present in the form of non-motor fluctuations with OFF periods (an episodic increase in symptoms evoked by a shift in levodopa levels). Therefore, most therapeutic targets have been explored using other pathways, including the ND system, and many more are under development (Freitas & Fox, 2016).

10.2 The Pathophysiological mechanisms of PD

The two major pathophysiological mechanisms of PD are the death of dopaminergic neurons in the substantia nigra pars compacta and the pathological aggregation of alpha-synuclein, which causes Lewy formation (Asuku, Ayinla, Olajide, Oyerinde, et al., 2024; Pardo-Moreno et al., 2023). These neurons' death lowers the amount of dopamine present in the striatum, impacting the motor circuits of the basal ganglia. 50%–80% of the dopaminergic neurons of the substantia nigra have degenerated by the time motor symptoms appear (Vázquez-Vélez & Zoghbi, 2021).

Lewy pathology and cell death, are not limited to the substantia nigra. According to the six-stage Braak scheme, alpha-synuclein pathology begins in the olfactory bulb or even the enteric nervous system, which is outside the central nervous system (CNS), and then moves up to the brain stem (Ye et al., 2023). By the sixth stage, Lewy body disease has spread to areas of the brain involved in emotions and higher thinking, starting in the substantia nigra during the third stage. Lewy pathology in about 50% of patients is non-uniform as per the model predicted, though Braak stage forms a good foundation for PD development (Henderson et al., 2019). In fact, Lewy pathology is very sporadic and can be completely absent in certain patients with PD.

For nearly 70 years, the dopaminergic system has been a focus of research, and therapies based on this system continue to serve as symptomatic treatments aimed at improving the quality of life for individuals suffering from Parkinson's disease (PD). However, as more evidence shows that Parkinson's disease is not just a movement disorder caused by problems with the dopaminergic system, there has been growing interest in other systems in the brain, even beyond neurotransmission. In fact, the disease is such that it arises in stages, preceded by damage to other regions and neurochemical systems before the deterioration of dopaminergic neurons within the SN (Miguelez et al., 2020).

The other involved systems participate in the so-called prodromal or pre-symptomatic phases, which affect the motor and non-motor circuits. Currently, it is better recognised that non-motor symptoms are present in PD patients. Since they are usually more disabling than the motor ones and are not treated well with dopaminergic-based therapy, they significantly impair the quality of life of the patients. Research into how antiparkinsonian drugs work found that non-dopaminergic mechanisms were responsible for both their benefits and side effects (Miguelez et al., 2020).

Paredes-Rodriguez et al. (2020) reported on the status of the noradrenergic system in PD, one of the traditional non-dopaminergic systems of the disease. According to the disease-spreading hypothesis between caudal and rostral regions of the brainstem, the noradrenergic system innervated by the locus coeruleus may exhibit extensive damage in the disease, supposedly before dopaminergic neurons. Researchers explain that damage to the noradrenergic system can worsen the disease because it helps protect dopaminergic neurones and reduce inflammation. Although the noradrenergic system has a role in the mechanism of action of L-DOPA, more studies should be conducted to firmly establish this connection.

Mallet et al. (2019) carried out a study on acetylcholine, another classic non-dopaminergic neurotransmitter implicated in PD before dopamine. Their study addresses the striatal cholinergic interneurons, which have specific electrophysiological properties but difficult to understand because of their dispersed distribution. The benefits of adopting optogenetic techniques, potentially in conjunction with computational research, to examine the function of cholinergic interneurons in the physiology and pathology of motor behavior and cognition are reported by researchers based on recent work.

The serotonergic system has been perhaps the most extensively studied non-dopaminergic neurotransmitter system over the last decade because it has been shown to play a significant part in the dyskinesia caused by L-DOPA (Mallet et al., 2019).

Multiple neurotransmitter imbalances in the brain are partly caused by degenerative events that occur outside of the substantial nigra compacta (SNc). According to Chambers et al. (2020), PD causes the neurons of pedunculopontine nucleus, a complex structure that contains glutamatergic, cholinergic, and GABAergic neurons to degenerate. Because the pedunculopontine nucleus connects to other parts of the brain besides the SNc, the loss of neurones there is believed to cause non-motor symptoms such as trouble sleeping and issues with movement, especially walking. Murueta-Goyena et al. (2019) discuss changes in the GABAergic system and non-motor symptoms in PD. They reported how GABAergic mechanisms are involved in a range of pre-symptomatic disruptions, such as changes in vision, gastrointestinal irregularities, emotional and cognitive problems, and loss of smell. Additionally, they observe that sleep behavior disorder is characterized by rapid eye movements.

10.3 Types of non-dopaminergic therapies

10.3.1 Anticholinergics

Anticholinergics were the only medications used to treat PD and were strictly for Parkinsonism prior to the discovery of levodopa. The mechanisms of action of trihexyphenidyl (Artane) and biperiden (Akineton) have not been well understood, though it is predicted that anticholinergic inhibition of the muscarinic acetylcholine receptors reduces asymmetry between dopamine and acetylcholine within the striatum (Table 10.1). However, the use of anticholinergic drugs is limited because of the potential for unwanted central and peripheral antimuscarinic effects. Negative neuropsychiatric consequences are common, particularly among the elderly. Severe side effects such as confusion, hallucinations, delirium, falls, and fractures can be induced by central toxic effects. Elevated risk of dementia is one long-term negative consequence of the anticholinergic therapies (Kawabata & Masahisa Katsuno, 2022, pp. 3333–3340).

10.4 Acetylcholinesterase inhibitors

A lack of cholinergic activity in Alzheimer's disease (AD) has been linked to the development of psychosis, backed by findings from brain imaging and chemical studies. Cholinergic deficits have also been linked with the onset of psychosis in PD and Dementia with Lewy Bodies (DLB) (d'Angremont et al., 2023). Cortical processing of movement and task signals to the striatum disruption is thought to

Table 10.1 Classes, Examples and the mechanisms of actions of non-dopaminergic therapies for PD.

Classes	Examples	Mechanisms of actions
Acetylcholinesterase inhibitors	Donepezil Rivastigmine	Inhibit acetylcholinesterase thereby elevating acetylcholine levels, and enhancing cognition in Parkinson's dementia
Anticholinergics	Biperiden Trihexyphenidyl Benztropine	Block muscarinic acetylcholine receptors to cause the restoration of balance in dopamine and acetylcholine
Adenosine A2A receptor antagonists	Istradefylline	Inhibit basal ganglia A2A receptors, modulate motor activities and decrease ''off'' time
Antagonists of NMDA receptor	Amantadine	Causes inhibition of the NMDA glutamate receptors, decrease excitotoxicity and improve motor symptoms
COMT inhibitors	Tolcapone Entacapone Opicapone	Suppress and block COMT, prolong the effect of levodopa (indirect dopaminergic support)
MGluR5 antagonists	Dipraglurant	Decrease the over activity of glutamate, improve dyskinesia and motor symptoms
Adrenergic Agents (β-adrenergic receptor agonists)	Salbutamol Salmeterol Indacaterol Vilanterol	Decreases inflammation
Noradrenergic Agents	Droxidopa	Control the activity of norepinephrine to improve orthostatic hypotension symptom
MAO-B inhibitors	Rasagiline Selegiline Safinamide	Suppress and block MAO-B, elevate the expression of neurotrophic factors, suppress apoptosis, and reduce dopaminergic breakdown (indirect dopaminergic support)

underlie the significant gait impairment and risk of falls observed in preclinical Parkinsonism mice lesioned in cortical cholinergic neurons (Sarter et al., 2014). As Morris et al. (2019) noted, more likely than cognitive deficits, gait disorder in PD would be caused by dysfunction of the brainstem cholinergic neurons; pedunculopontine nucleus (PPN), and laterodorsal tegmental nucleus (LDT). Furthermore, in this two-lesioned model, the symptoms were relieved to some extent by augmenting the cholinergic effect with either donepezil or rivastigmine (Koshy Cherian et al., 2019).

One common treatment for AD and vascular dementia is the use of cholinesterase inhibitors (ChEIs). Rivastigmine by itself currently has an evidence-based therapeutic benefit in PD dementia (Sarter et al., 2014). While numerous studies have been carried out on how ChEIs affect PD patients, most have concentrated on dementia and cognitive function (Sawada et al., 2018). Cholinesterase inhibitors (ChEIs) are therefore better tolerated than antipsychotics and benzodiazepines and effective in the symptomatic treatment of psychotic symptoms of AD, PD, and DLB. Open-label studies, post hoc analysis, and a variety of case series have shown that ChEI medication greatly reduced delusions and hallucinations in AD, PD, and DLB (d'Angremont et al., 2023).

10.5 Glutamate modulators

Using a range of receptor proteins, which are mainly found on pre- and post-synaptic neurons in almost all regions of the CNS, glutamate is essential for brain function. On the basis of pharmacological strategies, ionotropic (iGluRs) and metabotropic (mGluRs) glutamate receptors were the two general classes into which they were first separated. Fast excitatory transmission in the central nervous system of humans is mediated through the multimeric ion channels known as iGluRs (Zhang et al., 2019). iGluRs convert impulses into postsynaptic neuron activity on a millisecond timescale by binding the presynaptically released glutamate. The process creates a synaptic current that is essential to brain function and regulates memory and learning. N-methyl-D-aspartate (NMDA) receptors, α-amino-3-hydroxy-5-methyl-4-isoxazolepropionic acid (AMPA) receptors, and kainate receptors are different types of ionotropic glutamate receptors (iGluRs). Long-lasting alterations in synaptic activity are facilitated by the slow glutamate responses mediated by the mGluRs, which are members of the superfamily of G-protein receptors (Zhang et al., 2019). There are eight receptor subtypes within the mGluRs family. These subtypes are divided based on their pharmacological characteristics into three categories: signal transduction pathways and sequence homology. Group I receptors, such as mGluR1 and mGluR5, are associated with polyphosphoinositide hydrolysis mediated by phospholipase C. On the other hand, in recombinant mechanisms, group II receptors, such as mGluR2 and mGluR3, have a negative relationship with adenylate cyclase. Members of Group III are mGluR4, −6, −7, and −8. They are also negatively coupled to adenylate cyclase or linked to ion channels (Zhang et al., 2019). Some loci of the basal ganglia have disrupted glutamate receptor regulation in PD's pathogenesis. LID also alters the glutamate receptors (Jourdain et al., 2015).

Three areas can be noted concerning therapy of PD by blockade of glutamate receptors: (1) reduction of motor symptoms in PD, (2) enhancement of effectiveness of dopaminergic drugs for their anti-Parkinsonian activity, and (3) nigral neuroprotection. Glutamate receptors are present in nearly every brain cell type. Subunit expression patterns and composition differ significantly across cell types and brain regions. In addition, as PD is developing, the levels of subunit and variant expression are altered. NMDA receptor antagonists are involved in reducing motor symptoms, alleviating LIDs, and inhibiting neurodegeneration that progress in preclinical PD models (Zhang et al., 2019). AMPA receptors exert several effects; their agonist can serve as a neuroprotectant, and LID can be effectively treated with their antagonists. Because mGluRs can modulate neurotransmission, pharmacological control of these receptors is much more promising for PD therapy. In numerous PD animal models, pharmacological efficacy has been demonstrated for mGluR5 blockade and stimulation of mGluR2 and mGluR4. The types of therapeutic interventions, using agonists and antagonists, are in a position to counteract motor diseases and have neuroprotective actions. However, because past treatments for PD have always failed, there are some challenges faced in clinical practice for the drugs that act on these glutamate receptors (Zhang et al., 2019).

10.6 MAO-B inhibitors

There is a protein of riboflavin known as monoamine oxidase (MAO), which is situated on the mitochondrial outer membrane. Dopamine, phenethylamine, 5-hydroxytryptamine, and norepinephrine are among the monoamine and tyramine neurotransmitters that MAO catalyzes to undergo oxidative deamination (Shih, 2018). There are two MAO isoenzymes: MAO-A and MAO-B. Found mostly in the CNS, platelets, and the GI tract, MAO-A can help the body metabolize tyramine-rich foods such that they will no longer cause hypertensive crisis brought on by tyramine buildup (also called a "cheese reaction"). Catecholaminergic neurons like norepinephrine, the locus coeruleus' neurons, and dopaminergic neurons of the SN also possess MAO-A. About 20% of overall MAO activity in the brain is performed by MAO-A, and 80% is performed by MAO-B, which is found mostly in platelets and glial cells (Carradori et al., 2018). Dopamine is one of the amine neurotransmitters regulated by both MAO-A and MAO-B. MAO-B degrades released dopamine in the synaptic cleft and is taken up by glial cells, whereas MAO-A degrades dopamine within presynaptic neurons. Age has been proven to enhance glial cell counts, and as predictable, MAO-B activity also increased in neurodegenerative disorders (Heo et al., 2020). MAO-B drugs selectively raise dopamine within synaptic clefts, block catabolism of dopamine, increase dopamine signaling, and decrease MAO-B activity in the brain (Table 10.1). By their inhibition of the synthesis of harmful metabolites like hydrogen peroxide and dihydroxy acetaldehyde, MAO-B inhibitors may possibly safeguard neurons from harm caused by MAO-B metabolism of dopamine. Independently of their MAO-B inhibition, selegiline and rasagiline are also neuroprotectants linked to their propargylamine backbone. In order to exert a neuroprotective effect, rasagiline and selegiline can potentially elevate the level of expression of different nerve growth factors, such as neurotrophic factor generated from the brain or glial cells, among others (Alborghetti & Nicoletti, 2019). Rasagiline may suppress apoptosis by triggering anti-apoptotic proteins like Bcl-2 and Bcl-xL, either directly or indirectly, and suppressing the way pro-apoptotic factors like Bax, are expressed (Badinter et al., 2015). Rasagiline may be more neuroprotective than selegiline as a result of a distinctive metabolic pathway. For instance, in PC12 cell lines, selegiline and rasagiline may both suppress the oxygen-glucose deprivation-induced cell mortality. But instead of aminoindan, the primary metabolite of rasagiline, L-methamphetamine, a selegiline metabolite, enhanced the cell death induced by oxygen-glucose deprivation by 70%. Additionally, rasagiline stabilized regional cerebral blood flow perfusion in PD patients, as shown by brain SPECT scans, suggesting a neuroprotective effect (Im et al., 2019). Safinamide reduces excitotoxicity to dopaminergic neurons, modifies glutamate release, and blocks sodium and calcium channels differently from selegiline and rasagiline. Safinamide inhibits dopaminergic neurons from degenerating and microglial cells from being activated as shown by animal studies (Sadeghian et al., 2015).

10.7 COMT inhibitors

Entacapone, tolcapone, and opicapone are the catechol O-methyl transferase (COMT) inhibitors (Table 10.1) that were developed especially to treat wearing-off because they block levodopa from the COMT enzyme's primary peripheral pathway of metabolism. Tolcapone has been demonstrated to block central COMT; however, its therapeutic effect appears to be privately mediated through peripheral suppression of COMT and is contingent on concurrent administration of exogenous levodopa (Jenner et al., 2021). As they were introduced in the 1990s, tolcapone and entacapone were utilized primarily in more severe cases with persistent motor abnormalities. Neither has been perfect; entacapone has a plasma half-life that is short and needs to be dosed with each administration of levodopa, and tolcapone causes hepatic toxicity (Jenner et al., 2021). In comparison to the earlier COMT inhibitors, opicapone belongs to the third-generation COMT antagonists that were logically developed to optimize peripheral tissue selectivity, minimize toxicity risk, and improve COMT inhibitory action (Kiss & Soares-da-Silva, 2014).

The therapeutic goal of using a COMT inhibitor is to keep concentrations over the ON threshold because OFF symptoms are directly associated with declines in levodopa levels in plasma occurring in between dosages (Jenner et al., 2021). By not necessarily elevating levodopa dosage or frequency, a COMT inhibitor may be employed to prolong the activity of each levodopa dose and prevent the variations of oral levodopa therapy (Jenner et al., 2021).

10.8 Serotonergic agents

Tryptophan is converted into the bioactive molecule serotonin (5-hydroxytryptamine, 5-HT), which exists in the brain and in most peripheral tissues (Ohno et al., 2015). 5-HT is an inflammatory reaction chemical mediator, which causes platelet coagulation, stimulates vasoconstriction, and controls peripheral gastrointestinal system functions. Despite its very low brain concentrations (approximately 2%) compared to the peripheral concentrations, 5-HT is very important in the control of several CNS functions, including cognitive functions, sensory-motor integration, psycho-emotional expression, and endocrine and autonomic system regulation (Ohno et al., 2015). Multiple lines of data demonstrated that the serotonergic system is involved also in modulating non-motor symptoms associated with PD, like cognitive deterioration and psycho-emotional disorders, as well as extrapyramidal motor functions (Ohno et al., 2015).

Despite preclinical findings suggesting that the majority of the serotonergic medications employed, when examined, had the potential to decrease the severity of dyskinesia (Lanza & Bishop, 2018), they are not practically helpful because they can decrease L-DOPA's prokinetic implications or even produce additional unwanted adverse effects (Fidalgo et al., 2015). U.S. Food and Drug Administration (FDA)-approved antidepressant vilazodone, is a drug that has been under the spotlight for recent attention. Vilazodone possesses both 5-HT1A receptor partial agonist activity and SSRI characteristics (Cruz, 2012). Recent studies indicate that vilazodone given in addition to L-DOPA was effective in substantially reducing dyskinesia ratings without compromising the prokinetic effects of L-DOPA. Vilazodone's 5-HT1A partial agonist property evoked at least some of these anti-dyskinetic effects (Meadows et al., 2018).

10.9 Adrenergic therapies

Several cell types have adrenergic receptors (AR), seven-transmembrane receptors that act as adrenoreceptors for catecholamines like norepinephrine (NE) and epinephrine. Neurons, immunological cells, and astrocytes are a few of the cells in the CNS that have AR. There are numerous organs within the human body that contain adrenergic receptors, which control various physiological processes (Sharma & M. Flood, 2019). Treatment with long-acting agonists to the β2-AR is among the most effective and successful therapies for dopaminergic neurological toxicity caused by inflammation. Human β2-AR is found to be ubiquitously distributed on numerous cells, including brain cells, epithelial cells, immune cells such as eosinophils, mast cells, macrophages, and adaptive immune cells, as well as endothelial cells, and even the smooth muscles of the airway

(Sharma & M. Flood, 2019). Since NE is the most prevalent catecholamine in the CNS, β1-and β2-AR expression on microglial cells means that NE regulates microglia, the immune cells residing in the brain. On the other hand, epinephrine is believed to regulate mainly peripheral immune cells like T cells and macrophages, which also exhibit elevated concentrations of β1 and β-2 AR (Sharma & M. Flood, 2019).

A number of earlier studies on the etiology of PD have identified the inflammatory microglial cell as having a significant part in its pathogenesis. Targeting microglia-mediated neuroinflammation could therefore be therapeutically beneficial in the treatment of PD. The search for more potent neuroprotective drugs that act on the disease cause is now attracting a lot of attention because the traditional treatment of PD merely includes relief from its symptoms. Research on neuroinflammation is directed toward assisting the creation of a new therapeutic strategy and also facilitating the search for new drugs to cure PD. The activation of the β2-AR by drugs and natural products has been demonstrated to be a successful anti-inflammatory tactic in preventing dopaminergic neurodegeneration. Researchers have profiled and studied implications of β2-AR agonists, such as the effects of salbutamol, salmeterol, indacaterol, and vilanterol on neuroinflammation in neurotoxicity and inflammatory models of PD in vitro and in vivo (Sharma & M. Flood, 2019). The short-acting agonists were neuroprotective and may decrease inflammation in vitro at higher concentrations, whereas the long-acting agonist showed beneficial effects at low doses (10^{-9} M) in neurotoxicity and inflammatory models of PD.

10.10 GABAergic modulators

The CNS shows high levels of GABA, an inhibitory neurotransmitter (Elekhnawy & Negm, 2022). In peripheral nervous system, CNS, and non-neuronal tissues, GABA performs several roles (Al-Kuraishy et al., 2021). GABA modulates the GABA receptors, such as GABAA, GABAB, and GABAC. GABAA and GABAC are Cl^--gated channels, whereas GABAB is a G-protein metabotropic receptor. The enzyme glutamic acid decarboxylase (GAD) decarboxylates glutamate to produce GABA, which is conveyed to the presynaptic terminals and is sequestered in specific vesicles (Huang & Huang, 2024). GAD is bound to GABA neurons and is greatly expressed in inhibitory neurons of the brain. Epilepsy and schizophrenia are correlated with GAD dysregulation (Lee et al., 2019). GABA is released into the synaptic space upon depolarization of presynaptic GABergic neurons, which is followed by postsynaptic inhibition and post-GABA receptor stimulation (Huang & Huang, 2024). Furthermore, tonic inhibition may result from GABA leaking out of the synaptic cleft and triggering extra-synaptic GABA receptors (Lee et al., 2019). To avert over-activation of the cerebral cortex, the GABA system is required for the regulation of inhibitory tone on the thalamus, substantia nigra pars compacta (SNpc) and globus pallidus (GP) (Alrouji et al., 2023). Dyskinesia or bradykinesia results from neuronal hyper-excitability induced by dysregulation of the GABA pathway in PD. The progression and the exacerbation of PD symptoms, both motor and non-motor, may be attributable to the dysregulation of the GABA pathway (Al-kuraishy et al., 2022). The major causes of PD burden, according to Padilla-Godínez et al. (2021), is non-motor manifestations like sleep disorders, cognitive difficulties, olfactory deficit, gastrointestinal disease, and visual disturbances. These signs normally occur years before the appearance of motor difficulties and exacerbation. GABAergic dysfunction may be the core cause of these symptoms (Jing et al., 2022). Since GABA and dopamine are co-released within the striatum, it is revealed that injury to GABAergic neurons plays a role in the appearance of non-motor symptoms in early PD. Thus, GABAergic neurotransmission is disrupted by dopaminergic neurons death within the SNpc (Murueta-Goyena et al., 2019).

The PD symptoms, both motor and non-motor, are associated with cognitive failure (Verma et al., 2022). Notably, cortical networks underlying neuronal regulation are excitatory to GABAergic neurons expressing somatostatin (Prévot & Sibille, 2020). Cognitive impairment onset thus correlates with GABAergic neuron dysfunction. According to reports, PD patients' expression levels of GAD were lower, which in turn lowered the rate of GABA release and neuronal formation (Alharbi et al., 2024). Furthermore, cognitive and behavioral impairments result from the lowered GABA response of PD patients to dopamine agonists (Alharbi et al., 2024). The implications of these findings are that the evolution of cognitive decline in PD is linked to GABAergic dysfunction. Therefore, the increase in GABAergic activity caused by GABAA agonists might be of use in reducing cognitive impairment in PD.

Zolpidem helps PD patients having insomnia by modulating the GABAergic pathway and reducing the latency for NREM sleep (Brickley et al., 2018). Because zolpidem is short-acting and does not cause daytime sleepiness, it has also been found to be particularly useful in the management of insomnia in PD patients (Ray & Agarwal, 2020). Likewise, a clinical study revealed that the daily administration of eszopiclone, a benzodiazepine receptor agonist, enhances sleep in PD patients by augmenting GABA effects in the brain (Iwasawa et al., 2019). Therefore, the findings showed that GABAergic pathway disruption is a major cause of the occurrence of sleep problems in PD and that initiation of the GABA system controls sleep patterns and suppresses the occurrence of sleep disorders.

10.11 Challenges and future directions

In opposition to the conventional understanding of PD as a single disease condition, there has been conjecture that it may actually be a group of several disorders with a shared phenotype. It is not known whether the disease's genetic, chemical, and environmental expressions are all components of a common pathway to the disease or whether there are multiple types of diseases with differing characteristics that ultimately result in the same outcome. It may not be a one-size-fits-all treatment if the latter is the case. It also calls into question the assumption that the whole population of PD patients is inevitably the ideal test population for clinical trials and whether genetic testing and customized medications should be the final steps in the therapy test and diagnosis process. The presence of Lewy bodies and/or alpha-synuclein demonstrates that PD development involves a constellation of factors acting together or as "multiple hits." In this multiple-hit hypothesis, PD is the consequence of the combined action of a constellation of risk factors such as aging, exposure to toxins, genetic susceptibility, and potentially additional unidentified variables, coupled with mechanisms like oxidative stress, excitotoxicity, inflammation, etc (Stayte & Vissel, 2014). Further clinical trial design enhancements, particularly in the diagnosis and monitoring of PD and PD progression, will also be required to identify more effective medications for the treatment of its symptoms and/or neurodegeneration prevention. By enabling more appropriately defined patient groups to be included in clinical trials and by enabling more accurate measurement of new drugs versus accurate staging, biomarker identification associated with specific stages of disease can significantly advance treatment.

The effectiveness of any particular disease-modifying treatment in any particular patient is likely to be contingent on the cause and stage of the disease. It is, as Stayte and Vissel (2014) stated that PD is not diagnosed on a regular basis until there are approximately 80% lost DA neurons. If Braak staging (subsection beyond the midbrain dopamine system) is on average right, then loss of other areas will have commenced prior to DA loss. In a patient population with PD, each with his or her own etiology of the disease and at his or her own stage of the disease, it is therefore likely to remain challenging to achieve a clean-cut disease-modifying effect on particular outcomes within a short 6–12-month trial. Lack of proper mechanisms for early disease detection makes matters worse, probably suggesting that pharmacotherapy are administered too late to actually be useful. Ultimately, the current trial design to verify effective symptomatic as well as true disease-altering drugs is going to become a major question until issues with disease diversity and stage, as well as follow-up, is properly addressed.

10.12 Conclusion

Overall, ND drugs have recently been the focus of extensive studies with major progress. Adenosine A2A receptor antagonists have demonstrated superiority over controls in randomized controlled trials and are also promising as adjuncts for wearing off. Amantadine and other glutamate antagonists can decrease LID, but side effects continue to be an issue. The use of metabotropic glutamate receptor antagonists has been stopped because they failed to demonstrate a measurable therapeutic gain. Tolerability and effectiveness of AMPA receptor antagonists were extremely unsatisfactory. Furthermore, antiepileptic medications like levetiracetam and topiramate were not found to decrease LID in patients with PD. Buspirone and eltoprazine, commercially available serotonergic anxiolytics, have the ability to decrease LID, but further research on their mechanisms of action on PD should be carried out (Freitas & Fox, 2016). In all other clinical contexts, ND drugs used to manage non-dopaminergic symptoms were not specifically created for PD but instead were taken from therapeutically available drugs in non-PD disorders. Cholinesterase inhibitors for PDD and botulinum toxin for sialorrhea, are recent success stories. Research in the pathophysiology of PD non-motor problems has increased more recently, but there is limitation on motor symptom research, limiting the scope of developing medicines, particularly ND medications for PD. In summary, ND medications are currently being thoroughly investigated and are still regarded as promising treatments for motor and non-motor symptoms of PD.

References

Ajagun, E.J., Asuku, A.O., Ayinla, M.T., Abdulsalam, T.A., Ajibare, A.J., Olajide, T.S., Hamza, Y.O., Ganiyu, K. O., 2024. Pharmacotherapy of parkinson's disease and their limitations. In: Mohamed, W. (Ed.), Zebrafish as a model for parkinson's disease. Taylor and Francis. https://doi.org/10.1201/9781003402893-17. CRC.

Al-kuraishy, H.M., Al-Gareeb, A.I., Elekhnawy, E., Batiha, G.E.-S., 2022. Dipyridamole and adenosinergic pathway in Covid-19: A juice or holy grail. Egyptian Journal of Medical Human Genetics 23 (1). https://doi.org/10.1186/s43042-022-00354-1.

Al-Kuraishy, H.M., Hussian, N.R., Al-Naimi, M.S., Al-Gareeb, A.I., Al-Mamorri, F., Al-Buhadily, A.K., 2021. The potential role of pancreatic γ-Aminobutyric acid (GABA) in diabetes mellitus: A critical reappraisal. International Journal of Preventive Medicine 12, 19. https://doi.org/10.4103/ijpvm.IJPVM_278_19.

Alborghetti, M., Nicoletti, F., 2019. Different generations of Type-B monoamine oxidase inhibitors in parkinson's disease: From bench to bedside. Current Neuropharmacology 17 (9), 861–873. https://doi.org/10.2174/1570159x16666180830100754.

Alharbi, B., Al-kuraishy, H.M., Al-Gareeb, A.I., Engy, E., Alharbi, H., Alexiou, A., Papadakis, M., Gaber, E.-S.B., 2024. Role of GABA pathway in motor and non-motor symptoms in Parkinson's disease: A bidirectional circuit. European Journal of Medical Research 29 (1). https://doi.org/10.1186/s40001-024-01779-7.

Alrouji, M., Al-kuraishy, H.M., Al-buhadily, A.K., Al-Gareeb, A.I., Elekhnawy, E., El-Saber Batiha, G., 2023. DPP-4 inhibitors and type 2 diabetes mellitus in Parkinson's disease: A mutual relationship. Pharmacological Reports 75 (4), 923–936. https://doi.org/10.1007/s43440-023-00500-5.

Asuku, A.O., Adeyemo, M.B., Adeyemo, R.O., Agoro, S.A., Odugbesan, O.A., 2022. The physiology and neuroprotective role of melatonin in neurodegenerative diseases. International Journal of Medical Science and Research 4 (1), 54–60.

Asuku, A.O., Adeyemo, M.B., Adeyemo, R.O., Agoro, S.A., Odugbesan, O.A., Ayoola, S.A., 2022. Applications of stem cell therapy in neurodegenerative diseases. European Journal of Biotechnology and Bioscience 10 (2), 2321–9122, 17-24.

Asuku, A.O., Ayinla, M.T., Olajide, T.S., Ajagun, E.J., Ganiyu, K.O., Hamza, Y.O., Ajibare, A.J., Abdulsalam, T. A., 2024. Diagnosis and biomarkers of parkinson's disease. In: Mohamed, W. (Ed.), Zebrafish as a model for parkinson's disease. Taylor and Francis. https://doi.org/10.1201/9781003402893-15. CRC.

Asuku, A.O., Ayinla, M.T., Olajide, T.S., Oyerinde, T.O., Yusuf, J.A., Bayo-Olugbami, A.A., Fajemidagba, G.A., 2024. Coffee and Parkinon's disease. In: Moradikor, N., Chatterjee, I. (Eds.), Progress in Brain Research, 289: Neuroscience of Coffee. Elsevier. https://doi.org/10.1016/bs.pbr.2024.06.001.

Badinter, F., Amit, T., Bar-Am, O., Youdim, M.B.H., Weinreb, O., 2015. Beneficial behavioral, neurochemical and molecular effects of 1-(R)-aminoindan in aged mice. Neuropharmacology 99, 264–272. https://doi.org/10.1016/j.neuropharm.2015.05.041.

Brickley, S.G., Franks, N.P., Wisden, W., 2018. Modulation of GABA A receptor function and sleep. Current Opinion in Physiology 2, 51–57. https://doi.org/10.1016/j.cophys.2017.12.011.

Carradori, S., Secci, D., Petzer, J.P., 2018. MAO inhibitors and their wider applications: A patent review. Expert Opinion on Therapeutic Patents 28 (3), 211–226. https://doi.org/10.1080/13543776.2018.1427735.

Chambers, N.E., Lanza, K., Bishop, C., 2020. Pedunculopontine Nucleus degeneration contributes to both motor and non-motor symptoms of parkinson's disease. Frontiers in Pharmacology 10. https://doi.org/10.3389/fphar.2019.01494.

Cruz, M.P., 2012. Vilazodone HCl (Viibryd): A serotonin partial agonist and reuptake inhibitor for the treatment of major depressive disorder. Pharmacy and Therapeutics 37 (1), 28. https://pmc.ncbi.nlm.nih.gov/articles/PMC3278186/.

d'Angremont, E., Begemann, M.J.H., van, Sommer, I., 2023. Cholinesterase inhibitors for treatment of psychotic symptoms in alzheimer disease and parkinson disease. JAMA Neurology 80 (8). https://doi.org/10.1001/jamaneurol.2023.1835, 813–813.

Elekhnawy, E., Negm, W.A., 2022. The potential application of probiotics for the prevention and treatment of COVID-19. Egyptian Journal of Medical Human Genetics 23 (1). https://doi.org/10.1186/s43042-022-00252-6.

Fidalgo, C., Ko, W.K.D., Tronci, E., Li, Q., Stancampiano, R., Chuan, Q., Bezard, E., Carta, M., 2015. Effect of serotonin transporter blockade on L-DOPA-induced dyskinesia in animal models of Parkinson's disease. Neuroscience 298, 389–396. https://doi.org/10.1016/j.neuroscience.2015.04.027.

Freitas, M.E., Fox, S.H., 2016. Nondopaminergic treatments for Parkinson's disease: Current and future prospects. Neurodegenerative Disease Management 6 (3), 249–268. https://doi.org/10.2217/nmt-2016-0005.

Henderson, M.X., Trojanowski, J.Q., Lee, V.M.-Y., 2019. α-Synuclein pathology in Parkinson's disease and related α-synucleinopathies. Neuroscience Letters 709, 134316. https://doi.org/10.1016/j.neulet.2019.134316.

Heo, J.Y., Nam, M.-H., Yoon, H.H., Kim, J., Hwang, Y.J., Won, W., Woo, D.H., Lee, J.A., Park, H.-J., Jo, S., Lee, M.J., Kim, S., Shim, J.-E., Jang, D.-P., Kim, K.I., Huh, S.H., Jeong, J.Y., Kowall, N.W., Lee, J., Im, H., 2020. Aberrant tonic inhibition of dopaminergic neuronal activity causes motor symptoms in animal models of parkinson's disease. Current Biology 30 (2), 276–291.e9. https://doi.org/10.1016/j.cub.2019.11.079.

Huang, Y.-H., Huang, C.-Y., 2024. The complexed crystal structure of dihydropyrimidinase reveals a potential interactive link with the neurotransmitter γ-aminobutyric acid (GABA). Biochemical and Biophysical Research Communications 692, 149351. https://doi.org/10.1016/j.bbrc.2023.149351.

Im, J.J., Jeong, H., Chung, Y., Park, J., Heo, Y., Oh, J.K., Song, I., 2019. Neuroprotective effects of rasagiline in parkinson's disease: A regional cerebral blood flow Study. Journal of Neuroimaging 29 (6), 707–711. https://doi.org/10.1111/jon.12661.

Iwasawa, C., Kuzumaki, N., Suda, Y., Kagawa, R., Oka, Y., Hattori, N., Okano, H., Narita, M., 2019. Reduced expression of somatostatin in GABAergic interneurons derived from induced pluripotent stem cells of patients with parkin mutations. Molecular Brain 12 (1). https://doi.org/10.1186/s13041-019-0426-7.

Jenner, P., Rocha, J.-F., Ferreira, J.J., Rascol, O., Soares-da-Silva, P., 2021. Redefining the strategy for the use of COMT inhibitors in Parkinson's disease: The role of opicapone. Expert Review of Neurotherapeutics 21 (9), 1019–1033. https://doi.org/10.1080/14737175.2021.1968298.

Jing, X.-Z., Yuan, X.-Z., Luo, X., Zhang, S.-Y., Wang, X.-P., 2022. An Update on Nondopaminergic Treatments for Motor and Non-motor symptoms of Parkinson's disease. Current Neuropharmacology 20. https://doi.org/10.2174/1570159x20666220222150811.

Jourdain, V.A., Morin, N., Grégoire, L., Morissette, M., Di Paolo, T., 2015. Changes in glutamate receptors in dyskinetic parkinsonian monkeys after unilateral subthalamotomy. Journal of Neurosurgery 123 (6), 1383–1393. https://doi.org/10.3171/2014.10.jns141570.

Kawabata, K., Masahisa Katsuno, 2022. Trihexyphenidyl, biperiden, and other anticholinergics in the treatment of parkinson's disease. Springer EBooks. https://doi.org/10.1007/978-3-030-62059-2_221.

Kiss, L.E., Soares-da-Silva, P., 2014. Medicinal chemistry of Catechol O-Methyltransferase (COMT) inhibitors and their therapeutic utility. Journal of Medicinal Chemistry 57 (21), 8692–8717. https://doi.org/10.1021/jm500572b.

Koshy Cherian, A., Kucinski, A., Wu, R., de Jong, I.E.M., Sarter, M., 2019. Co-treatment with rivastigmine and idalopirdine reduces the propensity for falls in a rat model of falls in Parkinson's disease. Psychopharmacology 236 (6), 1701–1715. https://doi.org/10.1007/s00213-018-5150-y.

Lanza, K., Bishop, C., 2018. Serotonergic targets for the treatment of l-DOPA-induced dyskinesia. Journal of Neural Transmission 125 (8), 1203–1216. https://doi.org/10.1007/s00702-017-1837-1.

Lee, S.-E., Lee, Y., Lee, G.H., 2019. The regulation of glutamic acid decarboxylases in GABA neurotransmission in the brain. Archives of Pharmacal Research 42 (12), 1031–1039. https://doi.org/10.1007/s12272-019-01196-z.

Mallet, N., Leblois, A., Maurice, N., Beurrier, C., 2019. Striatal cholinergic interneurons: How to elucidate their function in health and disease. Frontiers in Pharmacology 10, 1488. https://doi.org/10.3389/fphar.2019.01488.

Meadows, S.M., Conti, M.M., Gross, L., Chambers, N.E., Avnor, Y., Ostock, C.Y., Lanza, K., Bishop, C., 2018. Diverse serotonin actions of vilazodone reduce l-3,4-dihidroxyphenylalanine-induced dyskinesia in hemi-parkinsonian rats. Movement Disorders 33 (11), 1740–1749. https://doi.org/10.1002/mds.100.

Miguelez, C., De Deurwaerdère, P., Sgambato, V., 2020. Editorial: Non-dopaminergic systems in parkinson's disease. Frontiers in Pharmacology 11, 593822. https://doi.org/10.3389/fphar.2020.593822.

Morris, R., Martini, D.N., Madhyastha, T., Kelly, V.E., Grabowski, T.J., Nutt, J., Horak, F., 2019. Overview of the cholinergic contribution to gait, balance and falls in Parkinson's disease. Parkinsonism & Related Disorders 63, 20–30. https://doi.org/10.1016/j.parkreldis.2019.02.017.

Murueta-Goyena, A., Andikoetxea, A., Gómez-Esteban, J.C., Gabilondo, I., 2019. Contribution of the GABAergic System to non-motor manifestations in premotor and early stages of parkinson's disease. Frontiers in Pharmacology 10, 1294. https://doi.org/10.3389/fphar.2019.01294.

National Institute of Neurological Disorders and Stroke. (November 15, 2024). Parkinson's disease. National Institute of Neurological Disorders and Stroke. https://www.ninds.nih.gov/health-information/disorders/parkinsons-disease.

Ohno, Y., Shimizu, S., Tokudome, K., Kunisawa, N., Sasa, M., 2015. New insight into the therapeutic role of the serotonergic system in Parkinson's disease. Progress in Neurobiology 134, 104–121. https://doi.org/10.1016/j.pneurobio.2015.09.005.

Padilla-Godínez, F.J., Ramos-Acevedo, R., Martínez-Becerril, H.A., Bernal-Conde, L.D., Garrido-Figueroa, J.F., Hiriart, M., Hernández-López, A., Argüero-Sánchez, R., Callea, F., Guerra-Crespo, M., 2021. Protein misfolding and aggregation: The relatedness between parkinson's disease and hepatic endoplasmic reticulum storage disorders. International Journal of Molecular Sciences 22 (22), 12467. https://doi.org/10.3390/ijms222212467.

Pardo-Moreno, T., García-Morales, V., Suleiman-Martos, S., Rivas-Domínguez, A., Mohamed-Mohamed, H., Ramos-Rodríguez, J.J., Melguizo-Rodríguez, L., González-Acedo, A., 2023. Current treatments and new, tentative therapies for parkinson's disease. Pharmaceutics 15 (3), 770. https://doi.org/10.3390/pharmaceutics15030770.

Paredes-Rodriguez, E., Vegas-Suarez, S., Morera-Herreras, T., De Deurwaerdere, P., Miguelez, C., 2020. The noradrenergic System in parkinson's disease. Frontiers in Pharmacology 11. https://doi.org/10.3389/fphar.2020.00435.

Prévot, T., Sibille, E., 2020. Altered GABA-mediated information processing and cognitive dysfunctions in depression and other brain disorders. Molecular Psychiatry. https://doi.org/10.1038/s41380-020-0727-3.

Ray, S., Agarwal, P., 2020. Depression and anxiety in parkinson disease. Clinics in Geriatric Medicine 36 (1), 93–104. https://doi.org/10.1016/j.cger.2019.09.012.

Sadeghian, M., Mullali, G., Pocock, J.M., Piers, T., Roach, A., Smith, K.J., 2015. Neuroprotection by safinamide in the 6-hydroxydopamine model of Parkinson's disease. Neuropathology and Applied Neurobiology 42 (5), 423–435. https://doi.org/10.1111/nan.12263.

Sarter, M., Albin, R.L., Kucinski, A., Lustig, C., 2014. Where attention falls: Increased risk of falls from the converging impact of cortical cholinergic and midbrain dopamine loss on striatal function. Experimental Neurology 257, 120–129. https://doi.org/10.1016/j.expneurol.2014.04.032.

Sawada, H., Oeda, T., Kohsaka, M., Umemura, A., Tomita, S., Park, K., Mizoguchi, K., Matsuo, H., Hasegawa, K., Fujimura, H., Sugiyama, H., Nakamura, M., Kikuchi, S., Yamamoto, K., Fukuda, T., Ito, S., Goto, M., Kiyohara, K., Kawamura, T., 2018. Early use of donepezil against psychosis and cognitive decline in Parkinson's disease: A randomised controlled trial for 2 years. Journal of Neurology, Neurosurgery & Psychiatry 89 (12), 1332–1340. https://doi.org/10.1136/jnnp-2018-318107.

Sharma, M., M. Flood, P., 2019. Adrenergic receptors as pharmacological targets for neuroinflammation and neurodegeneration in parkinson's disease. Neuroprotection. https://doi.org/10.5772/intechopen.81343.

Shih, J.C., 2018. Monoamine oxidase isoenzymes: Genes, functions and targets for behavior and cancer therapy. Journal of Neural Transmission 125 (11), 1553–1566. https://doi.org/10.1007/s00702-018-1927-8.

Stayte, S., Vissel, B., 2014. Advances in non-dopaminergic treatments for Parkinson's disease. Frontiers in Neuroscience 8 (113). https://doi.org/10.3389/fnins.2014.00113.

Vázquez-Vélez, G.E., Zoghbi, H.Y., 2021. Parkinson's disease genetics and pathophysiology. Annual Review of Neuroscience 44 (1), 87–108. https://doi.org/10.1146/annurev-neuro-100720-034518.

Verma, G., Bhardwaj, A., Aledavood, T., De Choudhury, M., Kumar, S., 2022. Examining the impact of sharing COVID-19 misinformation online on mental health. Scientific Reports 12 (1), 8045. https://doi.org/10.1038/s41598-022-11488-y.

Villalba, R.M., Mathai, A., Smith, Y., 2015. Morphological changes of glutamatergic synapses in animal models of Parkinson's disease. Frontiers in Neuroanatomy 9 (117). https://doi.org/10.3389/fnana.2015.00117.

Ye, H., Robak, L.A., Yu, M., Cykowski, M., Shulman, J.M., 2023. Genetics and pathogenesis of parkinson's syndrome. Annual Review of Pathology: Mechanisms of Disease 18 (1), 95–121. https://doi.org/10.1146/annurev-pathmechdis-031521-034145.

Zhang, Z., Zhang, S., Fu, P., Zhang, Z., Lin, K., Ko, J.K.-S., Yung, K.K.-L., 2019. Roles of glutamate receptors in parkinson's disease. International Journal of Molecular Sciences 20 (18), 4391. https://doi.org/10.3390/ijms20184391.

Further reading

Butterworth, R.F., 2020. Amantadine for the treatment of parkinson's disease and its associated Dyskinesias. J Parkinsons Dis Alzheimer Dis August 7 (1), 1. https://www.avensonline.org/wp-content/uploads/JPA-2376-922X-07-0031.pdf.

Sharma, M., Patterson, L., Chapman, E., Flood, P.M., 2017. Salmeterol, a long-acting β2-Adrenergic receptor agonist, inhibits macrophage activation by lipopolysaccharide from *Porphyromonas gingivalis*. Journal of Periodontology 88 (7), 681–692. https://doi.org/10.1902/jop.2017.160464.

CHAPTER

Management of motor symptoms 11

Yasser Mecheri[1,2]

[1]*Department of Neurology, Dr Benbadis University Hospital, Constantine, Algeria;* [2]*Department of Medicine, Salah Boubnider Constantine 3 University, Constantine, Algeria*

11.1 Introduction

Parkinson's disease is the second most frequent cause of motor handicap in the population after stroke; it is also the second most frequent neurodegenerative disorder in the world (Pringsheim et al., 2014). The disease prevalence is growing worldwide; this can be explained by the increasing life expectancy and aging (Reeve et al., 2014), increased diagnostic awareness of the disease, improved access to care and possibly the effect of increased exposure to environmental factors like pesticides (Ben-Shlomo et al., 2024; Savica et al., 2016; Willis et al., 2022).

In addition to environmental factors, genetic factors play an important role in the disease's development. Five to 10 percent of patients have a familial form of the disease, carrying rare pathogenic variants in one of the causal genes with Mendelian monogenic inheritance, the number of causal genes is growing steadily, with more than 10 genes unequivocally linked to the disease and many others that remain uncertainly implicated (Blauwendraat et al., 2020; Lange et al., 2022; Shadrina & Slominsky, 2023). The cumulative effect of common genetic variation in sporadic forms of the disease can explain up to 36% of the disease heritability. Ninety genome-wide significant risk signals across 78 genomic regions, including 38 novel independent risk signals, have been identified by Nalls and collaborators (Nalls et al., 2019). However, only a fraction of disease heritability is uncovered, with a large gap in knowledge to be filled, larger multi-ancestry efforts aim to include historically under-represented populations, yielding the possibility of new discoveries.

Parkinson's disease motor symptoms are caused by progressive degeneration of dopaminergic neurons in the substantia nigra pars compacta reducing dopamine concentration in the striatum, resulting in the appearance of classical motor symptoms, including bradykinesia, rigidity, postural instability and rest tremor (Jankovic, 2008). The onset of motor features occurs after significant depletion of dopaminergic neurons and is often preceded by many years by the appearance of classical prodromal symptoms like Rapid eye movement sleep behavioral disorder, hyposmia, constipation and depression.

The updated and validated 2019 web-based Movement Disorders Society Research Criteria for Prodromal Parkinson's Disease allow statistical estimation of prodromal PD likelihood

Pharmacological Foundations of Parkinson's Disease. https://doi.org/10.1016/B978-0-443-27702-3.00026-1

(Heinzel et al., 2019). These prodromal non-motor symptoms (NMS) become more apparent with disease progression and account for a significant part of disease burden in later stages of the disease. NMS occurrence can be explained by the involvement of noradrenergic, glutamatergic, serotonergic and adenosine circuits (Aarsland et al., 2017; Chaudhuri & Sauerbier, 2016; Kalia et al., 2013).

Dopamine substitution therapy using levodopa remains the gold standard treatment after more than 50 years of its discovery, it allows immediate alleviation of classical motor features without having a disease modifying effect that can alter the disease course or the appearance of motor complications (Segura-Aguilar et al., 2014; Zhou et al., 2023). However, newer pharmacological therapies were progressively developed and used in conjunction with levodopa. Those included Anticholinergics, Antiglutamatergics, Monoamine oxidase inhibitors, Catechol-O-methyl transferase inhibitors, dopamine agonists (DA), Adenosine A2 receptor antagonists and new formulations of levodopa (extended release, intranasal forms). In addition, advanced therapies like deep brain stimulation (DBS), Apomorphine pumps, Duodopa pumps and Foslevodopa pumps have significantly changed the management of severe forms of the disease. However, in late-stage PD arises dopa-resistant symptoms like dysarthria and freezing of gate that represent a major challenge for management. There is no disease-modifying therapy (DMTs) and the treatment remains purely symptomatic.

In this chapter, we will provide a brief overview of the available therapies, considerations for managing motor features, and proposed strategies to address motor symptoms and complications.

11.2 Pharmacotherapeutic options

We will go briefly over the therapeutic arsenal available for the clinician.

11.2.1 Levodopa formulations

Dopamine's role in Parkinson's disease was first suspected and confirmed by Carlson's work in late 1950s (Carlsson, 1959; Carlsson, 2002; Carlsson & Hillarp, 1958; Carlsson et al., 1957), Levodopa was first tested intravenously and proved efficacious with severe gastrointestinal side effects (Birkmayer & Hornykiewicz, 1961). In 1967 Cotzias tested Levodopa in adjunction with dopa-decarboxylase inhibitor orally and with high doses with significant motor improvement but the appearance of dyskinesias (Cotzias, 1971; Cotzias et al., 1967, 1969; Papavasiliou et al., 1972). Nowadays many formulations exist for Levodopa including classical oral immediate release (IR), extended-release (ER) forms used for night-time reduction of clinical symptoms, oral soluble forms and inhalers for quick and consistent relief of off-phenomena like early morning dystonia and wearing-off. Of note, the inhaled form lacks a decarboxylase inhibitor and needs to be used in conjunction with oral levodopa. levodopa-induced dyskinesia (LIDs) and fluctuations in advanced PD can be prevented by continuous dopaminergic receptor stimulation using ER forms of Levodopa as well as continuous delivery of Levodopa (Poewe & Antonini, 2015) as an intestinal gel infusion (Duodopa) (Nyholm, 2012) or a subcutaneous formulation (Foslevodopa/Foscarbidopa) approved in 2024 (Blair, 2025; Soileau et al., 2022).

Common side effects include nausea and vomiting, orthostatic hypotension, dyskinesia, impulse control disorders and drowsiness.

11.2.2 Anticholinergics

Due to the risk of increased dementia incidence and cognitive decline (Pieper et al., 2020), anticholinergics should be avoided unless necessary to treat levodopa-resistant tremor. Side effects also include confusion, dry mouth, blurred vision, constipation, urinary retention, dizziness, and tachycardia. They are contraindicated with narrow-angle glaucoma, tachycardia, and benign prostatic hypertrophy.

11.2.3 Antiglutamatergics

Amantadine is an anti-NMDA receptor that was used initially as an antiviral for influenza A and also used to manage LIDs in Parkinson's patients. Common side effects include dizziness, confusion, and insomnia. Amantadine is available in immediate- and extended-release forms (Rascol, Fabbri and Poewe, 2021).

11.2.4 Monoamine oxidase inhibitors (IMAO-B)

IMAO-B prolongs and increases synaptic dopamine concentrations and can be used as monotherapy for early PD or in combination with Levodopa for treatment of fluctuations. Selegiline or Rasagiline seem to be largely equivalent in efficacy (Marconi & Zwingers, 2014; Peretz et al., 2016). Unlike rasagiline and Selegiline, Safinamide is a reversible IMAO-B and not approved as monotherapy and is used only in conjunction with Levodopa for treating fluctuations. Side effects include nausea, hallucinations, confusion, and impulsive control behaviors when combined with other dopaminergic drugs. Its interaction with anti-serotonin antidepressants like IRSS may trigger serotonin syndrome, and consuming tyramine-rich foods could provoke severe hypertensive crises (Dezsi & Vecsei, 2017).

11.2.5 Dopamine agonists (DA)

DA induces less pulsatile striatal dopamine receptor stimulation than Levodopa with a reduced risk of motor complications but, overall, a less potent effect. Prioritization among DA is mainly based on side effects and toxicity; the most frequent side effects are sleepiness, hallucinations, dyskinesias, lower limb edema, and, most importantly, impulse control behaviors (ICBs). Pramipexole should be prioritized in liver failure, as it is mainly eliminated by the kidneys. The other DA is preferred in renal failure (Ceravolo et al., 2016). There is no scientific evidence of why piribedil should be preferred for tremor while being a solid clinical observation (Millan, 2010; Pirker et al., 2023). Ropinirole and pramipexol are both available in extended-release oral forms, and rotigotine is provided in 24-hour transdermal patches (Trenkwalder et al., 2011). Apomorphine has the advantage of equipotency to levodopa because of a similar receptor activation profile. It is available as subcutaneous injections and sublingual formulations that are used as rescue medication for OFF periods (Chen & Obering, 2005; Olanow et al., 2020). Apomorphine pumps allow continuous delivery, preventing motor fluctuations (Kukkle et al., 2023).

11.2.6 Catechol-O-methyl transferase inhibitors (I-COMT)

I-COMTs prevent peripheral metabolism of dopamine; they are used to treat motor fluctuations and wearing-off episodes by increasing Levodopa half-life and bioavailability by 20%–30% for entacapone and up to 50% with Opicapone (Schrag, 2005; Vokurka et al., 2020). While both molecules are largely equivalent, Opicapone has the advantage of being taken once daily, causing less diarrhea and liver enzyme elevation and having greater OFF-time reduction and UPDRS III score improvement compared to entacapone (Lew et al., 2020). Tolcapone is a second-line treatment because it needs rigorous monitoring for liver function due to potential severe hepatotoxicity.

11.2.7 Adenosine A2 receptor antagonist

Istradefylline was approved in 2013 and is used in combination with levodopa in patients experiencing the wearing-off phenomenon. Side effects include nausea, constipation, impulse control behavior, dyskinesia and visual hallucination. Psychiatric symptoms are present in less than 5% of patients (Hauser et al., 2021).

11.2.8 Zonisamide

Zonisamide is an antiseizure drug first approved in Japan and authorized since 2009 as adjunctive therapy with other dopaminergic medications (Yang & Perry, 2009), it has a favorable effect on motor symptoms in patients with wearing off (Essam et al., 2024).

Table 11.1 provides a brief summary of the most used pharmacological therapies available for the treatment of PD motor symptoms.

11.3 Considerations when managing motor features

Parkinson's disease age of onset and symptoms are variable from one patient to another, with significant variability in progression rates and severity. Therefore, the therapeutic strategy needs to be tailored depending on the patient's age, predominant symptoms, disease stage, severity of symptoms, motor complications of the disease and socio-professional needs of the patient. No unique strategy can be employed in all patients, and no treatment combination can be maintained throughout the disease's history. However, general treatment rules should be followed to optimize treatment responses and limit side effects. Additionally, specific management strategies should be employed to manage motor complications appearing with disease progression.

11.3.1 Age of onset and age at presentation

Parkinson's disease usually has an onset around 50–60 years of age. However, the age of onset is extremely variable; early-onset Parkinson's disease (EOPD) is defined by an onset before the age of 50 years (Mehanna et al., 2022) with some patients having juvenile onset before the age of 21 years. EOPD is associated with a higher risk of dyskinesias, more bradykinesia and rigidity, and more dystonia. Dystonia often appears early, especially in the feet. Some of those patients may have a

Table 11.1 Pharmacological options available for the treatment of motor symptoms.

Drug/Class	Year of Approval	Indications	Posology	Intake form
Levodopa	1967	First-line for motor symptoms Wearing-off, morning akinesia	Initial: 300 mg/day in divided doses; combined with carbidopa/ benserazide	Oral (IR/ER) Inhaler Intestinal gel infusion
Levodopa dispersible	1988	Wearing-off, morning akinesia	50–100 mg levodopa +12.5–25 mg benserazide	Oral (dispersible in water)
Foslevodopa	2024	Motor fluctuations	Continuous infusion; max 3525 mg/day (≈2500 mg levodopa equivalent)	Subcutaneous pump infusion
Anticholinergics				
Trihexyphenidyl	1949	Tremor-predominant disease	1–15 mg/day	Oral
Antiglutamatergics				
Amantadine	1966	Dyskinesia Early monotherapy or adjunct	100–400 mg/day	Oral (IR/ER) Syrup
Dopamine agonists				
Piribedil	1969	Early monotherapy or adjunct in fluctuating disease	150–250 mg/day	Oral
Pramipexole	1997		IR: 0.125–1.5 mg 3×/day ER: Up to 4.5 mg/ day	Oral (IR/ER)
Ropinirole	2000		IR: 0.25–8 mg 3×/ day ER: Up to 24 mg/ day	Oral (IR/ER)
Rotigotine	2007		2–8 mg/24h	Transdermal patch
Apomorphine	2004 (injection), 2020 (sublingual film)	Rescue therapy for off episodes and early morning off	Injection: 2–6 mg per dose; Sublingual: 10–30 mg per OFF episode	Subcutaneous injection, sublingual

Continued

Table 11.1 Pharmacological options available for the treatment of motor symptoms.—cont'd

Drug/Class	Year of Approval	Indications	Posology	Intake form
Monoamine oxidase inhibitors				
Selegiline Rasagiline	1989 2006	Early monotherapy or adjunct in fluctuating disease	5–10 mg/day 1 mg/day	Oral Oral
Safinamide	2017	Adjunct to levodopa in fluctuating disease	50–100 mg/day	Oral
Catechol-O-methyl transferase inhibitors				
Tolcapone	1997	Adjunct for wearing-off motor fluctuations	100–200 mg 3×/day (requires liver monitoring)	Oral
Entacapone	1999		200 mg with each levodopa dose	Oral
Opicapone	2016		50 mg once daily	Oral
Adenosine A2 receptor antagonist				
Istradefylline	2013	Adjunct for wearing-off motor fluctuations	20–40 mg once daily	Oral
Carbonic anhydrase inhibitor (off-label)				
Zonisamide	2009	Adjunct in fluctuating disease, reduces off time	100–600 mg/day	Oral

IR Immediate release, ER Extended release.

genetic cause of the disease. On the other hand, patients with a later age of onset after 70 years have more prominent tremors and may have increased polymedication, increased medication side effect risk, and fragile cognitive status (Wickremaratchi et al., 2011).

11.3.2 Clinical form and predominant symptoms

Parkinson's disease patients can be divided depending on clinical features into subgroups, and many studies suggest that these subtypes can determine the phenotype, natural disease history, progression rate, and distinct underlying pathogenic mechanisms. The two main subtypes proposed are tremor-dominant and postural-instability-gait-disorder (PIGD) with the latter considered to have a more severe at diagnosis, more rapid progression, marked cognitive decline, more hallucinations and psychosis and more frequent Levodopa-induced dyskinesias (LIDs) (Aleksovski et al., 2018; Savica et al., 2019). However, it has been shown that these subtypes can change with disease progression and under treatment effects (Luo et al., 2019; Mestre et al., 2018).

Tremor can be very debilitating for patients, causing embarrassment and affecting performance or confidence; it can draw unwanted attention, leading to acute self-awareness and fear of judgment.

11.3.3 Disease stage

Parkinson's disease is a neurodegenerative disorder with a progressive course of worsening of motor and non-motor features. The natural history of the disease can be divided into four stages: the prodromal stage, where only non-motor features are present; the early stage, where cardinal motor features like tremor, rigidity and bradykinesia are progressively worsening; mid-stage disease, or advanced PD when motor complications appear like LIDs and motor fluctuations; and finally, late-stage disease with the onset of dopa-resistant features like dysarthria, freezing of gait and axial instability and a significant worsening of non-motor symptoms and the appearance of psychosis and dementia (Poewe et al., 2017). Treatment needs vary depending on disease stage and predominant symptoms, bearing in mind the dynamic progression and change in predominant symptoms and complaints over time.

11.3.4 Disease severity and rate of progression evaluation

Disease severity and progression are important factors to take into account for the choice of PD medication and the posology used. Some patients have a relatively benign disease course and slow progression of symptoms, and others that have quick progression and early onset of motor complications, often needing many medications with increased risk of side effects and interactions and early need for advanced therapies. Many tools can be used to acquire a more objective evaluation of disease severity, and many scales and auto-questionnaires collecting data on motor symptoms, motor complications, autonomy and quality of life are validated in Parkinson's disease in many languages and include the Movement Disorder Society-Unified Parkinson's Disease Rating Scale (MDS-UPDRS), wearing-off questionnaires (WOQ-9, WOQ-19), the Unified Dyskinesia Rating Scale (UDysRS), the Schwab and England Activities of Daily Living Scale and Parkinson's Disease Questionnaire (PDQ-39).

Patient diaries were classically used when motor fluctuations and LIDs appear and serve to better identify the type of complication and the exact reason and timing of occurrence (peak of dose, end of dose ...). Review of homemade videos can be very useful for complicated patterns of fluctuations and unclear cases. A more objective alternative is kinematic sensors and different tracking devices that allow real-time monitoring and tracking of patients' state to be reviewed by clinicians.

11.3.5 Motor complications associated with advanced disease

The neurodegenerative character of the disease implies a continuous worsening of symptoms and the appearance of new ones in more advanced stages of the disease. Disease progression is associated with a change in the pharmacokinetics of levodopa. Initially, levodopa is being absorbed and then stored in dopaminergic neurons which allows a continuous baseline availability of dopamine in the brain. However, with a progressively reduced number of neurones, presynaptic storage capacity is reduced, and levodopa plasma concentration will follow intake patterns with progressively reduced half-life plasma availability and treatment effect duration and more marked drops and highs in plasma concentration. This discontinuous drug delivery, along with the variability in its gastrointestinal absorption and blood–brain barrier transport capacity, is linked to advanced disease complications (Poewe & Antonini, 2015).

The wearing-off phenomenon is an earlier than expected reappearance of motor features after levodopa intake due to a shorter half-life. Peak dose dyskinesias, on the other hand, are due to rapid and excessive increases in levodopa plasma concentrations resulting in excessive motor activation and the appearance of choreo-dystonic movements. Dyskinetic movements can be extremely disruptive in the most severe forms and harbor a significant risk of falls, stigma and alteration of self-image, causing further social isolation and professional limitations.

11.3.6 Socio-professional setting and patient's needs

Patients' perceptions of motor handicaps are variable depending on professional needs, daily activity, and social settings. The social burden of the disease is a significant factor to consider, particularly for early-onset forms that affect the most active individuals who have numerous social and professional commitments. Motor symptoms of the disease can significantly limit the capacity of women as main carers of the household in low socioeconomic and more traditional social settings. On the other hand, families in low socioeconomic settings typically expect young males to be the primary breadwinners, without the support of governmental and social security systems. Limited functionality can significantly reduce their earnings and negatively impact their economic status and access to health care. Manual work, driving, and artistic and ultra-specialized activities are the most impacted and should be considered in setting common treatment goals with patients.

11.3.7 Associated non-motor features

Associated non-motor symptoms should be considered in the choice of medication and the titration. DA should be prescribed with caution in patients with a history of ICBs like gambling and obsessive behavior (Claassen et al., 2011; Driver-Dunckley et al., 2003; Grosset et al., 2011; Sinha et al., 2013; Weintraub et al., 2006). They can be very useful in patients with depression and apathy (Bogdan et al., 2020; Liu et al., 2019; Maher et al., 2024; Pagonabarraga et al., 2015) but can cause more gastrointestinal signs, sedation and daytime sleepiness, orthostatic hypotension (HTO), hallucinations and psychosis than Levodopa (Ecker et al., 2009; Kujawa et al., 2000; O'Suilleabhain & Dewey, 2002). Sedation and HTO with DA can be managed by splitting the morning dose and adding an evening intake.

Psychosis in advanced disease can be exacerbated by polymedication; the drugs that are more prone to cause psychosis and are less potent to treat parkinsonism should be reduced or stopped without causing a significant aggravation of motor symptoms. Medications should be discontinued in the following order: anticholinergics, Amantadine, I-COMT, IMAO-B, DA, and finally carbidopa. Intake at bedtime should be reduced or stopped to reduce nighttime hallucination (Chen, 2017; Kuzuhara, 2001; Weiss & Adler, 2014).

11.4 Management strategy

11.4.1 Management strategy depending on age

The drug to use initially is also affected by the patient's age; usually after 70 years, the risk of medication side effects is increased. Therefore, the number of medications used needs to be reduced, and the most effective ones with fewer side effects, like levodopa are prioritized. Anticholinergics can usually cause visual hallucinations, sedation and confusion. Dopamine agonists cause more psychiatric symptoms and orthostatic hypotension than levodopa. DBS is usually performed before the age of 70 years due to the risk of induced cognitive decline and the risk of aggravated postural instability. Selected patients aged more than 70 years with excellent cognitive states can benefit from DBS if they pass a stricter cognitive assessment. The preferred initial and main therapy after the age of 70 years is levodopa, DA and other treatments can be used in low doses and with prudence when needed and for the treatment of specific symptoms like restless leg syndrome and apathy for DA. Before the age of 70 years, the strategy will depend on other factors like patients' needs and severity of symptoms.

11.4.2 The management strategy should be based on the predominant motor symptoms

Levodopa is the gold standard and most efficacious treatment of motor symptoms of PD (Fox et al., 2018). Bradykinesia and rigidity show more consistent responses to treatment than tremor (Fishman, 2008). Tremor is treated first by Levodopa as it is the most efficacious treatment, and tremor is typically very dopa-responsive but may need high unitary doses to be well-controlled. For off-period tremors, the strategy is the adjunction of add-on therapies like DA, IMAO-B, I-COMT, and infusion therapies (Lew, 2013). Tremor can be drug-resistant to high doses of Levodopa, in this case, DBS and focused ultrasound should be considered even in patients without motor fluctuations. Apomorphine is the only antiparkinsonian agent with an effect size on motor symptoms that is equivalent to that of levodopa (Kempster et al., 1990). Other DA have a weaker overall effect on motor symptoms, and there is no quality data comparing their specific effect on tremor versus Levodopa (Stowe et al., 2008). This includes Piribedil despite solid clinical observations of its specific tremor effect (Millan, 2010; Pirker et al., 2023). Anticholinergics' effect on PD tremor did not exceed the effect of levodopa or apomorphine and may be even lower (Schrag et al., 1999) and their usage is limited to selected young patients due to their side effect profile. Levodopa is effective on both rest and postural tremor (Tedeschi et al., 1990). Beta blockers have been shown to be also effective on both types of tremor and may be used as adjunct therapy to levodopa when its effect is insufficient to control tremor in PD (Koller & Herbster, 1987).

11.4.3 Management strategy depending on available therapies

The treatment strategy is also dependent on available therapies and tools for the clinician depending on his work setting. A limited-resource setting without access to advanced therapies will impose the need for a prolonged reliance on dopatherapy with an increased need for higher doses and an increased risk of induced dyskinesia without the possibility of using advanced infusion therapies and surgery. In such cases the therapeutic objectives need to be changed, and optimal symptom controls may be compromised in order to limit side effects and LIDs.

11.4.4 Management strategy depending on disease stage

11.4.4.1 Prodromal stage

At this stage, motor symptoms are absent, and the patient mainly has non-motor features. This patient population is interesting for inclusion in clinical trials for disease-modifying therapies.

11.4.4.2 Early stage

No consensus exists on a common strategy to follow even in the earliest stages of the disease. Most patients will require levodopa therapy within 2 years of symptoms' onset to control their symptoms. The introduction of levodopa is frequently delayed despite numerous pieces of high-quality scientific evidence showing no priming effect for levodopa on the appearance of dyskinesias and disease progression and that delaying its initiation doesn't postpone the onset of dyskinesia (Cilia et al., 2014; Fahn et al., 2004; Verschuur et al., 2019). A 9-month study, called the earlier versus later levodopa trial, compared 150, 300 and 600 mg daily doses of levodopa with a placebo and found no evidence of levodopa effect on dyskinesia onset time but a dose-dependent effect, with 16.5% of patients in the 600 mg group developing dyskinesia (Fahn et al., 2004). Additionally, a more recent delayed-start trial showed no disease-modifying effect when using levodopa in early PD and comparing the rate of progression between early- or delayed-start patients (Verschuur et al., 2019).

However, the general sentiment of levodopaphobia is still widespread, and many clinicians are still reluctant to introduce levodopa to their patients despite them clearly having poorly controlled symptoms under alternative therapeutic options. This attitude is most problematic in younger patients who are more prone to earlier and more severe motor complications and LIDs (Bjornestad et al., 2016; Cabreira et al., 2019; Espay et al., 2018) resulting in poor quality of life and lost years of good motor function control in the early disease phase before the onset of motor complications, often coinciding with the late decision of finally starting levodopa.

11.4.5 When to start symptomatic treatment

The question of when to start the treatment after a positive diagnosis of PD can be answered by knowing that all treatments lack a negative or positive disease-modifying effect, including levodopa (Olanow et al., 2009; Schapira et al., 2013; Verschuur et al., 2019).Therefore, all treatments are symptomatic, and the decision to initiate treatment is closely linked to patients' needs. It is wise to adopt a wait-and-see strategy and closely monitor the patient and start the treatment when symptoms impact the patient's quality of life and motor function.

11.4.6 Initial therapy choice

In patients older than 70 years or having comorbidities or cognitive impairment, or when motor impairment is significant, levodopa is the preferred initial therapy. However, quality of life and patient social and professional needs are the priority when considering the treatment choice in patients younger than 70 years. A strategy of starting with IMAO-B in the first months, then adding dopamine agonists after a few months and levodopa a little bit after seems acceptable in patients younger than 70 years and without cognitive impairment and presenting in early disease with mild symptoms (Schapira, 2007). The most important element is to quickly add sufficient doses of levodopa when symptoms are no longer controlled or when DA posology can't be increased further because of side effects. The rationale here emerges from recognizing that levodopa is the most potent drug among the three classes, followed by DA and IMAO-B at last. Therefore, a sequential introduction of the three drugs to fill patients' increased needs over time will strike a balance of avoiding using high doses of DA with many side effects that can limit social and professional activity and avoiding using unnecessarily high doses of levodopa more prone to cause LIDs while maintaining an overall control of motor symptoms because of the early adjunction of add-on therapies.

A more common and solid strategy widely adapted nowadays with the wider availability of advanced therapies is to start with levodopa regardless of patient age and to gradually increase doses following the patient's needs. The reasoning is that despite the fact that levodopa causes more LIDs than DA, it still has a better tolerance profile, more motor benefit and, most importantly, most of LIDs in the first 5 years are unlikely to be troublesome (Pringsheim et al., 2021). The next step is to use management strategies suggested below to manage motor fluctuations and LIDs over time. Afterward, advanced therapies will be discussed with the patient, and the better option chosen depending on his needs, risk factors and age will be implemented when motor complications are no longer satisfactorily controlled with a significant impact on QoL and professional activities. The 5-2-1 rule can be very useful to determine the need for advanced therapies; the patient needs to have at least one of the three: Five or more levodopa intakes are needed to control symptoms; the patient is having 2 hours or more of OFF time; the patient is having 1 hour or more of troublesome dyskinesias (Aldred et al., 2020). Advanced therapies have allowed for a significant increase in the quality of life and lifespan of patients with a significant reduction of motor fluctuations and LIDs, DBS, apomorphine subcutaneous pumps, intestinal levodopa pumps and, more recently, subcutaneous foslevodopa/foscarbidopa pump have significantly changed PD patients' care and management strategy.

11.5 Advanced-stage disease: levodopa-related motor complications

With disease advancement, the initial relief provided by chronic oral levodopa medication will be limited by the progressive appearance of motor and nonmotor complications, including motor and nonmotor fluctuations (NMFs) and LIDs. Up to 30% of patients will develop these complications within the first 2 years, and most patients will have at least one of them after more than 5 years of treatment (Fahn et al., 2004; Stocchi et al., 2014). While LIDs and on-off fluctuations both significantly impair the quality of life and cause significant disability, most patients prefer to stay in the on state with non-disabling dyskinesia rather than an off state (Hung et al., 2010). This can be linked to reduced motor function and mobility, rigidity, painful off dystonia and non-motor fluctuations that cause depressive mood, shortness of breath and impaired quality of life. The management strategy is tailored for each complication and includes the modification of Levodopa dosage and intake time and frequency, the introduction of new forms of oral levodopa like extended-release and soluble forms, the introduction of new classes of medications and extended-release forms and the use of advanced therapies like infusion therapy and DBS. Therefore, at this stage the patient is more progressed and more fragile, with the appearance of many NMS like orthostatic hypotension and cognitive decline, and is taking more medications and higher dosages, increasing the risk of medication interaction and side effects that will need to be considered in the management of motor complications.

11.5.1 Levodopa-induced dyskinesias (LIDs)

Levodopa-induced dyskinesias have been studied in many clinical trials; their frequency grows with disease duration from 16% in the first year of Levodopa treatment introduction to between 33% and 54% after 3–6 years (Holloway et al., 2004; Holloway et al., 2009; Stocchi et al., 2010). LIDs description and management will be detailed further in the specific chapter. Briefly, LIDs usually appear before the onset of motor fluctuations and include a variety of movements, mainly choreic movements of limbs and the trunk in peak of dose dyskinesia usually appearing 30–90 min after a dose of levodopa. Biphasic dyskinesias occurring after levodopa intake and at the end of dose wearing-off have a mixture of dystonic and phasic violent movements. Wearing-off dystonia causes end-of-dose painful dystonia of limbs.

Not all peak-dose LIDs require medication adjustment; a study found that only 17% of patients with LIDs by 5 years and 43% by 10 years needed treatment adjustment (Van Gerpen et al., 2006). The strategy to reduce troublesome peak-dose LIDs is to first reduce high unitary doses of levodopa. Increasing the number of levodopa intakes by reducing intake intervals is recommended if wearing-off appears with unitary dose reduction, as the objective is to limit the fluctuation in levodopa availability and remain below the threshold of LIDs appearance. This strategy is usually called levodopa dose fractionation (Nyholm & Stepien, 2014).

Continuous delivery of treatment allows maintaining a stable levodopa plasma concentration. Oral extended-release forms of levodopa, dopa agonists, IMAO-B (E.g. Rasagiline) and I-COMT (E.g. Tolcapone) can be used initially, but they can quickly cause an exacerbation of LIDs when low unitary normal release levodopa becomes insufficient to provide significant relief of symptoms with disease progression, making the management tricky in order to avoid crossing the threshold of LIDs without developing motor fluctuations and wearing-off periods. Another limitation of oral intake medications is that their pharmacokinetics change with the development of gastroparesis. The gastric void becomes unpredictable and negatively affected by the type of food ingested (like proteins). Therefore, the absorption of medications becomes fluctuating and Levodopa plasma concentrations unstable. Infusion therapies provide an interesting solution to this problem; Duodopa pumps, apomorphine and, most notably and recently, Foslevodopa/Foscarbidopa pumps short-circuit this issue, allowing direct intestinal (Duodopa) or subcutaneous systemic delivery. Amantadine on the other hand, can reduce LIDs and should be used when available. Amantadine immediate release can be titrated as tolerated up to 400 mg daily, divided into two to four doses a day. The extended-release formulation allows once-a-day intake without compromising on efficacy.

11.5.2 Motor fluctuations

Motor fluctuations are shifts between an on-state, where parkinsonian symptoms are relieved, and an off-state, where parkinsonian symptoms reemerge. They occur in 50% or more of PD subjects treated for longer than 5 years (Poewe et al., 1986; Schrag & Quinn, 2000; Stocchi et al., 2014). They are linked to Levodopa plasma concentration fluctuation, causing the quick fluctuation between on and off states in on-off fluctuations.

Types of motor fluctuations include the following.

- **'Wearing-off'** refers to the early end of levodopa's action due to its shortened half-life, which leads to an increase in off periods. This phenomenon is typically very predictable and first appears after 3–4 h of treatment intake, with intervals progressively shorter over time. Wearing-off is the most common type of motor fluctuation, and a significant proportion of patients may experience wearing-off before developing dyskinesias (Hauser et al., 2006).
- Early end of levodopa action because of shortened half-life, causing an increase of off periods. Wearing-off is usually very predictable and initially appears after 3–4 h of treatment intake with a progressive shortening of intervals. Wearing-off is the most frequent motor fluctuation, and a considerable proportion of patients may first develop wearing-off before dyskinesias arise (Hauser et al., 2006).
- **Morning off:** A recent survey involving 320 patients has found early morning off in 44% of patients in early disease stages and an overall prevalence of 60% (Rizos et al., 2014). It is linked to low Levodopa concentration in the plasma after sleep due to absent intake at night.
- **Early morning dystonia:** Dystonia in the morning-off period with painful dystonic cramping of the foot is a common and severe form of morning-off. (Lees et al., 1977; Poewe et al., 1988)
- **Delayed on, partial on, and dose failure refer to the inability to transition from an "off" parkinsonian state to an "on" response after taking a dose of levodopa.**includes failure to transition from an "off" parkinsonian state to an "on" response following a dose of levodopa. Such failure can be linked to the apparition of gastroparesis, with disease progression causing delayed emptying of gastric content, delayed absorption of medicaments and a delayed action of therapy. Levodopa absorption is duodenal and competitive with other amino acids. Therefore, a rich protein regimen can limit levodopa treatment absorption. A significant proportion of daily off time is attributable to delays in switching on after oral doses that can be managed by medications that provide rapid onset of effect after dosing.
- **Paradoxical OFF periods:** Are sudden off without an obvious relationship to levodopa or dopaminergic therapy dosing but may be precipitated by a relative excess of levodopa or gastroparesis.

General management of on-off fluctuation: The International Parkinson and Movement Disorder Society Evidence-Based Medicine in Movement Disorders Committee recently updated their review to establish recommendations on treatments for Parkinson's disease motor fluctuations. A total of 102 studies were evaluated to gather evidence on different interventions' efficacy on motor fluctuation reduction. The interventions were categorized into three groups—efficacious, likely efficacious, and limited evidence—based on the quality of studies, risk of bias, and available data. The interventions were categorized into three groups—efficacious, likely efficacious, and limited evidence—based on the quality of studies, risk of bias, and available data (de Bie et al., 2025). The interventions were grouped according to the quality of studies, risk of bias and the data available into efficacious, likely efficacious and limited evidence.

Efficacious interventions: Levodopa extended release, Pramipexole immediate release and extended release, Ropinirole immediate release, Rotigotine, Opicapone, Safinamide, and bilateral subthalamic nucleus DBS (STN-DBS) were assessed as efficacious because of the high quality of evidence available.

Levodopa Carbidopa Extended Release (IPX066) was efficacious for reducing off-time and increasing on-time without troublesome dyskinesia (Hauser et al., 2013). Ropinirole immediate release was assessed for the reduction of off-time and showed a statistically significant meaningful reduction of off-time (Barone et al., 2007; Lieberman et al., 1998; Mizuno et al., 2007; Rascol et al., 1996). Pramipexole immediate release and extended release were tested in various trials and were found to significantly reduce off-time in PD patients (Mizuno et al., 2003; Mizuno et al., 2012; Möller et al., 2005; Poewe et al., 2007; Schapira et al., 2011; Wong et al., 2003). Rotigotine was deemed efficacious with clear statistical significance in reducing off-time when compared to placebo; also, it had significant effect on disability and improvement of quality of life (LeWitt et al., 2007; Mizuno et al., 2014; Nomoto et al., 2014; Poewe et al., 2007). Opicapone efficacy in reducing off-time duration was statistically significant and clinically meaningful (Ferreira et al., 2016; Lees et al., 2017; Takeda et al., 2021)and Safinamide was found to be efficacious in treating motor fluctuations (Borgohain et al., 2014; Hattori, Tsuboi, et al., 2020; Schapira et al., 2017; Wei et al., 2022). STN-DBS improved motor impairment in PD patients experiencing motor fluctuations and disability (Anderson et al., 2005; Deuschl et al., 2006; Fonoff et al., 2016; Li et al., 2017; Schuepbach et al., 2013; Schüpbach et al., 2007; Vitek et al., 2020).

Likely efficacious interventions: Ropinirole prolonged release (Pahwa et al., 2007; Zesiewicz et al., 2017; Zhang et al., 2013), ropinirole patch (Hattori, Mochizuki, et al., 2020), 1 mg per day rasagiline (Hattori et al., 2018; Rascol et al., 2005; Schwid, 2005; Zhang et al., 2018) and istradefylline (Hauser et al., 2008; Hauser et al., 2003; LeWitt et al., 2008; Mizuno et al., 2010; Pourcher et al., 2012; Stacy et al., 2008) were found to likely reduce off-time and improve motor fluctuations.

Entacapone (Brooks & Sagar, 2003; Fénelon et al., 2003; Kieburtz, 1997; Poewe et al., 2002; Reichmann et al., 2005; Rinne et al., 1998), Amantadine extended release (not immediate release) (Oertel et al., 2017; Ory-Magne et al., 2014; Pahwa et al., 2017) and Zonisamide (Essam et al., 2024; Murata et al., 2007, 2015) as an add-on therapy were evaluated for treating motor fluctuations in PD patients and were considered to be likely efficacious to treat motor fluctuations in PD patients.

Advanced infusion therapies, including Levodopa/Carbidopa intestinal gel (Chung et al., 2022; Olanow et al., 2014), continuous subcutaneous Foslevodopa/Foscarbidopa(Soileau et al., 2022), continuous subcutaneous apomorphine infusion (Hattori et al., 2014) are likely efficacious for the treatment of motor fluctuations in PD patients. Bilateral internal globus pallidus (GPi) DBS (Odekerken et al., 2016; Weaver et al., 2012), unilateral pallidotomy are likely efficacious in treating motor fluctuations (Esselink et al., 2006; Vitek et al., 2020) (, 2004).

Limited evidence: Levodopa Carbidopa Controlled Release (Hutton et al., 1988; Wolters et al., 1992; Wolters & Tesselaar, 1996), Apomorphine intermittent sublingual film and apomorphine subcutaneous pen.

As rescue therapy (Hattori et al., 2014; Olanow et al., 2020), Nicotine (Villafane et al., 2018), the eradication of Helicobacter pylori (Pierantozzi et al., 2006) and perampanel (Eggert et al., 2010; Lees et al., 2012) all had insufficient evidence to support their efficacy in reducing motor fluctuations.

11.6 Specific management of motor fluctuations

- **Wearing off:** Early end of levodopa action because of shortened half-life can be specifically managed by either progressively reducing the intervals between levodopa intakes or by the adjunction of I-COMT, which can increase Levodopa action duration by 20%–50% depending on agent used.

- **Morning off:** Low Levodopa concentration in the plasma after sleep due to absent intake at night can be managed by either providing long-acting agents at bedtime, like extended-release levodopa, or extended-release DA. Another strategy to provide quick release is to provide quick-acting agents when the patient awakes, like soluble levodopa formulations that can provide relief of symptoms much quicker than classical Levodopa formulations.
- **Early morning dystonia:** The management is similar to morning-off, with the possibility to use botulinum toxin injections when dystonia is persistent or debilitating.
- **Delayed on, partial on and dose failure:** The gastroparesis effect can be managed by taking levodopa on an empty stomach (30–60 min before or 60–90 min after a meal), reducing protein intake at the time of drug intake and moving it from the day to the evening and reducing the quantity of food at each food intake (Karstaedt & Pincus, 1992; Riley & Lang, 1988). Levodopa soluble formulations can help, but subcutaneous or sublingual Apomorphine are a preferable rescue medication.
- **Paradoxical OFF periods:** They are hard to manage and may need rescue medication or advanced therapies like infusions and DBS in addition to managing gastroparesis.

11.7 Late-stage disease: dopa-resistant motor symptoms

11.7.1 Freezing of gait (FOG)

FOG is an episodic inability to step and advance in any direction occurring when initiating walking, turning or upon passing a door or transitioning between two different places. It can be levodopa-responsive when occurring as a transient "off" phenomenon, and it can be managed like other end-of-dose wearing-off phenomena by reducing levodopa doses intervals. Additionally, FOG can be Levodopa-related also called "on" FOG, occurring in advanced PD randomly at variable frequency and duration in the "on" state with poor response to dopaminergic therapy and to surgical and infusion therapies (Tosserams et al., 2025). However, if FOG occurs at the levodopa peak effect, reducing the dose of the potentially associated DA and of levodopa can be useful. Physical therapy in this case is the main therapeutic intervention, involving planning movement strategies or using visual imagery and cues like simulating an obstacle or using a regular cane or special laser cane may also be of use in FOG (McCandless et al., 2016).

11.7.2 Dysarthria and dysphagia

Dysarthria and dysphagia are often treated by speech and voice therapists. Pharmacological treatments have little effect on severe forms occurring in late-stage disease (Megna et al., 2012).

11.7.3 Persistent dystonic symptoms can benefit from botulinum toxin

Blepharospasm may precede PD motor symptoms or be associated with eyelid opening apraxia. It can be treated by Levodopa and fluctuate with other motor symptoms. It has a good response to botulinum toxin injections (Rana et al., 2012; Yoon et al., 2005). Torticollis is the most frequent cervical dystonia reported in PD. It usually does not respond to levodopa but has a good response to botulinum toxin (Papapetropoulos & Singer, 2006).

Camptocormia is an anteflexion of the trunk that improves in the supine position with a geste antagonist and botulinum toxin injections (Azher & Jankovic, 2005; von Coelln et al., 2008). Anterocollis is seen in more advanced cases of PD and usually does not respond to sensory tricks or to botulinum toxin injections (Van De Warrenburg et al., 2007). Pisa syndrome is a lateral flexion of the trunk when standing. Unlike kyphoscoliosis, it disappears when lying down. It sometimes responds to botulinum toxin injections or DBS (Bonanni et al., 2007; Umemura et al., 2010). Some reports suggest that camptocormia, Pisa syndrome and Anterocollis can be caused by changes in the treatment or the introduction of DA and may regress with drug withdrawal (Cannas et al., 2009; Mano, 2018; Prakash & Lang, 2007).

Focal dystonia of the limbs is more frequently seen in the foot than the upper limbs; it can be task-specific or triggered by walking. They can be linked to idiopathic PD or genetic forms of the PARKIN, PINK1, *PARKIN, PINK1* and *DJ1* mutations (Wickremaratchi et al., 2011). Deformities of the limbs, also called striatal postures, like striatal hand and striatal toe, persist at rest and during sleep and may have a dystonic origin; they can rarely respond to levodopa and other anti-parkinsonian drugs (Ashour et al., 2005). Alternatively, botulinum toxin injection can be used successfully (Cordivari et al., 2001; Giladi et al., 1994; Jankovic, 2004) to provide functional improvement, pain relief and limit injuries. DBS also was reported to be efficacious (Morishita et al., 2008). Orthopedic surgical interventions can be performed if the above therapies are unsuccessful (Moore et al., 1998).

11.8 Conclusion

In this chapter we highlighted the main pharmacological options available to treat motor symptoms in Parkinson's disease. We explained the different factors to consider in the management of motor symptoms, like the age of the patients and the disease stage. We also laid down the main strategies employed to manage on-off fluctuations and LIDs. The therapeutic strategy for motor symptom disease is dynamic; no standard protocol can be used for all patients. The strategy needs to be tailored to patients' age, patients' socio-professional needs, disease stage, disease prominent features and many other factors. Many advancements over the years allowed the use of new medication classes, new medication formulations like inhaled and extended-release formulations, and new delivery mechanisms like subcutaneous or intraduodenal pumps for infusion therapies. Future perspectives include the hope of the development of disease-modifying therapies that can slow the progression of the disease and limit the development of treatment-resistant complications.

AI Disclosure

During the preparation of this work the author(s) used Copilot in order to The tool was used to collate data and generate Table 01. After using this tool/service, the author(s) reviewed and edited the content as needed and take (s) full responsibility for the content of the publication.

References

Aarsland, D., Creese, B., Politis, M., Chaudhuri, K.R., Ffytche, D.H., Weintraub, D., Ballard, C., 2017. Cognitive decline in Parkinson disease. Nature Reviews Neurology 13 (4), 217–231. https://doi.org/10.1038/nrneurol.2017.27.

Aldred, J., Anca-Herschkovitsch, M., Antonini, A., Bajenaru, O., Bergmann, L., Bourgeois, P., Cubo, E., Davis, T. L., Iansek, R., Kovács, N., Kukreja, P., Onuk, K., Pontieri, F.E., Robieson, W., Siddiqui, M.S., Simu, M., Standaert, D.G., Ray Chaudhuri, K., 2020. Application of the '5-2-1' screening criteria in advanced Parkinson's disease: Interim analysis of DUOGLOBE. Neurodegenerative Disease Management 10 (5), 309–323. https://doi.org/10.2217/nmt-2020-0021.

Aleksovski, D., Miljkovic, D., Bravi, D., Antonini, A., 2018. Disease progression in Parkinson subtypes: The PPMI dataset. Neurological Sciences 39 (11), 1971–1976. https://doi.org/10.1007/s10072-018-3522-z.

Anderson, V.C., Burchiel, K.J., Hogarth, P., Favre, J., Hammerstad, J.P., 2005. Pallidal vs subthalamic nucleus deep brain stimulation in Parkinson disease. Archives of Neurology 62 (4), 554–560. https://doi.org/10.1001/archneur.62.4.554.

Ashour, R., Tintner, R., Jankovic, J., 2005. Striatal deformities of the hand and foot in Parkinson's disease. The Lancet Neurology 4 (7), 423–431. https://doi.org/10.1016/s1474-4422(05)70119-8.

Azher, S.N., Jankovic, J., 2005. Camptocormia: Pathogenesis, classification, and response to therapy. Neurology 65 (3), 355–359. https://doi.org/10.1212/01.wnl.0000171857.09079.9f.

Barone, P., Lamb, J., Ellis, A., Clarke, Z., 2007. Sumanirole versus placebo or ropinirole for the adjunctive treatment of patients with advanced Parkinson's disease. Movement Disorders 22 (4), 483–489. https://doi.org/10.1002/mds.21191.

Ben-Shlomo, Y., Darweesh, S., Llibre-Guerra, J., Marras, C., San Luciano, M., Tanner, C., 2024. The epidemiology of Parkinson's disease. The Lancet 403 (10423), 283–292. https://doi.org/10.1016/S0140-6736(23)01419-8.

Birkmayer, W., Hornykiewicz, O., 1961. The L-3,4-dioxyphenylalanine (DOPA)-effect in parkinson-akinesia. Wiener Klinische Wochenschrift 73, 787–788.

Bjornestad, A., Forsaa, E.B., Pedersen, K.F., Tysnes, O.B., Larsen, J.P., Alves, G., 2016. Risk and course of motor complications in a population-based incident Parkinson's disease cohort. Parkinsonism & Related Disorders 22, 48–53. https://doi.org/10.1016/j.parkreldis.2015.11.007.

Blair, H.A., 2025. Foslevodopa/Foscarbidopa: A review in advanced parkinson's disease. CNS Drugs 39 (6), 621–632. https://doi.org/10.1007/s40263-025-01179-3.

Blauwendraat, C., Nalls, M.A., Singleton, A.B., 2020. The genetic architecture of Parkinson's disease. The Lancet Neurology 19 (2), 170–178. https://doi.org/10.1016/S1474-4422(19)30287-X.

Bogdan, A., Manera, V., Koenig, A., David, R., 2020. Pharmacologic approaches for the management of apathy in neurodegenerative disorders. Frontiers in Pharmacology 10. https://doi.org/10.3389/fphar.2019.01581.

Bonanni, L., Thomas, A., Varanese, S., Scorrano, V., Onofrj, M., 2007. Botulinum toxin treatment of lateral axial dystonia in parkinsonism. Movement Disorders 22 (14), 2097–2103. https://doi.org/10.1002/mds.21694.

Borgohain, R., Szasz, J., Stanzione, P., Meshram, C., Bhatt, M., Chirilineau, D., Stocchi, F., Lucini, V., Giuliani, R., Forrest, E., Rice, P., Anand, R., 2014. Randomized trial of safinamide add-on to levodopa in Parkinson's disease with motor fluctuations. Movement Disorders 29 (2), 229–237. https://doi.org/10.1002/mds.25751.

Brooks, D.J., Sagar, H., 2003. Entacapone is beneficial in both fluctuating and non-fluctuating patients with Parkinson's disease: A randomised, placebo controlled, double blind, six month study. Journal of Neurology Neurosurgery and Psychiatry 74 (8), 1071–1079. https://doi.org/10.1136/jnnp.74.8.1071.

Cabreira, V., Soares-da-Silva, P., Massano, J., 2019. Contemporary options for the management of motor complications in parkinson's disease: Updated clinical review. Drugs 79 (6), 593–608. https://doi.org/10.1007/s40265-019-01098-w.

Cannas, A., Solla, P., Floris, G., Tacconi, P., Serra, A., Piga, M., Marrosu, F., Marrosu, M.G., 2009. Reversible Pisa syndrome in patients with Parkinson's disease on dopaminergic therapy. Journal of Neurology 256 (3), 390–395. https://doi.org/10.1007/s00415-009-0072-6.

Carlsson, A., 1959. The occurrence, distribution and physiological role of catecholamines in the nervous system. Pharmacological Reviews 11 (2), 490–493. https://doi.org/10.1016/s0031-6997(25)07428-9.

Carlsson, A., 2002. Treatment of Parkinson's with L-DOPA. The early discovery phase, and a comment on current problems. Journal of Neural Transmission 109 (5–6), 777–787. https://doi.org/10.1007/s007020200064.

Carlsson, A., Hillarp, N., 1958. On the State of the Catechol amines of the adrenal medullary granules. Acta Physiologica Scandinavica 44 (2), 163–169. https://doi.org/10.1111/j.1748-1716.1958.tb01618.x.

Carlsson, A., Lindqvist, M., Magnusson, T., 1957. 3,4-Dihydroxyphenylalanine and 5-hydroxytryptophan as reserpine antagonists [16]. Nature 180 (4596), 1200. https://doi.org/10.1038/1801200a0.

Ceravolo, R., Rossi, C., Del Prete, E., Bonuccelli, U., 2016. A review of adverse events linked to dopamine agonists in the treatment of Parkinson's disease. Expert Opinion on Drug Safety 15 (2), 181–198. https://doi.org/10.1517/14740338.2016.1130128.

Chaudhuri, K.R., Sauerbier, A., 2016. Parkinson disease: Unravelling the nonmotor mysteries of Parkinson disease. Nature Reviews Neurology 12 (1), 10–11. https://doi.org/10.1038/nrneurol.2015.236.

Chen, J.J., 2017. Treatment of psychotic symptoms in patients with Parkinson disease. Mental Health Clinician 7 (6), 262–270. https://doi.org/10.9740/mhc.2017.11.262.

Chen, J.J., Obering, C., 2005. A review of intermittent subcutaneous apomorphine injections for the rescue management of motor fluctuations associated with advanced Parkinson's disease. Clinical Therapeutics 27 (11), 1710–1724. https://doi.org/10.1016/j.clinthera.2005.11.016.

Chung, S.J., Calopa, M., Ceravolo, M.G., Tambasco, N., Antonini, A., Chaudhuri, K.R., Robieson, W.Z., Sánchez-Soliño, O., Zadikoff, C., Jin, M., Barbato, L.M., 2022. Effects of levodopa-carbidopa intestinal gel compared with optimized medical treatment on nonmotor symptoms in advanced Parkinson's Disease: INSIGHTS Study. Parkinson's Disease 2022. https://doi.org/10.1155/2022/1216975.

Cilia, R., Akpalu, A., Sarfo, F.S., Cham, M., Amboni, M., Cereda, E., Fabbri, M., Adjei, P., Akassi, J., Bonetti, A., Pezzoli, G., 2014. The modern pre-levodopa era of Parkinson's disease: Insights into motor complications from Sub-Saharan Africa. Brain 137 (10), 2731–2742. https://doi.org/10.1093/brain/awu195.

Claassen, D.O., van den Wildenberg, W.P.M., Ridderinkhof, K.R., Jessup, C.K., Harrison, M.B., Wooten, G.F., Wylie, S.A., 2011. The risky business of dopamine agonists in Parkinson disease and impulse control disorders. Behavioral Neuroscience 125 (4), 492–500. https://doi.org/10.1037/a0023795.

Cordivari, C., Misra, V.P., Catania, S., Lees, A.J., 2001. Treatment of dystonic clenched fist with botulinum toxin. Movement Disorders 16 (5), 907–913. https://doi.org/10.1002/mds.1186.

Cotzias, G.C., 1971. Levodopa in the treatment of parkinsonism. JAMA, the Journal of the American Medical Association 218 (13), 1903–1908. https://doi.org/10.1001/jama.1971.03190260019005.

Cotzias, G.C., Papavasiliou, P.S., Gellene, R., 1969. Modification of Parkinsonism–chronic treatment with L-dopa. New England Journal of Medicine 280 (7), 337–345. https://doi.org/10.1056/NEJM196902132800701.

Cotzias, G.C., Van Woert, M.H., Schiffer, L.M., 1967. Aromatic amino acids and modification of parkinsonism. New England Journal of Medicine 276 (7), 374–379. https://doi.org/10.1056/NEJM196702162760703.

de Bie, R.M.A., Katzenschlager, R., Swinnen, B.E.K.S., Peball, M., Lim, S.Y., Mestre, T.A., Perez Lloret, S., Coelho, M., Aquino, C., Tan, A.H., Bruno, V., Dijk, J.M., Heim, B., Lin, C.H., Kauppila, L.A., Litvan, I., Spijker, R., Seppi, K., Costa, J., Silverdale, M.A., 2025. Update on treatments for Parkinson's Disease motor fluctuations – An international parkinson and movement disorder Society evidence-based medicine review. Movement Disorders 40 (5), 776–794. https://doi.org/10.1002/mds.30162.

Deuschl, G., Schade-Brittinger, C., Krack, P., Volkmann, J., Schäfer, H., Bötzel, K., Daniels, C., Deutschländer, A., Ulrich, D., Eisner, W., Gruber, D., Hamel, W., Herzog, J., Hilker, R., Klebe, S., Kloß, M., Koy, J., Krause, M., Kupsch, A., Voges, J., 2006. A randomized trial of deep-brain stimulation for Parkinson's Disease. New England Journal of Medicine 355 (9), 896–908. https://doi.org/10.1056/nejmoa060281.

Dezsi, L., Vecsei, L., 2017. Monoamine oxidase B inhibitors in Parkinson's Disease. CNS & Neurological Disorders - Drug Targets 16 (4). https://doi.org/10.2174/1871527316666170124165222.

Driver-Dunckley, E., Samanta, J., Stacy, M., 2003. Pathological gambling associated with dopamine agonist therapy in Parkinson's disease. Neurology 61 (3), 422–423. https://doi.org/10.1212/01.wnl.0000076478.45005.ec.

Ecker, D., Unrath, A., Kassubek, J., Sabolek, M., 2009. Dopamine Agonists and their risk to induce psychotic episodes in Parkinson's disease: A case-control study. BMC Neurology 9 (1). https://doi.org/10.1186/1471-2377-9-23.

Eggert, K., Squillacote, D., Barone, P., Dodel, R., Katzenschlager, R., Emre, M., Lees, A.J., Rascol, O., Poewe, W., Tolosa, E., Trenkwalder, C., Onofrj, M., Stocchi, F., Nappi, G., Kostic, V., Potic, J., Ruzicka, E., Oertel, W., 2010. Safety and efficacy of perampanel in advanced Parkinson's disease: A randomized, placebo-controlled study. Movement Disorders 25 (7), 896–905. https://doi.org/10.1002/mds.22974.

Espay, A.J., Morgante, F., Merola, A., Fasano, A., Marsili, L., Fox, S.H., Bezard, E., Picconi, B., Calabresi, P., Lang, A.E., 2018. Levodopa-induced dyskinesia in Parkinson disease: Current and evolving concepts. Annals of Neurology 84 (6), 797–811. https://doi.org/10.1002/ana.25364.

Essam, M., Hamid, E., Abushady, E., El-Balkimy, M., Antonini, A., Ali, S., 2024. Role of zonisamide in advanced Parkinson's disease: A randomized placebo-controlled study. Neurological Sciences 45 (4), 1725–1734. https://doi.org/10.1007/s10072-024-07396-w.

Esselink, R.A.J., de Bie, R.M.A., de Haan, R.J., Steur, E.N.H.J., Beute, G.N., Portman, A.T., Schuurman, P.R., Bosch, D.A., Speelman, J.D., 2006. Unilateral pallidotomy versus bilateral subthalamic nucleus stimulation in Parkinson's disease: One year follow-up of a randomised observer-blind multi centre trial. Acta Neurochirurgica 148 (12), 1247–1255. https://doi.org/10.1007/s00701-006-0907-1.

Fénelon, G., Giménez-Roldán, S., Montastruc, J.L., Bermejo, F., Durif, F., Bourdeix, I., Péré, J.-J., Galiano, L., Schadrack, J., 2003. Efficacy and tolerability of entacapone in patients with Parkinson's disease treated with levodopa plus a dopamine agonist and experiencing wearing-off motor fluctuations. A randomized, double-blind, multicentre study. Journal of neural transmission (Vienna, Austria: 1996) 110 (3), 239–251.

Fahn, S., Oakes, D., Shoulson, I., Kieburtz, K., Rudolph, A., Marek, K., Seibyl, J., Lang, A., Olanow, C.W., Tanner, C., Schifitto, G., Zhao, H., Reyes, L., Shinaman, A., Comella, C., Goetz, C., Blasucci, L., Samanta, J., Stacy, M., Wernette, K., 2004. Levodopa and the progression of parkinson's disease. New England Journal of Medicine 351 (24), 2498–2508. https://doi.org/10.1056/NEJMoa033447.

Ferreira, J.J., Lees, A., Rocha, J.F., Poewe, W., Rascol, O., Soares-da-Silva, P., 2016. Opicapone as an adjunct to levodopa in patients with Parkinson's disease and end-of-dose motor fluctuations: A randomised, double-blind, controlled trial. The Lancet Neurology 15 (2), 154–165. https://doi.org/10.1016/S1474-4422(15)00336-1.

Fishman, P.S., 2008. Paradoxical aspects of parkinsonian tremor. Movement Disorders 23 (2), 168–173. https://doi.org/10.1002/mds.21736.

Fonoff, E.T., Azevedo, A., Dos Angelos, J.S., Martinez, R.C.R., Navarro, J., Reis, P.R., Sepulveda, M.E.S.M., Cury, R.G., Ghilardi, M.G.D.S., Teixeira, M.J., Lopez, W.O.C., 2016. Simultaneous bilateral stereotactic procedure for deep brain stimulation implants: A significant step for reducing operation time. Journal of Neurosurgery 125 (1), 85–89. https://doi.org/10.3171/2015.7.JNS151026.

Fox, S.H., Katzenschlager, R., Lim, S.Y., Barton, B., de Bie, R.M.A., Seppi, K., Coelho, M., Sampaio, C., 2018. International Parkinson and movement disorder society evidence-based medicine review: Update on treatments for the motor symptoms of Parkinson's disease. Movement Disorders 33 (8), 1248–1266. https://doi.org/10.1002/mds.27372.

Giladi, N.I.R., Meer, J., Honigman, S., 1994. The use of botulinum toxin to treat 'striatal' toes [2]. Journal of Neurology Neurosurgery and Psychiatry 57 (5), 659. https://doi.org/10.1136/jnnp.57.5.659.

Grosset, D.G., Cardoso, F., Lees, A., 2011. Dopamine agonists vs levodopa in impulse control disorders. Archives of Neurology 68 (4), 544–545. https://doi.org/10.1001/archneurol.2011.41.

Hattori, N., Mochizuki, H., Hasegawa, K., Nomoto, M., Uchida, E., Terahara, T., Okawa, K., Fukuta, H., 2020a. Ropinirole patch versus placebo, ropinirole extended-release tablet in advanced Parkinson's Disease. Movement Disorders 35 (9), 1565–1573. https://doi.org/10.1002/mds.28071.

Hattori, N., Nomoto, M., Kimura, T., Kikuchi, S., Enomoto, H., Yoshizawa, K., Tamaoka, A., Hatano, T., Murata, M., Hasegawa, K., Tanaka, K., Arahata, Y., Kanda, F., Kashihara, K., Yamamoto, M., Nishikawa, N., Tsuboi, Y., Ohya, Y., 2014. Sustained efficacy of apomorphine in Japanese patients with advanced Parkinson's disease. Parkinsonism & Related Disorders 20 (8), 819–823. https://doi.org/10.1016/j.parkreldis.2014.04.008.

Hattori, N., Takeda, A., Takeda, S., Nishimura, A., Kato, M., Mochizuki, H., Nagai, M., Takahashi, R., 2018. Efficacy and safety of adjunctive rasagiline in Japanese Parkinson's disease patients with wearing-off phenomena: A phase 2/3, randomized, double-blind, placebo-controlled, multicenter study. Parkinsonism & Related Disorders 53, 21–27. https://doi.org/10.1016/j.parkreldis.2018.04.025.

Hattori, N., Tsuboi, Y., Yamamoto, A., Sasagawa, Y., Nomoto, M., 2020b. Efficacy and safety of safinamide as an add-on therapy to L-DOPA for patients with Parkinson's disease: A randomized, double-blind, placebo-controlled, phase II/III study. Parkinsonism & Related Disorders 75, 17–23. https://doi.org/10.1016/j.parkreldis.2020.04.012.

Hauser, R.A., Hattori, N., Fernandez, H., Isaacson, S.H., Mochizuki, H., Rascol, O., Stocchi, F., Li, J., Mori, A., Nakajima, Y., Ristuccia, R., Lewitt, P., 2021. Efficacy of istradefylline, an adenosine A2A receptor antagonist, as adjunctive therapy to levodopa in Parkinson's Disease: A pooled analysis of 8 phase 2b/3 trials. Journal of Parkinson's Disease 11 (4), 1663–1675. https://doi.org/10.3233/jpd-212672.

Hauser, R.A., Hsu, A., Kell, S., Espay, A.J., Sethi, K., Stacy, M., Ondo, W., O'Connell, M., Gupta, S., 2013. Extended-release carbidopa-levodopa (IPX066) compared with immediate-release carbidopa-levodopa in patients with Parkinson's disease and motor fluctuations: A phase 3 randomised, double-blind trial. The Lancet Neurology 12 (4), 346–356. https://doi.org/10.1016/S1474-4422(13)70025-5.

Hauser, R.A., Hubble, J.P., Truong, D.D., 2003. Randomized trial of the adenosine A2A receptor antagonist istradefylline in advanced PD. Neurology 61 (3), 297–303. https://doi.org/10.1212/01.WNL.0000081227.84197.0B.

Hauser, R.A., McDermott, M.P., Messing, S., 2006. Factors associated with the development of motor fluctuations and dyskinesias in Parkinson disease. Archives of Neurology 63 (12), 1756–1760. https://doi.org/10.1001/archneur.63.12.1756.

Hauser, R.A., Shulman, L.M., Trugman, J.M., Roberts, J.W., Mori, A., Ballerini, R., Sussman, N.M., 2008. Study of istradefylline in patients with Parkinson's disease on levodopa with motor fluctuations. Movement Disorders 23 (15), 2177–2185. https://doi.org/10.1002/mds.22095.

Heinzel, S., Berg, D., Gasser, T., Chen, H., Yao, C., Postuma, R.B., 2019. Update of the MDS research criteria for prodromal Parkinson's disease. Movement Disorders 34 (10), 1464–1470. https://doi.org/10.1002/mds.27802.

Holloway, R., Marek, K., Biglan, K., Dick, A., Fahn, S., Julian-Baros, E., Kamp, C., Kieburtz, K., Lang, A., McDermott, M., Seibyl, J., Shinaman, A., Shoulson, I., Weiner, W., 2009. Long-term effect of initiating Pramipexole vs Levodopa in early Parkinson disease. Archives of Neurology 66 (5), 563–570. https://doi.org/10.1001/archneurol.2009.32.

Holloway, Shoulson, Fahn, Kieburtz, Lang, Marek, McDermott, Seibyl, Weiner, Musch, Kamp, Welsh, Shinaman, Pahwa, Barclay, Hubble, LeWitt, Miyasaki, Suchowersky, Stacy, Russell, Ford, Hammerstad, Riley, Standaert, Wooten, Factor, Jankovic, Atassi, Kurlan, Panisset, Rajput, Rodnitzky, Shults, Petsinger, Waters, Pfeiffer, Biglan, Borchert, Montgomery, Sutherland, Weeks, DeAngelis, Sime, Wood, Pantella, Harrigan, Fussell, Dillon, Alexander-Brown, Rainey, Tennis, Rost-Ruffner, Brown, Evans, Berry, Hall, Shirley, Dobson, Fontaine, Pfeiffer, Brocht, Bennett, Daigneault, Hodgeman, Connell, Ross, Richard, Watts, 2004. Pramipexole vs levodopa as initial treatment for Parkinson disease: A 4-year randomized controlled trial. Archives of Neurology 61, 1044–1053. https://doi.org/10.1001/archneur.61.7.1044.

Hung, S.W., Adeli, G.M., Arenovich, T., Fox, S.H., Lang, A.E., 2010. Patient perception of dyskinesia in Parkinson's disease. Journal of Neurology, Neurosurgery & Psychiatry 81 (10), 1112–1115. https://doi.org/10.1136/jnnp.2009.173286.

Hutton, J.T., Morris, J.L., Roman, G.C., Imke, S.C., Elias, J.W., 1988. Treatment of chronic Parkinson's Disease with controlled-release Carbidopa/Levodopa. Archives of Neurology 45 (8), 861–864. https://doi.org/10.1001/archneur.1988.00520320047014.

Jankovic, J., 2004. Botulinum toxin in clinical practice. Journal of Neurology, Neurosurgery & Psychiatry 75 (7), 951–957. https://doi.org/10.1136/jnnp.2003.034702.

Jankovic, J., 2008. Parkinson's disease: Clinical features and diagnosis. Journal of Neurology, Neurosurgery & Psychiatry 79 (4), 368–376. https://doi.org/10.1136/jnnp.2007.131045.

Kalia, L.V., Brotchie, J.M., Fox, S.H., 2013. Novel nondopaminergic targets for motor features of Parkinson's disease: Review of recent trials. Movement Disorders 28 (2), 131–144. https://doi.org/10.1002/mds.25273.

Karstaedt, P.J., Pincus, J.H., 1992. Protein redistribution diet remains effective in patients with fluctuating parkinsonism. Archives of Neurology 49 (2), 149–151. https://doi.org/10.1001/archneur.1992.00530260049018.

Kempster, P.A., Frankel, J.P., Stern, G.M., Lees, A.J., 1990. Comparison of motor response to apomorphine and levodopa in Parkinson's disease. Journal of Neurology, Neurosurgery and Psychiatry 53 (11), 1004–1007. https://doi.org/10.1136/jnnp.53.11.1004.

Kieburtz, 1997. Entacapone improves motor fluctuations in levodopa-treated Parkinson's disease patients. Annals of Neurology 42 (5), 747–755. https://doi.org/10.1002/ana.410420511.

Koller, W.C., Herbster, G., 1987. Adjuvant therapy of Parkinsonian tremor. Archives of Neurology 44 (9), 921–923. https://doi.org/10.1001/archneur.1987.00520210023013.

Kujawa, K., Leurgans, S., Raman, R., Blasucci, L., Goetz, C.G., 2000. Acute orthostatic hypotension when starting dopamine agonists in Parkinson's disease. Archives of Neurology 57 (10), 1461–1463. https://doi.org/10.1001/archneur.57.10.1461.

Kukkle, P.L., Garg, D., Merello, M., 2023. Continuous subcutaneous infusion delivery of apomorphine in Parkinson's Disease: A systematic review. Movement Disorders Clinical Practice 10 (9), 1253–1267. https://doi.org/10.1002/mdc3.13810.

Kuzuhara, S., 2001. Drug-induced psychotic symptoms in Parkinson's disease. Problems, management and dilemma. Journal of Neurology 248 (S3), 28–31. https://doi.org/10.1007/pl00007823.

Lange, L.M., Gonzalez-Latapi, P., Rajalingam, R., Tijssen, M.A.J., Ebrahimi-Fakhari, D., Gabbert, C., Ganos, C., Ghosh, R., Kumar, K.R., Lang, A.E., Rossi, M., van der Veen, S., van de Warrenburg, B., Warner, T., Lohmann, K., Klein, C., Marras, C., 2022. Nomenclature of genetic movement disorders: Recommendations of the international parkinson and movement disorder Society task force – An update. Movement Disorders 37 (5), 905–935. https://doi.org/10.1002/mds.28982.

Lees, A., Fahn, S., Eggert, K.M., Jankovic, J., Lang, A., Micheli, F., Maral Mouradian, M., Oertel, W.H., Olanow, C.W., Poewe, W., Rascol, O., Tolosa, E., Squillacote, D., Kumar, D., 2012. Perampanel, an AMPA antagonist, found to have no benefit in reducing "off" time in Parkinson's disease. Movement Disorders 27 (2), 284–288. https://doi.org/10.1002/mds.23983.

Lees, A.J., Ferreira, J., Rascol, O., Poewe, W., Rocha, J.F., McCrory, M., Soares-Da-Silva, P., 2017. Opicapone as adjunct to levodopa therapy in patients with Parkinson disease and motor fluctuations a randomized clinical trial. JAMA Neurology 74 (2), 197–206. https://doi.org/10.1001/jamaneurol.2016.4703.

Lees, A.J., Shaw, K.M., Stern, G.M., 1977. "Off period" dystonia and "on period" choreoathetosis in levodopa-treated patients with Parkinson's disease. The Lancet 310 (8046), 1034. https://doi.org/10.1016/s0140-6736(77)92939-7.

Lew, M.F., 2013. Rasagiline treatment effects on parkinsonian tremor. International Journal of Neuroscience 123 (12), 859–865. https://doi.org/10.3109/00207454.2013.812085.

Lew, M., Hauser, R., Isaacson, S., Ferreira, J., Serbin, M., Farahmand, K., Olson, K., Klepitskaya, O., Rocha, F., Soares-da-Silva, P., Liang, G., 2020. Efficacy of Opicapone Compared to Entacapone in Parkinson's Patients with Motor Fluctuations and ON Hoehn & Yahr ≤ 2.5: A Post Hoc Analysis of BIPARK-1 (4429). Neurology 94 (15_Suppl. ment). https://doi.org/10.1212/wnl.94.15_supplement.4429.

LeWitt, P.A., Guttman, M., Tetrud, J.W., Tuite, P.J., Mori, A., Chaikin, P., Sussman, N.M., 2008. Adenosine A2A receptor antagonist istradefylline (KW-6002) reduces off time in Parkinson's disease: A double-blind, randomized, multicenter clinical trial (6002-US-005). Annals of Neurology 63 (3), 295–302. https://doi.org/10.1002/ana.21315.

LeWitt, P.A., Lyons, K.E., Pahwa, R., 2007. Advanced Parkinson disease treated with rotigotine transdermal system: PREFER Study. Neurology 68 (16), 1262–1267. https://doi.org/10.1212/01.wnl.0000259516.61938.bb.

Li, D., Zhang, C., Gault, J., Wang, W., Liu, J., Shao, M., Zhao, Y., Zeljic, K., Gao, G., Sun, B., 2017. Remotely programmed deep brain stimulation of the bilateral subthalamic nucleus for the treatment of primary parkinson disease: A randomized controlled trial investigating the safety and efficacy of a novel deep brain stimulation System. Stereotactic and Functional Neurosurgery 95 (3), 174–182. https://doi.org/10.1159/000475765.

Lieberman, A., Olanow, C.W., Sethi, K., Swanson, P., Waters, C.H., Fahn, S., Hurtig, H., Yahr, M., 1998. A multicenter trial of ropinirole as adjunct treatment for Parkinson's disease. Neurology 51 (4), 1057–1062. https://doi.org/10.1212/wnl.51.4.1057.

Liu, J., Cooper, C.A., Weintraub, D., Dahodwala, N., 2019. Pharmacological treatment of apathy in Lewy body disorders: A systematic review. Parkinsonism & Related Disorders 60, 14–24. https://doi.org/10.1016/j.parkreldis.2018.11.002.

Luo, L., Andrews, H., Alcalay, R.N., Poyraz, F.C., Boehme, A.K., Goldman, J.G., Xie, T., Tuite, P., Henchcliffe, C., Hogarth, P., Amara, A.W., Frank, S., Sutherland, M., Kopil, C., Naito, A., Kang, U.J., 2019. Motor phenotype classification in moderate to advanced PD in BioFIND study. Parkinsonism & Related Disorders 65, 178–183. https://doi.org/10.1016/j.parkreldis.2019.06.017.

Möller, J.C., Oertel, W.H., Köster, J., Pezzoli, G., Provinciali, L., 2005. Long-term efficacy and safety of pramipexole in advanced Parkinson's disease: Results from a European multicenter trial. Movement Disorders 20 (5), 602–610. https://doi.org/10.1002/mds.20397.

Maher, S., Donlon, E., Mullane, G., Walsh, R., Lynch, T., Fearon, C., 2024. Treatment of apathy in parkinson's disease and implications for underlying pathophysiology. Journal of Clinical Medicine 13 (8), 2216. https://doi.org/10.3390/jcm13082216.

Mano, T., 2018. Camptocormia induced by a dopaminergic agonist. Clinical Neuropharmacology 41 (2), 70–72. https://doi.org/10.1097/wnf.0000000000000266.

Marconi, S., Zwingers, T., 2014. Comparative efficacy of selegiline versus rasagiline in the treatment of early Parkinson's disease. European Review for Medical and Pharmacological Sciences 18 (13), 1879–1882.

McCandless, P.J., Evans, B.J., Janssen, J., Selfe, J., Churchill, A., Richards, J., 2016. Effect of three cueing devices for people with Parkinson's disease with gait initiation difficulties. Gait & Posture 44, 7–11. https://doi.org/10.1016/j.gaitpost.2015.11.006.

Megna, M., Cortese, R., Dellomonaco, A., Bellomo, R., Salonna, I., Cristella, G., Ranieri, G., 2012. Pharmacological aspects and neurological speech therapy: Target of dysphony, dysarthria and Dysphagia. International Journal of Immunopathology and Pharmacology 25 (1_Suppl. l), 29–33. https://doi.org/10.1177/03946320120250s105.

Mehanna, R., Smilowska, K., Fleisher, J., Post, B., Hatano, T., Pimentel Piemonte, M.E., Kumar, K.R., McConvey, V., Zhang, B., Tan, E.K., Savica, R., Mehanna, R., Smilowska, K., Marras, C., Ross, O., Fleisher, J., McConvey, V., Wu, Y.R., Zhang, B., Salari, M., 2022. Age cutoff for early-onset Parkinson's

Disease: Recommendations from the international parkinson and movement disorder Society task force on early onset Parkinson's Disease. Movement Disorders Clinical Practice 9 (7), 869–878. https://doi.org/10.1002/mdc3.13523.

Mestre, T.A., Eberly, S., Tanner, C., Grimes, D., Lang, A.E., Oakes, D., Marras, C., 2018. Reproducibility of data-driven Parkinson's disease subtypes for clinical research. Parkinsonism & Related Disorders 56, 102–106. https://doi.org/10.1016/j.parkreldis.2018.07.009.

Millan, M.J., 2010. From the cell to the clinic: A comparative review of the partial D2/D3 receptor agonist and α2-adrenoceptor antagonist, piribedil, in the treatment of Parkinson's disease. Pharmacology & Therapeutics 128 (2), 229–273. https://doi.org/10.1016/j.pharmthera.2010.06.002.

Mizuno, Y., Abe, T., Hasegawa, K., Kuno, S., Kondo, T., Yamamoto, M., Nakashima, M., Kanazawa, I., 2007. Ropinirole is effective on motor function when used as an adjunct to levodopa in Parkinson's disease: STRONG study. Movement Disorders 22 (13), 1860–1865. https://doi.org/10.1002/mds.21313.

Mizuno, Y., Hasegawa, K., Kondo, T., Kuno, S., Yamamoto, M., Sakou, K., Shoji, M., Abe, T., Nomura, H., Maeda, T., Shintani, S., Tamaoka, A., Hirata, K., Hishida, R., Nakano, I., Okamoto, K., Asahina, M., Shimura, H., Hashida, H., Ishigaki, Y., 2010. Clinical efficacy of istradefylline (KW-6002) in Parkinson's disease: A randomized, controlled study. Movement Disorders 25 (10), 1437–1443. https://doi.org/10.1002/mds.23107Japan.

Mizuno, Y., Nomoto, M., Hasegawa, K., Hattori, N., Kondo, T., Murata, M., Takeuchi, M., Takahashi, M., Tomida, T., 2014. Rotigotine vs ropinirole in advanced stage Parkinson's disease: Adouble-blind study. Parkinsonism & Related Disorders 20 (12), 1388–1393. https://doi.org/10.1016/j.parkreldis.2014.10.005.

Mizuno, Y., Yamamoto, M., Kuno, S., Hasegawa, K., Hattori, N., Kagimura, T., Sarashina, A., Rascol, O., Schapira, A.H.V., Barone, P., Hauser, R.A., Poewe, W., 2012. Efficacy and safety of extended-versus immediate-release pramipexole in Japanese patients with advanced and L-dopa-undertreated Parkinson disease: A double-blind, randomized trial. Clinical Neuropharmacology 35 (4), 174–181. https://doi.org/10.1097/WNF.0b013e31825f77b9.

Mizuno, Y., Yanagisawa, N., Kuno, S., Yamamoto, M., Hasegawa, K., Origasa, H., Kowa, H., Tamaki, S., Koh, M., Kachi, T., Hazama, M., Kawamura, H., Nakamuro, K., Nakajima, A., Sunada, T., Yoshinaga, Y., Yamada, F., Moriwaka, B., Toyoshima, A., Mizuno, O., 2003. Randomized, double-blind study of pramipexole with placebo and bromocriptine in advanced Parkinson's disease. Movement Disorders 18 (10), 1149–1156. https://doi.org/10.1002/mds.10508.

Moore, T.J., Evans, W., Murray, D., 1998. Operative management of foot and ankle equinovarus associated with focal dystonia. Foot & Ankle International 19 (4), 229–231. https://doi.org/10.1177/107110079801900408.

Morishita, T., Katayama, Y., Kobayashi, K., Oshima, H., Fukaya, C., Yamamoto, T., 2008. Effect of subthalamic nucleus stimulation on severe striatal hand deformity in Parkinson's disease: A case report. Neuromodulation 11 (2), 124–127. https://doi.org/10.1111/j.1525-1403.2008.00153.x.

Murata, M., Hasegawa, K., Kanazawa, I., Aizawa, H., Kimura, T., Kikuchi, S., Baba, M., Chida, K., Hisanaga, K., Toyoshima, I., Kurita, K., Suzuki, Y., Yoshizawa, K., Shoji, S., Nakano, I., Hirata, K., Kamakura, K., Shimizu, T., Nogawa, S., Kawamura, M., 2007. Zonisamide improves motor function in Parkinson disease: A randomized, double-blind study. Neurology 68 (1), 45–50. https://doi.org/10.1212/01.wnl.0000250236.75053.16.

Murata, M., Hasegawa, K., Kanazawa, I., Fukasaka, J., Kochi, K., Shimazu, R., 2015. Zonisamide improves wearing-off in Parkinson's disease: A randomized, double-blind study. Movement Disorders 30 (10), 1343–1350. https://doi.org/10.1002/mds.26286.

Nalls, M.A., Blauwendraat, C., Vallerga, C.L., Heilbron, K., Bandres-Ciga, S., Chang, D., Tan, M., Kia, D.A., Noyce, A.J., Xue, A., Bras, J., Young, E., von Coelln, R., Simón-Sánchez, J., Schulte, C., Sharma, M., Krohn, L., Pihlstrøm, L., Siitonen, A., Zhang, F., 2019. Identification of novel risk loci, causal insights, and heritable risk for Parkinson's disease: A meta-analysis of genome-wide association studies. The Lancet Neurology 18 (12), 1091–1102. https://doi.org/10.1016/S1474-4422(19)30320-5.

Nomoto, M., Mizuno, Y., Kondo, T., Hasegawa, K., Murata, M., Takeuchi, M., Ikeda, J., Tomida, T., Hattori, N., 2014. Transdermal rotigotine in advanced Parkinson's disease: A randomized, double-blind, placebo-controlled trial. Journal of Neurology 261 (10), 1887–1893. https://doi.org/10.1007/s00415-014-7427-3.

Nyholm, D., 2012. Duodopa® treatment for advanced Parkinson's disease: A review of efficacy and safety. Parkinsonism & Related Disorders 18 (8), 916–929. https://doi.org/10.1016/j.parkreldis.2012.06.022.

Nyholm, D., Stepien, V., 2014. Levodopa fractionation in Parkinson's Disease. Journal of Parkinson's Disease 4 (1), 89–96. https://doi.org/10.3233/jpd-130244.

O'Suilleabhain, P.E., Dewey Jr., R.B., 2002. Contributions of dopaminergic drugs and disease severity to daytime sleepiness in parkinson disease. Archives of Neurology 59 (6), 986. https://doi.org/10.1001/archneur.59.6.986.

Odekerken, V.J.J., Boel, J.A., Schmand, B.A., de Haan, R.J., Figee, M., van den Munckhof, P., Richard Schuurman, P., de Bie, R.M.A., 2016. GPi vs STN deep brain stimulation for Parkinson disease. Neurology 86 (8), 755–761. https://doi.org/10.1212/WNL.0000000000002401.

Oertel, W., Eggert, K., Pahwa, R., Tanner, C.M., Hauser, R.A., Trenkwalder, C., Ehret, R., Azulay, J.P., Isaacson, S., Felt, L., Jean Stempien, M., 2017. Randomized, placebo-controlled trial of ADS-5102 (amantadine) extended-release capsules for levodopa-induced dyskinesia in Parkinson's disease (EASE LID 3). Movement Disorders 32 (12), 1701–1709. https://doi.org/10.1002/mds.27131.

Olanow, C.W., Factor, S.A., Espay, A.J., Hauser, R.A., Shill, H.A., Isaacson, S., Pahwa, R., Leinonen, M., Bhargava, P., Sciarappa, K., Navia, B., Blum, D., xx, x., 2020. Apomorphine sublingual film for off episodes in Parkinson's disease: A randomised, double-blind, placebo-controlled phase 3 study. The Lancet Neurology 19 (2), 135–144. https://doi.org/10.1016/S1474-4422(19)30396-5.

Olanow, C.W., Kieburtz, K., Odin, P., Espay, A.J., Standaert, D.G., Fernandez, H.H., Vanagunas, A., Othman, A. A., Widnell, K.L., Robieson, W.Z., Pritchett, Y., Chatamra, K., Benesh, J., Lenz, R.A., Antonini, A., 2014. Continuous intrajejunal infusion of levodopa-carbidopa intestinal gel for patients with advanced Parkinson's disease: A randomised, controlled, double-blind, double-dummy study. The Lancet Neurology 13 (2), 141–149. https://doi.org/10.1016/S1474-4422(13)70293-X.

Olanow, C.W., Rascol, O., Hauser, R., Feigin, P.D., Jankovic, J., Lang, A., Langston, W., Melamed, E., Poewe, W., Stocchi, F., Tolosa, E., 2009. A double-blind, delayed-start trial of rasagiline in Parkinson's disease. New England Journal of Medicine 361 (13), 1268–1278. https://doi.org/10.1056/NEJMoa0809335.

Ory-Magne, F., Corvol, J.-C., Azulay, J.-P., Bonnet, A.-M., Brefel-Courbon, C., Damier, P., Dellapina, E., Destee, A., Durif, F., Galitzky, M., Lebouvier, T., Meissner, W., Thalamas, C., Tison, F., Salis, A., Sommet, A., Viallet, F., Vidailhet, M., Rascol, O., 2014. Withdrawing amantadine in dyskinetic patients with Parkinson disease: The amandysk trial. Neurology 82 (4), 300–307. https://doi.org/10.1212/WNL.0000000000000050.

Pagonabarraga, J., Kulisevsky, J., Strafella, A.P., Krack, P., 2015. Apathy in Parkinson's disease: Clinical features, neural substrates, diagnosis, and treatment. The Lancet Neurology 14 (5), 518–531. https://doi.org/10.1016/S1474-4422(15)00019-8.

Pahwa, R., Stacy, M.A., Factor, S.A., Lyons, K.E., Stocchi, F., Hersh, B.P., Elmer, L.W., Truong, D.D., Earl, N.L., 2007. Ropinirole 24-hour prolonged release: Randomized, controlled study in advanced Parkinson disease. Neurology 68 (14), 1108–1115. https://doi.org/10.1212/01.wnl.0000258660.74391.c1.

Pahwa, R., Tanner, C.M., Hauser, R.A., Isaacson, S.H., Nausieda, P.A., Truong, D.D., Agarwal, P., Hull, K.L., Lyons, K.E., Johnson, R., Stempien, M.J., 2017. ADS-5102 (Amantadine) extended-release capsules for levodopa-induced dyskinesia in Parkinson Disease (EASE LID Study): A randomized clinical trial. JAMA Neurology 74 (8), 941–949. https://doi.org/10.1001/jamaneurol.2017.0943.

Papapetropoulos, S., Singer, C., 2006. Cervical dystonia as a presenting symptom of Parkinson's disease. Parkinsonism & Related Disorders 12 (8), 514–516. https://doi.org/10.1016/j.parkreldis.2006.05.031.

Papavasiliou, P.S., Cotzias, G.C., Düby, S.E., Steck, A.J., Fehling, C., Bell, M.A., 1972. Levodopa in parkinsonism: Potentiation of central effects with a peripheral inhibitor. New England Journal of Medicine 286 (1), 8–14. https://doi.org/10.1056/NEJM197201062860102.

Peretz, C., Segev, H., Rozani, V., Gurevich, T., El-Ad, B., Tsamir, J., Giladi, N., 2016. Comparison of selegiline and rasagiline therapies in parkinson disease: A real-life Study. Clinical Neuropharmacology 39 (5), 227–231. https://doi.org/10.1097/wnf.0000000000000167.

Pieper, N.T., Grossi, C.M., Chan, W.Y., Loke, Y.K., Savva, G.M., Haroulis, C., Steel, N., Fox, C., Maidment, I.D., Arthur, A.J., Myint, P.K., Smith, T.O., Robinson, L., Matthews, F.E., Brayne, C., Richardson, K., 2020. Anticholinergic drugs and incident dementia, mild cognitive impairment and cognitive decline: A meta-analysis. Age and Ageing 49 (6), 939–947. https://doi.org/10.1093/ageing/afaa090.

Pierantozzi, M., Pietroiusti, A., Brusa, L., Galati, S., Stefani, A., Lunardi, G., Fedele, E., Sancesario, G., Bernardi, G., Bergamaschi, A., Magrini, A., Stanzione, P., Galante, A., 2006. Helicobacter pylori eradication and l-dopa absorption in patients with PD and motor fluctuations. Neurology 66 (12), 1824–1829. https://doi.org/10.1212/01.wnl.0000221672.01272.ba.

Pirker, W., Katzenschlager, R., Hallett, M., Poewe, W., 2023. Pharmacological treatment of tremor in parkinson's disease revisited. Journal of Parkinson's Disease 13 (2), 127–144. https://doi.org/10.3233/jpd-225060.

Poewe, W., Antonini, A., 2015. Novel formulations and modes of delivery of levodopa. Movement Disorders 30 (1), 114–120. https://doi.org/10.1002/mds.26078.

Poewe, W.H., Deuschl, G., Gordin, A., Kultalahti, E.-R., Leinonen, M., 2002. Efficacy and safety of entacapone in Parkinson's disease patients with suboptimal Levodopa response: A 6-month randomized placebo-controlled double-blind study in Germany and Austria (Celomen study). Acta Neurologica Scandinavica 105 (4), 245–255. https://doi.org/10.1034/j.1600-0404.2002.1o174.x.

Poewe, W.H., Lees, A.J., Stern, G.M., 1986. Low-dose L-dopa therapy in parkinson's disease: A 6-year follow-up study. Neurology 36 (11), 1528–1530. https://doi.org/10.1212/wnl.36.11.1528.

Poewe, W.H., Lees, A.J., Stern, G.M., 1988. Dystonia in Parkinson'S disease: Clinical and pharmacological features. Annals of Neurology 23 (1), 73–78. https://doi.org/10.1002/ana.410230112.

Poewe, W.H., Rascol, O., Quinn, N., Tolosa, E., Oertel, W.H., Martignoni, E., Rupp, M., Boroojerdi, B., 2007. Efficacy of pramipexole and transdermal rotigotine in advanced Parkinson's disease: A double-blind, double-dummy, randomised controlled trial. Lancet Neurology 6 (6), 513–520. https://doi.org/10.1016/S1474-4422(07)70108-4.

Poewe, W., Seppi, K., Tanner, C.M., Halliday, G.M., Brundin, P., Volkmann, J., Schrag, A.E., Lang, A.E., 2017. Parkinson disease. Nature Reviews Disease Primers 3, 1–21. https://doi.org/10.1038/nrdp.2017.13.

Pourcher, E., Fernandez, H.H., Stacy, M., Mori, A., Ballerini, R., Chaikin, P., 2012. Istradefylline for Parkinson's disease patients experiencing motor fluctuations: Results of the KW-6002-US-018 study. Parkinsonism & Related Disorders 18 (2), 178–184. https://doi.org/10.1016/j.parkreldis.2011.09.023.

Prakash, K.M., Lang, A.E., 2007. Reversible dopamine agonist induced anterocollis in a multiple system atrophy patient [2]. Movement Disorders 22 (15), 2292–2293. https://doi.org/10.1002/mds.21729.

Pringsheim, T., Day, G.S., Smith, D.B., Rae-Grant, A., Licking, N., Armstrong, M.J., De Bie, R.M.A., Roze, E., Miyasaki, J.M., Hauser, R.A., Espay, A.J., Martello, J.P., Gurwell, J.A., Billinghurst, L., Sullivan, K., Fitts, M. S., Cothros, N., Hall, D.A., Rafferty, M., Lang, A.E., 2021. Dopaminergic therapy for motor symptoms in early Parkinson disease practice Guideline summary. Neurology 97 (20), 942–957. https://doi.org/10.1212/WNL.0000000000012868.

Pringsheim, T., Jette, N., Frolkis, A., Steeves, T.D.L., 2014. The prevalence of Parkinson's disease: A systematic review and meta-analysis. Movement Disorders 29 (13), 1583–1590. https://doi.org/10.1002/mds.25945.

Rana, A.Q., Kabir, A., Dogu, O., Patel, A., Khondker, S., 2012. Prevalence of blepharospasm and apraxia of eyelid opening in patients with parkinsonism, cervical dystonia and essential tremor. European Neurology 68 (5), 318–321. https://doi.org/10.1159/000341621.

Rascol, O., Brooks, D.J., Melamed, E., Oertel, W., Poewe, W., Stocchi, F., Tolosa, E., 2005. Rasagiline as an adjunct to levodopa in patients with Parkinson's disease and motor fluctuations (LARGO, lasting effect in Adjunct therapy with rasagiline Given Once daily, study): A randomised, double-blind, parallel-group trial. Lancet 365 (9463), 947–954. https://doi.org/10.1016/S0140-6736(05)71083-7.

Rascol, O., Fabbri, M., Werner, P., 2021. Amantadine in the treatment of Parkinson's disease and other movement disorders. The Lancet. Neurology 20 (12), 1048–1056.

Rascol, O., Lees, A.J., Senard, J.M., Pirtosek, Z., Montastruc, J.L., Fuell, D., 1996. Ropinirole in the treatment of levodopa-induced motor fluctuations in patients with Parkinson's Disease. Clinical Neuropharmacology 19 (3), 234–245. https://doi.org/10.1097/00002826-199619030-00005.

Reeve, A., Simcox, E., Turnbull, D., 2014. Ageing and Parkinson's disease: Why is advancing age the biggest risk factor? Ageing Research Reviews 14 (1), 19–30. https://doi.org/10.1016/j.arr.2014.01.004.

Reichmann, H., Boas, J., MacMahon, D., Myllyla, V., Hakala, A., Reinikainen, K., 2005. Efficacy of combining levodopa with entacapone on quality of life and activities of daily living in patients experiencing wearing-off type fluctuations. Acta Neurologica Scandinavica 111 (1), 21–28. https://doi.org/10.1111/j.1600-0404.2004.00363.x.

Riley, D., Lang, A.E., 1988. Practical application of a low-protein diet for Parkinson's disease. Neurology 38 (7), 1026–1031. https://doi.org/10.1212/wnl.38.7.1026.

Rinne, U.K., Larsen, J.P., Siden, A., Worm-Petersen, J., 1998. Entacapone enhances the response to levodopa in parkinsonian patients with motor fluctuations. Neurology 51 (5), 1309–1314. https://doi.org/10.1212/WNL.51.5.1309.

Rizos, A., Martinez-Martin, P., Odin, P., Antonini, A., Kessel, B., Kozul, T.K., Todorova, A., Douiri, A., Martin, A., Stocchi, F., Dietrichs, E., Chaudhuri, K.R., 2014. Characterizing motor and non-motor aspects of early-morning off periods in Parkinson's disease: An international multicenter study. Parkinsonism & Related Disorders 20 (11), 1231–1235. https://doi.org/10.1016/j.parkreldis.2014.09.013.

Savica, R., Grossardt, B.R., Bower, J.H., Eric Ahlskog, J., Rocca, W.A., 2016. Time trends in the incidence of parkinson disease. JAMA Neurology 73 (8), 981–989. https://doi.org/10.1001/jamaneurol.2016.0947.

Savica, R., Turcano, P., Bower, J.H., Ahlskog, J.E., Mielke, M.M., 2019. Survival and progression in synucleinopathy phenotypes with parkinsonism: A population-based Study. Mayo Clinic Proceedings 94 (9), 1825–1831. https://doi.org/10.1016/j.mayocp.2019.04.010.

Schüpbach, W.M.M., Maltête, D., Houeto, J.L., Du Montcel, S.T., Mallet, L., Welter, M.L., Gargiulo, M., Béhar, C., Bonnet, A.M., Czernecki, V., Pidoux, B., Navarro, S., Dormont, D., Cornu, P., Agid, Y., 2007. Neurosurgery at an earlier stage of Parkinson disease: A randomized, controlled trial. Neurology 68 (4), 267–271. https://doi.org/10.1212/01.wnl.0000250253.03919.fb.

Schapira, A.H.V., 2007. Treatment options in the modern management of Parkinson disease. Archives of Neurology 64 (8), 1083–1088. https://doi.org/10.1001/archneur.64.8.1083.

Schapira, A.H.V., Barone, P., Hauser, R.A., Mizuno, Y., Rascol, O., Busse, M., Salin, L., Juhel, N., Poewe, W., 2011. Extended-release pramipexole in advanced Parkinson disease: A randomized controlled trial. Neurology 77 (8), 767–774. https://doi.org/10.1212/WNL.0b013e31822affdb.

Schapira, A.H.V., Fox, S.H., Hauser, R.A., Jankovic, J., Jost, W.H., Kenney, C., Kulisevsky, J., Pahwa, R., Poewe, W., Anand, R., 2017. Assessment of safety and efficacy of safinamide as a levodopa adjunct in patients with Parkinson disease and motor fluctuations a randomized clinical trial. JAMA Neurology 74 (2), 216–224. https://doi.org/10.1001/jamaneurol.2016.4467.

Schapira, A.H.V., McDermott, M.P., Barone, P., Comella, C.L., Albrecht, S., Hsu, H.H., Massey, D.H., Mizuno, Y., Poewe, W., Rascol, O., Marek, K., 2013. Pramipexole in patients with early Parkinson's disease (PROUD): A randomised delayed-start trial. The Lancet Neurology 12 (8), 747–755. https://doi.org/10.1016/S1474-4422(13)70117-0.

Schrag, A., 2005. Entacapone in the treatment of Parkinson's disease. The Lancet Neurology 4 (6), 366–370. https://doi.org/10.1016/s1474-4422(05)70098-3.

Schrag, A., Quinn, N., 2000. Dyskinesias and motor fluctuations in Parkinson's disease: A community-based study. Brain 123 (11), 2297–2305. https://doi.org/10.1093/brain/123.11.2297.

Schrag, A., Schelosky, L., Scholz, U., Poewe, W., 1999. Reduction of parkinsonian signs in patients with Parkinson's disease by dopaminergic versus anticholinergic single-dose challenges. Movement Disorders 14 (2), 252–255. https://doi.org/10.1002/1531-8257(199903)14:2<252::AID-MDS1009>3.0.CO;2-N.

Schuepbach, W.M.M., Rau, J., Knudsen, K., Volkmann, J., Krack, P., Timmermann, L., Hälbig, T.D., Hesekamp, H., Navarro, S.M., Meier, N., Falk, D., Mehdorn, M., Paschen, S., Maarouf, M., Barbe, M.T., Fink, G.R., Kupsch, A., Gruber, D., Schneider, G.-H., Deuschl, G., 2013. Neurostimulation for Parkinson's Disease with early motor complications. New England Journal of Medicine 368 (7), 610–622. https://doi.org/10.1056/NEJMoa1205158.

Schwid, S.R., 2005. A randomized placebo-controlled trial of rasagiline in levodopa-treated patients with Parkinson disease and motor fluctuations: The PRESTO study. Archives of Neurology 62 (2), 241–248. https://doi.org/10.1001/archneur.62.2.241.

Segura-Aguilar, J., Paris, I., Muñoz, P., Ferrari, E., Zecca, L., Zucca, F.A., 2014. Protective and toxic roles of dopamine in Parkinson's disease. Journal of Neurochemistry 129 (6), 898–915. https://doi.org/10.1111/jnc.12686.

Shadrina, M.I., Slominsky, P.A., 2023. Genetic Architecture of parkinson's disease. Biochemistry (Moscow) 88 (3), 417–433. https://doi.org/10.1134/S0006297923030100.

Sinha, N., Manohar, S., Husain, M., 2013. Impulsivity and apathy in Parkinson's disease. Journal of Neuropsychology 7 (2), 255–283. https://doi.org/10.1111/jnp.12013.

Soileau, M.J., Aldred, J., Budur, K., Fisseha, N., Fung, V.S., Jeong, A., Kimber, T.E., Klos, K., Litvan, I., O'Neill, D., Robieson, W.Z., Spindler, M.A., Standaert, D.G., Talapala, S., Vaou, E.O., Zheng, H., Facheris, M.F., Hauser, R.A., 2022. Safety and efficacy of continuous subcutaneous foslevodopa-foscarbidopa in patients with advanced Parkinson's disease: A randomised, double-blind, active-controlled, phase 3 trial. The Lancet Neurology 21 (12), 1099–1109. https://doi.org/10.1016/S1474-4422(22)00400-8.

Stacy, M., Silver, D., Mendis, T., Sutton, J., Mori, A., Chaikin, P., Sussman, N.M., 2008. A 12-week, placebo-controlled study (6002-US-006) of istradefylline in Parkinson disease. Neurology 70 (23), 2233–2240. https://doi.org/10.1212/01.wnl.0000313834.22171.17.

Stocchi, F., Antonini, A., Barone, P., Tinazzi, M., Zappia, M., Onofrj, M., Ruggieri, S., Morgante, L., Bonuccelli, U., Lopiano, L., Pramstaller, P., Albanese, A., Attar, M., Posocco, V., Colombo, D., Abbruzzese, G., 2014. DEEP study group, Early DEtection of wEaring off in Parkinson disease: The DEEP study. Parkinsonism & Related Disorders 20 (2), 204–211. https://doi.org/10.1016/j.parkreldis.2013.10.027.

Stocchi, F., Rascol, O., Kieburtz, K., Poewe, W., Jankovic, J., Tolosa, E., Barone, P., Lang, A.E., Olanow, C.W., 2010. Initiating levodopa/carbidopa therapy with and without entacapone in early Parkinson disease: The STRIDE-PD study. Annals of Neurology 68 (1), 18–27. https://doi.org/10.1002/ana.22060Italy.

Stowe, R.L., Ives, N.J., Clarke, C., Van Hilten, J., Ferreira, J., Hawker, R.J., Shah, L., Wheatley, K., Gray, R., 2008. Dopamine agonist therapy in early Parkinson's disease. Cochrane Database of Systematic Reviews (2). https://doi.org/10.1002/14651858.CD006564.pub2.

Takeda, A., Takahashi, R., Tsuboi, Y., Nomoto, M., Maeda, T., Nishimura, A., Yoshida, K., Hattori, N., 2021. Randomized, controlled Study of opicapone in Japanese parkinson's patients with motor fluctuations. Movement Disorders 36 (2), 415–423. https://doi.org/10.1002/mds.28322.

Tedeschi, G., Sasso, E., Marshall, R.W., Bonavita, V., 1990. Tremor in Parkinson disease: Acute response to oral levodopa. The Italian Journal of Neurological Sciences 11 (3), 259–263. https://doi.org/10.1007/bf02333855.

Tosserams, A., Fasano, A., Gilat, M., Factor, S.A., Giladi, N., Lewis, S.J.G., Moreau, C., Bloem, B.R., Nieuwboer, A., Nonnekes, J., 2025. Management of freezing of gait — Mechanism-based practical recommendations. Nature Reviews Neurology 21 (6), 327–344. https://doi.org/10.1038/s41582-025-01079-6.

Trenkwalder, C., Kies, B., Rudzinska, M., Fine, J., Nikl, J., Honczarenko, K., Dioszeghy, P., Hill, D., Anderson, T., Myllyla, V., Kassubek, J., Steiger, M., Zucconi, M., Tolosa, E., Werner, P., Surmann, E., Whitesides, J., Boroojerdi, B., Kallol Ray Chaudhuri, the RECOVER Study Group, 2011. Rotigotine effects on early morning motor function and sleep in Parkinson's disease: A double-blind, randomized, placebo-controlled study (RECOVER). Movement Disorders 26 (1), 90–99. https://doi.org/10.1002/mds.23441.

Umemura, A., Oka, Y., Ohkita, K., Yamawaki, T., Yamada, K., 2010. Effect of subthalamic deep brain stimulation on postural abnormality in Parkinson disease. Journal of Neurosurgery 112 (6), 1283–1288. https://doi.org/10.3171/2009.10.jns09917.

Van De Warrenburg, B.P.C., Cordivari, C., Ryan, A.M., Phadke, R., Holton, J.L., Bhatia, K.P., Hanna, M.G., Quinn, N.P., 2007. The phenomenon of disproportionate antecollis in Parkinson's disease and multiple system atrophy. Movement Disorders 22 (16), 2325–2331. https://doi.org/10.1002/mds.21634.

Van Gerpen, J.A., Kumar, N., Bower, J.H., Weigand, S., Ahlskog, J.E., 2006. Levodopa-associated dyskinesia risk among Parkinson disease patients in Olmsted County, Minnesota, 1976-1990. Archives of Neurology 63 (2), 205–209. https://doi.org/10.1001/archneur.63.2.205.

Verschuur, C.V.M., Suwijn, S.R., Boel, J.A., Post, B., Bloem, B.R., Van Hilten, J.J., Van Laar, T., Tissingh, G., Munts, A.G., Deuschl, G., Lang, A.E., Dijkgraaf, M.G.W., De Haan, R.J., De Bie, R.M.A., 2019. Randomized delayed-start trial of levodopa in Parkinson's disease. New England Journal of Medicine 380 (4), 315–324. https://doi.org/10.1056/NEJMoa1809983.

Villafane, G., Thiriez, C., Audureau, E., Straczek, C., Kerschen, P., Cormier-Dequaire, F., Van Der Gucht, A., Gurruchaga, J.-M., Quéré-Carne, M., Evangelista, E., Paul, M., Defer, G., Damier, P., Remy, P., Itti, E., Fénelon, G., 2018. High-dose transdermal nicotine in Parkinson's disease patients: A randomized, open-label, blinded-endpoint evaluation phase 2 study. European Journal of Neurology 25 (1), 120–127. https://doi.org/10.1111/ene.13474.

Vitek, J.L., Jain, R., Chen, L., Tröster, A.I., Schrock, L.E., House, P.A., Giroux, M.L., Hebb, A.O., Farris, S.M., Whiting, D.M., Leichliter, T.A., Ostrem, J.L., San Luciano, M., Galifianakis, N., Verhagen Metman, L., Sani, S., Karl, J.A., Siddiqui, M.S., Tatter, S.B., Starr, P.A., 2020. Subthalamic nucleus deep brain stimulation with a multiple independent constant current-controlled device in Parkinson's disease (INTREPID): A multicentre, double-blind, randomised, sham-controlled study. The Lancet Neurology 19 (6), 491–501. https://doi.org/10.1016/S1474-4422(20)30108-3.

Vokurka, P., Barron, A., Sumaria, S., Stockford, L., Jarman, P., Bhatia, K., Farmer, S., Saifee, T., Warner, T., Weil, R., Gandhi, S., Limousin, P., Korlipara, P., Foltynie, T., 2020. Opicapone efficacy and tolerability in Parkinson's Disease patients reporting insufficient Benefit/Failure of entacapone. Movement Disorders Clinical Practice 7 (8), 955–960. https://doi.org/10.1002/mdc3.13094.

von Coelln, R., Raible, A., Gasser, T., Asmus, F., 2008. Ultrasound-guided injection of the iliopsoas muscle with botulinum toxin in camptocormia. Movement Disorders 23 (6), 889–892. https://doi.org/10.1002/mds.21967.

Weaver, F.M., Follett, K.A., Stern, M., Luo, P., Harris, C.L., Hur, K., Marks, W.J., Rothlind, J., Sagher, O., Moy, C., Pahwa, R., Burchiel, K., Hogarth, P., Lai, E.C., Duda, J.E., Holloway, K., Samii, A., Horn, S., Bronstein, J.M., Reda, D.J., 2012. Randomized trial of deep brain stimulation for Parkinson disease: Thirty-six-month outcomes. Neurology 79 (1), 55–65. https://doi.org/10.1212/WNL.0b013e31825dcdc1.

Wei, Q., Tan, Y., Xu, P., Tao, E., Lu, Z., Pan, X., Wang, B., Liu, C., Dong, X., Tian, Y., Sun, X., Cattaneo, C., Chen, S., Shang, H., Chen, S., Shang, H., Tao, E., Liu, C., Wu, Y., Pan, X., 2022. The XINDI Study: A randomized phase III clinical trial evaluating the efficacy and safety of safinamide as Add-On therapy to levodopa in Chinese patients with parkinson's disease with motor fluctuations. CNS Drugs 36 (11), 1217–1227. https://doi.org/10.1007/s40263-022-00958-6.

Weintraub, D., Siderowf, A.D., Potenza, M.N., Goveas, J., Morales, K.H., Duda, J.E., Moberg, P.J., Stern, M.B., 2006. Association of dopamine agonist use with impulse control disorders in Parkinson disease. Archives of Neurology 63 (7), 969–973. https://doi.org/10.1001/archneur.63.7.969.

Weiss, H.D., Adler, S., 2014. Management of psychosis in Parkinson disease. Psychiatric Times 31 (4).

Wickremaratchi, M.M., Knipe, M.D.W., Sastry, B.S.D., Morgan, E., Jones, A., Salmon, R., Weiser, R., Moran, M., Davies, D., Ebenezer, L., Raha, S., Robertson, N.P., Butler, C.C., Ben-Shlomo, Y., Morris, H.R., 2011. The motor phenotype of Parkinson's disease in relation to age at onset. Movement Disorders 26 (3), 457–463. https://doi.org/10.1002/mds.23469.

Willis, A.W., Roberts, E., Beck, J.C., Fiske, B., Ross, W., Savica, R., Van Den Eeden, S.K., Tanner, C.M., Marras, C., Alcalay, R., Schwarzschild, M., Racette, B., Chen, H., Church, T., Wilson, B., Doria, J.M., 2022. Incidence of Parkinson disease in North America. Npj Parkinson's Disease 8 (1). https://doi.org/10.1038/s41531-022-00410-y.

Wolters, E.C., Horstink, M.W.I.M., Roos, R.A.C., Jansen, E.N.H., 1992. Clinical efficacy of sinemet CR 50/200 versus sinemet 25/100 in patients with fluctuating Parkinson'S disease. An open, and a double-blind, double-dummy, multicenter treatment evaluation. Clinical Neurology and Neurosurgery 94 (3), 205. https://doi.org/10.1016/0303-8467(92)90090-P.

Wolters, E.C., Tesselaar, H.J., 1996. International (NL-UK) double-blind study of Sinemet CR and standard Sinemet (25/100) in 170 patients with fluctuating Parkinson's disease. Journal of neurology 243 (3), 235–240.

Wong, K.S., Lu, C.S., Shan, D.E., Yang, C.C., Tsoi, T.H., Mok, V., 2003. Efficacy, safety, and tolerability of pramipexole in untreated and levodopa-treated patients with Parkinson's disease. Journal of the Neurological Sciences 216 (1), 81–87. https://doi.org/10.1016/S0022-510X(03)00217-X.

Yang, L.P.H., Perry, C.M., 2009. Zonisamide: In Parkinsons disease. CNS Drugs 23 (8), 703–711. https://doi.org/10.2165/00023210-200923080-00007.

Yoon, W.T., Chung, E.J., Lee, S.H., Kim, B.J., Lee, W.Y., 2005. Clinical analysis of blepharospasm and apraxia of eyelid opening in patients with parkinsonism. Journal of Clinical Neurology 1 (2), 159. https://doi.org/10.3988/jcn.2005.1.2.159.

Zesiewicz, T.A., Chriscoe, S., Jimenez, T., Upward, J., Davy, M., VanMeter, S., 2017. A randomized, fixed-dose, dose-response study of ropinirole prolonged release in advanced Parkinson's disease. Neurodegenerative Disease Management 7 (1), 61–72. https://doi.org/10.2217/nmt-2016-0038.

Zhang, Z., Wang, J., Chen, S., Liu, C., Zhang, B., Peng, R., Sun, S., Sun, X., Zhao, G., Qu, Q., Li, Y., Zhu, S., Pan, X., Shao, M., Wang, Y., 2018. Efficacy and safety of rasagiline in Chinese patients with early Parkinson's disease: A randomized, double-blind, parallel, placebo-controlled, fixed-dose study. Translational Neurodegeneration 7 (1). https://doi.org/10.1186/s40035-018-0137-5.

Zhang, Z., Wang, J., Zhang, X., Chen, S., Wang, Z., Zhang, B., Liu, C., Qu, Q., Cheng, Y., Li, J., Cao, H., Cai, M., Zhu, R., 2013. The efficacy and safety of ropinirole prolonged release tablets as adjunctive therapy in Chinese subjects with advanced Parkinson's disease: A multicenter, double-blind, randomized, placebo-controlled study. Parkinsonism & Related Disorders 19 (11), 1022–1026. https://doi.org/10.1016/j.parkreldis.2013.07.009.

Zhou, Z.D., Yi, L.X., Wang, D.Q., Lim, T.M., Tan, E.K., 2023. Role of dopamine in the pathophysiology of Parkinson's disease. Translational Neurodegeneration 12 (1). https://doi.org/10.1186/s40035-023-00378-6.

CHAPTER

12 Non-motor symptoms of parkinson's disease and their pharmacological management

Shaimaa El-Jaafary
Cairo University, Cairo, Egypt

12.1 Introduction

Parkinson's disease (PD) has been classically described as a motor disorder, with the hallmark characteristic symptoms being bradykinesia, resting tremor, muscular rigidity, and postural instability. These motor features, along with their typically favorable response to dopaminergic therapy such as levodopa (L-dopa), have long served as the cornerstone for clinical diagnosis. However, a deeper understanding of the disease's complexity increasingly challenges this motor-centric view (Simonet et al., 2021).

Now Parkinson's disease is recognized as a heterogonous syndrome of motor and non-motor symptoms (NMS) (Ray Chaudhuri et al., 2019; Marinus et al., 2018). These non-motor symptoms reflect a multisystem pathology, that can either precede the onset of motor symptoms in the prodromal phase, progress over the course of the disease or appear and advance in the late stages with a higher burden (Sardar et al., 2023; Rukavina et al., 2021). This shift has brought more focus on the non-motor symptoms of Parkinson's disease, leading to extensive research, especially in the early stages of the disease (Radad et al., 2023).

The identification of the NMS is highly appreciated and should be screened in every patient with PD at any stage, as these symptoms increase the disease burden both socially and financially and impair the quality of life of the affected individuals (Schapira et al., 2017). Recognizing prodromal non-motor symptoms early on is crucial for mitigating disease progression, improving patient outcomes, and enhancing their quality of life. The task is also challenging in the era of developing disease-modifying therapies for PD with the continuous search for prodromal biomarkers (Li et al., 2024).

Some recent reports highlight sex-based differences in non-motor symptoms (NMS) associated with Parkinson's disease (PD). Depression, fatigue, pain, and sleep disturbances tend to be more prevalent and more severe in females, whereas male patients more frequently exhibit hypersexuality and sexual dysfunction (Santos-García et al., 2023; Kang et al., 2022; Maas et al., 2024). It was also reported that NMS burden is greater in women compared to men, with higher non-motor fluctuations (Picillo et al., 2017). Further research is needed to determine the factors that contribute to these sex differences, like hormonal differences and environmental exposures (Goldman, 2025; Murueta-Goyena et al., 2025).

Pharmacological Foundations of Parkinson's Disease. https://doi.org/10.1016/B978-0-443-27702-3.00019-4

The aim of this chapter is to give a comprehensive overview of the non-motor functions of Parkinson's disease, discuss their clinical implications for the management and quality of life of the patients, and review current and future therapeutic options to reduce the burden of these symptoms.

12.2 Classification of non-motor symptoms in parkinson's disease and their prevalence

The non-motor manifestations can be grouped into neuropsychiatric symptoms, autonomic dysfunction, disorders of sleep and wakefulness, and sensory manifestations (Seppi et al., 2019). The neuropsychiatric manifestations primarily include depression, anxiety, apathy, psychosis, impulse control disorders, dementia, and mild cognitive impairment, which is a form of cognitive impairment that does not involve dementia. The autonomic dysfunction includes drooling, excessive sweating, orthostatic hypotension, gastrointestinal dysfunction, urinary impairment, and erectile dysfunction. Disorders of sleep and wakefulness manifest as rapid eye movement, sleep behavior disorder (RBD), sleep fragmentation, insomnia, and excessive daytime sleepiness. Sensory manifestations include mainly olfactory dysfunction, ophthalmologic dysfunction, pain, and fatigue (Goldman, 2025; Seppi et al., 2019).

Regarding the prevalence of NMS, olfactory dysfunction occurs in 90% of early-stage PD cases. Neuropsychiatric manifestations include depression in 40%–55% of cases; it can occur in the early stage and advances with the disease progression. Anxiety is in 20%–40%; psychosis can be detected in 20%–70%. Apathy is present in 39.8%. Sleep disorders: some are early manifestations, while others appear later in the disease course. RBD is a prodromal symptom that can occur in 23.6% of patients and manifest even decades before the motor symptoms. Insomnia and EDS each occur in about 55% of cases. Fatigue is a common symptom that can be manifested in 33%–80% of cases. Cognitive impairment: SCS 28.1%, MCI 25%–30%, PDD 90%, Autonomic dysfunctions: Constipation is a common symptoms that is also considered a prodromal marker, that occur decades before the motor onset in 5%–80% of PD, OH 30%–40%, Bladder disturbances 50%, Sexual dysfunction 68% in men and 53% in women, Gastrointestinal disturbances Sialorrhea (10%–84%), dysphagia (11%–81%), gastroparesis (70%–100%), Small intestine bacterial overgrowth (54%–67%), Pain is also common in about 30%–50% (Radad et al., 2023)

12.3 Pathophysiology of non-motor symptoms

The symptom profile observed in Parkinson's disease (PD)—including hyposmia, constipation, rapid eye movement sleep behavior disorder (RBD), autonomic dysfunction, and neuropsychiatric manifestations such as depression and anxiety—reflects its multisystemic nature. Such clinical heterogeneity has urged researchers to investigate extranigral regions as potential sites of early PD pathology. Neuropathological studies unravel the origins of PD-related neurodegeneration in extranigral regions (Schapira et al., 2017). As explained by Braak and colleagues (Braak et al., 2003), Lewy bodies, which are α-synuclein pathology, were shown to be deposited in the olfactory bulb, the dorsal motor nucleus of the vagus, and autonomic ganglia in the early stages of disease progression. The hypothesis provided insights into why hyposmia, REM sleep behavior disorder, and autonomic failure frequently manifest decades before motor symptoms. However, it could not further explain the progression of non-motor symptoms (NMS) and their correlation with the severity of motor symptoms; such evidence indicates that the Braak staging model requires additional validation through clinical research (Ray Chaudhuri et al., 2023).

The recently proposed α-Synuclein Origin and Connectome (SOC) Model by Borghammer (2021) introduces a compelling framework for understanding the heterogeneity of Parkinson's disease (PD). This model delineates two distinct phenotypes—brain-firstandbody-first—based on the initial site of α-synuclein pathology and the symmetry of motor symptoms.

The brain-first phenotype is thought to originate within subcortical brain regions, such as the olfactory bulb or amygdala. Clinically, this subtype is associated with asymmetric motor symptoms, lateralized dopaminergic denervation, and a slower progression of both motor and cognitive decline. Patients with this phenotype typically exhibit fewer autonomic disturbances, less REM sleep behavior disorder, and milder hyposmia, suggesting a more localized and gradual disease spread.

In contrast, the body-first phenotype is hypothesized to begin in the enteric nervous system, with pathology ascending via the vagus nerve to the brain. This subtype is characterized by symmetrical motor symptoms, more widespread dopaminergic degeneration, and a faster disease progression, particularly in terms of cognitive decline and autonomic dysfunction. Non-motor symptoms such as constipation, sleep disturbances, and anxiety often precede motor signs in these patients, highlighting the importance of early recognition and intervention.

This dual-pathway model has gained significant traction recently, as it offers a biologically plausible explanation for the variability in symptom presentation and progression among PD patients. Moreover, it underscores the critical role of non-motor symptoms not only in diagnosis but also in stratifying patients for personalized therapeutic approaches. The SOC model is increasingly supported by imaging studies, postmortem analyses, and longitudinal clinical data, reflecting a paradigm shift in PD research toward a more holistic understanding of disease mechanisms (Voruz et al., 2025).

Parkinson's disease (PD) also affects multiple non-dopaminergic neurotransmitter systems. These transmitters include the cholinergic, adenosinergic, glutamatergic, GABAergic, noradrenergic, serotonergic, and histaminergic systems (Kalia et al., 2013).

There is a great overlap between the molecular hallmarks of brain aging (such as oxidative stress, mitochondrial dysfunction, impaired protein homeostasis, neuroinflammation, genomic instability, and defective stress responses) and the key mechanisms driving neurodegeneration in Parkinson's disease (PD). Age-related deterioration in these pathways increases neuronal susceptibility to environmental and genetic risk factors associated with PD, thereby amplifying cellular dysfunction and promoting the accumulation of pathological α-synuclein (Coleman & Ian, 2022).

Aging plays a pivotal role in the pathogenesis of Parkinson's disease (PD), particularly due to the vulnerability of dopaminergic neurons in the substantia nigra. These neurons are metabolically demanding due to their extensive axonal arborization and sustained activity, which makes them susceptible to age-related mitochondrial dysfunction, impaired protein turnover, and oxidative stress. The accumulation of toxic dopamine metabolites exacerbates this cellular stress, ultimately disrupting neuronal homeostasis. Other mechanisms included changes in the immune system and deterioration of the blood-brain barrier with age, as explained by the authors in their review (Kalia et al., 2013).

In the pathogenesis of NMS, we concluded that impairments in both dopaminergic and non-dopaminergic pathways are the major contributors. This is why some non-motor symptoms (NMS), such as pain and depression, respond to dopamine treatment, particularly when they fluctuate and become more pronounced during the off state; in contrast, symptoms like orthostatic hypotension and dopamine dysregulation syndrome worsen with dopamine therapy (Janz et al., 2024). Therefore, it's crucial to identify the NMS in every patient with PD to assure proper management.

12.4 Screening and assessment of non-motor symptoms (NMS)

Proper screening and assessment of NMS in patients with PD becomes crucial for adequate management and patient stratification. Some specific tools are validated and available even in different languages for this purpose. The Unified Parkinson's Disease Rating Scale (UPDRS) includes a few items for NMS, but its application is limited (Disease, 2003). Additionally, the Movement Disorders Society-Unified Parkinson's Rating Scale contains items specifically designed to identify NMS (Goetz et al., 2008). Another battery of assessments for PD is the Scale for Outcomes in Parkinson's Disease (SCOPA), which consists of seven sub-rating scales that widely cover multiple PD domains. It's short, practical, and can be either self-assessed or observer-administered with subscales to screen for cognition, sleep, and autonomic dysfunction (Martinez-Martin, 2013). The Non-Motor Symptoms Questionnaire (NMSQ) is a self-administered screening instrument comprising 30 items designed to identify the presence of non-motor symptoms (NMS) for further clinical evaluation (Chaudhuri et al., 2006). In contrast, the Non-Motor Symptoms Scale (NMSS) is an observer-rated assessment tool of 30 items across nine distinct domains, which was developed to quantify clinically relevant NMS by evaluating both the frequency and severity (Chaudhuri & Martinez-Martin, 2008). The International Parkinson and Movement Disorder Society (MDS)-Non-Motor Rating Scale is a revised, clinician-rated version of the Non-Motor Symptoms Scale (NMSS) (Chaudhuri et al., 2020). It quantifies both the frequency and severity of non-motor symptoms across 13 domains in 53 items. The scale includes an additional subscale to assess non-motor NMS fluctuations. Other global rating scales and symptom-focused scales (e.g., specific rating scales for depression, anxiety, sleep, and constipation) can also be used to assess the NMS, as endorsed by the MDS (Rukavina et al., 2021).

12.5 Pharmacological management of non-motor symptoms (NMS)

In this section, we will explore the pharmacological management of non-motor symptoms (NMS) throughout the progression of Parkinson's disease (PD), navigating them from the prodromal phase until the advanced stages. In 2019, the International Parkinson and Movement Disorder Society (MDS) Evidence-Based Medicine committee developed evidence-based treatment guidelines for managing NMS; a few years later, in 2023, van Wamelen and colleagues updated these management guidelines (Seppi et al., 2019; Wamelen et al., 2022). We will be referring to these guidelines when discussing individual NMS management throughout this chapter.

12.5.1 Autonomic dysfunctions

Autonomic dysfunction usually manifests early in the prodromal PD. It affects over 90% of patients and frequently precedes motor onset. The dysfunction affects the gastrointestinal system, cardiovascular control, thermoregulation, and urinary function (Chen et al., 2020).

Gastrointestinal (GI) manifestations are wide, including constipation, drooling, swallowing dysfunction, delayed gastric emptying, gastroparesis, bloating, and defecatory troubles, which are the most common non-motor symptoms in PD (Peña-Zelayeta et al., 2025). They will be discussed briefly, with main emphasis on the updated and evidence-based management.

12.5.1.1 Constipation

Constipation is one of the earliest and most common non-motor symptoms of PD. It is considered a prodromal biomarker that manifests decades before motor signs. It affects up to 63% of patients, with increasing prevalence and severity as the disease progresses (Peña-Zelayeta et al., 2025). The constipation is managed mainly by lifestyle and dietary modifications (with a high-fiber diet and increased fluid intake). The medications used are laxatives (e.g., polyethylene glycol), bulking agents (e.g., psyllium), and stool softeners, followed by groups of prokinetic (e.g., prucalopride) and prosecretory (e.g., lubiprostone) drugs in resistant cases (Safarpour et al., 2024).

Prokinetics act mainly on the gut microbiome; they are especially useful in cases of colonic hypomotility. Under this category, prucalopride is a selective 5-HT4 receptor agonist that improved the mobility of the stomach and colon in small studies without cardiovascular side effects, so it's given a recommendation for use when other measures fail to improve constipation. Pyridostigmine is a cholinesterase inhibitor that can improve chronic constipation by improving colonic motility; it was also reported to be effective in cases of colonic atonia associated with PD (Safarpour et al., 2024; Ly et al., 2022).

As a secretory drug, lubiprostone increases intestinal fluid secretion and gut motility with proven efficacy in PD; it is "likely efficacious" and "possibly useful" in an evidence-based review (Seppi et al., 2019; Safarpour et al., 2024).

Some ongoing clinical trials investigate a novel agents (ENT-01), which improved constipation by inhibiting the formation of alpha-synuclein aggregates in enteric neurons (Camilleri et al., 2022)

In cases when constipation is linked to motor fluctuation, adding opicapone – a third-generation COMT inhibitor – is helpful to improve the symptoms (Seppi et al., 2019)

Emerging evidence indicates a link between gut microbiota composition and Parkinson's disease-associated constipation. It was reported that the imbalance in gut flora is a significant player in the development and progression of PD-related constipation. This research prompted a shift in therapeutic strategies toward microecological interventions like the fecal microbiota transplantation (FMT). This novel intervention has demonstrated encouraging outcomes in alleviating constipation associated with Parkinson's disease (Yuan et al., 2024).

12.5.1.2 Orthostatic hypotension

Orthostatic hypotension (OH) is defined as a sustained decrease in systolic blood pressure (SBP) of at least 20 mmHg, diastolic blood pressure (DBP) of at least 10 mmHg, or both within 3 minutes of standing (Grosu et al., 2025). It is present in up to 30% and now recognized as a diagnostic marker of prodromal PD (Heinzel et al., 2019). The presentation of OH ranges from being asymptomatic to having symptoms such as light-headedness, dizziness, or even falls upon standing. It often goes untreated and can significantly increase the disability and dependence in PwP (Grosu et al., 2025).

Accumulating evidence showed association between OH and impaired cognitive function and cognitive decline in PD (Loureiro et al., 2023)

Pharmacological therapies include agents that increase vascular tone or expand plasma volume; examples are midodrine, droxidopa, and fludrocortisone, which are commonly prescribed. A balance should be maintained to prevent supine hypertension upon elevating standing BP, which increases the risk of cardiovascular complications during rest or sleep (Grosu et al., 2025). The MDS Evidence-Based Medicine Committee classified droxidopa, fludrocortisone and midodrine as 'possibly useful', with droxidopa only categorized as efficacious in the short term (Seppi et al., 2019; Wamelen et al., 2022).

Ampreloxetine, a norepinephrine reuptake inhibitor, which is currently under investigations to treat OH (Eisenhofer & Goldstein, 2021)

12.5.1.3 Sialorrhea/drooling

Sialorrhea/drooling is a serious clinically significant non-motor manifestation of Parkinson's disease. It's reported in up to 84% of patients, increasing morbidity and impacting the quality of life, and it can lead to social isolation (van Wamelen et al., 2020). It progresses with advanced stages of the disease and becomes associated with dry mouth, speech difficulties, and dehydration (van Wamelen et al., 2020; Reynolds et al., 2018). The mechanism of sialorrhea mainly involves the brainstem nuclei, with orofacial bradykinesia and cholinergic deficits that lead to decreased clearance of saliva (Peña-Zelayeta et al., 2025). It can be the leading cause of death in PD due to the significant risk of aspiration pneumonia.

Management of sialorrhea/drooling requires multidisciplinary approaches involving neurologists, speech therapists, and nutritionists. Anticholinergic drugs, either sublingual (atropine, ipratropium) or oral (glycopyrrolate) can be used for drooling that is not severe. Another drug investigated in sialorrhea is oral dihydroergotoxine mesylate, which showed a reduction in sialorrhea scores (Wamelen et al., 2022). Severe or refractory drooling can be managed with botulinum toxin injection into the salivary glands at regular intervals (Seppi et al., 2019; Safarpour et al., 2024). Other interventions, including dietary modifications, swallowing rehabilitation, and compensatory strategies, are essential (Safarpour et al., 2024).

12.5.1.4 Urinary dysfunction

Urinary dysfunction is estimated to affect approximately 61% of patients with PD. Though it's very common, it's a frequently underrecognized non-motor manifestation of PD that significantly impacts the quality of life (Li et al., 2022). Urinary symptoms often emerge during the premotor phase; in advanced stages, lower urinary tract symptoms (LUTS) may include urgency, frequency, nocturia, incontinence, and urinary retention. With disease progression, urinary dysfunction tends to correlate with greater motor impairment and more extensive dopaminergic denervation. Detrusor overactivity is the most common urinary disturbance in PD, and it's manifested as urgency, nocturia and incontinence (Peña-Zelayeta et al., 2025; Li et al., 2022).

The accumulation of α-synuclein, which spreads widely not only in the basal ganglia but also in the pontine center of micturition, sympathetic neurones, sacral parasympathetic nuclei, and pelvic plexus, disrupts the balance between excitatory and inhibitory control of the bladder, resulting in a wide range of urinary dysfunctions that evolve with disease severity (Li et al., 2022).

12.5.1.5 For treatment

Solifenacin (a muscarinic antagonist) is recommended medical therapy in the published guidelines as possibly useful for symptoms of overactive bladder (Seppi et al., 2019). Muscarinic receptor blockade can cause adverse effects at non-target sites, including blurred vision, dry mouth, constipation, and acute cognitive disturbances like confusion and hallucinations. Antimuscarinic agents may also impair gastrointestinal motility, leading to disruption of medication absorption like levodopa. These agents are contraindicated in individuals with narrow-angle glaucoma or severe constipation (Barrett et al., 2021).

It's important to emphasize that anticholinergic side effects tend to be more pronounced in the context of polypharmacy. Individuals with Parkinson's disease (PD) are frequently prescribed multiple medications with anticholinergic properties, both for PD-specific symptoms (e.g., trihexyphenidyl for tremor) and for other unrelated conditions (e.g., oral hypoglycemic and beta blockers). This cumulative exposure increases the risk of adverse effects, especially in the elderly who are sensitive to the effect of anticholinergics, especially on cognition (De Vreese et al., 2018).

Mirabegron, a beta-3 agonist, is a secure and efficacious treatment for overactive bladder. In a randomized controlled trial assessing the use of mirabegron in patients over the age of 65 with overactive bladder, the medication demonstrated significant efficacy with a favorable safety profile, with no observed decline in cognitive function over a 12-week follow-up period. Potential adverse effects associated with mirabegron include the exacerbation of palpitations, urinary retention, and worsening of pre-existing hypertension (Wagg et al., 2020).

Opicapone also showed improved urinary symptoms (Seppi et al., 2019). Safinamide, a monoamine oxidase-B inhibitor, was found to improve urinary urgency, incontinence, frequency and nocturia in a retrospective analysis of patients with PD (Gómez-López et al., 2021)

Botulinum toxin injections into the detrusor also provide benefit. A recent study investigated the effect of behavioral therapy compared to drug therapy to control bladder symptoms due to overactive bladder. The results showed noninferiority compared with drug therapy with clinically important treatment outcomes, including fewer symptoms and improved quality of life. Behavioral therapy seems to be a good option for people with PD even with cognitive impairment, with good adherence to therapy (Vaughan et al., 2025).

Obstructive urinary symptoms due to prostatic hypertrophy can be treated with alpha-adrenergic antagonists (e.g., tamsulosin, terazosin, and doxazosin) or 5-alpha reductase inhibitors (such as dutasteride or finasteride) (Rukavina et al., 2021).

12.5.1.6 Sexual dysfunction

Despite being common, sexual dysfunction is rarely reported in people with Parkinson's disease, especially in females. Previous reports indicated that up to 87% of PwPD experience sexual difficulties (Vafaeimastanabad et al., 2023). These difficulties are various, including but not limited to decreased sexual arousal, erectile dysfunction and premature ejaculation in males, and dry vagina and painful intercourse in females, with difficulty reaching orgasm or orgasmic dissatisfaction. Erectile dysfunction is the most common symptom, especially in the context of depression; it's also a known side effect of some antidepressants. Hypersexuality is also reported as a symptom of ICD and is more related to dopaminergic drugs (Vafaeimastanabad et al., 2023; Groote Clara et al., 2024). Sexual symptoms are mainly manifestations of autonomic dysfunction, but they can also be attributed to disability associated with PD or as side effects of medications or result from non-neurological comorbidity (Urso et al., 2022). Management of sexual dysfunction begins with screening and identification of the symptoms and requires careful review of the patient's medications, symptomatic treatment, and patient education. Phosphodiesterase-5 inhibitors, e.g., sildenafil and vardenafil, are the first-line treatment for erectile dysfunction in PD (Vaughan, 2019).

12.5.2 Neuropsychiatric symptoms

Depression, anxiety, and apathy are common neuropsychiatric symptoms in PD, and they are reported to precede motor onset by several years in the premotor phase, making them considered prodromal biomarkers (Berg et al., 2015).

12.5.2.1 Depression

Depression is the most common non-motor symptom across all stages of Parkinson's disease (PD) and has a profound impact on the quality of life for both patients and caregivers. Depressive symptoms may precede the onset of motor manifestations (in the prodromal phase) and worsen with disease progression. Methods to report depressive and depression-like symptoms in PD complicate the prevalence of depression, which varies from study to study (Ahmad et al., 2023). It's worth mentioning that the most frequent and clinically significant depression-like symptoms occur in between 40% and 50% of all PD cases at some time during the course of PD (Cong et al., 2022). The diagnosis of depression in PD can be very challenging due to the overlapping features with the symptoms of the disease itself, like slowness, hypomimia, changes in appetite, sleep disturbance and fatigue, and the subsyndromic nature of the depressive symptoms that don't fully meet the criteria of the DSM-5 to diagnose depression (Ahmad et al., 2023).

Studies to explore the neurobiology of depression in PD have demonstrated dysregulation of the hypothalamic-pituitary-adrenal (HPA) axis, along with deficits in serotoninergic, dopaminergic, and noradrenergic innervation in the limbic system and basal ganglia. This is reflected in the treatment of depression using selective serotonin reuptake inhibitors, serotonin/norepinephrine reuptake inhibitors, and dopamine agonists (Jankovic & Tan, 2020). Despite being common and prevalant, depression is only treated in up to 26% of patients with PD, with lower screening rates even in a specialized clinic for movement disorders (Marras et al., 2024).

12.5.2.2 Pharmacological management of depression in Parkinson's disease (PD)

Antidepressants such as selective serotonin reuptake inhibitors (SSRIs) and serotonin-norepinephrine reuptake inhibitors (SNRIs) are the main pillars and a first-line treatment of depression in PD. They are well known for their favorable efficacy and safety profiles. According to the Movement Disorder Society's evidence-based medicine review, venlafaxine is classified as "efficacious" and "clinically useful," while citalopram, sertraline, paroxetine, and fluoxetine are classified as "possibly useful" due to limited supporting evidence (Seppi et al., 2019). Tricyclic antidepressants show comparable efficacy to SSRIs, and they are considered possibly useful, but their use is not always recommended because of the adverse effects, such as confusion, cardiac arrhythmias, and orthostatic hypotension.

Drugs acting on the dopaminergic transmitter, such as levodopa, dopaminergic agonists, and monoamine oxidase B (MAO-B) inhibitors, also show antidepressant effects (Angelopoulou et al., 2023).

Dopaminergic agents: levodopa and dopamine agonists (pramipexole, ropinirole, and rotigotine). Pramipexole has been rated as "efficacious" and "clinically useful". Recently, this drug has shown efficacy in treating resistant major depression as an adjuvant outside the context of Parkinson's disease (Browning et al., 2025). Monoamine oxidase B (MAO-B) inhibitors (selegiline, rasagiline, and safinamide) can have antidepressant effects. MAO-B inhibitors may be particularly effective in early PD (Kulisevsky et al., 2024).

Non-pharmacological treatments for depression include cognitive behavioral therapy (CBT), exercise, repetitive transcranial magnetic stimulation (rTMS), deep brain stimulation (DBS), acupuncture, and electroconvulsive therapy (ECT).

12.5.2.3 Anxiety

Anxiety is highly prevalent in PD, with up to 40% affected, especially in the prodromal stage. About one-third of patients reported having more than one anxiety symptom. In many patients, anxious and depressive symptoms co-exist. The spectrum of anxiety in PD includes a generalized anxiety disorder, panic disorder, phobias, depression, obsessive-compulsive disorder, and situational anxiety. It's important to consider that mood disorders such as dysphoria, anxiety, and panic symptoms can occur as off-period non-motor fluctuation symptoms in up to 40% of patients with PD (Goldman, 2025).

Clinical drug trials on PD-related anxiety are still needed. The medications commonly used in clinical practice to treat anxiety are generally SSRIs or SNRIs; buspirone is also a possible option. Benzodiazepines can also be used carefully due to their unpleasant side effects. Mirtazapine also showed some benefits with a safe profile, especially in older patients with depression. Adjustment of the dopaminergic medication is very advantageous during the fluctuation to manage anxiety in the off state (Goldman, 2025).

12.5.2.4 Apathy

Apathy is a highly prevalent and disabling symptom in Parkinson's Disease (PD) that can occur at any stage of the disease and tends to increase with disease progression. It is linked to early-onset motor symptoms and cognitive decline and often occurs without depression (De Waele et al., 2022). It's higher among patients with Rapid Eye Movement Sleep Behavior Disorder (RBD), pointing to either a shared pathophysiological mechanism or playing a role in sleep disruption. Early deficits in the serotonergic as well as the dopaminergic pathways could be implicated, as reported in some studies (Angelopoulou et al., 2023; Maher et al., 2024). Apathy is still underrecognized and often attributed to depression or cognitive decline, leading to diagnostic confusion and improper management. Comprehensive screening and early identification are important in approaching apathy that is still unsatisfactory and challenging to manage. Dopaminergic drugs, e.g., levodopa and dopamine agonists, are advantageous. Piribedil, a dopamine agonist, is "possibly useful" in apathy following deep brain stimulation; rotigotine also shows some benefits but is still investigational. Rivastigmine (acetylcholinesterase inhibitor) is possibly useful (Seppi et al., 2019). Other drugs that showed promise in improving apathy are SSRIs, memantine, and methylphenidate, but more studies are needed. Vortioxetine modulates serotonergic, dopaminergic and catecholaminergic neurotransmission and shows greater efficacy than other SSRIs and SNRIs in affective apathy. A novel small-molecule compound, Pirepemat (IRL-752), is currently under investigation. The molecule is classified as a cortical enhancer that demonstrated a significant reduction in apathy severity scores in the phase 2b clinical trial (Maher et al., 2024).

12.5.2.5 Hallucinations and psychosis

Minor hallucinatory phenomena in PD previously reported by various studies include presence and passage hallucinations; they tend to occur in up to 40% of untreated patients in the early stages of Parkinson's disease. Presence hallucinations are defined as in the absence of external sensory stimuli, where there is a vivid sensation of another person being nearby, while passage hallucinations are formed mainly of brief visual perceptions of a person, animal, or object passing by. Visual illusions, or pareidolia, are also common, in which misinterpretations of real objects or forms occur to an individual. The patients usually have the insight to recognize the hallucinations as unreal, and they don't consider them distressing. PwPs, particularly the elderly and those with severe REM sleep-behavior disorder (RBD), may experience minor hallucinations in the prodromal phase (Amstutz et al., 2025).

Visual hallucinations are the most frequent symptoms of PD psychosis; it affects 27%–50%. Its presence usually indicates rapid progression to cognitive dysfunction and dementia, with increased mortality and the need for institutional care. The pathophysiology of visual hallucinations is attributed to disturbance in dopaminergic and cholinergic pathways (Ignatavicius et al., 2025)

A comprehensive approach is required while managing hallucination and psychosis in Parkinson's disease. This includes the identification and treatment of underlying medical conditions, such as delirium, infections, and any metabolic disturbances, as well as screening for potential contributing factors like medication effects and sensory deprivation. Adjustment of dopaminergic therapies used for motor symptom control may be necessary, either by dose reduction or discontinuation (Amstutz et al., 2025). Other drugs that act centrally, such as anticholinergics, analgesics, benzodiazepines, and medications for neurogenic bladder, should be carefully revised and adjusted. Pharmacologic management may include the use of antipsychotics or cholinesterase inhibitors. Antipsychotics with significant anti-dopaminergic effects should be avoided (e.g., haloperidol, risperidone, and olanzapine) because of the risk of exacerbating motor symptoms. Pimavanserin, a selective 5-HT2A inverse agonist, is approved in the United States for the treatment of PD psychosis. Clozapine has demonstrated efficacy without worsening motor function. Although quetiapine is frequently used in clinical practice, evidence is still needed to support its efficacy. Cholinesterase inhibitors can also be used for managing hallucinations and delusions in PD (Goldman, 2025; Ignatavicius et al., 2025). Ulotaront (SEP-363,856), a trace amine-associated receptor one agonist with 5-HT1A activity, is under investigation (Isaacson et al., 2023).

12.5.2.6 Cognitive impairment

Cognitive impairment in PD is one of the most disabling aspects of NMS, which adds much to the disease burden and greatly impacts the quality of life of patients and their caregivers. The spectrum of cognitive dysfunction in PD patients is multifaceted, ranging from subjective cognitive impairment to frank dementia. The most affected domains are typically executive functions, visual-spatial abilities, memory, and attention. At earlier stages of the disease, patients often report difficulties in concentration, reduced organizational skills, multitasking problems, and a tip-of-the-tongue phenomenon; these symptoms progress with the advancement of the disease. Subjective cognitive decline (SCD) in Parkinson's disease refers to a self-reported reduction in cognitive abilities, despite normal performance on standardized cognitive assessments adjusted for age, sex, and educational background, indicating preserved objective cognitive function (Oedekoven et al., 2022).

Mild cognitive impairment (MCI), representing a transitional phase between normal cognition, subjective cognitive decline (SCD), and dementia, may manifest at any stage of Parkinson's disease (PD). Its reported prevalence among PD patients ranges from 19% to 62% (Aarsland et al., 2021). MCI is characterized by a progressive decline in cognitive performance, affecting one or multiple domains, particularly during the execution of complex tasks, yet the activities of daily living are still preserved in contrast to dementia, in which the activities of daily living are impaired.

Parkinson's disease MCI (PD-MCI) exhibits considerable heterogeneity in terms of severity, progression rate, and the specific cognitive domains affected, putting the individuals at a higher risk of developing frank Parkinson's disease dementia (PDD) (Carceles-Cordon et al., 2023). It's worth mentioning that the prevalence of subjective cognitive decline (SCD), and particularly mild cognitive impairment (MCI), in individuals with Parkinson's disease (PD) is significantly higher than in age-matched control populations. However, reported frequencies vary widely due to inconsistencies in diagnostic criteria and differences in neuropsychological assessment methodologies (Jellinger, 2024).

Previous studies reported that up to 50% of patients with PD develop dementia after 10 years, rising to 80% after 20 years (Amstutz et al., 2025). The temporal relationship is important to differentiate Parkinson's disease dementia from dementia with Lewy bodies. If the symptoms of dementia develop 1 year or more after the onset of motor symptoms of PD, it is classified as Parkinson's disease dementia; however, if cognitive impairment occurs within 1 year of motor symptom onset or precedes it, the diagnosis is dementia with Lewy bodies (DLB) (McKeith et al., 2017).

Cognitive dysfunction in Parkinson's disease (PD) is heterogenous, reflecting the complexity of the underlying neuropathological and neuropharmacological mechanisms. Parkinson's disease (PD) implicates both the nigrostriatal and mesocorticolimbic dopaminergic pathways, as well as cortical and subcortical regions. Moreover, multiple neurotransmitter systems, including glutamatergic, serotonergic, cholinergic, and noradrenergic, are affected, with the resultant differential involvement of distinct cortico-subcortical circuits that add to the complexity of the cognitive profile observed in PD (Schneider & Kortagere, 2022).

The risk factors for cognitive impairment in PD are multiple, including male sex, REM sleep behavior disorder (RBD), mood disorders, hypertension, diabetes mellitus, cardiovascular disease, hyperuricemia, and orthostatic hypotension. Environmental factors are also involved, including head trauma and pesticides, as well as genetic factors such as the Apolipoprotein E (APOE) ε4 allele, microtubule-associated protein tau (MAPT) H1/H1 haplotype, mutations in the glucocerebrosidase gene (GBA1), and comorbid conditions such as Alzheimer's disease (AD) (Degirmenci et al., 2023). Precise management of cognitive impairment in Parkinson's disease (PD) necessitates objective assessments of cognitive and functional abilities using appropriate neuropsychological tools. Unfortunately, there is currently no consensus on the optimal testing protocols. The Movement Disorder Society (MDS) has recommended several instruments for global cognitive screening, e.g., the Montreal Cognitive Assessment (MoCA) and also proposed criteria to diagnose mild cognitive impairment (MCI) and Parkinson's disease dementia in PDD (Litvan et al., 2012). Premorbid cognitive function: the functional impact of cognitive symptoms should be considered due to their impact on cognition.

Currently, effective and well-tolerated pharmacological treatments for PD-related mild cognitive impairment (PD-MCI) and Parkinson's disease dementia (PDD) remain limited. With the unclear effect of cholinesterase inhibitors (ChIs). Rivastigmine, a cholinesterase inhibitor, is the only agent with Level A evidence and FDA approval for the treatment of PDD. Other cholinesterase inhibitors, such as donepezil and galantamine, have been classified as "possibly useful" according to MDS evidence-based reviews (Seppi et al., 2019). The effect of memantine is still debatable, and further studies are needed; the current evidence showed some effect when it's combined with other ChIs to improve cognition in PD (Cani et al., 2025).

Results from a recent randomized clinical trial showed that ambroxol was safe and well-tolerated in PDD, with target engagement, but its effect on cognition was not confirmed (Silveira et al., 2025). For PD-MCI, clinical trials evaluating the effect of rivastigmine, rasagiline, and atomoxetine showed no significant cognitive benefits compared to placebo (Goldman, 2025). Despite ongoing trials and extensive research, there is still no disease-modifying therapy to prevent or delay the cognitive impairment associated with PD (Bayram et al., 2023).

There are some non-pharmacological interventions to improve cognitive abilities in PD. These include, but are not limited to, cognitive interventions, physical exercises; and brain stimulation. Cognitive interventions in Parkinson's disease can be broadly categorized into three types: cognitive training, cognitive rehabilitation, and cognitive stimulation (Bahar-Fuchs et al., 2019). Cognitive training and rehabilitation are particularly well-suited for individuals with PD-related mild cognitive impairment (PD-MCI), given their targeted complexity and therapeutic objectives. In contrast, cognitive stimulation is more commonly indicated for patients with advanced cognitive decline or dementia (Kalbe et al., 2024).

In their systematic review and meta-analysis, Kim and colleagues indicated that physical exercise interventions are effective in enhancing global cognitive function in patients with Parkinson's disease (PD), with a modest impact observed on executive function. We recommend a minimum of 60 min per day of combined exercise modalities, performed on as many days per week as feasible, as a non-pharmacological therapeutic strategy to support cognitive health in this population (Kim et al., 2023).

Non-invasive brain stimulation has been studied for its effect on cognition in Parkinson's disease. Findings of a systematic review showed that the efficacy of non-invasive brain stimulation (NIBS) appears to be domain-specific and should be considered for targeted applications aimed at modest improvements in working memory or attentional processes (Begemann et al., 2020). These findings were supported by another systematic review by Zhang et al., evaluating the effect of repetitive transcranial magnetic stimulation (rTMS) on motor and non-motor symptoms of PD; they concluded there is a lack of sufficient evidence to support cognitive improvement with transcranial magnetic stimulation, and they stressed the need for further studies to optimize the parameters, frequency, and duration of the stimulation (Zhang et al., 2022). Transcranial direct current stimulation (tDCS) and vagus nerve stimulation (VND) are also considered promising techniques that require further studies (Moshayedi et al., 2025).

It is worth mentioning that emerging therapies targeting alpha-synuclein pathology have been investigated with two experimental agents, namely prasinezumab and minzasolmin. The former didn't show improvements in global cognitive functions, while the results of minzasolmin are still pending (Abdelnour et al., 2025).

12.5.3 Sleep disorders

Sleep disorders comprise a large and heterogeneous group of pathologies, including insomnia, nighttime sleep fragmentation, excessive daytime sleepiness, sleep-disordered breathing disorders (SDB), reduced sleep efficiency, rapid eye movements (REM), sleep behavior disorders (RBD), sleep-related movement disorders, and disturbances of circadian rhythm (Liu et al., 2018). Sleep disturbances in Parkinson's disease (PD) are commonly associated with, or exacerbated by, comorbid conditions such as anxiety and mood disorders, the severity of motor symptoms, the duration of the disease, and dopaminergic therapy. These disorders are often present in the prodromal and early stages of PD, with increasing prevalence in the later stages. They may occur in isolation or in combination, with potentiation of their clinical impact on quality of life for the patients and caregivers (Iranzo et al., 2024; Dodet et al., 2024).

12.5.3.1 Rapid eye movement (REM) sleep behavior disorder (RBD)

REM sleep behavior disorder (RBD) affects approximately 42% of all PD patients and often precedes motor PD symptoms by decades. RBD is linked to an increased severity of motor symptoms and higher rates of depression, hallucinations, and cognitive decline (Marafioti et al., 2023). RBD is a type of parasomnia characterized by the loss of normal REM sleep atonia, which results in dream enactment behaviors as well as complex motor and vocal actions. It can happen at any point between sleep onset and awakening; patients usually complain of non-restorative sleep, EDS, and nightmares, and many are unaware of their abnormal behaviors during sleep (Schütz et al., 2022). Idiopathic RBD is highly perceived as a prodromal marker of neurodegenerative synucleinopathies; it's more common in males than females. The prevalence reported in patients with Parkinson's disease (33%–50%) is the highest; in multiple system atrophy, it reaches 80%–95%; and in dementia with Lewy bodies, it's approximately 80% (Martinez-Nunez et al., 2025). For a definitive diagnosis of RBD, polysomnographic (PSG) confirmation is required. The findings include a loss of normal REM sleep atonia, which is detected by sustained or intermittent elevations in muscle tone, as reported by electromyography (EMG) (Maggi et al., 2023).

Concerning pharmacological management Melatonin is the first-line treatment for REM sleep behavior disorder (RBD) in patients with Parkinson's disease (PD). Dopamine agonists, such as rotigotine and pramipexole, have shown potential efficacy as well. Clonazepam is the best treatment for idiopathic RBD, but it should be used with caution and only when other treatments fail due to its association with an increased risk of falls in PD patients (Liu et al., 2018). Rivastigmine may be advantageous, while sodium oxybate still needs further studies to prove its efficacy (Goldman, 2025).

12.5.3.2 Insomnia

Insomnia is a sleep disorder with difficulty initiating or maintaining sleep; it can also present as early morning awakenings that occur at least three times a week for a minimum duration of 3 months. Sleep fragmentation is the most prevalent form of insomnia in PwP, affecting up to 81% of patients. Insomnia, in some cases, may precede the onset of motor symptoms in PD (Iranzo et al., 2024; Duan et al., 2025). Insomnia is more prevalent in advanced PD disease, and the female gender is more affected; other risk factors include inadequate sleep habits and quality, together with REM sleep latency. Insomnia is a clinical diagnosis; sleep questionnaires can be used for screening, and a polysomnography is required if another sleep disorder is suspected (Dodet et al., 2024). It has a slower rate of progression; some investigators found insomnia to have almost the same prevalence over time. Insomnia in PD could stem from a multifactorial interplay of motor symptoms, non-motor manifestations, and mood affection. For effective management, the underlying contributing factors should be targeted. A multimodal therapeutic approach is required, matching the stage and progression of the disease to achieve satisfactory results. For medical treatment, eszopiclone and melatonin have been reported to improve some of the clinical measures of insomnia and marked as possibly useful (Seppi et al., 2019). Doxepin is likely efficacious in improving insomnia in patients with PD; rotigotine and rasaligine may improve sleep efficiency by reducing sleep onset latency and overnight fragmentation (Liu et al., 2018).

12.5.3.3 Excessive daytime sleepiness (EDS)

Excessive daytime sleepiness (EDS) can happen in up to 46% of individuals with Parkinson's disease (PD), with its prevalence and severity increasing with disease progression and the use of dopaminergic medications, namely dopamine agonists. EDS can lead to difficulty in concentration, with impaired attention, and catastrophic consequences with a higher risk of accidents, e.g., falls (Peña-Zelayeta et al., 2025).

Pathophysiology involves neurodegeneration in the arousal centers, including the locus coeruleus, the tuberomammillary nucleus, and orexin-producing neurones in the lateral hypothalamus that disrupt wakefulness regulation. Exacerbation of this dysfunction can be induced by medications. Fragmented nocturnal sleep contributes to daytime sleepiness (Liu et al., 2018). Management of EDS is mainly by treating the underlying cause (e.g., depression, sedating medications, nocturnal disturbances, .). Medications that promote alertness, such as modafinil or caffeine, may improve EDS with insufficient evidence. Solriamfetol, sodium oxybate, and atomoxetine showed promise in clinical trials, but further investigations are needed (Goldman, 2025).

12.5.4 Sensory manifestations

These manifestations include pain, fatigue and hyposmia.

12.5.4.1 Pain

Pain is prevalent in PD in all stages, affecting up to 85% of individuals with Parkinson's disease, and may present as an early non-motor symptom and become worse in the late stages (Rukavina et al., 2021) (Nardelli et al., 2024). In 5% of cases, pain can be the first clinical symptom that signals the onset of PD. It's present in chronic or fluctuating form, with its burden usually underestimated. Chronic pain is heterogeneous; the common types include **musculoskeletal pain** (affecting up to 75% of patients), dystonic pain (up to 50%), radicular and neuropathic pain (up to 50%), visceral pain (up to 24%), orofacial pain (up to 24%) and central pain (around 10%). Each type has peculiar characteristics and underlying mechanisms (Nardelli et al., 2024). It's reported more frequently in women with PD, with negative impacts on quality of life in both sexes. Pain management in PD is still challenging with a few high-quality, controlled studies and a low level of evidence with frequent patient disappointment. Many pharmacological options are commonly used, among them dopaminergic therapies, antidepressants (e.g., serotonin-norepinephrine reuptake inhibitors and tricyclic antidepressants), anticonvulsants (gabapentin, pregabalin), non-steroidal anti-inflammatory drugs (NSAIDs), and opioids. The effectiveness of these treatments is not yet established, with high risks of adverse effects and even dependency. Acetaminophen, opioids, antidepressants, and antiepileptics are commonly used in PD patients more than usual in the general population (Buhmann et al., 2020).

Dopaminergic dysfunction in the nigrostriatal pathway can result in lower pain thresholds in Parkinson's disease, so optimizing dopaminergic therapy has a major effect on reducing pain. Safinamide is considered probably efficacious, while rotigotine is possibly efficacious in pain management (Wamelen et al., 2022). A recent clinical trial to investigate the efficacy of prolonged-release oxycodone-PR, or high doses of levodopa, in alleviating pain failed to demonstrate any superiority compared to placebo (Brefel-Courbon et al., 2024).

12.5.4.2 Fatigue

Fatigue is a common, under-recognized non-motor symptom associated with Parkinson's disease (PD) that can affect up to 80% of patients across different stages of the disease, with a prevalence of 30% in the prodromal phase (Siciliano et al., 2018). Some meta-analyses estimated the overall prevalence of fatigue in PD to be about 50%, with a significant negative impact on patients' quality of life (Sarmento et al., 2024). It is primarily characterized by extreme mental and physical exhaustion during daily activities. Recent studies hypothesized that the widely spread hypodominergic state is the cause of fatigue that often leads to reduced initiation and persistence in task performance (Amstutz et al., 2025). Although fatigue exhibits strong correlations with apathy and depression, accumulating evidence supports that fatigue is a distinct neuropsychiatric condition (Amstutz et al., 2025; Siciliano et al., 2018).

Depression is a common comorbidity in Parkinson's disease (PD) and can independently contribute to fatigue. Effective management requires identifying the underlying cause of fatigue, as depression, which is a common comorbidity in PD, can cause fatigue and necessitates different therapeutic strategies (Friedman & Friedman, 2001).

MAO-B Inhibitors Rasagiline is marked as possibly useful to treat fatigue in PD (Seppi et al., 2019); however, there are no standardized guidelines for the treatment of fatigue in Parkinson's disease (PD). This variation could be attributed to the variability in fatigue assessment methodologies across studies and the challenges of comorbid symptoms like depression and apathy. Further studies are needed to enhance diagnostic tools, establish uniform screening and assessment protocols, and develop effective therapeutic strategies for fatigue in Parkinson's disease (PD) through objective evaluation.

Stimulant medications such as modafinil and methylphenidate have been investigated for fatigue in Parkinson's disease. Methylphenidate functions as a dopamine transporter inhibitor, blocking the reuptake of both dopamine and norepinephrine at presynaptic sites. A placebo-controlled trial demonstrated a statistically significant reduction in fatigue scores, while clinical outcome measurements have been inconsistent, with some patients reporting noticeable improvement and others experiencing minimal benefit. These stimulants are not currently approved for the treatment of PD-related fatigue, and there is still a need for further well-designed studies to establish their efficacy and safety (Pitton Rissardo et al., 2025).

12.5.4.3 Hyposmia

Hyposmia, defined as a decrease in the sense of smell, is a common symptom of PD and significantly impacts quality of life (Fullard et al., 2017). It occurs early in the course of the disease and often precedes the motor onset by at least 4 years; therefore, it's considered a prodromal biomarker. Up to 68% of PD patients are unaware of the severity of their olfactory loss (Torres-Pasillas et al., 2023).

12.6 Non-motor fluctuations (NMFs)

Non-motor fluctuations (NMFs) in Parkinson's disease (PD) refer to the dynamic variations in non-motor symptoms (NMSs) that often correlate with the pharmacokinetics of dopaminergic therapies. They are still underrecognized, and they are suboptimally managed in clinical settings. They are not always linked to motor fluctuations (MFs), as emerging evidence suggests that NMFs represent distinct clinical entities that partially overlap with motor fluctuation but with independent pathophysiological mechanisms. These fluctuations involve a range of neuropsychiatric, sensory, and autonomic symptoms, each of which has a variable contribution and impact on the overall burden and quality of life (QoL) in PwP (Mujahid et al., 2025).

Recognizing non-motor fluctuations (NMFs) in routine clinical practice is crucial for guiding treatment strategies. They should also be differentiated from motor symptoms (NMSs) that are not influenced by motor fluctuation. The management of NMFs should adopt the approach used for motor fluctuations, aiming to adjust and optimize dopaminergic replacement therapy (DRT) to achieve continuous, non-pulsatile stimulation (Rukavina et al., 2021).

In conclusion, it's important to screen for and identify the non-motor symptoms in Parkinson's disease that could even be experienced by the affected individuals in the prodromal phase, sometimes decades before the onset of motor symptoms. Physicians and patients should be aware of these symptoms and how to manage them, as they can be difficult to treat. Left untreated, these NMS add to the burden of PD and negatively impact the quality of life of patients and their carers, so adequate screening and proper treatment are crucial.

12.7 Challenges and considerations in pharmacological management

12.7.1 Polypharmacy

Polypharmacy is commonly defined as the regular use of five or more medications. It has become a significant medical concern due to its association with increased drug-related complications, frequent hospitalizations, higher risks of morbidity and mortality, and increased healthcare costs. For example, the elderly are at increased risk of injurious falls; this risk significantly increases with polypharmacy (Masnoon et al., 2017).

Older adults tend to exhibit more profound Parkinson's disease (PD) symptoms at the time of diagnosis compared to younger individuals. In this population, motor symptoms progress more rapidly, and the incidence of neuropsychiatric complications such as hallucinations and dementia is significantly higher. For them, levodopa is often the drug of choice to treat the symptoms, given its superior efficacy in alleviating motor symptoms and its relatively favorable side effect profile (McLean et al., 2017). Patients with Parkinson's disease (PD) commonly incorporate adjunctive anti-PD therapies alongside a baseline dose of levodopa, regardless of age group. This happens especially when the dose is equal to or higher than 300 mg/day, aiming to mitigate motor complications associated with higher levodopa dosages (Seki et al., 2023).

Polypharmacy represents a significant concern in the geriatric population, particularly among individuals with Parkinson's disease (PD), where excessive pharmacological intervention may precipitate adverse clinical outcomes. Given that multiple pharmacological agents modulate the equilibrium of various neurotransmitter systems in PD, the introduction of an additional drug has the potential to disrupt the neuronal network's homeostasis. Therefore, prioritizing deprescribing strategies in routine clinical practice may be more beneficial than initiating new medications in response to emerging symptoms or adverse drug reactions. In light of these considerations, minimizing pharmaceutical burdens is imperative whenever they are clinically feasible. Careful medication review and judicious prescription practices could achieve these objectives (Yamaguchi et al., 2024).

12.7.2 Individualized treatment strategies

It is essential to address the presence of non-motor symptoms (NMS) when managing Parkinson's disease (PD) and to customize management plans for each individual, particularly given the absence of standardised regimens. The heterogeneity of NMS in Parkinson's disease (PD) presents a significant challenge in evaluating the efficacy of treatment strategies. Due to the wide variation in nature, severity, and duration of NMS, it's difficult to design clinical studies with generalizable findings across a diverse patient population. Another caveat is the dynamic interplay between motor and non-motor symptoms, which adds more complexity. So a personalized approach in the management of NMS is inevitable; incorporating symptom-specific treatment strategies, patient preferences, and outcome monitoring through validated assessment tools is recommended (Liu & Wang, 2024).

Individualized therapy necessitates consideration of age, comorbidities, social factors, neuropsychiatric symptoms, and any reported adverse effects. Overmedication with dopaminergic therapy should be avoided, while the doses and interactions of the non-dopaminergic agents managing the present NMS should be considered. Non-pharmacological strategies to alleviate the NMS can maximize therapeutic efficacy and patient adherence (Regensburger et al., 2025). To avoid the complications of fluctuation and off periods, on-demand therapy is a good option. They are used when the patients anticipate fluctuation in the drug response while the optimum function is needed; examples include fast-acting levodopa preparations (e.g., inhaled powder) and subcutaneous apomorphine (Pahwa et al., 2023). Patients require good education to identify the best therapeutic options, recognize their symptoms, and determine effective administration methods. These on-demand therapies should be discussed with the patients individually, allowing them to choose the therapy according to patient preferences, symptom profiles, severity and timing of the off periods (Isaacson et al., 2024).

Multidisciplinary care in Parkinson's disease (PD) provides a comprehensive and individualized approach to care, addressing the multifaceted needs of patients across physical, cognitive, emotional, and social domains. By integrating the expertise of various healthcare professionals—including neurologists, physiotherapists, occupational therapists, speech-language pathologists, psychologists, and social workers—this collaborative model enhances symptom management, supports functional independence, and contributes to improved overall quality of life for individuals living with PD (Weise et al., 2024).

12.7.3 Balancing efficacy and side effects in elderly populations

Advancing age significantly influences pharmacological decision-making in PD. The scarcity of geriatric-specific clinical trials and the under-representation of older adults in existing studies result in a less robust evidence base for treatment strategies in such a population. Moreover, older patients exhibit increased susceptibility to adverse drug reactions, which, in certain cases, may outweigh the therapeutic benefits (Mouchaileh & Hughes, 2020). It's important to consider geriatric comorbidities (falls, delirium, cognitive impairment), polypharmacy, sarcopenia, and frailty when prescribing drugs. It's recommended to avoid complex treatment regimens and unnecessary medications. Dopamine agonists and MAO-B inhibitors should be used with caution in older adults because they are more likely to cause neuropsychiatric problems when medications are reviewed often and drug interactions are taken into account. Controlling NMS shouldn't cause hazardous consequences, as in treating sleep disturbances with benzodiazebine, which can lead to an increased risk of falls. Non-pharmacological interventions should be encouraged with frequent education and counseling.

12.7.4 Emerging therapies and future directions

Emerging therapeutic strategies for Parkinson's disease are increasingly focused on disease modification, with particular emphasis on targeting pathological mechanisms such as α-synuclein aggregation and genetic contributors including leucine-rich repeat kinase 2 (LRRK2), parkin, and glucocerebrosidase. Despite substantial research efforts, no disease-modifying agents have yet demonstrated the ability to halt or reverse disease progression. Several investigational compounds are currently being evaluated for their potential to rescue neuronal function through specific molecular pathways. Additionally, novel pharmacological therapies have shown promise in improving symptomatic management of PD. These include agents in phase 2 or later clinical trials, such as ambroxol, which targets glucocerebrosidase and has demonstrated potential benefits in PD-related dementia, and TAK-071, an acetylcholine M1 receptor positive allosteric modulator, which is being studied for cognitive impairment in PD (Chhetri et al., 2023).

Therapeutic research targeting α-synuclein in Parkinson's disease (PD) has primarily focused on monoclonal antibodies and small-molecule inhibitors. Selective anti-α-synuclein antibodies have shown that they can lower the buildup of harmful proteins and mitochondrial dysfunction in astrocytes, which helps protect dopaminergic neurones from dying. Agents such as PRX002, P21, and P22 have shown potential disease-modifying effects in preclinical and early clinical studies. Beyond α-synuclein, other emerging pharmacological strategies include Nurr1 activators (e.g., IRX4204, bexarotene, amodiaquine), which aim to enhance dopaminergic neuron survival and function. Additionally, compounds that improve glucocerebrosidase (GCase) activity, such as ambroxol and S-181, are being investigated for their neuroprotective properties. Drugs originally developed for diabetes management, including exenatide, terazosin, metformin, thiazolidinediones (TZDs), and vildagliptin, have also shown promise in modulating neurodegenerative pathways relevant to PD (Ullah et al., 2024).

12.7.5 Role of digital tools and biomarkers to monitor NMS

As mentioned earlier in this chapter, some non-motor symptoms can appear during the prodromal phase of PD, which makes them potentially sensitive biomarkers for disease progression. This sensitivity enhances their utility in disease-modifying clinical trials, particularly for identifying and enrolling individuals in prodromal or at-risk stages. NMS may also serve as important diagnostic indicators in conventional clinical practice. Integrating digital biomarkers allows for objective and remote monitoring of NMS across varying stages of disease severity, offering more patient-centered and unobtrusive outcome measures in clinical research (van Wamelen et al., 2021).

In a recent review by Janssen Daalen discussing the digital biomarkers for NMS, they indicated that sleep-related symptoms represent some of the most promising biomarkers for the prodromal phase of Parkinson's disease (PD). Digital biomarkers for REM sleep -behavior disorder (RBD) and excessive daytime sleepiness have already been validated in prodromal cohorts, with both conditions serving as reliable predictors of future conversion to clinically manifest PD. These features make them suitable candidates for selection and progression biomarkers in disease-modifying trials. They also pointed out the role of accelerometry-derived sleep metrics such as reduced sleep efficiency and decreased turn velocity, which have demonstrated strong correlations with polysomnography and have been validated across multiple PD cohorts. They concluded that these parameters have shown predictive value for PD onset several years prior to diagnosis and may continue to reflect disease progression throughout its course (Janssen Daalen et al., 2024).

12.8 Conclusion

Nonmotor symptoms are now recognized as integral parts of PD. These symptoms increase the disease burden and impair the quality of life of the affected individuals. Some NMS appear very early in the prodromal stage of PD, even decades before the onset of the motor symptoms. NMS should be addressed in every patient to ensure satisfactory management of Parkinson's disease. Adapting well-integrated multidisciplinary care to PD with NMS is crucial. Development in the methods of screening and monitoring of NMS is highly required to characterize these symptoms for their use as prodromal markers. Such developments are highly important for patient stratification and enrollment in clinical trials targeting PD in its very early stages. There is also a pressing need for clinical trials investigating new drugs for the management of NMS, especially in the geriatric population, considering the co-existing aging comorbidities.

References

Aarsland, D., Batzu, L., Halliday, G. M., Geurtsen, G. J., Ballard, C., Ray Chaudhuri, K., et al. (2021). Parkinson disease-associated cognitive impairment. *Nature Reviews Disease Primers, 7*(1), 47. https://doi.org/10.1038/s41572-021-00280-3

Abdelnour, C., Gibson, L. L., Batzu, L., & Aarsland, D. (2025). How to advance the pharmacological management of cognitive impairment in Parkinson's disease. *Journal of Parkinson's Disease.*. https://doi.org/10.1177/1877718X251315645. Epub ahead of print. PMID: 39973493.

Ahmad, M. H., Rizvi, M. A., Ali, M., & Mondal, A. C. (2023). Neurobiology of depression in parkinson's disease: Insights into epidemiology, molecular mechanisms and treatment strategies. *Ageing Research Reviews, 85*, Article 101840. https://www.sciencedirect.com/science/article/pii/S1568163722002823.

Amstutz, D., Sousa, M., Maradan-Gachet, M. E., Debove, I., Lhommée, E., & Krack, P. (2025). Psychiatric and cognitive symptoms of parkinson's disease: A life's tale. *Revue Neurologique, 181*, 265–283. Elsevier Masson s.r.l.

Angelopoulou, E., Stanitsa, E., Karpodini, C. C., Bougea, A., Kontaxopoulou, D., Fragkiadaki, S., et al. (2023). Pharmacological and non-pharmacological treatments for depression in parkinson's disease: An updated review. *Medicina (B Aires), 59*(8). https://www.mdpi.com/1648-9144/59/8/1454.

Bahar-Fuchs, A., Martyr, A., Goh, A. M. Y., Sabates, J., & Clare, L. (2019). Cognitive training for people with mild to moderate dementia. *Cochrane Database of Systematic Reviews*, (3)https://doi.org/10.1002/14651858.CD013069.pub2

Barrett, M. J., Sargent, L., Nawaz, H., Weintraub, D., Price, E. T., & Willis, A. W. (2021). Antimuscarinic anticholinergic medications in parkinson disease: To prescribe or deprescribe? *Movement Disorders Clinical Practice, 8*(8), 1181–1188. https://movementdisorders.onlinelibrary.wiley.com/doi/abs/10.1002/mdc3.13347.

Bayram, E., Batzu, L., Tilley, B., Gandhi, R., Jagota, P., Biundo, R., et al. (2023). Clinical trials for cognition in Parkinson's disease: Where are we and how can we do better? *Parkinsonism Relat Disord, 112*. https://doi.org/10.1016/j.parkreldis.2023.105385

Begemann, M. J., Brand, B. A., Ćurčić-Blake, B., Aleman, A., & Sommer, I. E. (2020). Efficacy of non-invasive brain stimulation on cognitive functioning in brain disorders: A meta-analysis. *Psychol Med, 50*(15), 2465–2486. https://www.cambridge.org/core/product/014F47EDEC0BD2B10A8B13DB0D3D9343.

Berg, D., Postuma, R. B., Adler, C. H., Bloem, B. R., Chan, P., Dubois, B., et al. (2015). MDS research criteria for prodromal Parkinson's disease. *Movement Disorders, 30*(12), 1600–1611. https://movementdisorders.onlinelibrary.wiley.com/doi/abs/10.1002/mds.26431.

Borghammer, P. (2021). The α-Synuclein origin and connectome model (SOC model) of parkinson's disease: Explaining motor asymmetry, non-motor phenotypes, and cognitive decline. *Journal of Parkinson's Disease, 11*(2), 455–474. https://journals.sagepub.com/action/showAbstract.

Braak, H., Tredici, K Del, Rüb, U., de Vos, R. A. I., Jansen Steur, E. N. H., & Braak, E. (2003). Staging of brain pathology related to sporadic parkinson's disease. *Neurobiology of Aging, 24*(2), 197–211. https://www.sciencedirect.com/science/article/pii/S0197458002000659.

Brefel-Courbon, C., Harroch, E., Marques, A., Devos, D., Thalamas, C., Rousseau, V., et al. (2024). Oxycodone or higher dose of levodopa for the treatment of parkinsonian central pain: OXYDOPA trial. *Movement Disorders, 39*(9), 1533–1543. https://movementdisorders.onlinelibrary.wiley.com/doi/abs/10.1002/mds.29878.

Browning, M., Cowen, P. J., Galal, U., Baldwin, A., Cleare, A. J., Evans, J., et al. (2025). Pramipexole augmentation for the acute phase of treatment-resistant, unipolar depression: A placebo-controlled, double-blind, randomised trial in the UK. *The Lancet Psychiatry, 12*(8), 579–589. https://doi.org/10.1016/S2215-0366(25)00194-4

Buhmann, C., Kassubek, J., & Jost, W. H. (2020). Management of pain in parkinson's disease. *Journal of Parkinson's Disease, 10*(s1), S37–S48. https://doi.org/10.3233/JPD-202069

Camilleri, M., Subramanian, T., Pagan, F., Isaacson, S., Gil, R., Hauser, R. A., et al. (2022). Oral ENT-01 targets enteric neurons to treat constipation in parkinson disease. *Annals of Internal Medicine, 175*(12), 1666–1674. https://doi.org/10.7326/M22-1438

Cani, I., Grotteschi, N., Calandra-Buonaura, G., Guarino, M., Guaraldi, P., Giannini, G., et al. (2025). Efficacy of cholinesterase inhibitors and memantine on symptoms not responsive to levodopa in patients affected by parkinson's disease without dementia: A systematic review. *BMJ Neurol Open, 7*(2), Article e001079. https://doi.org/10.1136/bmjno-2025-001079

Carceles-Cordon, M., Weintraub, D., & Chen-Plotkin, A. S. (2023). Cognitive heterogeneity in Parkinson's disease: A mechanistic view. *Neuron, 111*(10), 1531–1546. https://doi.org/10.1016/j.neuron.2023.03.021

Chaudhuri, K. R., & Martinez-Martin, P. (2008). Quantitation of non-motor symptoms in Parkinson's disease. *European Journal of Neurology, 15*(s2), 2–8. https://doi.org/10.1111/j.1468-1331.2008.02212.x

Chaudhuri, K. R., Martinez-Martin, P., Schapira, A. H. V., Stocchi, F., Sethi, K., Odin, P., et al. (2006). International multicenter pilot study of the first comprehensive self-completed nonmotor symptoms questionnaire for parkinson's disease: The NMSQuest study. *Movement Disorders, 21*(7), 916–923. https://doi.org/10.1002/mds.20844

Chaudhuri, K. R., Schrag, A., Weintraub, D., Rizos, A., Rodriguez-Blazquez, C., Mamikonyan, E., et al. (2020). The movement disorder Society nonmotor rating Scale: Initial validation Study. *Movement Disorders, 35*(1), 116–133. https://doi.org/10.1002/mds.27862

Chen, Z., Li, G., & Liu, J. (2020). Autonomic dysfunction in parkinson's disease: Implications for pathophysiology, diagnosis, and treatment. *Neurobiology of Disease, 134*, Article 104700. https://www.sciencedirect.com/science/article/pii/S0969996119303754.

Chhetri, J. K., Mei, S., Wang, C., & Chan, P. (2023). New horizons in parkinson's disease in older populations. *Age and Ageing, 52*(10), Article afad186. https://doi.org/10.1093/ageing/afad186

Coleman, C., & Ian, M. (2022). Unraveling parkinson's disease neurodegeneration: Does aging hold the clues? *Journal of Parkinson's Disease, 12*(8), 2321–2338. https://journals.sagepub.com/action/showAbstract.

Cong, S., Xiang, C., Zhang, S., Zhang, T., Wang, H., & Cong, S. (2022). Prevalence and clinical aspects of depression in parkinson's disease: A systematic review and meta-analysis of 129 studies. *Neuroscience & Biobehavioral Reviews, 141*, Article 104749. https://www.sciencedirect.com/science/article/pii/S014976342200238X.

De Vreese, L. P., Mantesso, U., De Bastiani, E., Marangoni, A., Weger, E., & Gomiero, T. (2018). Anticholinergic burden in adult and elderly people with intellectual disabilities: Results from an Italian multicenter cross-sectional study [cited 2025 Oct 15]T. van Amelsvoort (Ed.). *PLoS One, 13*(10), Article e0205897 https://dx.plos.org/10.1371/journal.pone.0205897.

De Waele, S., Cras, P., & Crosiers, D. (2022). Apathy in parkinson's disease: Defining the Park apathy subtype. *Brain Sciences, 12*(7). https://www.mdpi.com/2076-3425/12/7/923.

Degirmenci, Y., Angelopoulou, E., Georgakopoulou, V. E., & Bougea, A. (2023). Cognitive impairment in parkinson's disease: An updated overview focusing on emerging pharmaceutical treatment approaches. *Medicina (B Aires), 59*(10). https://www.mdpi.com/1648-9144/59/10/1756.

Disease MDSTF on RS for P. (2003). The unified parkinson's disease rating scale (UPDRS): Status and recommendations. *Movement Disorders, 18*(7), 738–750. https://doi.org/10.1002/mds.10473

Dodet, P., Houot, M., Leu-Semenescu, S., Corvol, J. C., Lehéricy, S., Mangone, G., et al. (2024). Sleep disorders in Parkinson's disease, an early and multiple problem. *npj Parkinson's Disease, 10*(1), 46. https://doi.org/10.1038/s41531-024-00642-0

Duan, X., Liu, H., Hu, X., Yu, Q., Kuang, G., Liu, L., et al. (2025). Insomnia in parkinson's disease: Causes, consequences, and therapeutic approaches. *Molecular Neurobiology, 62*, 2292–2313. Springer.

Eisenhofer, G., & Goldstein, D. S. (2021). Norepinephrine reuptake blockade to treat neurogenic orthostatic hypotension. *Clinical Autonomic Research, 31*(3), 351–353. https://doi.org/10.1007/s10286-021-00808-3

Friedman, J. H., & Friedman, H. (2001). Fatigue in parkinson's disease: A nine-year follow-up. *Movement Disorders, 16*(6), 1120–1122. https://movementdisorders.onlinelibrary.wiley.com/doi/abs/10.1002/mds.1201.

Fullard, M. E., Morley, J. F., & Duda, J. E. (2017). Olfactory dysfunction as an early biomarker in parkinson's disease. *Neuroscience Bulletin, 33*(5), 515–525. https://doi.org/10.1007/s12264-017-0170-x

Gómez-López, A., Sánchez-Sánchez, A., Natera-Villalba, E., Ros-Castelló, V., Beltrán-Corbellini, Á., Fanjul-Arbós, S., et al. (2021). SURINPARK: Safinamide for urinary symptoms in parkinson's disease. *Brain Sciences, 11*(1). https://www.mdpi.com/2076-3425/11/1/57.

Goetz, C. G., Tilley, B. C., Shaftman, S. R., Stebbins, G. T., Fahn, S., Martinez-Martin, P., et al. (2008). Movement Disorder Society-sponsored revision of the unified parkinson's disease rating scale (MDS-UPDRS): Scale presentation and clinimetric testing results. *Movement Disorders, 23*(15), 2129–2170. https://doi.org/10.1002/mds.22340

Goldman, J. G. (2025). Non-motor symptoms and treatments in parkinson's disease. *Neurologic Clinics, 43*, 291–317. W.B. Saunders.

Groote Clara, De, Kathy, D., Luc, D., Bérengère, F., Virginie, H., Nicolas, C., et al. (2024). Development of a screening tool for assessing sexual difficulties among patients with parkinson's disease: The PD-SDS. *Journal of Parkinson's Disease, 14*(5), 1015–1025. https://doi.org/10.3233/JPD-240063

Grosu, C., Noea, O., Mastaleru, A., Ignat, E. B., & Leon, M. M. (2025). Neurogenic orthostatic hypotension in parkinson Disease—A narrative review of diagnosis and management. *Journal of Clinical Medicine, 14*. Multidisciplinary Digital Publishing Institute (MDPI).

Heinzel, S., Berg, D., Gasser, T., Chen, H., Yao, C., Postuma, R. B., et al. (2019). Update of the MDS research criteria for prodromal Parkinson's disease. *Movement Disorders, 34*(10), 1464–1470. https://doi.org/10.1002/mds.27802

Ignatavicius, A., Matar, E., & Lewis, S. J. G. (2025). Visual hallucinations in Parkinson's disease: Spotlight on central cholinergic dysfunction. *Brain, 148*, 376–393. Oxford University Press.

Iranzo, A., Cochen De Cock, V., Fantini, M. L., Pérez-Carbonell, L., & Trotti, L. M. (2024). Sleep and sleep disorders in people with Parkinson's disease. *Lancet Neurology, 23*(9), 925–937. https://doi.org/10.1016/S1474-4422(24)00170-4

Isaacson, S. H., Goldstein, M., Pahwa, R., Singer, C., Klos, K., Pucci, M., et al. (2023). Ulotaront, a trace amine-associated receptor 1/Serotonin 5-HT1A agonist, in patients with parkinson disease psychosis A pilot Study. *Neurology. Clinical Practice, 13*(4). https://www.scopus.com/inward/record.uri?eid=2-s2.0-85165881640&doi=10.1212%2fCPJ.0000000000200175&partnerID=40&md5=d184df75d7fd25c9fb19c5c2556c7a52.

Isaacson, S., Phillips, O., & Jimenez-Shahed, J. (2024). <em>Hope vs. Hype III:</em> Rescue/on-demand therapies are preferable to device-assisted therapies in Parkinson disease. *Parkinsonism Relat Disord, 126*. https://doi.org/10.1016/j.parkreldis.2024.106079

Jankovic, J., & Tan, E. K. (2020). Parkinson's disease: Etiopathogenesis and treatment. *Journal of Neurology Neurosurgery and Psychiatry, 91*(8), 795–808.

Janssen Daalen, J. M., van den Bergh, R., Prins, E. M., Moghadam, M. S. C., van den Heuvel, R., Veen, J., et al. (2024). Digital biomarkers for non-motor symptoms in Parkinson's disease: The state of the art. *Npj Digital Medicine, 7*. Nature Research.

Janz, C., Timpka, J., Rosqvist, K., Paul, G., Storch, A., & Odin, P. (2024). Non-Motor symptom management: Insights into adherence to treatment guidelines in parkinson's disease patients. *Journal of Parkinson's Disease, 14*(2), 297–312.

Jellinger, K. A. (2024). Mild cognitive impairment in parkinson's disease: Current view. *Frontiers in Cognition, 3*. Frontiers Media SA.

Kalbe, E., Folkerts, A. K., Witt, K., Buhmann, C., & Liepelt-Scarfone, I. (2024). German society of neurology guidelines for the diagnosis and treatment of cognitive impairment and affective disorders in people with Parkinson's disease: New spotlights on diagnostic procedures and non-pharmacological interventions. *Journal of Neurology, 271*(11), 7330–7357.

Kalia, L. V., Brotchie, J. M., & Fox, S. H. (2013). Novel nondopaminergic targets for motor features of parkinson's disease: Review of recent trials. *Movement Disorders, 28*(2), 131–144.

Kang, K. W., Choi, S. M., & Kim, B. C. (2022). Gender differences in motor and non-motor symptoms in early Parkinson disease. *Medicine, 101*(3). https://journals.lww.com/md-journal/fulltext/2022/01210/gender_differences_in_motor_and_non_motor_symptoms.59.aspx.

Kim, R., Lee, T. L., Lee, H., Ko, D. K., Lee, J. H., Shin, H., et al. (2023). Effects of physical exercise interventions on cognitive function in Parkinson's disease: An updated systematic review and meta-analysis of randomized controlled trials. *Parkinsonism Relat Disord, 117*, Article 105908. https://www.sciencedirect.com/science/article/pii/S1353802023009872.

Kulisevsky, J., Ferraz, H. B., Suppa, A., & Reichmann, H. (2024). Effects of safinamide on motor and non-motor symptoms in patients with parkinson's disease and motor fluctuations. *European Neurology, 87*(5–6), 291–305.

Li, X., Chen, C., Pan, T., Zhou, X., Sun, X., Zhang, Z., et al. (2024). Trends and hotspots in non-motor symptoms of Parkinson's disease: A 10-year bibliometric analysis. *Frontiers in Aging Neuroscience, 16*. Frontiers Media SA.

Li, F. F., Cui, Y. S., Yan, R., Cao, S. S., & Feng, T. (2022). Prevalence of lower urinary tract symptoms, urinary incontinence and retention in Parkinson's disease: A systematic review and meta-analysis. *Frontiers in Aging Neuroscience, 14*, Article 977572.

Litvan, I., Goldman, J. G., Tröster, A. I., Schmand, B. A., Weintraub, D., Petersen, R. C., et al. (2012). Diagnostic criteria for mild cognitive impairment in Parkinson's disease: Movement disorder society task force guidelines. *Movement Disorders, 27*(3), 349–356. https://movementdisorders.onlinelibrary.wiley.com/doi/abs/10.1002/mds.24893.

Liu, H., & Wang, X. P. (2024). Alternative therapies for non-motor symptoms in parkinson's disease: A mini review. *Neuropsychiatric Disease and Treatment, 20*, 2585–2591. Dove Medical Press Ltd.

Liu, C. F., Wang, T., Zhan, S. Q., Geng, D. Q., Wang, J., Liu, J., et al. (2018). Management recommendations on sleep disturbance of patients with parkinson's disease. *Chinese Medical Journal, 131*(24). https://journals.lww.com/cmj/fulltext/2018/12200/management_recommendations_on_sleep_disturbance_of.12.aspx.

Loureiro, D., Bilbao, R., Bordet, S., Grasso, L., Otero-Losada, M., Capani, F., et al. (2023). A systematic review and meta-analysis on the association between orthostatic hypotension and mild cognitive impairment and dementia in Parkinson's disease. *Neurological Sciences, 44*(4), 1211–1222. https://doi.org/10.1007/s10072-022-06537-3

Ly, A., Rahman, M., & Song, D. (2022). Pyridostigmine as an effective treatment for atonic Colon in parkinson's disease (P13-11.007). *Neurology, 98*(18_Suppl. ment), 1539. https://doi.org/10.1212/WNL.98.18_supplement.1539

Maas, B. R., Göttgens, I., Tijsse Klasen, H. P. S., Kapelle, W. M., Radder, D. L. M., Bloem, B. R., et al. (2024). Age and gender differences in non-motor symptoms in people with Parkinson's disease. *Frontiers in Neurology, 15*, 2024. https://www.frontiersin.org/journals/neurology/articles/10.3389/fneur.2024.1339716.

Maggi, G., Vitale, C., Cerciello, F., & Santangelo, G. (2023). Sleep and wakefulness disturbances in Parkinson's disease: A meta-analysis on prevalence and clinical aspects of REM sleep behavior disorder, excessive daytime sleepiness and insomnia. *Sleep Medicine Reviews, 68*, Article 101759. https://www.sciencedirect.com/science/article/pii/S1087079223000151.

Maher, S., Donlon, E., Mullane, G., Walsh, R., Lynch, T., & Fearon, C. (2024). Treatment of apathy in parkinson's disease and implications for underlying pathophysiology. *Journal of Clinical Medicine, 13*(8). https://www.mdpi.com/2077-0383/13/8/2216.

Marafioti, G., Corallo, F., Cardile, D., Di Lorenzo, G., Quartarone, A., & Lo Buono, V. (2023). REM sleep behavior disorder and cognitive functions in parkinson's patients: A systematic review. *Journal of Clinical Medicine, 12*(23). https://www.mdpi.com/2077-0383/12/23/7397.

Marinus, J., Zhu, K., Marras, C., Aarsland, D., & van Hilten, J. J. (2018). Risk factors for non-motor symptoms in Parkinson's disease. *Lancet Neurology, 17*(6), 559–568. https://doi.org/10.1016/S1474-4422(18)30127-3

Marras, C., Meyer, Z., Liu, H., Luo, S., Mantri, S., Allen, A., et al. (2024). Improving parkinson's disease care through systematic screening for depression. *Movement Disorders Clinical Practice, 11*(10), 1212–1222. https://doi.org/10.1002/mdc3.14163

Martinez-Martin, P. (2013). Instruments for holistic assessment of parkinson's disease. *Journal of Neural Transmission, 120*(4), 559–564. https://doi.org/10.1007/s00702-013-1005-1

Martinez-Nunez, A. E., Hutchinson, H., Coutinho, P., Sarmento, F. P., Lavu, V. S., Yuan, Q., et al. (2025). Clinically probable RBD is an early predictor of malignant non-motor parkinson's disease phenotypes. *npj Parkinson's Disease, 11*(1), 25. https://doi.org/10.1038/s41531-025-00874-8

Masnoon, N., Shakib, S., Kalisch-Ellett, L., & Caughey, G. E. (2017). What is polypharmacy? A systematic review of definitions. *BMC Geriatrics, 17*(1), 230. https://doi.org/10.1186/s12877-017-0621-2

McKeith, I. G., Boeve, B. F., Dickson, D. W., Halliday, G., Taylor, J. P., Weintraub, D., et al. (2017). Diagnosis and management of dementia with lewy bodies. *Neurology, 89*(1), 88–100. https://www.scopus.com/inward/record.uri?eid=2-s2.0-85021876617&doi=10.1212%2fWNL.0000000000004058&partnerID=40&md5=4cd7ed7df77df8e07f5dfbf9cd7d27af.

McLean, G., Hindle, J. V., Guthrie, B., & Mercer, S. W. (2017). Co-morbidity and polypharmacy in Parkinson's disease: Insights from a large scottish primary care database. *BMC Neurology, 17*(1), 126. https://doi.org/10.1186/s12883-017-0904-4

Moshayedi, A. J., Mokhtari, T., & Emadi Andani, M. (2025). Brain stimulation techniques in research and clinical practice: A comprehensive review of applications and therapeutic potential in parkinson's disease. *Brain Sciences, 15*(1). https://www.mdpi.com/2076-3425/15/1/20.

Mouchaileh, N., & Hughes, A. J. (2020). Pharmacological management of Parkinson's disease in older people. *Journal of Pharmacy Practice and Research, 50*(5), 445–454. https://onlinelibrary.wiley.com/doi/abs/10.1002/jppr.1683.

Mujahid, B. I. M., Holla, V. V., Kamble, N., Yadav, R., Pal, P. K., & Mahale, R. R. (2025). Non-motor fluctuations in parkinson's disease: Frequency and clinical correlate. *Journal of Neural Transmission*. https://doi.org/10.1007/s00702-025-02908-0

Murueta-Goyena, A., Del Pino, R., Carmona-Abellán, M., Tijero, B., Ruiz-Lopez, M., Acera, M., et al. (2025). Effect of sex on the progression of non-motor symptoms in parkinson's disease: A registry-based cohort study. *Neurologia*.

Nardelli, D., Gambioli, F., De Bartolo, M. I., Mancinelli, R., Biagioni, F., Carotti, S., et al. (2024). Pain in Parkinson's disease: A neuroanatomy-based approach. *Brain Communications, 6*. Oxford University Press.

Oedekoven, C., Egeri, L., Jessen, F., Wagner, M., & Dodel, R. (2022). Subjective cognitive decline in idiopathic parkinson's disease: A systematic review. *Ageing Research Reviews, 74*, Article 101508. https://www.sciencedirect.com/science/article/pii/S1568163721002555.

Pahwa, R., Pagan, F. L., Kremens, D. E., & Saint-Hilaire, M. (2023). Clinical use of On-Demand therapies for patients with parkinson's disease and OFF periods. *Neurol Ther, 12*(4), 1033–1049. https://doi.org/10.1007/s40120-023-00486-5

Peña-Zelayeta, L., Delgado-Minjares, K. M., Villegas-Rojas, M. M., León-Arcia, K., Santiago-Balmaseda, A., Andrade-Guerrero, J., et al. (2025). Redefining non-motor symptoms in parkinson's disease. *Journal of Personalized Medicine, 15*. Multidisciplinary Digital Publishing Institute (MDPI).

Picillo, M., Nicoletti, A., Fetoni, V., Garavaglia, B., Barone, P., & Pellecchia, M. T. (2017). The relevance of gender in Parkinson's disease: A review. *Journal of Neurology, 264*(8), 1583–1607. https://doi.org/10.1007/s00415-016-8384-9

Pitton Rissardo, J., Jayasinghe, M., Gadelmawla, A. F., Rashidi, M., Rashidi, F., Moharam, H., et al. (2025). Exploring fatigue in parkinson's disease: A comprehensive literature review. *Cureus*.

Radad, K., Moldzio, R., Krewenka, C., Kranner, B., & Rausch, W. D. (2023). Pathophysiology of non-motor signs in Parkinson's disease: Some recent updating with brief presentation. *Exploration of Neuroprotective Therapy, 3*, 24–46. Open Exploration Publishing Inc.

Ray Chaudhuri, K., Antonini, A., Robieson, W. Z., Sanchez-Soliño, O., Bergmann, L., Poewe, W., et al. (2019). Burden of non-motor symptoms in parkinson's disease patients predicts improvement in quality of life during treatment with levodopa-carbidopa intestinal gel. *European Journal of Neurology, 26*(4). https://doi.org/10.1111/ene.13847

Ray Chaudhuri, K., Leta, V., Bannister, K., Brooks, D. J., & Svenningsson, P. (2023). The noradrenergic subtype of Parkinson disease: From animal models to clinical practice. *Nature Reviews Neurology, 19*, 333–345. Nature Research.

Regensburger, M., Csoti, I., Jost, W. H., Kohl, Z., Lorenzl, S., Pedrosa, D. J., et al. (2025). Motor and non-motor fluctuations in Parkinson's disease: The knowns and unknowns of current therapeutic approaches. *Journal of Neural Transmission, 133*(2), 309–324. https://doi.org/10.1007/s00702-025-02990-4

Reynolds, H., Miller, N., & Walker, R. (2018). Drooling in parkinson's disease: Evidence of a role for divided attention. *Dysphagia, 33*(6), 809–817. https://doi.org/10.1007/s00455-018-9906-7

Rukavina, K., Batzu, L., Boogers, A., Abundes-Corona, A., Bruno, V., & Chaudhuri, K. R. (2021). Non-motor complications in late stage parkinson's disease: Recognition, management and unmet needs. *Expert Review of Neurotherapeutics, 21*, 335–352. Taylor and Francis Ltd.

Safarpour, D., Stover, N., Shprecher, D. R., Hamedani, A. G., Pfeiffer, R. F., Parkman, H. P., et al. (2024). Consensus practice recommendations for management of gastrointestinal dysfunction in Parkinson disease. *Parkinsonism Relat Disord, 124*. https://doi.org/10.1016/j.parkreldis.2024.106982

Santos-García, D., Laguna, A., Hernández-Vara, J., de Deus Fonticoba, T., Cores Bartolomé, C., Feal Painceiras, M. J., et al. (2023). Sex differences in motor and non-motor symptoms among Spanish patients with parkinson's disease. *Journal of Clinical Medicine, 12*(4). https://www.mdpi.com/2077-0383/12/4/1329.

Sardar, Z., Liaquat, S., Yousaf, Q., Bano, S., & Numan, A. (2023). Non-motor symptoms burden in early stages of parkinson's disease. *Annals of Indian Academy of Neurology, 26*(1), 39–43.

Sarmento, F., Lamp, G., Lavu, V. S., Madamangalam, A. S., Reddy Dwarampudi, J. M., Yuan, Q., et al. (2024). Exploring the layers of fatigue in Parkinson's disease: A comprehensive analysis of its prevalence and contributing factors. *Clin Park Relat Disord, 11*, Article 100288. https://www.sciencedirect.com/science/article/pii/S2590112524000598.

Schütz, L., Sixel-Döring, F., & Hermann, W. (2022). Management of sleep disturbances in parkinson's disease. *Journal of Parkinson's Disease, 12*(7), 2029–2058. https://doi.org/10.3233/JPD-212749

Schapira, A. H. V., Chaudhuri, K. R., & Jenner, P. (2017). Non-motor features of Parkinson disease. *Nature Reviews Neuroscience, 18*(7), 435–450. https://doi.org/10.1038/nrn.2017.62

Schneider, J. S., & Kortagere, S. (2022). Current concepts in treating mild cognitive impairment in Parkinson's disease. *Neuropharmacology, 203*, Article 108880. https://www.sciencedirect.com/science/article/pii/S0028390821004354.

Seki, M., Kawata, Y., Hayashi, A., Arai, M., & Fujimoto, S. (2023). Prescribing patterns and determinants for elderly patients with parkinson's disease in Japan: A retrospective observational study using insurance claims databases. *Frontiers in Neurology, 14*. https://www.frontiersin.org/journals/neurology/articles/10.3389/fneur.2023.1162016.

Seppi, K., Ray Chaudhuri, K., Coelho, M., Fox, S. H., Katzenschlager, R., Perez, L. S., et al. (2019). Update on treatments for nonmotor symptoms of parkinson's disease—an evidence-based medicine review. *Movement Disorders, 34*, 180–198. John Wiley and Sons Inc.

Siciliano, M., Trojano, L., Santangelo, G., De Micco, R., Tedeschi, G., & Tessitore, A. (2018). Fatigue in Parkinson's disease: A systematic review and meta-analysis. *Movement Disorders, 33*(11), 1712–1723. https://doi.org/10.1002/mds.27461

Silveira, C. R. A., Coleman, K. K. L., Borron, K., Tirona, R. G., Rupar, C. A., Zou, G., et al. (2025). Ambroxol as a treatment for parkinson disease dementia: A randomized clinical trial. *JAMA Neurology, 82*(8), 797–807. https://doi.org/10.1001/jamaneurol.2025.1687

Simonet, C., Schrag, A., Lees, A. J., & Noyce, A. J. (2021). The motor prodromes of parkinson's disease: From bedside observation to large-scale application. *Journal of Neurology, 268*, 2099–2108. Springer Science and Business Media Deutschland GmbH.

Torres-Pasillas, G., Chi-Castañeda, D., Carrillo-Castilla, P., Marín, G., Hernández-Aguilar, M. E., Aranda-Abreu, G. E., et al. (2023). Olfactory dysfunction in parkinson's disease, its functional and neuroanatomical correlates. *NeuroSci, 4*(2), 134–151. https://www.mdpi.com/2673-4087/4/2/13.

Ullah, I., Wang, X., & Li, H. (2024). Novel and experimental therapeutics for the management of motor and non-motor Parkinsonian symptoms. *Neurological Sciences, 45*(7), 2979–2995. https://doi.org/10.1007/s10072-023-07278-7

Urso, D., Leta, V., & Rukavina, K. (2022). Chapter five - Management strategies of sexual dysfunctions in parkinson's disease. In K. R. Chaudhuri, C. Falup-Pecurariu, & M. Parry (Eds.), *International review of neurobiology* (pp. 97–116). Academic Press. https://www.sciencedirect.com/science/article/pii/S0074774221001100.

Vafaeimastanabad, M., Salemi, M. H., Jodki, T., Sabri, V., Talab, E. K., Babaei, F. N., et al. (2023). Sexual dysfunction among patients with Parkinson's disease: A systematic review and meta-analysis. *Journal of Clinical Neuroscience, 117*, 1–10. https://www.sciencedirect.com/science/article/pii/S0967586823002424.

van Wamelen, D. J., Leta, V., Johnson, J., Ocampo, C. L., Podlewska, A. M., Rukavina, K., et al. (2020). Drooling in parkinson's disease: Prevalence and progression from the Non-motor International Longitudinal Study. *Dysphagia, 35*(6), 955–961.

van Wamelen, D. J., Sringean, J., Trivedi, D., Carroll, C. B., Schrag, A. E., Odin, P., et al. (2021). Digital health technology for non-motor symptoms in people with Parkinson's disease: Futile or future? *Parkinsonism Relat Disord, 89*, 186–194. https://doi.org/10.1016/j.parkreldis.2021.07.032

Vaughan, C. P. (2019). Treatment of urinary and sexual dysfunction in parkinson's disease. In S. G. Reich, & S. A. Factor (Eds.), *Therapy of movement disorders: A case-based approach* (pp. 59–63). Cham: Springer International Publishing. https://doi.org/10.1007/978-3-319-97897-0_14

Vaughan, C. P., Morley, J. F., Lehosit, J., McGwin, G., Muirhead, L., Khakharia, A., et al. (2025). Behavioral compared with drug therapy for overactive bladder symptoms in parkinson disease: A randomized non-inferiority trial. *JAMA Neurology, 82*(9), 925–931. https://doi.org/10.1001/jamaneurol.2025.1904

Voruz, P., Guérin, D., & Péron, J. A. (2025). Impact of motor symptom asymmetry on non-motor outcomes in Parkinson's disease: A systematic review. *npj Parkinson's Disease, 11*(1).

Wagg, A., Staskin, D., Engel, E., Herschorn, S., Kristy, R. M., & Schermer, C. R. (2020). Efficacy, safety, and tolerability of mirabegron in patients aged ≥65yr with overactive bladder wet: A phase IV, double-blind, randomised, placebo-controlled study (PILLAR). *European Urology, 77*(2), 211–220. https://www.sciencedirect.com/science/article/pii/S0302283819307687.

Wamelen, DJ Van, Rukavina, K., Podlewska, A. M., & Chaudhuri, K. R. (2022). Advances in the pharmacological and non-pharmacological management of non-motor symptoms in parkinson's disease: An update since 2017. *Current Neuropharmacology, 21*(8), 1786–1805.

Weise, D., Claus, I., Dresel, C., Kalbe, E., Liepelt-Scarfone, I., Lorenzl, S., et al. (2024). Multidisciplinary care in Parkinson's disease. *Journal of Neural Transmission, 131*(10), 1217–1227. https://doi.org/10.1007/s00702-024-02807-w

Yamaguchi, T., Aihara, A., Mashiko, S., Kurosawa, E., Oizumi, T., Yamagata, T., et al. (2024). Exacerbation of delirium and epileptic seizures in an older man with idiopathic Parkinson's disease due to multiple prescriptions: A case report. *Frontiers of Medicine, 11*. https://www.frontiersin.org/journals/medicine/articles/10.3389/fmed.2024.1415988.

Yuan, X. Y., Chen, Y. S., & Liu, Z. (2024). Relationship among Parkinson's disease, constipation, microbes, and microbiological therapy. *World Journal of Gastroenterology, 30*(3), 225–237. https://www.wjgnet.com/1007-9327/full/v30/i3/225.htm.

Zhang, W., Deng, B., Xie, F., Zhou, H., Guo, J. F., Jiang, H., et al. (2022). Efficacy of repetitive transcranial magnetic stimulation in Parkinson's disease: A systematic review and meta-analysis of randomised controlled trials. *EClinicalMedicine, 52*. https://doi.org/10.1016/j.eclinm.2022.101589

CHAPTER

Clinical case studies and practical applications 13

Nada Fath[1], Ismail Louragli[2], Muhammad Aminu[3] and Mohammad Ammar Qaed[4]

[1]School of Basic Medical Sciences, Fujian Medical University, Fuzhou, China; [2]Higher Institute of Nursing and Health Techniques, Ministry of Health and Social Protection, Dakhla, Morocco; [3]School of Public Health, Fujian Medical University, Fuzhou, Fujian, China; [4]School of Health Management, Fujian Medical University, Fuzhou, Fujian, China

13.1 Introduction

Parkinson's disease (PD) is a progressive neurodegenerative disorder with primary effects on motor control (Tenchov et al., 2025). The pathophysiology of the disease is complex, involving not just the central nervous system (CNS) but also the enteric nervous system (ENS) (Gao et al., 2025). The proposed underlying mechanisms of PD are multiple and diverse, but the pathogenesis has been long attributed to the loss of dopaminergic neurons in the substantia nigra, and the resulting motor dysfunction manifested by tremor, bradykinesia, rigidity, and postural instability (Pitton (Rissardo et al., 2025). Its pathophysiology is further characterized by non-motor features such as cognitive decline, anxiety, depression, and sleep disorders. Furthermore, at the cellular level, the pathophysiology includes α-synuclein protein deposit forming lewy bodies, mitochondrial disease, neuroinflammation, and oxidative stress (Tenchov et al., 2025). Clinical manifestations of PD have been attributed to dopaminergic dysfunction, and even though some of the symptoms are relieved by dopamine replacement therapy, these medications do not treat the non-motor manifestations of the disease (Pitton (Rissardo et al., 2025). Treatment of PD nowadays consists of dopaminergic therapy with levodopa and dopamine agonists, and monoamine oxidase B (MAO-B) inhibitors, catechol-O-methyl transferase (COMT) inhibitors, and surgery such as deep brain stimulation (DBS). They provide relief from some of the symptoms but do not halt the disease process. Therefore, research has been aimed at the creation of disease-modifying treatments, drug repurposing, novel targets, and stable biomarkers, like genetic markers, cerebrospinal fluid (CSF) proteins, and biomarkers for diagnosis, disease progression, and treatment response (Tenchov et al., 2025). Clinical trials and case reports offer valuable data on the efficacy, safety, and side effects of different pharmacologic therapies, which can also be highly variable in different individuals. For instance, the response to dopaminergic therapy with levodopa can differ based on the stage of illness, genetic influences, and comorbid illnesses. Case reports help to bring such differences to light and to develop more personalized treatment strategies. PD clinical pharmacotherapy targets both motor and non-motor symptoms with its drugs. The dopaminergic medications are the most commonly utilized drugs for improving the functioning of the motor system and treating motor symptoms. COMT inhibitors and MAO-B inhibitors are used to

Pharmacological Foundations of Parkinson's Disease. https://doi.org/10.1016/B978-0-443-27702-3.00016-9

prolong the action of levodopa, whereas drugs like amantadine and anticholinergics are used to treat dyskinesias and tremor, respectively. Additionally, treating non-motor symptoms, like using antidepressants for depression and cholinesterase inhibitors for memory problems, is an important part of a comprehensive treatment plan for Parkinson's disease (Tenchov et al., 2025).

The Parkinson's Progression Markers Initiative (PPMI) has played a significant role in tracking drug administration and its effects on the progression of the disease, while its findings have been beneficial in clinical setting research (Spott et al., 2025). The study identifies the necessity for accurate and standardized reporting of drug use that is essential in determining the effect of new therapeutic agents in clinical trial settings. These drugs are intended to enhance motor symptoms, quality of life (QoL), and prevent disease progression. Nevertheless, issues such as medication heterogeneity, off-label prescribing, and the necessity for standardized documentation indicate the continuous work that is needed to optimize pharmacotherapy in PD (Spott et al., 2025). The objective is to optimize medication regimens in order to improve QoL and functional independence in PD patients. The chapter provides valuable insights into treating Parkinson's disease by discussing clinical cases and trials that focus on both early and advanced stages of the disease, along with managing non-motor symptoms like cognitive issues and mental health problems. The chapter also delves into basic principles of pharmacotherapy in clinical practice, symptom-based treatment, and use of notable drugs. We also discuss the clinical relevance of these principles to practical settings, with an emphasis on treatment individualization, and examine emerging trends and new therapies and their effects on clinical practice.

13.2 Clinical trials and case studies in parkinson's disease management

13.2.1 Early-stage parkinson's disease

Hasan et al. (2023) reported a case study of Mr. Smith, a 65-year-old patient who was diagnosed with PD 5 years earlier than the time when the study was conducted, and the patient had the early-stage motor features (tremor, rigidity, bradykinesia, and loss of balance). Despite a history of PD in his family (affected father) and comorbid hypertension and hyperlipidemia, the diagnosis of the patient was made using dopamine transporter (DaT) imaging, which showed decreased uptake of dopamine, along with clinical assessment. Initial pharmacotherapy with levodopa-carbidopa—selected due to symptom severity impacting daily function—and physical therapy with individualized exercise program resulted in only incomplete improvement. With time, Mr. Smith evolved into patient with dyskinetic fluctuations, which is a classic side effects of long-term levodopa therapy. The treatment was changed by lowering the amount of levodopa and adding entacapone to help the body use it better, demonstrating how adjusting the treatment plan can be effective in early Parkinson's disease (Hasan et al., 2023). When pharmacotherapy was insufficient, multidisciplinary intervention led to referral for DBS, with dramatic alleviation of symptoms and functional improvement. This case shows several key things: the need for quick and personalized diagnosis, considering the benefits and long-term side effects of levodopa, and starting advanced treatments like DBS when standard treatments don't work (Hasan et al., 2023). Combined levodopa therapy with carbidopa was also investigated in a Levodopa in Early Parkinson's Disease (LEAP) trial. It's a landmark multicenter, double-blind, placebo-controlled delayed-start trial Verschuur (Verschuur et al., 2019). Researchers determined if early levodopa therapy (100 mg three times daily with carbidopa) has disease-modifying effects in early PD. Patients received either early treatment with levodopa for 80 weeks (early-start group), or a placebo for 40 weeks, followed by levodopa treatment for 40 weeks (delayed-start group). The study showed that the main endpoint, as assessed by the Unified Parkinson's Disease Rating Scale (UPDRS), did not differ significantly between groups at the 80-week time point (mean change: −1.0 vs. −2.0 points; $P = .44$), which suggests that levodopa does not have disease-modifying activity. The additional analyses showed that symptom progression was similar during the placebo-controlled phase (weeks 4–40), but they did not prove that starting treatment early was just as good during the follow-up phase (weeks 44–80), which further supports that there is no disease-modifying effect. Dyskinesia and motor fluctuation rates did not differ significantly between groups. Thus, the role of levodopa in early PD is exclusively symptomatic, with no evidence of altering the disease process. Clinically, the evidence shows the importance of the timing of treatment initiation in early-stage management and justifies delaying levodopa initiation until the onset of motor symptoms (Verschuur et al., 2019). In addition, the benefits of neurostimulation for patients with early motor complications have been investigated earlierin a randomized, controlled trial, known as the EARLYSTIM study by (Schuepbach et al., 2013). Researchers randomized 251 PD and early motor complication patients to subthalamic nucleus stimulation and medical therapy or medical therapy alone and compared their effectiveness. The primary result was QoL as assessed by the Parkinson's Disease Questionnaire (PDQ-39) summary index. Overall, the results showed a big improvement in quality of life for the neurostimulation group, with an average score increase of 7.8 points, while the medical therapy group had a small decrease of 0.2 points ($P = .002$). In addition, neurostimulation was linked to significant improvements in motor disability, activities of daily living, and motor complications triggered by levodopa. The research demonstrated that subthalamic nucleus stimulation not only benefitted motor symptoms but also enhanced global QoL, indicating that neurostimulation may be an effective treatment option at an earlier stage of PD than has traditionally been considered. The finding contradicts the traditional practice of reserving neurostimulation for late stages of the disease and reveals the possibility of early intervention greatly enhancing patient outcomes (Schuepbach et al., 2013).

13.2.2 Progression, motor complications and advanced-stage PD

A phase II, double-blind, placebo-controlled study assessed the efficacy and tolerability of a new D1/D5 dopamine receptor partial agonist, PF-06,649,751, in patients with early PD for 15 weeks (Riesenberg et al., 2020). Even though the study ended early, it found that PF-06,649,751 led to a notable improvement in motor symptoms, showing an average decrease of 9.0 points in the Movement Disorder Society-UPDRS (MDS-UPDRS) Part III score, while the placebo group only had a decrease of 4.3 points ($P = .0407$). The effect was observed on the first visit, week 3, and sustained until week 15, indicating rapid onset of action. The overall safety profile was positive, with nausea, headache, and dry mouth being common adverse events. Importantly, the drug did not have a notable risk of inducing orthostatic hypotension or other major cardiovascular events. The results indicate that PF-06,649,751 could be a helpful and safe early treatment for Parkinson's disease and should be tested in bigger and longer studies. This research highlights the continuous quest for therapeutic alternatives capable of enhancing motor complications and enhancing QoL in PD patients (Riesenberg et al., 2020).

In addition, a review by (Olanow et al., 2021) provides a comprehensive overview of on-demand therapies for managing OFF episodes. OFF episodes, defined as a return of parkinsonian features during times in between doses of levodopa, are a major cause of disability for PD patients. These episodes can worsen movement problems and cause painful muscle contractions, along with many other non-movement issues, greatly limiting the quality of life. Three currently available on-demand therapies are reviewed, namely subcutaneous injection of apomorphine, sublingual apomorphine film and inhaled levodopa. While subcutaneous apomorphine is effective, its use has been limited because of injection administration and side effects. Sublingual apomorphine is easy to take, avoids the body's initial breakdown, and works quickly and lasts a long time; however, it can cause problems in the mouth and throat. While inhaled levodopa provides a discrete responsive dose, the established dose and cough response may potentially compromise its efficacy. These therapies provide patients and clinicians with the ability to quickly and reliably resolve OFF episodes, with potential benefits for functional outcomes and quality of life (Olanow et al., 2021). Besides, long-term levodopa treatment has been associated with levodopa-induced dyskinesias (LIDs), a common and disabling side effect of PD. Its clinical presentation is chorea, dystonia, and other abnormal movements that have a tendency to occur during peak-dose periods or at the onset and offset of levodopa effects. In a review by Calabresi et al. (2010), authors elucidated the pathophysiological mechanisms behind LIDs, underscoring the role of pulsatile stimulation of dopamine receptors and the critical role of D1 dopamine receptors in the genesis of these dyskinesias. This also highlights the complexity of LIDs and the interminable challenge toward formulating viable therapies, implicating that a multi-pronged approach comprising of drug and surgical interventions may be required to control it in these afflicted individuals with advanced PD (Calabresi et al., 2010). Furthermore, a recent study has assessed the role of opicapone, a third-generation catechol-O-methyltransferase (COMT) inhibitor, in levodopa therapy optimization (Ferreira et al., 2022). The open-label phase 2 trial looked at how taking opicapone once a day affects how the body processes levodopa and how well it helps with movement in patients with fluctuating Parkinson's disease. This phase involved 24 patients from the original study who took levodopa/carbidopa (LD/CD) 500/125 mg for 2 weeks, and then were randomly chosen to take LD/CD 400/100 mg along with opicapone 50 mg four or five times a day for another 2 weeks. The main effect was levodopa 12-hour pharmacokinetics. Combination of opicapone with the standard regimen dramatically extended levodopa plasma half-life and reduced its fluctuation. The better absorption of the medication led to less time when symptoms were not controlled (OFF time) and more time when symptoms were managed (ON time), showing that opicapone can make levodopa work better without needing to increase the total daily amount of levodopa taken (Ferreira et al., 2022). Another study by (Aldred et al., 2023) has shown useful data on the safety and efficacy of foslevodopa/foscarbidopa continuous subcutaneous infusion in advanced PD. The 52-week, open-label, phase 3 trial compared continuous 24-hour/day infusion of foslevodopa/foscarbidopa, in advanced PD patients with motor fluctuations despite oral medication. Patients taking foslevodopa/foscarbidopa had less OFF time and more ON time without bothersome dyskinesia at every visit after the first check-up, and this effect was noticeable right from the first check-up after starting treatment. At week 52, patients experienced a mean reduction of 3.5 h in OFF time and a 3.8-hour increase in ON time without troublesome dyskinesia. In addition, the treatment had beneficial effects on sleep quality, morning akinesia and overall QoL. Safety profile was acceptable, with infusion site events being most frequent adverse events, the majority of which were mild to moderate in severity. These results suggest that foslevodopa/foscarbidopa could be a safe and effective non-surgical choice for treating movement problems in advanced Parkinson's disease and should be looked at more closely in medical practice (Aldred et al., 2023). Moreover (Bovenzi et al., 2024), reported the data on the actual use of safinamide, a dual-site antiparkinsonian drug with action on dopaminergic and glutamatergic systems. The study includes a detailed look at the Italian group from the SYNAPSES study, which looked at how well and safely safinamide works for patients with changing motor symptoms in regular medical settings. It involved 616 patients across 52 centers, with 86.0% completing the 12-month follow-up. The results showed that safinamide greatly helped with movement problems and changes in symptoms, based on the UPDRS III and IV scores, and there were no major safety issues. Significantly, the drug exerted an impact on the reduction of unpredictable OFF periods and early morning OFF phenomena, with responses occurring as early as the initial 3 months of treatment. Furthermore, safinamide positively influenced the non-motor signs of depression, sleep, and pain, which paralleled an overall gain in QoL. The study upholds safinamide's good safety profile even in riskier patient groups such as elderly patients above the age of 75 years and those with psychiatric disease. These results indicate that safinamide might be a helpful option for treating both movement and non-movement symptoms in Parkinson's disease patients, especially those who experience changes in their movement (Bovenzi et al., 2024).

13.2.3 Non-motor symptoms

Parkinson's disease isn't just about shaking palsy and movement dysfunctions, but there's a whole combination of challenges that come with it. In a clinical case study, a 65-year-old male with a 10-year history of PD started showing signs that went far beyond the typical motor symptoms, highlighting the multifaceted nature of psychiatric complications in PD. The patient wasn't only struggling with movement troubles; but he also had mood disorders, showing clear signs of depression, apathy, and impulse control disorders (ICDs). Interestingly, the usual dopaminergic treatment, such as levodopa and a dopamine agonist, largely controlled his movement issues. Yet, as it is often the case, while his motor control got better, those same drugs seemed to exacerbate his psychiatric issues. This case demonstrates the challenges in balancing motor and nonmotor symptom management, as dopaminergic medications, while effective for motor symptoms, can worsen psychiatric conditions such as impulsivity and compulsive behaviors—a kind of double-edged sword. The patient was eventually given an antidepressant, venlafaxine, which demonstrated clinical utility in managing his depressive symptoms without significant adverse effects, illustrating the importance of pharmacotherapy tailored to nonmotor symptoms (Seppi et al., 2019). Moreover, a cognitive-behavioral therapy (CBT) that was implemented for the management of impulse control problems displayed first steps toward changing damaging behaviors and bringing about a general improvement in the level of activity. This particular clinical case is a good illustration of the idea of the necessity of a complete treatment strategy, which includes pharmacotherapy and psychological therapy, for the correct treatment of PD psychiatric disorders. Additionally, a comprehensive meta-analysis of case–control studies (Molde et al., 2018), explored the incidence of ICDs in PD. The survey with data from 2371 PD patients and 2168 people without the disease showed a striking link between PD and different ICDs, namely gambling, hypersexuality, eating disorders, compulsive spending (pounding), and hobbyism. The relative odds of these ICDs were higher for PD patients as compared to healthy controls. The research established two decisive mediators: being medically treated for PD and disease duration. It was in this case that the use of dopaminergic agents by patients was a clear risk factor with the neurotransmitter therapy being the most direct path to these behaviors. The results put a significant emphasis on the necessity of regular check-ups for ICDs in PD patients, in particular, in the context of the medication with dopaminergic drugs, which makes monitoring an effective way to keep these mental disorders at least under control (Molde et al., 2018). Moreover, in a recent study by (Akbar & Friedman, 2022), the long-term effects of pimavanserin treatment for psychosis in PD was investigated through the review of 54 patients' charts. The findings showed that pimavanserin, which is the only FDA-approved drug for PD psychosis, was the medication that provided some initial improvement to 47% of the subjects, the majority (50%) of the patients with dementia of Lewy bodies were amenable to it. Nevertheless, just a small fraction (15%) of patients with pimavanserin monotherapy was taking it all the way to a successful treatment after a median of 52 weeks. According to the study, the long-term response rate of pimavanserin was lower than that reported from various clinical trials even though the drug was found safe and well tolerated (Akbar & Friedman, 2022). The findings suggest that pimavanserin may require concomitant antipsychotic medication for sustained efficacy in many patients, emphasizing the need for further research to identify ideal candidates and develop more effective treatments for PD psychosis. In a groundbreaking study called VOPARK, researchers looked at vortioxetine, an antidepressant that works in different ways, in 30 patients with Parkinson's disease and major depression over 12 weeks (Santos García et al., 2022). A 53% decrease in depression symptoms was found as the primary outcome using the 17-item Hamilton Depression Rating Scale (HAM-D17) test, with 50% of the patients reaching a $\geq$50% response and 43.3% being in remission. The tool PD Cognitive Rating Scale (PD-CRS) was used to measure the cognitive function, and it presented significant positive changes mainly in the late verbal memory domain as well as with other certain trends related to fronto-subcortical and posterior cortical areas. The result of this is that the QoL as well as the affected aspects, such as apathy, and fatigue, have been improved, and the PDQ-39 (a health-related QoL instrument) score was 24% better. However, there were 33.3% of patients experiencing side effects, the most prevalent of which were gastrointestinal, and in general, they were quite tolerable. Demonstrating PD's dependence on its impact on both mood and cognitive abilities, the results of this analysis of vortioxetine's serotonin and choline effects are strong. While it has an open label design and a small sample size, the study underscores vortioxetine as a possible auxiliary drug in the pharmacotherapy of PD especially for patients with comorbid depression and cognitive impairment (Santos García et al., 2022). Additional research is needed so that the results can be confirmed in extensive controlled studies. Moreover, a twofold mechanism of action targeting the dopaminergic and glutamatergic systems has confirmed safinamide as a pioneering PD treatment. The results of various clinical studies have shown that it is effective in improving movement problems and other symptoms in PD patients who are at a moderate to advanced stage. The most notable effect was when it was combined with levodopa therapy, which had benefits for at least 2 years. The follow-up review of the data shows it may help with non-motor symptoms such as pain and mood, likely due to its effect on glutamate levels (Abbruzzese et al., 2021). Safinamide's safety profile is favorable, with adverse events comparable to placebo and no significant drug-drug interactions (Abbruzzese et al., 2021). Movement disorder specialists have looked at how safinamide helps treat Parkinson's disease, especially its effectiveness in handling both movement and non-movement symptoms, like mental health issues (Stocchi et al., 2022). The research, which was carried out among 90 professionals from 8 European nations, gave a clear agreement about safinamide's success in controlling the symptoms of movement, motor fluctuations, and QoL. A good opinion was also formed about the absence of non-motor symptoms such as sleep/fatigue, mood, and pain. However, there was a lack of consensus regarding its efficacy in improving cognition, urinary, and sexual functions, while there was the opposite for orthostatic hypotension. The study noted that safinamide's effect on the glutamatergic system by temporarily blocking MAO-B, along with its role as a new modulator for glutamate release, probably helps explain the clinical benefits seen in both motor and non-motor symptoms (Stocchi et al., 2022).

13.3 Key pharmacotherapy principles in practice

In PD, the primary dysfunction in the basal ganglia circuitry involves overactivity of Medium Spiny Neurons (MSNs)—the striatum's main projection neurons—particularly those of the D2-receptor-expressing indirect pathway. Hyperactivity of this pathway leads to excessive suppression of movement by reinforcing thalamic inhibition (Calabresi et al., 2014). Therefore, regulation of receptors on MSNs of this pathway to tone down its activity would yield several therapeutic windows for the disease. Indirect-pathway MSNs overactivity reinforces GABAergic inhibition of the external globus pallidus (GPe). This diminishes GPe inhibition of the subthalamic nucleus (STN), resulting in STN disinhibition. In combination with hyperactivity of excitatory cortico-subthalamic (hyperdirect pathway) projections, this results in overactivity of STN output. The STN over-excites the globus pallidus interna (GPi) and substantia nigra pars reticulata (SNr), reinforcing their inhibitory GABAergic output to the thalamus and inhibiting movement (Song et al., 2023). Pharmacological manipulation at any point in this circuitry downstream of the striatum appears able to alleviate parkinsonism. Also, while it may not be as significant, the lack of activity in the direct pathway also plays a role in causing parkinsonian symptoms. As with overactivity of the indirect pathway, this leads to overactivity of the GPi/SNr (Song et al., 2023). Reducing indirect pathway overactivity may exert anti-parkinsonian effects and/or potentiate therapies targeting this pathway. In Parkinson's disease, the indirect pathway becomes too active because there is less inhibition from D2 receptors, which supports the use of dopamine-replacing treatments, especially D2 receptor agonists (Gerfen, 2023; Zha et al., 2024).

Although all current dopaminergic treatments stimulate D2 receptors to some degree, their other drug properties also influence how well they work. For instance, activating the D1 receptor can enhance the benefits of D2 stimulation by improving the direct pathway function, which is why L-DOPA is preferred over D2 agonists for treatment. For instance, activating the D1 receptor can enhance the benefits of the D2-mediated pathway by restoring direct pathway function, which is why L-DOPA is preferred for treatment over D2 agonists. L-DOPA raises dopamine levels, activating both D1 and D2-like receptors at once, making it more effective than drugs that only target D2 receptors (Gerfen, 2023). Furthermore, L-DOPA's conversion to noradrenaline may provide supplementary benefits beyond dopamine receptor activation (Antonini et al., 2023). However, too much stimulation of D1 receptors can cause movement problems, showing that it's important to balance how we activate different receptors (Chhetri et al., 2023; Isaacson et al., 2021). Furthermore, the absence of D2 receptor activation in PD impairs dopaminergic regulation of cholinergic interneurons, leading to their hyperactive acetylcholine output. This cholinergic enhancement respectively depolarizes indirect pathway MSNs via M1 muscarinic receptor stimulation. The acknowledged but not widely performing muscarinic antagonists' anti-parkinsonian action is probably due to the blocking of the above-cited process (LeWitt et al., 2024; Myslivecek, 2021; Pasquini et al., 2021). However, their modest therapeutic efficacy probably reflects two key limitations: (1) poor selectivity for M1 receptors over other muscarinic receptor subtypes, and (2) inability to specifically target M1 receptors on indirect-pathway MSNs versus those on direct-pathway neurons. Furthermore, impairment of the D2 receptor can disrupt numerous neurotransmitter systems beyond the cholinergic system. The other unforeseen effects of D2 receptors blockade account for the excessive activity of the indirect pathway and as such it would be beneficial to explore these effects further in terms of finding targets for new therapeutic strategies.

Dopamine is incapable of crossing the blood–brain barrier (BBB), and it must be produced within the central nervous system to act in the striatum (Zha et al., 2024). It is primarily synthesized in dopaminergic neurons within the brain, with small amounts of dopamine also being produced in the medulla of the adrenal glands. In the classical biosynthetic pathway of dopamine, the immediate precursor is L-dihydroxyphenylalanine (levodopa or L-DOPA), synthesized from tyrosine (a non-essential amino acid) or indirectly from phenylalanine (an essential amino acid). In the liver, phenylalanine is changed into tyrosine by an enzyme called phenylalanine hydroxylase (PH), which needs oxygen, iron, and tetrahydrobiopterin to work. Tyrosine is then actively transported into dopaminergic neurons, where it undergoes hydroxylation by tyrosine hydroxylase (TH) to form L-DOPA. Next, L-3,4-dihydroxyphenylalanine decarboxylase (also known as DOPA decarboxylase or aromatic-L-amino acid decarboxylase, AADC) removes a part of L-DOPA to produce dopamine (Tai et al., 2024). A small alternative route, controlled by CYP2D6 in the substantia nigra, changes tyramine (which comes from tyrosine through AADC) into dopamine. Dopamine metabolism occurs after neuronal or glial reuptake. Oxidative deamination by MAO generates the reactive intermediate 3,4-dihydroxyphenylacetaldehyde (DOPAL), which is further metabolized by alcohol dehydrogenase (ADH) to 3,4-dihydroxyphenylethanol (DOPET) or by aldehyde dehydrogenase (ALDH) to 3,4-dihydroxyphenylacetic acid (DOPAC). DOPAC is then changed by catechol-O-methyl transferase (COMT) into homovanillic acid (HVA), which is the main substance that gets removed from the body. Alternatively, dopamine can first be methylated by COMT to 3-methoxytyramine, which is subsequently deaminated by MAO and converted to HVA via ALDH (Tai et al., 2024). These enzymatic steps—particularly TH, AADC, MAO, and COMT—serve as critical targets for pharmacotherapy in PD, guiding the use of levodopa, MAO inhibitors, and COMT inhibitors, which aims to restore dopaminergic tone while minimizing motor and non-motor complications. Pharmacotherapy remains the cornerstone of Parkinson's disease (PD) management, aiming to address the underlying dopamine deficiency responsible for motor and non-motor symptoms. In practice, pharmacological treatment is usually started when symptoms become disabling or disrupt daily activities. While optimizing regimens often requires iterative adjustments, the carbidopa-levodopa combination remains the gold standard for symptomatic control (Lees et al., 2023).

PD pharmacotherapy requires tailored strategies balancing efficacy, side effects, and disease stage. Dosing and selecting the most effective medicines with the least side effects while considering the stage of the illness are the two most important strategies used by pharmaceutical management to maximize patient's health. The symptomatology treatment is started as the beginning of a functional impairment. There is no evidence of neuroprotective therapies, but the symptoms of the disease become a reason for using it. Despite the lack of proven neuroprotective therapies, we initiate symptomatic management when functional impairment emerges. Younger patients often start with MAO-B inhibitors such as selegiline, or rasagiline to delay levodopa use, mitigating early motor fluctuations and dyskinesias (Jost, 2022). Conversely, older patients or those who have cognitive decline usually go for levodopa/carbidopa first owing to not only shorter life expectancy but also the more urgent need for rapid symptom control. The gold standard is still levodopa (300–600 mg/day) and it as well demands to be titrated carefully in order to prevent dyskinesias; peripheral decarboxylase inhibition by carbidopa increases CNS delivery and causes a decrease in nausea (Lees et al., 2023). Recently, using COMT inhibitors like entacapone can make levodopa work longer in advanced Parkinson's disease, but using them too soon can raise the chance of dyskinesia (Reichmann, 2023). Dopamine agonists (pramipexole, ropinirole) can help with symptoms early on and have a lower risk of causing dyskinesia, but they are more likely to lead to problems with impulse control and hallucinations (Soileau et al., 2024). Cognitive side effects limit the use of anticholinergics like trihexyphenidyl for tremor-dominant PD (LeWitt et al., 2024). For late-stage movement problems (like wearing-off and dyskinesias), options include a steady flow of levodopa (Duodopa), adenosine A2A blockers (istradefylline), or amantadine, which helps with dyskinesias (Karakulova & Golchenko, 2024). Non-motor symptoms (depression, psychosis, orthostatic hypotension) significantly impact quality of life and are managed with targeted therapies (e.g., SSRIs, pimavanserin), per AAN guidelines. Evidence supports sildenafil for erectile dysfunction, polyethylene glycol for constipation, and modafinil for daytime somnolence. If someone has hallucinations, they might need pimavanserin (which works on a specific brain receptor), and if they have depression, they should consider taking SSRIs or SNRIs (Janz et al., 2024; Saini et al., 2024).

13.4 Practical applications in clinical settings

13.4.1 Tailoring pharmacotherapy to individual Parkinson's disease patients

In Parkinson's disease (PD), pharmacotherapy should be tailored to the patient's unique characteristics, including symptoms, age, comorbidities, and disease progression. A patient-centered approach ensures the selection of the most effective treatment with the fewest side effects. Recent studies emphasize personalized pharmacotherapy, where therapies are adjusted to maximize outcomes for each individual (Chaudhuri, 2023). Incorporating individual patient covariates allows for personalized drug comparisons, optimizing treatment efficacy while minimizing adverse effects. This approach significantly enhances quality of life for PD patients.

13.4.2 Importance of patient education and adherence

Patient education is critical for promoting medication adherence in PD. Thus, understanding the disease, treatment regimens, and potential side effects helps patients manage their condition and reduces fear—a major barrier to adherence. A Latin American multicenter study identified high non-adherence rates due to cognitive decline, motor complications, and complex medication schedules (Castro et al., 2021). Key barriers included limited education, side effect concerns, and perceptions of overtreatment. Therefore, strategies such as individualized education, caregiver involvement, and shared decision-making are essential for improving adherence and patient experience. Moreover, effective patient education enhances adherence by clarifying PD and its treatments. Clear communication, visual aids, and ongoing support help patients navigate disease progression, treatment options, and medication impacts (Pitts et al., 2022). Highlighted the importance of adjusted communication methods, such as simplified language, pictograms, and confirmation of understanding, to reduce cognitive burden. Building trusting therapeutic relationships further improves adherence by ensuring patients feel supported and informed. Such tailored consultations are particularly crucial for patients with cognitive or motor deficits.

13.4.3 Providing resources and support for patients and caregivers

PD patients and caregivers benefit from community resources, support groups, and educational materials (Portillo et al., 2021). These resources alleviate caregiver stress and provide emotional and practical support, empowering patients to engage in their treatment. These networks enhance disease management and QoL. In addition, encouraging patient involvement in care improves adherence and QoL. Thomsen et al. (2024) found that co-created self-management programs—incorporating patient and healthcare professional input—enhanced engagement and symptom control. These programs help patients set goals, track symptoms, and develop personalized action plans. Education fosters active participation in care decisions, leading to better outcomes, increased satisfaction, and long-term disease control (Mathur & Mathur, 2024). Furthermore, optimal PD care requires multidisciplinary collaboration, including neurology, physical therapy, occupational therapy, and psychology (Goldman et al., 2024). Reported the need for structured team-based care, as no single discipline can address all PD complexities (Radder et al., 2020). Advocate for patient-centered care, where teams work closely with patients and caregivers to develop tailored plans. Open communication among providers ensures alignment on treatment goals.

13.4.4 Monitoring and optimizing treatment outcomes

Effective PD management relies on continuous monitoring and personalized adjustments (Stocchi et al., 2022). Recommend integrating biomarkers and novel technologies to track progression and guide therapy for motor and non-motor symptoms; and (Nyholm & Bergquist, 2022) highlight the role of real-time sensor technology in optimizing dopaminergic therapies. Remote monitoring also enhances outcomes, as demonstrated by (Gharabaghi et al., 2025), reporting that internet-based deep brain stimulation (DBS) adjustments improved symptom control more effectively than in-clinic visits, enabling frequent and accessible optimization. Combining traditional tools with remote monitoring provides a comprehensive view of patient progress, allowing timely therapy adjustments as PD evolves.

13.4.5 Addressing drug-drug interactions in parkinson's disease

Polypharmacy in PD increases the risk of drug-drug interactions (DDIs), particularly when combining PD medications with comorbid treatments (Bitner et al., 2015). Advise cautious selection of antihypertensives, favoring ACE inhibitors or beta-blockers due to their lower interaction risk with PD drugs. Concurrent use of levodopa and diuretics may worsen orthostatic hypotension. Additionally (Müller et al., 2024), emphasize therapeutic drug monitoring (TDM) to optimize PD therapy by measuring plasma drug levels. TDM helps identify pharmacokinetic interactions, enabling dose adjustments to improve safety and efficacy. Common DDIs include 1) antipsychotics, which antagonize dopamine receptors and worsen motor symptoms; 2) iron supplements, which reduce levodopa absorption; and 3) dopamine agonists, which amplify antihypertensive effects, increasing orthostatic hypotension risk (Bhagavathula et al., 2022). Proactive medication selection and DDI monitoring are vital for successful PD management.

13.5 Future directions and emerging therapies

The treatment of Parkinson's disease (PD) is undergoing a revolution, driven by advances in molecular biology, neurology, and pharmacology. Current treatments for Parkinson's disease, mainly medications like levodopa, dopamine agonists, and MAO inhibitors, are essential but have challenges in controlling movement issues, other symptoms, and lasting effectiveness. Emerging therapies aim to address both PD pathophysiology and symptom control, offering hope for disease modification alongside symptomatic relief.

Highlight Several promising avenues have been proposed including stem-cell-based therapies and gene-editing techniques (e.g., siRNA, shRNA) to halt or reverse dopaminergic neurodegeneration; novel drug delivery systems, such as nanomedicine-enabled nose-to-brain delivery, which bypasses the blood-brain barrier noninvasively; AI and federated learning to accelerate drug discovery by analyzing large datasets without compromising privacy; and device-aided therapies, like focused ultrasound and neuromodulation which complement pharmacotherapy with targeted symptom control (Ahmad et al., 2022; Khanna et al., 2024; Serva et al., 2022).

13.5.1 Beyond dopamine: gene and stem cell therapies

Conventional therapies, though effective, often lack disease-modifying potential and carry significant side effects. Emerging approaches aim to overcome these challenges, including gene therapy, where viral vectors deliver enzymes to restore dopamine production directly, circumventing traditional drug limitations; stem cell therapies using induced pluripotent stem cells (iPSCs) and embryonic stem cells (ESCs) that can regenerate dopaminergic neurons in the striatum; and finally non-invasive adjuncts, such as electroceuticals and focused ultrasound modulating brain activity without surgery, offering alternatives to deep brain stimulation (DBS) (Patel et al., 2025). Furthermore, advances in biomarker discovery may enable earlier diagnosis and precision therapy, further personalizing treatment. These innovations could transform PD management by addressing critical gaps in current pharmacotherapy, such as levodopa-induced dyskinesias and neuropsychiatric complications and the lack of long-term neuroprotective effects (Stoker et al., 2018). Personalized medicine—guided by biomarkers and genetic profiling—may allow clinicians to tailor therapies to individual patient biology and adjust treatments in real time based on disease progression. These advances could improve safety, efficacy, and quality of life—potentially altering PD's trajectory rather than merely managing symptoms.

13.6 Conclusion

The management of Parkinson's disease requires a balanced integration of established therapeutic strategies and innovative approaches, all tailored to the individual patient's needs. A multidisciplinary framework—encompassing pharmacological optimization, rehabilitation therapies, and personalized care—remains fundamental for addressing both motor and non-motor symptoms while maximizing QoL. Current treatment paradigms must evolve to minimize polypharmacy risks and adapt dynamically to disease progression, guided by continuous monitoring and evidence-based adjustments. Meanwhile, emerging therapies such as gene therapy, stem cell transplantation, and advanced drug delivery systems hold immense potential to modify disease progression rather than merely alleviate symptoms, though challenges like biological barriers, ethical considerations, and technical limitations must still be overcome. As research advances, the integration of precision medicine, biomarker-guided therapies, and collaborative care models will be crucial in translating scientific breakthroughs into clinical practice. By uniting rigorous patient-centered care with cutting-edge innovation, the future of

PD management promises not only enhanced symptom control but also the potential to fundamentally alter the disease's trajectory, offering hope for improved long-term outcomes and QoL for patients worldwide.

References

Abbruzzese, G., Kulisevsky, J., Bergmans, B., Gomez-Esteban, J.C., Kägi, G., Raw, J., Stefani, A., Warnecke, T., Jost, W.H., Bergmans, B., Bourgeois, P., Cras, P., de Klippel, N., Dethy, S., Franco, G., Garraux, G., Geens, K., Jacquerye, P., Jeanjean, A., Silverdale, M., 2021. A european observational study to evaluate the safety and the effectiveness of safinamide in routine clinical practice: The SynapSES trial. Journal of Parkinson's Disease 11 (1), 187–198. https://doi.org/10.3233/JPD-202224.

Ahmad, J., Haider, N., Khan, M.A., Md, S., Alhakamy, N.A., Ghoneim, M.M., Alshehri, S., Sarim Imam, S., Ahmad, M.Z., Mishra, A., 2022. Novel therapeutic interventions for combating parkinson's disease and prospects of nose-to-brain drug delivery. Biochemical Pharmacology 195. https://doi.org/10.1016/j.bcp.2021.114849.

Akbar, U., Friedman, J.H., 2022. Long-term outcomes with pimavanserin for psychosis in clinical practice. Clinical Parkinsonism & Related Disorders 6, 100143. https://doi.org/10.1016/j.prdoa.2022.100143.

Aldred, J., Freire-Alvarez, E., Amelin, A.V., Antonini, A., Bergmans, B., Bergquist, F., Bouchard, M., Budur, K., Carroll, C., Chaudhuri, K.R., Criswell, S.R., Danielsen, E.H., Gandor, F., Jia, J., Kimber, T.E., Mochizuki, H., Robieson, W.Z., Spiegel, A.M., Standaert, D.G., Fung, V.S.C., 2023. Continuous subcutaneous foslevodopa/foscarbidopa in parkinson's disease: safety and efficacy results from a 12-Month, Single-Arm, Open-Label, phase 3 Study. Neurology and Therapy 12 (6), 1937–1958. https://doi.org/10.1007/s40120-023-00533-1.

Antonini, A., Emmi, A., Campagnolo, M., 2023. Beyond the dopaminergic system: lessons learned from levodopa resistant symptoms in parkinson's disease. Movement Disorders Clinical Practice 10 (S2). https://doi.org/10.1002/mdc3.13786.

Bhagavathula, A.S., Tesfaye, W., Vidyasagar, K., Fialova, D., 2022. Polypharmacy and hyperpolypharmacy in older individuals with parkinson's disease: a systematic review and meta-analysis. Gerontology 68 (10), 1081–1090. https://doi.org/10.1159/000521214.

Bitner, A., Zalewski, P., Klawe, J.J., Newton, J.L., 2015. Drug interactions in parkinson's disease: Safety of pharmacotherapy for arterial hypertension. Drugs - Real World Outcomes 2 (1), 1–12. https://doi.org/10.1007/s40801-015-0008-7.

Bovenzi, R., Liguori, C., Canesi, M., D'Amelio, M., De Pandis, M.F., Marini, C., Monge, A., Padovani, A., Tessitore, A., Stefani, A., Zappia, M., Abbruzzese, G., Aguggia, M., Avarello, T., Barone, P., Bentivoglio, A. R., Bosco, D., Calabresi, P., Callegarini, C., Zambito Marsala, S., 2024. Real-world use of safinamide in motor fluctuating parkinson's disease patients in Italy. Neurological Sciences 45 (2), 573–583. https://doi.org/10.1007/s10072-023-07001-6.

Calabresi, P., Filippo, M.D., Ghiglieri, V., Tambasco, N., Picconi, B., 2010. Levodopa-induced dyskinesias in patients with Parkinson's disease: Filling the bench-to-bedside gap. The Lancet Neurology 9 (11), 1106–1117. https://doi.org/10.1016/S1474-4422(10)70218-0.

Calabresi, P., Picconi, B., Tozzi, A., Ghiglieri, V., Di Filippo, M., 2014. Direct and indirect pathways of basal ganglia: a critical reappraisal. Nature Neuroscience 17 (8), 1022–1030.

Castro, G.S., Aguilar-Alvarado, C.M., Zúñiga-Ramírez, C., Sáenz-Farret, M., Otero-Cerdeira, E., Serrano-Dueñas, M., González-Usigli, H.A., Bernal, O., Leal-Ortega, R., Estrada-Bellmann, I., Meléndez-Flores, J. D., Miranda-Cabezas, M., Martínez-Hernández, H.R., Giugni, J.C., Mejía-Rojas, K.K., Mori, N., Raina, G.B., García Fernández, C.L., Pecci, C., Álvarez-Villalobos, N.A., Micheli, F., 2021. Adherence to treatment in parkinson's disease: a multicenter exploratory study with patients from six latin american countries. Parkinsonism & Related Disorders 93, 1–7. https://doi.org/10.1016/j.parkreldis.2021.10.028.

Chaudhuri, K.R., 2023. *Personalized medicine for Parkinson's disease*. MDPI-Multidisciplinary Digital Publishing Institute, p. 214.

Chhetri, J.K., Mei, S., Wang, C., Chan, P., 2023. New horizons in Parkinson's disease in older populations. Age and Ageing 52 (10). https://doi.org/10.1093/ageing/afad186.

Ferreira, J.J., Poewe, W., Rascol, O., Stocchi, F., Antonini, A., Moreira, J., Guimarães, B., Rocha, J.F., Soares-da-Silva, P., 2022. Effect of opicapone on levodopa pharmacokinetics in patients with fluctuating parkinson's Disease. Movement Disorders 37 (11), 2272–2283. https://doi.org/10.1002/mds.29193.

Gao, V., Crawford, C.V., Burré, J., 2025. The gut–brain axis in parkinson's disease. Cold Spring Harbor Perspectives in Medicine 15 (1), a041618. https://doi.org/10.1101/cshperspect.a041618.

Gerfen, C.R., 2023. Segregation of D1 and D2 dopamine receptors in the striatal direct and indirect pathways: An historical perspective. Frontiers in Synaptic Neuroscience 14. https://doi.org/10.3389/fnsyn.2022.1002960.

Gharabaghi, A., Groppa, S., Navas-Garcia, M., Schnitzler, A., Muñoz-Delgado, L., Marshall, V.L., Karl, J., Zhang, L., Alvarez, R., Feldman, M.S., Soileau, M.J., Luo, L., Zauber, S.E., Walter, B.L., Wu, C., Lei, H., Herz, D.M., Chung, M.H., Pathak, Y., Weiss, D., 2025. Accelerated symptom improvement in Parkinson's disease via remote internet-based optimization of deep brain stimulation therapy: A randomized controlled multicenter trial. Communications Medicine 5 (1). https://doi.org/10.1038/s43856-025-00744-7.

Goldman, J.G., Volpe, D., Ellis, T.D., Hirsch, M.A., Johnson, J., Wood, J., Aragon, A., Biundo, R., Di Rocco, A., Kasman, G.S., Iansek, R., Miyasaki, J., McConvey, V.M., Munneke, M., Pinto, S., Clair, K.A.S., Toledo, S., York, M.K., Todaro, R., Yarab, N., Wallock, K., 2024. Delivering multidisciplinary rehabilitation care in parkinson's disease: An international consensus statement. Journal of Parkinson's Disease 14 (1), 135–166. https://doi.org/10.3233/JPD-230117.

Hasan, M.Z., Hussain, M.Z., Anjum, K., Anwar, A., 2023. Case study (A and B): A patient with Parkinson's disease. Journal of Neuroscience and Neurological Disorders 7, 5–10.

Isaacson, S., Goldstein, M., Pahwa, R., Singer, C., Klos, K., Zhang, I., Crandall, D., Navia, B., 2021. Efficacy and safety of SEP-363856, a Non–D2-Receptor binding drug with antipsychotic activity, in patients with parkinson's disease psychosis (2102). Neurology 96 (15_Supplment). https://doi.org/10.1212/wnl.96.15_supplement.2102.

Janz, C., Timpka, J., Rosqvist, K., Paul, G., Storch, A., Odin, P., 2024. Non-Motor symptom management: insights into adherence to treatment guidelines in parkinson's disease patients. Journal of Parkinson's Disease 14 (2), 297–312. https://doi.org/10.3233/jpd-230263.

Jost, W.H., 2022. A critical appraisal of MAO-B inhibitors in the treatment of parkinson's disease. Journal of Neural Transmission 129 (5–6), 723–736. https://doi.org/10.1007/s00702-022-02465-w.

Karakulova, Y.V., Golchenko, E.A., 2024. Therapy for advanced stages of parkinson's disease. Perm Medical Journal 41 (4), 70–79. https://doi.org/10.17816/pmj41470-79.

Khanna, A., Adams, J., Antoniades, C., Bloem, B.R., Carroll, C., Cedarbaum, J., Cosman, J., Dexter, D.T., Dockendorf, M.F., Edgerton, J., Gaetano, L., Goikoetxea, E., Hill, D., Horak, F., Izmailova, E.S., Kangarloo, T., Katabi, D., Kopil, C., Lindemann, M., Jones, G.B., 2024. Accelerating parkinson's disease drug development with federated learning approaches. Npj Parkinson's Disease 10 (1). https://doi.org/10.1038/s41531-024-00837-5.

Lees, A., Tolosa, E., Stocchi, F., Ferreira, J.J., Rascol, O., Antonini, A., Poewe, W., 2023. Optimizing levodopa therapy, when and how? Perspectives on the importance of delivery and the potential for an early combination approach. Expert Review of Neurotherapeutics 23 (1), 15–24. https://doi.org/10.1080/14737175.2023.2176220.

LeWitt, P.A., Hong, L., Moehle, M.S., 2024. Anticholinergic drugs for parkinsonism and other movement disorders. Journal of Neural Transmission 131 (12), 1481–1494. https://doi.org/10.1007/s00702-024-02799-7.

Mathur, S., Mathur, S., 2024. Patient empowerment for those living with parkinson's disease. Journal of Parkinson's Disease 14 (s1), S173. https://doi.org/10.3233/jpd-230235.

Molde, H., Moussavi, Y., Kopperud, S.T., Erga, A.H., Hansen, A.L., Pallesen, S., 2018. Impulse-control disorders in Parkinson's Disease: A meta-analysis and review of case-control studies. Frontiers in Neurology 9 (MAY). https://doi.org/10.3389/fneur.2018.00330.

Müller, T., Gerlach, M., Hefner, G., Hiemke, C., Jost, W.H., Riederer, P., 2024. Therapeutic drug monitoring in Parkinson's disease. Journal of Neural Transmission 131 (10), 1247–1262. https://doi.org/10.1007/s00702-024-02828-5.

Myslivecek, J., 2021. Two players in the field: Hierarchical model of interaction between the dopamine and acetylcholine signaling systems in the striatum. Biomedicines 9 (1), 25. https://doi.org/10.3390/biomedicines9010025.

Nyholm, D., Bergquist, F., 2022. Optimizing treatment of parkinson's disease. Journal of Personalized Medicine 12 (2), 245. https://doi.org/10.3390/jpm12020245.

Olanow, C.W., Poewe, W., Rascol, O., Stocchi, F., 2021. On-demand therapy for OFF episodes in parkinson's disease. Movement Disorders 36 (10), 2244–2253. https://doi.org/10.1002/mds.28726.

Pasquini, J., Brooks, D.J., Pavese, N., 2021. The cholinergic brain in parkinson's disease. Movement Disorders Clinical Practice 8 (7), 1012–1026. https://doi.org/10.1002/mdc3.13319.

Patel, U.S., Sufi, A.J., Mehra, R.S., Patel, A.S., Noolvi, D.M.N., Rathod, M.N., 2025. A newer approach to parkinson's disease: Addressing therapeutic features, repurposing drugs and the latest concepts with future goals. World Journal of Biology Pharmacy and Health Sciences 21 (1), 568–588. https://doi.org/10.30574/wjbphs.2025.21.1.0098.

Pitts, E., Wylie, K., Loftus, A.M., Cocks, N., 2022. Communication strategies used by Parkinson's nurse specialists during healthcare interactions: A qualitative descriptive study. Journal of Advanced Nursing 78 (6), 1773–1786. https://doi.org/10.1111/jan.15196.

Portillo, M.C., Haahr, A., Navarta-Sánchez, M.V., 2021. Management, levels of support, quality of life, and social inclusion in parkinson's disease: Interventions, innovation, and practice development. Parkinson's Disease 2021. https://doi.org/10.1155/2021/4681251.

Radder, D.L.M., Nonnekes, J., Van Nimwegen, M., Eggers, C., Abbruzzese, G., Alves, G., Browner, N., Chaudhuri, K.R., Ebersbach, G., Ferreira, J.J., Fleisher, J.E., Fletcher, P., Frazzitta, G., Giladi, N., Guttman, M., Iansek, R., Khandhar, S., Klucken, J., Lafontaine, A.L., Bloem, B.R., 2020. Recommendations for the organization of multidisciplinary clinical care teams in parkinson's disease. Journal of Parkinson's Disease 10 (3), 1087–1098. https://doi.org/10.3233/JPD-202078.

Reichmann, H., 2023. Real-world considerations regarding the use of the combination of levodopa, carbidopa, and entacapone (Stalevo®) in parkinson's disease. European Journal of Neurology 30 (2), 15–20. https://doi.org/10.1111/ene.15992.

Riesenberg, R., Werth, J., Zhang, Y., Duvvuri, S., Gray, D., 2020. PF-06649751 efficacy and safety in early Parkinson's disease: A randomized, placebo-controlled trial. Therapeutic Advances in Neurological Disorders 13. https://doi.org/10.1177/1756286420911296.

Rissardo, K., Dway, A., Elhassan, W.A., Elbadawi, M.H., Sayad, R., Caprara. 2025. Exploring Fatigue in Parkinson's Disease: A Comprehensive Literature Review. https://doi.org/10.20944/preprints202501.2084.v1.

Saini, N., Singh, N., Kaur, N., Garg, S., Kaur, M., Kumar, A., Verma, M., Singh, K., Sohal, H.S., 2024. Motor and non-motor symptoms, drugs, and their mode of action in Parkinson's disease (PD): A review. Medicinal Chemistry Research 33 (4), 580–599. https://doi.org/10.1007/s00044-024-03203-5.

Santos García, D., Alonso Losada, M.G., Cimas Hernando, I., Cabo López, I., Yáñez Baña, R., Alonso Redondo, R., Paz González, J.M., Cores Bartolomé, C., Feal Painceiras, M.J., Íñiguez Alvarado, M.C., Labandeira, C., García Díaz, I., 2022. Vortioxetine improves depressive symptoms and cognition in parkinson's disease patients with major depression: An open-label prospective study. Brain Sciences 12 (11). https://doi.org/10.3390/brainsci12111466.

Schuepbach, W.M.M., Rau, J., Knudsen, K., Volkmann, J., Krack, P., Timmermann, L., Hälbig, T.D., Hesekamp, H., Navarro, S.M., Meier, N., Falk, D., Mehdorn, M., Paschen, S., Maarouf, M., Barbe, M.T., Fink, G.R., Kupsch, A., Gruber, D., Schneider, G.-H., Deuschl, G., 2013. Neurostimulation for parkinson's disease with early motor complications. New England Journal of Medicine 368 (7), 610–622. https://doi.org/10.1056/NEJMoa1205158.

Seppi, K., Ray Chaudhuri, K., Coelho, M., Fox, S.H., Katzenschlager, R., Perez Lloret, S., Weintraub, D., Sampaio, C., Chahine, L., Hametner, E.M., Heim, B., Lim, S.Y., Poewe, W., Djamshidian-Tehrani, A., 2019. Update on treatments for nonmotor symptoms of Parkinson's disease—an evidence-based medicine review. Movement Disorders 34 (2), 180–198. https://doi.org/10.1002/mds.27602.

Serva, S.N., Bernstein, J., Thompson, J.A., Kern, D.S., Ojemann, S.G., 2022. An update on advanced therapies for parkinson's disease: From gene therapy to neuromodulation. Frontiers in Surgery 9. https://doi.org/10.3389/fsurg.2022.863921.

Soileau, L.G., Talbot, N.C., Storey, N.R., Spillers, N.J., D'antoni, J.V., Carr, P.C., Galardo, C.M., Shilpadevi, P., Ahmadzadeh, S., Shekoohi, S., Kaye, A.D., 2024. Impulse control disorders in Parkinson's disease patients treated with pramipexole and ropinirole: A systematic review and meta-analysis. Neurological Sciences 45 (4), 1399–1408. https://doi.org/10.1007/s10072-023-07254-1.

Song, J., Lin, H., Liu, S., 2023. Basal ganglia network dynamics and function: Role of direct, indirect and hyper-direct pathways in action selection. Network: Computation in Neural Systems 34 (1–2), 84–121. https://doi.org/10.1080/0954898x.2023.2173816.

Spott, M., Javidnia, M., Pedata, A., Müller, M., Carrillo, L., Simuni, T., Pagano, G., Kwok, K., Romero, K., Stephenson, D., 2025. Addressing the need for standardization of symptomatic medication documentation in parkinson's disease clinical research: A call to action. Journal of Parkinson's Disease 15 (1), 227–235. https://doi.org/10.1177/1877718x241305711.

Stocchi, F., Antonini, A., Berg, D., Bergmans, B., Jost, W., Katzenschlager, R., Kulisevsky, J., Odin, P., Valldeoriola, F., Ray Chaudhuri, K., 2022. Safinamide in the treatment pathway of Parkinson's disease: A european Delphi consensus. Npj Parkinson's Disease 8 (1). https://doi.org/10.1038/s41531-022-00277-z.

Stoker, T.B., Torsney, K.M., Barker, R.A., 2018. Emerging treatment approaches for parkinson's disease. Frontiers in Neuroscience 12. https://doi.org/10.3389/fnins.2018.00693.

Tai, M.D.S., Gamiz-Arco, G., Martinez, A., 2024. Dopamine synthesis and transport: Current and novel therapeutics for parkinsonisms. Biochemical Society Transactions 52 (3), 1275–1291. https://doi.org/10.1042/BST20231061.

Tenchov, R., Sasso, J.M., Zhou, Q.A., 2025. Evolving landscape of parkinson's disease research: Challenges and perspectives. ACS Omega 10 (2), 1864–1892. https://doi.org/10.1021/acsomega.4c09114.

Thomsen, T.H., Skovbølling, S.L., Møller, M., Brønden, M., Grønlund, V., Ilsfort, D.N., Frederiksen, J., Biering-Sørensen, B., 2024. Empower-PD: Development of a self-management program in empowering people with Parkinson's disease: A qualitative study using a co-creation framework. International Journal of Nursing and Health Care Research 7 (4), 1541.

Verschuur, C.V.M., Suwijn, S.R., Boel, J.A., Post, B., Bloem, B.R., Van Hilten, J.J., Van Laar, T., Tissingh, G., Munts, A.G., Deuschl, G., Lang, A.E., Dijkgraaf, M.G.W., De Haan, R.J., De Bie, R.M.A., 2019. Randomized delayed-start trial of levodopa in parkinson's disease. New England Journal of Medicine 380 (4), 315–324. https://doi.org/10.1056/NEJMoa1809983.

Zha, S., Liu, H., Li, H., Li, H., Wong, K.L., All, A.H., 2024. Functionalized nanomaterials capable of crossing the blood-brain barrier. ACS Nano 18 (3), 1820–1845. https://doi.org/10.1021/acsnano.3c10674.

SECTION III

Adjunctive and advanced therapies

CHAPTER

Emergent therapeutic agents in the treatment of Parkinson's disease 14

Doaa S.R. Khafaga[1, a], Eman K. Abdelhadi[2], Ziad E. Farouk[3], Darin W. Aswa[3], Ahmed T. Elhendawy[4], Amera M. Ghazi[5], Radwa N. Selim[6], Ahmed Tharwat Al-Namrouti[3], Esraa A. Elgayar[7], Manar T. El-Morsy[6] and Salma K. Mohamed[3]

[1]*Department of Basic Medical Sciences, Health Sector, Galala University, New Galala City, Suez, Egypt;* [2]*Faculty of Pharmacy, Clinical Pharmacy Department, Suez Canal University, Ismailia, Egypt;* [3]*Faculty of Medicine, Galala University, New Galala City, Suez, Egypt;* [4]*Physics Department, Faculty of Science, Galala University, New Galala City, Suez, Egypt;* [5]*Faculty of Science, Microbiology and Chemistry Department, Al-Azhar University, Cairo, Egypt;* [6]*Biotechnology Department, Faculty of Postgraduate Studies for Nanotechnology, Cairo University, Giza, Egypt;* [7]*Faculty of Biotechnology, Nile University, Sheikh Zayed, Cairo, Egypt*

14.1 Introduction

PD is a distinct disease with a wide range of causes and clinical symptoms. PD is a fast-increasing neurological disorder; its rising global incidence holds many of the traits of a pandemic, with the exception of an infectious source (Bloem et al., 2021; Chopade et al., 2023). In most groups, genetic factors associated with known PD genes account for 3%–5% of PD, resulting in monogenic PD, whereas 90 genetic risk variants contribute for 16%–36% of the heritable risk of nonmonogenic PD. Additional causative associations include having a family with PD or tremor, constipation, and not smoking, all of which improve the chance of PD by at least double (Bloem et al., 2021; Chopade et al., 2023). The medical evaluation is primarily clinical, with additional testing reserved for atypical presentations. PD is currently characterized by bradykinesia in conjunction with resting tremors, rigidity, or both symptoms. The clinical presentation is complex, characterized by various nonmotor symptoms. Understanding disease subgroups provides prognostic assessments (Bloem et al., 2021; Chopade et al., 2023). AD is the most prevalent neurodegenerative disorder globally, progressively disrupts cognitive abilities, leading to dementia, disorientation, and a decline in mental function. These characteristic symptoms stem from brain shrinkage (atrophy) and abnormal neuronal activity in regions crucial for memory and cognition, including the cerebral cortex and hippocampus (Chopade et al., 2023). Thus, AD is characterized by the production of two types of insoluble protein aggregates in the brain: extracellular Aβ plaques and intraneuronal/extracellular tau neurofibrillary tangles (Chopade et al., 2023). Although the exact etiology of AD is unknown, the "amyloid hypothesis" suggests that Aβ aggregates play a key role in its development and progression. Nevertheless, there is a

[a]Contributions included supervising the chapter preparation, reviewing all submitted files, revising reviewer comments, following up on the peer-review process, and coordinating the submission of the chapter.

Pharmacological Foundations of Parkinson's Disease. https://doi.org/10.1016/B978-0-443-27702-3.00022-4

growing awareness of discontent that research needs to shift its attention away from the "amyloid hypothesis" and toward other possible pathogenic ideas. Despite this, the "amyloid hypothesis" is still up for debate; drugs given too late in the course of AD development are expected to have limited therapeutic impact, leading to clinical failures (Chopade et al., 2023). PD occurs throughout a potentially lengthy prodromal period. Currently, the existence of prodromal symptoms has no therapeutic implications other than symptom suppression, although diagnosis of prodromal parkinsonism will almost certainly have ramifications once disease-modifying drugs become available. Treatment objectives vary from person to person, emphasizing the significance of tailored management. There is no reason to delay symptomatic treatment in PD patients. Levodopa is the most frequently administered first-line therapy. Also, optimal management should begin with diagnosis and necessitate a multidisciplinary team approach, which includes an expanding range of nonpharmacological treatments. Currently, no treatment can halt or stop the progression of PD (Chopade et al., 2023). Aducanumab (Aduhelm), an anti-Aβ monoclonal antibody, was approved by the FDA in 2021 as the first plaque-reducing medication for AD. However, the usefulness of aducanumab is widely debated, as phase III clinical trials were inconclusive in proving therapeutic benefits, particularly improved cognitive function and dementia reduction. Patients in one research saw a reduction in AD-related cognitive loss, whereas those in another did not have a statistically significant reduction. Adunumab's therapeutic limitations include a number of treatment-emergent adverse events (TEAEs) reported during early phase clinical trials assessing its safety (Chopade et al., 2023; Dunn et al., 2021). Scientists have primarily focused on seven therapy strategies for fighting AD: antiaggregation, anti-inflammatory, antioxidant, antiexcitotoxicity, antiapoptotic, and regeneration. In contrast of the linked nature of several neurological disorders—including inflammation, oxidative stress, and excitotoxicity—we categorized treatment processes according to the primary intervention goal (Liu et al., 2020). Although viral vectors and cell therapy, which includes stem cells and different immune cells, are becoming more common, there are still a lot of potential therapies that are either still in clinical trials or are in the early stages of preclinical research. Immune system training against Aβ or tau in AD and alpha-synuclein (α-syn) in PD can be achieved using neurodegeneration vaccines. An mRNA vaccine that enhances its own Aβ production offers an alternate to conventional antigen/adjuvant methods for AD.

Nevertheless, both safety and effectiveness in terms of autoimmunity, increased inflammation, and early AD have yet to be investigated. With the potential of Clustered Regularly Interspaced Short Palindromic Repeats (CRISPR)/Cas9 intervention in Huntington disease, researchers are looking at CRISPR applications in AD and PD. The receptor for advanced glycation end products was altered via CRISPR/Cas9 technology. Mesenchymal stem cells sRAGE-MSCs decreased neuronal mortality and enhanced mobility in rotenone-induced PD rat models (Chopade et al., 2023). By applying adeno-associated viral vectors, Gyorgy et al. showed that CRISpen/Cas9 efficiently targeted and removed the APP Swedish mutant, hence minimizing Aβ buildup in transgenic mice built to overexpress this variation. An increasing body of research, meantime, emphasizes the function of extracellular vehicles (EVs) classified as exosomes or microvesicles depending on size—as possible biomarkers for tracking disease development in AD and PD. These vesicles are being studied more and more for potential diagnostic and therapeutic applications in neurodegenerative diseases. The complex functions that EVs produced from various donor cell sources play in cell-to-cell communication, as well as their ability to cross the blood-brain barrier and transport therapeutic cargo, have prompted their investigation as potential therapeutics. Additionally, as delivery mechanisms, EVs produced from mesenchymal stem cells (MSCs) show huge therapeutic promise. Using a 6-hydroxydopamine (6-OHDA)-induced PD rat model, intratracheal infusion of EVs derived from human dental stem cells restored gait function, therefore emphasizing their ability to address motor disorders. These results highlight the potential of MSC-derived EVs as novel neurodegenerative disease treatment agents. The growing prevalence of neurodegenerative diseases like Alzheimer and Parkinson, together with the lack of effective treatments, highlights the critical need for novel techniques to drug administration and innovative thought about methods of treatment to combat these conditions (György et al., 2018).

14.2 Pathophysiology of parkinson's disease: therapeutic targets

PD is the primary movement disorder globally and ranks as the second most common neurodegenerative disease, affecting approximately 2% of individuals aged 65 years and older. Pathologically, PD is defined by two key hallmarks: (1) the progressive degeneration of dopamine-producing neurons in the substantia nigra pars compacta (SNpc), causing a decline in dopamine (DA) levels within the basal ganglia, and (2) the accumulation of Lewy bodies—intracytoplasmic inclusions containing fibrillar α-syn (Mg et al., 1997). The substantia nigra pars compacta contains dopaminergic neurons. Motor symptoms such as akinesia/bradykinesia, tremor, rigidity, and postural instability are caused by a DA deficiency in the striatum. Nonmotor symptoms of PD patients include depression, autonomic disturbance, hyposmia, and rapid eye movement sleep behavior disorder (RBD), which arises before motor symptoms (Neuron-Astrocyte Interactions in Parkinson's Disease, 2020). In neurological disorders, synuclein aggregation encourages neurodegeneration. Numerous investigations have documented the dissemination of α-syn aggregates from neurone to neurone or neurone to astrocyte through a "prion-like" process in both cellular and animal models (Vargas et al., 2019; Tyson et al., 2016). Multiple system atrophy (MSA), dementia with Lewy bodies (DLB), and PD are examples of synucleinopathies, a class of neurodegenerative diseases with a wide range of clinical and pathological manifestations and an unclear etiology. Nonetheless, these disorders have certain common characteristics, the most important of which is the accumulation of α-syn, which is seen as cytoplasmic inclusion bodies in the cells of the afflicted brain areas (Mg et al., 1997; Papp & Lantos, 1992). Neuroinflammation has garnered more attention in recent years as a potential mechanism behind PD pathogenesis. As people age, their brain's equilibrium is compromised due to a decline in the activation of survival systems. Neuroinflammation may so arise in PD. To preserve the health of neurones in the central nervous system (CNS), neuroinflammation is a necessary immune response. However, its neurotoxicity can make the damage to the neurones worse (Marogianni et al., 2020; Wang et al., 2015). As a result of aging, neurodegenerative illness currently affects many communities. As of right now, neurodegenerative disorders can only be treated for their symptoms. Some medications used to treat PD have dangerous adverse effects (Pingale & Gupta, 2021).

14.3 Disease-modifying therapies

14.3.1 Alpha-synuclein-targeted therapies

The primary characteristic of PD, a neurodegenerative condition, is the destruction of dopaminergic neurones in the substantia nigra. Lewy bodies are aberrant aggregates found in degenerating neurones that are primarily made up of the protein α-syn that has been misfolded or altered. It is believed that cellular stress, inflammation, posttranslational changes, and gene alterations cause pathological misfolding and aggregation. A-syn pathology is closely linked to dopaminergic neuronal toxicity; therefore, methods to lessen its load should help delay the course of the disease (Xiao & Tan, 2025). Immunization against α-syn, both active and passive, is the most recent disease-modifying therapeutic strategy being researched for PD. In PD, three medications are presently being researched as active immunization modalities, while five distinct monoclonal antibodies are being investigated as passive immunization. By decreasing α-syn synthesis, enhancing α-syn degradation, and inhibiting aggregation and cell-to-cell propagation, these aim toward minimizing or preventing α-syn-driven neurotoxicity (Castonguay et al., 2020). The multifunctional protein leucine-rich repeat kinase 2 (LRRK2) controls a wide range of biological functions, including as autophagy, lysosome degradation, neurotransmission, mitochondrial activity, and vesicle transport. PD is caused by hyperactivation of LRRK2, which also causes vesicle transport problems, neuroinflammation, α-syn buildup, mitochondrial failure, and cilia loss. As a result, one intriguing treatment approach for PD is to target the LRRK2 protein (Hu et al., 2023).

14.3.2 Gene therapies

Recent conceptual and technological advances have resulted in several exciting novel engineered adeno-associated viral (AAV) vector variants. In the last decade, clinical trials in PD have shown that AAV is a safe and suitable vector for gene therapy; however, it might significantly improve with enhanced specificity and potency (Björklund et al., 2021). Genetic variations in the SNCA gene, responsible for the synthesis of the α-synuclein (α-syn) protein, are recognized as significant factors in hereditary in PD. The A53T variation in SNCA is a well-documented genetic mutation associated with PD. However, strategies for the selective eradication of the mutant SNCA gene in live animals have been limited. Recent developments applying the CRISPR-Cas9 technology have facilitated the elimination of A53T-SNCA in both experimental and live organisms. In vitro investigations indicated that adeno-associated viruses (AAVs) administering SaCas9-KKH and a guide RNA aimed at A53T-SNCA markedly reduced its expression. To evaluate therapeutic potential, researchers employed a PD rat model genetically modified to overexpress the A53T-SNCA gene. The elimination of this mutation significantly diminished clinical characteristics, including α-synuclein buildup, neuroinflammation (reactive microgliosis), depletion of neurons that produce dopamine, and motor impairments linked to PD. These findings highlight CRISPR-Cas9 as a viable technique for avoiding PD disease associated with the A53T-SNCA mutation, providing a focused approach to prevent disease progression (Yoon et al., 2022).

14.3.3 Neurotrophic factors and regenerative strategies

For many years, researchers have tried to use growth factors to heal the brain in a number of neurodegenerative illnesses, most notably PD, by employing glial cell line-derived neurotrophic factors (GDNFs). Discovered in 1993, this neurotrophic factor has been demonstrated to have specific effects on boosting the survival and regeneration of specific neuronal populations, such as the dopaminergic (Barker et al., 2020). GDNF is a protein consisting of 134 amino acids, enzymatically produced from a precursor sequence of 211 amino acids known as pre-pro-GDNF. Two GDNF monomers, connected by a disulfide bond to form a homodimer, serve as a powerful neurotrophic factor that promotes the survival of dopaminergic neurons. GDNF signaling is complex, including at least four distinct cell surface receptors. A crucial process is the interaction of GDNF family receptor 1α with RET, therefore activating Ret tyrosine kinase and subsequently launch intracellular signaling cascades that promote neurite growth, survival, differentiation, and synaptic plasticity (Gash et al., 2020). Recent advancements in stem cell research have improved options for therapy for people with neglected diseases and conditions. Human pluripotent stem cells (hPSCs) and multipotent MSCs are essential elements of regenerative medicine, serving as stem cell-based therapies that have gained prominence recently. hPSCs have the capacity for self-renewal and can differentiate into the three germ layers and many cellular phenotypes found in the human body (Hoang et al., 2022).

14.4 Symptomatic treatments: Beyond dopamine replacement

14.4.1 Nondopaminergic pharmacotherapies

In PD, the adenosine A-adrenergic receptor (A-aAR) has become a key target for treatment. It is co-expressed in striatopallidal neurones in conjunction with dopamine D_2 receptors, which form heterodimeric complexes with these receptors. While inhibiting A_2AAR with antagonists improves the therapeutic effects of L-DOPA and lessens L-DOPA-induced dyskinesia, studies have shown that A_2AAR stimulation decreases the affinity of D_2 receptor agonists. Furthermore, A-a antagonists have been shown to have neuroprotective properties, which may halt the advancement of PD. The combination of A_2AAR antagonists with L-DOPA has gained popularity as an alternative to DA replacement therapy alone as a result of these findings (Shao et al., 2018). Nondopaminergic receptors' involvement in the etiology of PD has come to light more and more in recent years. The A-A receptor is one of these that has drawn a lot of interest as a potential pharmaceutical target for easing motor symptoms. In striatopallidal neurones, A-A receptors are abundantly expressed and control inhibitory GABAergic activity. GABA release is regulated by blocking A-A receptors, most likely at the nerve terminals of recurrent collaterals, which lessens striatopallidal neurone overactivity. Parkinsonian symptoms may be lessened by using A-A antagonists to strengthen this feedback inhibition (Richardson, 2001). It is believed that the neuroprotective effects of A-A receptor antagonists are due to their influence on glutamate control. Quinolinic acid (QA)-induced glutamate outflow is decreased by blocking A_2AAR, which may also prevent QA-dependent NMDA receptor activation (Popoli et al., 2004). Additionally, pretreatment with the A_2A antagonist SCH 58,261 has been demonstrated to decrease the formation of reactive oxygen species (ROS) in response to hydrostatic pressure and suppress microglial proliferation (Aires et al., 2019). By reducing oxidative stress activation, reactive gliosis, microglial proliferation, and elevated proinflammatory cytokines brought on by environmental stress, the A_2A antagonist ZM241385 has shown neuroprotective properties (Gao et al., 2020). Levodopa's motor-activating effects are amplified by A-a receptor antagonists, allowing for the use of lower, nondyskinetic dosages. According to (Morelli et al., 2012), this could lessen or postpone maladaptive striatal alterations that cause dyskinesia. In animal models of PD, A-A receptor antagonists have been demonstrated to improve motor deficits when given in conjunction with low dosages of levodopa or DA agonists. More significantly, they may enhance motor function without worsening dyskinesia and delay the initiation of involuntary movements (Jenner, 2014). Istradefylline is one example of an A-A receptor antagonist that has shown encouraging outcomes in therapeutic settings. Istradefylline considerably decreased OFF time and enhanced ON-WoTD (wearing-off time with dyskinesia) in clinical trials when compared to a placebo (Hauser et al., 2021). No significant difference was seen between istradefylline and placebo in terms of tolerability, side effects, or UPDRS III scores, despite the fact that its effects on dyskinesia were statistically significant (Wang, Feng, et al., 2022). Research has demonstrated that istradefylline treatment resulted in a consistent decrease in OFF time over a 52-week period and was well tolerated by PD patients on levodopa (Kondo et al., 2015). 38.2% of patients reported less time off, 44.7% reported better or considerably better OFF-time symptoms, and 42.3% reported improvements in motor dysfunction, according to patient-reported results (Takahashi et al., 2018).

Even with these encouraging outcomes, patient variability in A_2A antagonist response is still a major drawback, requiring individualized treatment strategies to maximize therapeutic effectiveness (Zheng et al., 2019). According to recent study, combining A_2A and NR2B receptor antagonists may improve motor function in ways that go beyond the advantages of A_2A antagonists alone, potentially providing a combination therapy approach for PD (Michel et al., 2014). A promising approach to treating the disease's motor and nonmotor symptoms is the creation of dual-action medications that target both A_1 and A_2A receptors (Marucci et al., 2021). Excitotoxicity, oxidative stress, and calcium influx result from the overactivation of NMDA and AMPA receptors due to excess extracellular glutamate in PD. These factors contribute to dopaminergic neuron degeneration (Wang et al., 2020). While NMDA receptor hyperactivation in the basal ganglia selectively impairs motor control, AMPA receptor-mediated excitotoxicity increases neuronal sensitivity (Zheng et al., 2019).

Under normal conditions, astrocytes and microglia regulate glutamate clearance. However, in PD, their dysfunction leads to excessive glutamate in synapses, prolonged activation of NMDA receptors, and excitotoxicity (Iovino et al., 2020). Furthermore, motor neurons are more vulnerable to excitotoxic damage in neurodegenerative diseases like Parkinson due to increased calcium permeability, resulting from the downregulation of GluR2 subunits in AMPA receptors (Van Damme et al., 2002). Ultimately, the prolonged overactivation of NMDA and AMPA receptors in motor cortex neurons triggers oxidative stress, persistent intracellular calcium buildup, and neuronal apoptosis, contributing to neurodegeneration in PD (Young et al., 2007). Amantadine, an NMDA receptor antagonist, has been shown to modify glutamatergic transmission in the basal ganglia, thereby reducing levodopa-induced dyskinesia (LID) (Danysz et al., 1997). Moreover, a meta-analysis indicates that amantadine significantly, though temporarily, reduces the severity of dyskinesia in PD patients (Elahi et al., 2012). A primate model of PD corroborates its clinical use, showing a dose-dependent reduction in dyskinetic movements following amantadine administration (Blanchet et al., 1998). Another NMDA receptor antagonist, memantine, has demonstrated promise in neuroprotection and symptom relief in PD, but further research is required to assess its clinical efficacy (Rabey et al., 1992).

In the MPTP macaque model, dipraglurant, a selective mGluR5 receptor negative allosteric modulator, significantly reduced LID without diminishing the antiparkinsonian effects of levodopa (Bezard et al., 2014). According to a meta-analysis of randomized controlled trials, mGluR5 antagonists, such as mavoglurant and dipraglurant, appear to substantially reduce the severity of LID. However, due to variability in study designs, clinical benefits should be interpreted with caution (Wang et al., 2018). Targeting mGluR5 with negative allosteric modulators like mavoglurant and dipraglurant offers a promising approach to treating LID by modulating glutamatergic overactivity associated with dyskinesia development (Pourmirbabaei et al., 2019). The complexity of mGluR5 modulation in PD is evident, as subsequent clinical trials of mavoglurant for LID failed to meet efficacy endpoints, despite early-phase studies showing encouraging results (Petrov et al., 2014).

Perampanel has a generally neutral cognitive profile, with no significant cognitive declines or gains observed in the studies examined (Witt & Helmstaedter, 2022). It effectively reduces seizure frequency and shows a satisfactory responder rate. However, aggressive behavior was significantly affected, particularly in patients with preexisting psychiatric comorbidities, while cognitive function remained largely unaffected (Fong et al., 2022; Olanow et al., 2020). While combination therapies have the potential to improve therapeutic efficacy, they also come with drawbacks, such as increased toxicity and the need for meticulous clinical trial design to assess their mechanisms of action (Ascierto & Marincola, 2011). To overcome drug resistance and minimize side effects, the development of multitarget drugs is essential. This is because selectively targeting cancer cells may improve therapeutic efficacy while reducing off-target effects (Doostmohammadi et al., 2024). Additionally, understanding polypharmacology and the common targets of medications with similar side effect profiles is crucial to predict and mitigate adverse effects, which remain a major clinical challenge (Garcia-Serna & Mestres, 2010). The growing potential of polypharmacology lies in its ability to create drugs that target multiple pathways, overcoming the limitations of conventional single-target therapies and offering new therapeutic options (Ryszkiewicz et al., 2023). When administered or present up to 4 hours after stroke onset, isradipine has been shown to reduce infarct size, as assessed by magnetic resonance imaging (MRI) at 24 h and histological analysis at 5 days following MCA occlusion (Sauter & Rudin, 1990). Additionally, isradipine provides neuroprotection against brain ischemia and stroke in hypertensive rat models (Anekonda & Quinn, 2011). Beyond stroke, this specific calcium channel blocker may have therapeutic potential in AD, as demonstrated by its neuroprotective effects at clinically relevant concentrations both in vitro and in vivo (Anekonda et al., 2011).

However, in PD, the long-term use of immediate-release isradipine did not slow the clinical progression of early-stage PD (Simuni, 2020). The treatment effect was −0.27 (CI, −3.02 to 2.48) points ($P = .85$), and the adjusted least-squares mean changes in the total UPDRS score in the antiparkinsonian medication ON state over 36 months were 2.99 (95% CI, 0.95–5.03) points for the isradipine group and 3.26 (CI, 1.25–5.26) points for the placebo group (Simuni, 2020). In contrast, when used in conjunction with levodopa, rasagiline has been shown to significantly reduce OFF-time and alleviate motor symptoms such as bradykinesia and rigidity, thereby improving overall mobility (Gaines & Hinson, 2012). Additionally, emerging nondopaminergic therapies, such as adenosine A2A receptor antagonists, have demonstrated potential in enhancing motor function, particularly in reducing bradykinesia and rigidity when combined with dopaminergic treatments (Fox, 2013). More broadly, adjunctive oral therapies targeting both dopaminergic and nondopaminergic pathways have been effective in improving motor control by minimizing bradykinesia, rigidity, and motor fluctuations (Sisodia et al., 2024).

Despite their benefits, antiparkinsonian medications, particularly DA agonists and MAO-B inhibitors, frequently cause orthostatic hypotension, increasing the risk of syncope, dizziness, and falls. Given the high prevalence of blood pressure fluctuations in PD, routine cardiovascular monitoring is strongly recommended, especially in elderly patients or those with preexisting cardiovascular conditions (Nimmons et al., 2022). Levodopa, in particular, should be administered with caution in patients with cardiovascular comorbidities, as it has been associated with a significant decrease in mean arterial pressure—primarily due to its negative inotropic effect rather than direct vasodilation. Regular blood pressure monitoring is essential to mitigate the risk of hypotension-related complications, including falls and cerebral hypoperfusion (Noack et al., 2014). DA agonists play a crucial role as adjuncts to levodopa therapy by providing continuous dopaminergic stimulation (CDS) and reducing "off" periods, particularly in patients experiencing motor fluctuations. Their addition can enhance motor control and, in some cases, allow for a reduction in levodopa dosage, potentially decreasing the risk of long-term complications such as dyskinesia (Poewe, 1998). Adjunctive therapies, including DA agonists, MAO-B inhibitors, and COMT inhibitors, are valuable options for managing motor fluctuations and prolonging "on" time when levodopa alone is insufficient. The optimal choice of adjunct therapy should be individualized based on a patient's symptomatology, treatment response, and risk of adverse effects (Fabbri et al., 2018).

14.4.2 Advances in dopamine replacement

CDS aims to reduce the motor fluctuations and dyskinesias associated with pulsatile dopaminergic therapies by mimicking the physiological tonic release of dopamine. Intermittent administration of levodopa results in nonphysiological fluctuations in striatal DA levels, which exacerbate motor complications (Lee et al., 2023; Olanow et al., 2020). The concept of CDS is based on findings that continuous stimulation of DA receptors, as opposed to intermittent pulses, leads to more stable motor responses and a lower risk of motor complications. Restoring a steady dopaminergic flow has been proposed as a strategy to minimize PD-related fluctuations and dyskinesias (Wright & Waters, 2013). In patients with severe PD, continuous cerebroventricular DA administration has emerged as a novel approach to achieving stable dopaminergic stimulation while reducing motor complications. Compared to conventional oral levodopa regimens, research suggests that continuous infusion therapies provide a more physiological dopaminergic tone (Laloux et al., 2017). To stabilize dopaminergic stimulation and reduce motor fluctuations, several continuous drug delivery techniques have been developed, including transdermal rotigotine patches, intrajejunal levodopa infusion, and subcutaneous apomorphine infusion. Levodopa-carbidopa intestinal gel (LCIG) enables continuous infusion of levodopa into the small intestine, preventing delays in gastric emptying and reducing fluctuations in plasma drug levels (Van Wamelen et al., 2018). Additionally, extended-release (ER) formulations such as IPX066 provide longer plasma concentration durations compared to standard levodopa, potentially resulting in more consistent motor responses. Continuous subcutaneous apomorphine infusion (CSAI) has also been shown to improve motor fluctuations by maintaining a steady dopaminergic agonist effect throughout the day (Olanow et al., 2020). Collectively, transdermal delivery systems, infusion therapies, and ER oral levodopa formulations represent key advancements in CDS strategies. Notably, continuous levodopa infusion via a pump system has demonstrated promise in reducing both the severity of dyskinesia and OFF-time (Timpka et al., 2016).

Deep brain stimulation (DBS) of the subthalamic nucleus (STN) has been associated with a significant reduction in LID, often allowing for a considerable decrease in dopaminergic medication dosages. Patients undergoing DBS have reported improved symptom control, leading to fewer medication-related side effects, including motor fluctuations and dyskinesia (Bratsos et al., 2018). However, despite its benefits, DBS carries certain risks, with approximately 5%–10% of patients experiencing device-related complications such as infections, lead displacement, or hardware malfunctions. Additionally, some patients have reported nonmotor side effects post-DBS implantation, including mood changes, speech difficulties, and cognitive decline (Pouratian et al., 2012). Given these potential drawbacks, patient selection remains a crucial factor in the success of DBS, as individuals with severe cognitive impairment or psychiatric comorbidities may have poorer outcomes. Although DBS provides long-term symptom relief, disease progression may lead to the emergence of new motor and nonmotor symptoms that are not alleviated by stimulation (Pouratian et al., 2012).

Emerging drug delivery technologies and gene therapy approaches hold promise for advancing PD treatment. Exosome-based gene delivery systems have gained attention as a viable alternative to synthetic and viral carriers due to their biocompatibility, potential for personalized medicine, and ability to cross biological barriers (Duan et al., 2021). The development of nanocarriers, such as liposomes, polymeric nanoparticles (NPs), and dendrimers, has revolutionized gene therapy by enhancing transfection efficiency while reducing immune responses (Xu et al., 2014). Lipid nanoparticles (LNPs), which have demonstrated success in mRNA vaccine delivery, have also emerged as an effective platform for gene therapy, expanding the potential applications of nucleic acid-based treatments (Lee et al., 2023).

Despite these advancements, several challenges remain in the clinical translation of nanoparticle-based gene delivery, including issues related to stability, targeted delivery, and immunogenicity. Continued research into these novel delivery systems may further improve treatment strategies for PD and other neurological disorders.

Compared to the immediate-release formulation, ER pramipexole reduces motor fluctuations and improves adherence by maintaining a more consistent plasma concentration over a 24-hour period. As evidence of the benefits of CDS, patients on pramipexole ER reported fewer "off" periods and better overall symptom control (Eisenreich et al., 2010). To further address the limitations of pulsatile dopaminergic stimulation, polymeric NPs offer a promising approach for DA replacement therapy. These nanoparticle-based delivery systems enhance levodopa bioavailability and facilitate its passage through the blood-brain barrier, leading to better symptom management (Alabrahim & Azzazy, 2022; Metta et al., 2023).

Since pramipexole ER is taken once daily, it minimizes fluctuations in plasma concentration, resulting in better symptom control and improved adherence. This enhanced compliance leads to more effective long-term disease management. Similarly, the LCIG, delivered through an intrajejunal pump, provides continuous drug infusion, maintaining stable plasma levels while reducing motor fluctuations and dyskinesias. By simulating physiological DA release, LCIG addresses the limitations of oral levodopa and improves both motor and nonmotor symptoms in advanced PD (Thakkar et al., 2021). By continuously stimulating DA receptors over a 24-hour period, transdermal rotigotine reduces the motor fluctuations associated with pulsatile oral therapy. Patients using rotigotine patches reported better symptom control and a lower incidence of peak-dose dyskinesia compared to those on oral DA agonists (Güldenpfennig et al., 2005). In patients with advanced PD, CSAI significantly reduces "off" time by providing stable DA receptor stimulation. Apomorphine infusion serves as an effective alternative for patients with severe motor fluctuations who are not candidates for DBS (Henriksen & Staines, 2021). When administered subcutaneously over an extended period, apomorphine is generally well tolerated, with mild nausea and local skin reactions being the most common side effects—both of which can be managed with dose adjustments. Due to a reduction in erratic motor fluctuations, patients receiving apomorphine infusion therapy reported an overall improvement in quality of life (Metta et al., 2023). Compared to oral formulations, rotigotine transdermal patches provide a more stable pharmacokinetic profile by ensuring continuous drug absorption through the skin, thereby bypassing gastrointestinal (GI) metabolism. This steady DA delivery helps reduce fluctuations in DA levels, potentially lowering the risk of impulse control disorders commonly associated with oral DA agonists (Chen et al., 2009). To enhance drug delivery to affected brain regions in PD, NPs offer a promising method to cross the blood-brain barrier effectively. Advances in nanotechnology-based drug delivery systems have introduced novel neuroprotective strategies, which may enhance dopaminergic neuron survival and slow disease progression (Yadav et al., 2025). In addition to improving drug bioavailability, nanoparticle-based delivery systems help minimize systemic side effects, making them a viable future treatment option for PD. The integration of nanotechnology with regenerative medicine holds great potential for restoring neuronal function and improving the efficacy of treatments for neurodegenerative diseases (Pawar & Patil, 2024).

14.5 Personalized medicine in PD

Personalized medicine is used to treat individual patients based on their vital signs, genes and clinical characteristics, but it has not been fully applied currently due to the cost, but we need it to make the diagnosis clearer in terms of the individual's need for specific doses, and this varies from one person to another. In the cases of Parkinson patients who are detected early, they undergo surgical operations and need a suitable environment to live in, and some of them need exercise therapy (Mishima et al., 2021).

14.5.1 GBA1 and LRRK2 mutations

The GBA1 gene has revealed a novel approach to treating PD by administering GCase to the brain via gene therapy. GCase is employed to lower glycosphingolipids and has demonstrated efficacy in decreasing the accumulation of fat in the nerve cells of PD patients with a GBA1 gene mutation (Smith et al., 2022). The prevalence of PD caused by a mutation in LRRK2 varies with age, so a small-molecule LRRK2 kinase inhibitor was used because it has a strong effect on the nerves. They were found to be good and have no harmful effects when tested on mice. It does not affect body weight, food intake, or behavior, but it lacks vital indicators (Smith et al., 2022). In terms of cognitive and motor deterioration and impaired sense of smell, patients with PD who have a mutation in LRRK2 exhibit fewer symptoms than those with a mutation in GBA1. However, individuals with both mutations develop the disease at an early age (Smith et al., 2022). Research has been conducted in the European community and has confirmed that the genetic structure of PD differs according to the indigenous population and research in genetics is a matter of multiple ancestors is very important for developing successful treatment for this disease. Therefore, scientists aim to promote a treatment strategy that focuses on gene therapy because it causes success in treating this disease by 2.6 times compared to that which does not contain it (Jones et al., 2024).

14.5.2 Biomarkers for therapeutic selection and monitoring

Efforts should be made to detect the disease early in order to treat it better. Among the indicators that appear are motor dysfunction or nonvital symptoms such as rapid eye movement disorder during sleep, weakness in the sense of smell, constipation, and mood disorders. This is part of the early detection of PD. Most evidence indicates that the most common symptom is the dysfunction in the sense of smell, as the patient is affected by it before the weakness in movement occurs, for a period of 4–6 years. However, relying on nonvital indicators is not sufficient for the early diagnosis of PD, and therefore clinical vital indicators must be strengthened (Li & Le, 2020).

14.6 Innovate delivery mechanisms

There are many challenges to treat CNS diseases because of the blood-brain barrier (BBB) (Khatri et al., 2023; Song et al., 2021), BBB is a specialized semipermeable structure that highly regulates exchanges between the CNS parenchyma and blood vessels (Zha et al., 2024). It is the main barrier contributing to CNS protection and maintaining the brain homeostasis (Sanches et al., 2025). The BBB prevents almost 98% of small molecules and all therapeutically active large molecules from reaching the brain (Montegiove et al., 2022). That is because there are certain morphological, structural, and functional traits that distinguish brain microvascular endothelial cells from other vascular endothelial cells that line peripheral blood arteries (Pfau et al., 2024; Song et al., 2021). These consist of the following: One is the expression of tight junctions (TJs), which extremely close the paracellular pathways between neighboring endothelial cells and stop polar (water-soluble) molecules from moving freely between the blood and the brain; two is the lack of fenestrations; three is the absence of pinocytic activity; and four is the expression of active transport mechanisms, which control the movement of vital molecules, such as nutrients and essential amino acids (Khatri et al., 2023). The brain parenchyma is barred from the entry of blood-circulating macromolecules, including recombinant proteins, antibodies, and nucleic acids, as well as macromolecules such as trastuzumab, doxorubicin, or vincristine, by this superselective barrier (Banks et al., 2024). Regarding to all of this, effective therapeutic interventions are often rare or ineffectual.

PD is one of the most neurodegenerative diseases, PD models show a deficiency in DA transporters, which are responsible for DA uptake by dopaminergic neurons then progression of neuronal communications. Reduction in DA delivery during PD results in serious loss of neuronal functions. Another trademark of PD is accumulation of α-syn in the Lewy bodies (Tolosa et al., 2021). Despite there are some synthetic drugs that can delayed the progression of PD like levodopa drug (the precursor of dopamine) and was the most common one; still, it has been shown that the peripheral nervous system can be attack by the untargeted delivery of levodopa leading to dyskinesia and adverse cardiovascular (Islam et al., 2020; Morris et al., 2024). The treatment of Parkinson involves either reducing the concentration of DA inhibitors or increasing DA levels in the brain (Khatri et al., 2023), Therefore, it is advisable to use a suitable delivery system to carefully deliver neurotransmitters for PD treatment across the BBB and not allowing penetration into other peripheral vessels (Islam et al., 2020).

Although insight into active transport systems has advanced drug administration across the BBB into the CNS, major challenges remain. Many medications, particularly big molecules, either break down in the GI tract or are processed by the liver, therefore substantially lowering the active compound content by entering systemic circulation. Often impossible, raising oral doses to compensate can cause significant GI or systemic side effects. Similarly, this approach is difficult for therapies requiring regular dosing or self-administration at home, even though injections provide 100% bioactive medicines into the bloodstream. These constraints stimulated attraction in other ways, including intranasal (IN) delivery. For drugs with poor oral bioavailability, delayed absorption, or slow onset, this strategy avoids hepatic metabolism and GI breakdown and provides a potential path forward. Furthermore, since it allows direct access to the brain, the nasal route is especially helpful for drugs designed for the central nervous system that find difficulty crossing the BBB. Some formulations can even include active transport systems to improve the absorption of drugs from the bloodstream into the brain, therefore further applying IN delivery as a flexible and effective method for complex therapeutic conditions (Islam et al., 2020; Kamei et al., 2021; Tashima, 2020). Many benefits accrue to drug administration via the IN route compared to more traditional routes, particularly to the brain, where the olfactory bulb increases drug bioavailability. Furthermore, it limits drugs breakdown and waste via systemic clearance. The benefits of nasal-brain delivery of drugs relative to other drug administration methods have been extensively evaluated in clinical and pharmacological applications (Islam et al., 2020; Jeong et al., 2023). The physiology of the nasal cavity is the central premise behind IN delivery (Kiran et al., 2022). The nasal cavity can be structured into the respiratory, olfactory, and nasopharyngeal regions, as well as nasal vestibules (Jeong et al., 2023). The primary function of the nasal vestibules, which are situated in the anterior section of the nasal cavity, is to facilitate the expulsion of drugs and other substances. The respiratory and olfactory regions, which are situated in the middle and upper sections of the nasal cavity, are essential for the delivery of drugs. The olfactory region is predominantly responsible for olfactory perception, while the respiratory area is involved in the processing of multiple senses and respiration. The cribriform plate of the ethmoid bone is anatomically situated between the nasal cavity and the brain, which contains olfactory bulbs and sensory neurons. Additionally, the migration of cerebrospinal fluid toward the brain is dependent on the cribriform plate. The nasal mucosa is responsible for the lining of the nasal cavity (Jeong et al., 2023). The exact transport mechanism of drugs from the nasal mucosa to the brain is not well (Islam et al., 2020). However, there is currently limited practical study and data on nasal-brain medicine delivery, most likely because to a lack of knowledge about the mechanism and action in comparison to more frequently used drug administration channels such as oral and intravenous routes (Jeong et al., 2023).

The olfactory pathway is represented by two methods, transcellular and paracellular, another way of drug transport across olfactory epithelium cells is obtained through paracellular method via cell junctions and transcellular method like endocytosis and simple diffusion (Bahadur et al., 2020; Jeong et al., 2023). Naturally, drugs physicochemical characteristics may alter olfactory nerve and epithelial cell drug delivery. The path via the olfactory epithelium cells typically proceeds faster (Jeong et al., 2023). The nasal cavity, which is filled with capillaries, is mostly occupied by the respiratory region. As a result, the drugs delivered to the respiratory area is taken up by the blood and circulated throughout the body, potentially creating an indirect pathway for the drug to reach the brain via the BBB.

Each of the trigeminal nerve's three branches connects to the olfactory bulb and the brain stem. As a result, drugs transport from the nasal cavity to the brain may take place directly via the trigeminal nerve. Even though the majority of trigeminal nerves are located in the respiratory region, some have been discovered in the olfactory region of the nasal cavity. All medications that reach the trigeminal nerves in the olfactory and respiratory systems will thereafter be delivered directly to the brain. Similarly, drugs that exit the nasal cavity and travel into the stomach or airway are indirectly carried to the brain via the systemic circulation. Medications must, however, pass through the BBB before reaching the brain via the systemic circulation. Because of the BBB's thickness and the body's significant drug metabolism and/or clearance, the amount of medications given indirectly to the brain is likely to be less than that delivered directly from the nasal cavity (Jeong et al., 2023). Despite all the benefits that the IN route offers, drugs can face many challenges as it passes through the nasal passage (Khatri et al., 2023).

Mucociliary clearance can remove the drug from the nasal cavity, reducing the drug's residence period in the cavity. To overcome mucociliary clearance and lengthen the drug's residence time in the nasal cavity, mucoadhesive agents can be used. In order to anticipate medication uptake and design IN drug administration, a new advancement in computer analysis of a 3D mucociliary clearance model can be useful (Khatri et al., 2023). Peptidase and protease enzymes can restrict the translocation of peptide and protein medicines over the nasal mucosa, respectively. Also, glutathione s-transferases, epoxide hydrolases, esterase, and aldehyde dehydrogenase are just a few of the enzymes found in the nasal cavity that play an essential role in the breakdown of numerous medicines (Keller et al., 2022; Khatri et al., 2023). Levodopa, one of the small compounds used to treat PD, has a short half-life due to its significant first-pass catabolism. To prevent enzymatic breakdown, enzymatic breakdown can be prevented by administering a variety of enzyme inhibitors that block particular enzymes (Keller et al., 2022; Khatri et al., 2023). Various transporters in the respiratory and olfactory regions of the nasal cavity are engaged in the transfer of different lipophilic and amphiphilic compounds and have acquired resistance to multiple pharmaceuticals. The ciliated epithelium and submucosa of the olfactory region of the nasal cavity express P-glycoprotein. The latter facilitates the direct expulsion of drugs from the nasal mucosa into the lumen, hence diminishing drug absorption (Khatri et al., 2023).

When a drug is administered in its original form for IN administration, it encounters several challenges as previously elucidated. To address these difficulties, pharmaceuticals may be developed in various suitable formulations via diverse carriers (Khatri et al., 2023). NPs serve as optimal drug carriers, capable of either encapsulating pharmaceuticals inside or facilitating surface loading by absorption or chemical bonding with the polymer (Montegiove et al., 2022). Different NPs are effective in nose-to-brain drug transport, including nanocarriers liposomes, nano-emulsion, solid-lipid NPs, metal NPs, nanostructured lipid carriers, dendrimers, exosomes, nano micelles, and quantum dots (Butola & Nainwal, 2024). One of the most promising is biodegradable NPs as a molecule transporter for developing controlled-release systems (Montegiove et al., 2022). Drug-loaded nanocarriers offer multiple benefits for nose-to-brain delivery, including improved patient compliance compared to injections, the ability to bypass biological barriers such as intestinal breakdown, first-pass metabolism, and the BBB, as well as accelerated drug uptake and increased bioavailability. These systems enable the transport of hydrophobic drugs, shield unstable molecules from degradation, and enhance the stability of sensitive compounds. NPs are particularly effective for delivering therapeutic agents like drugs, nucleic acids, and proteins, demonstrating versatility in addressing challenges associated with conventional delivery methods (Kapoor et al., 2024; Montegiove et al., 2022). The basic prerequisite for using a biomaterial in this way is its biocompatibility, which includes its ability to be digested without causing adverse effects, dose reduction, brain targeting, stability, efficacy, and safety for drug-loaded nanocarriers (Calzoni et al., 2019; Kapoor et al., 2024). Natural polymers such as chitosan, sodium alginate, and gelatin can be used to fabricate biopolymer NPs for delivery of drugs in the central nervous system, as can synthetic polymers like polylactic acid (PLA), polyglycolic acid (PGA), polylactic-co-glycolic acid (PLGA), polybutyl cyanoacrylates (PBCA), and (PCL) (Getahun et al., 2024; Reddy et al., 2021).

The translocation of NPs across the BBB may be elucidated by two primary mechanisms: passive transport and active transport, which is the one requiring consumption of energy in the form of ATP (Hersh et al., 2022). Owing to their small size, NPs can cross the BBB by means of passive diffusion through the endothelial cells just like small lipophilic molecules. Furthermore, by incorporating lipid molecules and cationic charges onto the NP surface, their capacity to passively penetrate the membrane can be enhanced (Gosselet et al., 2021). Instead, receptor-mediated and adsorption-mediated endocytosis are the main active transport routes. Adsorption-mediated endocytosis relies on electrostatic interactions between nanoparticle surfaces and cell membranes, while receptor-mediated endocytosis involves ligands on NPs binding to endothelial cell membrane receptors. Both times the cell membrane folds inward to create vesicles that enclose and absorb the NPs for movement. These methods allow for targeted and effective nanoparticle absorption, with the main difference being their initiation procedures (molecular recognition vs. charge-based interactions) (Erickson & Banks,

2022). Since receptor-mediated endocytosis takes advantage of the receptors found on the apical surface of BBB endothelial cells, it is most likely the most popular transport method for the administration of NPs (Hao et al., 2019). There are several examples of polymeric formulations used to deliver therapeutic substances in vitro and in animal models (Montegiove et al., 2022). The delivery of PEG-PCL-GB NPs, approximately 90 nm in diameter and created via antisolvent precipitation, resulted in significantly improved pharmacokinetics compared to the drug in its unencapsulated condition. PEG is the most frequently used ligand to date because it stabilizes NPs in biological environments, including blood. According to studies, a PEG coating gives NPs a stealth property that allows them to avoid immune system responses, such as macrophage activity (Montegiove et al., 2022).

14.7 Emerging role of gut-brain axis in PD therapy

A complex communication network that connects the GI tract with the central nervous system, the gut-brain axis has a profound effect on both health and illness (Ullah et al., 2023). The start and progression of PD may be significantly influenced by gut flora, according to research (Scheperjans et al., 2015). According to a number of studies, PD patients' gut microbiomes have been found to shift, including variations in the quantity of particular bacterial species in comparison to healthy controls. Furthermore, the enteric nervous system (ENS) is where α-syn also accumulates (Holmqvist et al., 2014; Wang, Zhang, et al., 2022; Yang et al., 2024). The gut may be an early source of disease pathology since this accumulation can happen years before the typical motor symptoms of PD manifest. Knowing how the gut-brain axis functions in PD may lead to new opportunities for early detection and focused therapies that alter the gut microbiota or its metabolic products, which may reduce symptoms or halt the course of the disease.

Neurons of the sympathetic and parasympathetic nervous systems connect the CNS and ENS of the GI tract, facilitating bidirectional communication between them (Cryan et al., 2019; Quigley, 2017). This is known as the gut-brain axis. This network of two-way communication helps signals to affect the GI tract's motor, sensory, and secretory modalities from the brain, and vice versa, visceral signals from the GI tract can affect brain activity (O'Mahony et al., 2011). It is currently hypothesized that gut bacteria could play a major role in the two-way communication that occurs along the gut-brain axis. The microbiome population supports general health and equilibrium and performs critical metabolic and physiological tasks for the host (Ma et al., 2019; Rhee et al., 2009).

14.7.1 Probiotics and prebiotics

Probiotics are live microorganisms that help the host's health when given in sufficient quantities (Hill et al., 2014). The preventative and therapeutic benefits of taking probiotics are believed to be mediated by a broad range of processes, which are briefly outlined here and have been thoroughly characterized elsewhere (Hill et al., 2014; Sanders et al., 2019; Suez et al., 2019). Probiotic supplementation can affect the host gut microbiota through antagonism, cross-feeding, and competition for nutrients and adherence to the intestinal epithelium (Hill et al., 2014; Sanders et al., 2019). Probiotic bacteria evade harmful bacterial adhesion by forming biofilms, which are three-dimensional bacterial colonies embedded in extracellular matrix they manufacture themselves. This enhances colonization and prolonged permanence in the host's mucosa (Salas-Jara et al., 2016). The presence of α-syn structures in the colons of those with early-stage PD suggests that the disease may have started in the gut (Fricova, Harsanyiova and Kralova Trancikova, 2020). Prebiotics are nonviable food items that have been altered by the gut microbiota. They help the intestines absorb more minerals, including calcium, magnesium, and others (Gerritsen et al., 2011). Prebiotics may be based on polyunsaturated fatty acids, polyphenols, or carbohydrates. Bacteria that produce short-chain fatty acids (SCFAs) break down products based on polyunsaturated fatty acids, polyphenols, or carbs.

14.7.2 Microbiota-based interventions

As previously stated, the occurrence, progression, and development of PD, particularly in its early stages, are closely linked to the gut microbiota, an improved comprehension of the microbiome. Through altering the composition of the gut microbiota, the gut-brain axis in PD can offer a way to track a person's health. Numerous strategies, including the use of probiotics, psychobiotics, prebiotics, synbiotics, postbiotics, fecal microbiota transplantation (FMT), dietary changes, and Chinese medications, have been attempted to lessen the negative consequences of dysbiosis and slow the progression of PD (Zhu et al., 2022). Probiotics are live bacteria that help the host's health when given in appropriate quantities. A unique subclass of probiotics known as psychobiotics helps people's mental health (Dinan et al., 2013). Psychiatric and neurodevelopmental diseases are currently being studied with psychobiotics as direct and/or supplementary therapy, and potentially in the clinical treatment of brain problems, and they might provide novel therapeutic options for neurodegenerative illness. The majority of prebiotics are indigestible fibers.

Currently, research is being done on psychobiotics as direct and/or supplemental treatments for neurodevelopmental and mental illnesses, and they may in the clinical treatment of brain problems, and they might provide novel therapeutic options for neurodegenerative illness. The majority of prebiotics are indigestible fibers. Numerous neurotransmitters that are present in the human brain, including dopamine, serotonin, gamma aminobutyric acid, and norepinephrine, are produced by the gut microbiota (Luqman et al., 2018; Strandwitz, 2018; Strandwitz et al., 2018).

These neurotransmitters have been demonstrated to impact PD and other neurodegenerative diseases. The brain processes of emotion, movement, learning, and memory are all influenced by these neurotransmitters actively. In most cases, the gut microbiota either controls the host's manufacture of neurotransmitters using bacterial metabolites or directly generates neurotransmitters by encoding genes for certain enzymes (Y. Chen et al., 2021). Levodopa is frequently used to treat PD because it can pass across the BBB and be converted into DA in the brain, which reduces PD symptoms (Wang et al., 2021). Nonetheless, levodopa's bioavailability is necessary to guarantee that the brain will receive enough dopamine. There is mounting evidence that the gut microbiota can either directly or indirectly affect drug pharmacokinetics, which in turn can affect bioavailability, efficacy, or side effects.

14.7.3 Antiinflammatory agents targeting the gut

Antiinflammatory medications that are nanoencapsulated successfully address the issues of conventional medications' poor retention duration and nonspecific dispersion. The medications can be precisely transported to the site of gut inflammation by regulating the size of the nanocap capsules, surface charge, pH-responsive design, and particular ligands/antibodies on the carriers' surface. This achieves a more direct and effective therapeutic goal. By precisely controlling the size of the nanocapsule, nanocapsule technology can match the microenvironment of the gut inflammation site. This is especially true for small lesions, where the smaller size of the nanocapsule allows it to penetrate deeper. The size effect guarantees that the nanocapsule is precisely retained and released at the site of inflammation. Furthermore, the surface charge's design is also very important (Siegel et al., 2024). Positively charged proteins slow down when the intestinal mucosa swells, making it easier for drug delivery nanocarriers with a negative surface charge to attach onto it (Iqbal et al., 2018). To further improve the impact of targeted medication delivery, certain ligands or antibodies could be altered on the surface of nanomedicines to address the buildup of ROS brought on by gut inflammation. Additionally, antiinflammatory medications can be wrapped in nanocarriers using nanoencapsulation technology to create a stable nanodrug system, which greatly increases the stability and prevents oxidative degradation. It has been demonstrated that intestinal inflammation may be treated with ROS-responsive NPs B-ATK-T, which can regulate medication release in the presence of different hydrogen peroxide (H_2O_2) concentrations (X. Li et al., 2023).

14.8 Neuroprotection and lifestyle-based interventions

The bioactive chemicals contained in foods are appealing molecules for the creation of new medications with activity against a variety of disorders, including those connected with inflammatory processes that are frequently linked to oxidative stress. Many of these substances have a significant inhibitory effect on oxidative stress and inflammatory response, and they may help to enhance quality of life in a preventive manner by consuming a diet rich in them. For example, Eugenol is a natural chemical with a variety of pharmacological activity, effects on redox state, and applications in the food and pharmaceutical industries. Given the importance of this molecule, the current review covers its antiinflammatory and antioxidant capabilities, as well as its methods of action and therapeutic promise for the treatment of inflammatory illnesses (Barboza et al., 2018). Emerging research has identified disruptions in critical signaling pathways—specifically the IκB/NF-κB and KEAP1/Nrf2 systems—as key contributors to neurodegenerative processes. These pathways play vital roles in modulating neuroinflammation, oxidative stress, and mitochondrial efficiency. Despite the absence of curative treatments for neurodegenerative diseases, current therapies primarily target symptom management. However, such drugs offer only short-term relief and may lead to adverse effects with prolonged use. This challenge has spurred interest in plant-derived bioactive compounds, such as baicalein, a flavonoid extracted from *Scutellaria baicalensis*, which exhibits therapeutic potential by targeting these pathways. Baicalein mitigates neuroinflammation by suppressing NF-κB activity, thereby reducing the production of inflammatory cytokines (e.g., TNF-α, IL-1β, and IL-6) and the NLRP3 inflammasome, as well as enzymes like COX-2, LOX, and iNOS, which are critical to immune responses. Concurrently, it activates Nrf2 signaling, enhancing the expression of antioxidant enzymes such as HO-1, NQO1, GPx, and SOD to counteract oxidative damage. By addressing both inflammatory and oxidative pathways while improving mitochondrial function, baicalein emerges as a promising adjunct therapy. Its multifaceted action presents a safer, holistic alternative to conventional treatments, offering potential for more comprehensive management of neurodegenerative conditions (Kuwar & Kalia, 2025). Environmental and lifestyle variables may greatly impact PD, according to research. If established as causes, these variables might help prevent or manage PD at the individual and public health levels. Over the past decade, data have strengthened causal relationships and shown their complex dynamics. Physical exercise, pesticide and chemical exposure, food, chronic stress, brain trauma, and smoking have been studied, as have several gene-environment interactions. These findings emphasize the significance of addressing modifiable risk factors in PD prevention and treatment. To achieve this, certain low-risk yet potentially high-yield lifestyle modifications may be suggested for reducing the individual and communal burdens of PD, including dietary adjustments, enhanced physical activity, and the prevention of head injuries. Moreover, diminishing pesticide application could substantially affect global health, encompassing, but not restricted to, PD. Due to the disorder's increasing prevalence, prioritizing the development and dissemination of these recommendations is essential (Marras et al., 2019).

14.9 Digital health and technology in PD management

Digital health technology encompasses a wide range of technical applications, including devices worn on the body or the analysis of frequently used appliances. In theory, digital technologies offer the opportunity to monitor people for extended periods of time, and their use, some in conjunction with connected devices (e.g., smartphones), is increasing to improve the management of medical conditions, including PD (van Wamelen et al., 2021). Digital assessments are promising objective indicators for PD symptoms, such as bradykinesia, freezing of gait, decreased dexterity, balance, and speech issues, according to recent studies (Goñi et al., 2022).

14.9.1 Digital biomarkers and the role of wearable remote management tools

Digital biomarkers are objective, quantitative physiological and behavioral data obtained using digital sensors that are portable, wearable, implanted, or ingestible (Sun et al., 2024). There are three primary types of digital health devices used to measure digital biomarkers. First, wearable technology, including biometric skin patches, portable sensors, and accelerometers worn on the wrist. Secondly, smartphones or applications identify voice/speech metrics, cognitive assessments, typing patterns, and other related data. Thirdly, sensor-equipped environments utilize nonvisual technologies that provide passive measurement without requiring the subject to wear sensors (Dockendorf et al., 2021). These devices can be attached to various body regions or applied in sensor-equipped environments (e.g., smartwatches, wrist-worn accelerometers, forearm and footwear accelerometers, smart insoles, etc.), alongside instruments for assessing both motor and nonmotor symptoms across various body areas (e.g., smartphones, finger-tapping keyboards, facial monitoring cameras, etc.) and evaluating serial reaction time (Sun et al., 2024).

14.9.2 Telemedicine

Telemedicine can offer high-quality, affordable, and easily accessible healthcare services and is especially helpful for underserved and rural regions since it leverages information and communication technology (ICTs) to transcend geographic boundaries (Cubo & Delgado-López, 2022). According to surveys measuring satisfaction, most doctors and patients were content with using telemedicine overall (Houston et al., 2022). Since a large portion of the results of neurological examinations are visual, telemedicine is especially well-suited to evaluate patients with PD and other movement disorders. Neurological examinations can be conducted in part during teleconsultations, with results that are comparable to those of in-person assessments and evaluations of candidates for advanced PD therapy. These teleconsultations consisted of phone and e-consultations in addition to synchronous interactions (videoconferences) (Cubo & Delgado-López, 2022).

14.9.3 AI in drug discovery

Pharmaceutical research could be expedited by machine learning/artificial intelligence (AI/ML) by gleaning new and significant information from the massive volume of intricate data produced throughout the drug discovery process. The most difficult area of drug discovery, CNS therapies, has showed promise in the creation of AI/ML systems. Preclinical development, lead generation and optimization, and target identification are the three phases of the early drug discovery process where AI/ML has been applied (Vatansever et al., 2021). Models of ML and AI have been linked to the diagnosis, prognosis, and management of PD. The use of AI and ML models in the classification of PD based on neuroimaging techniques, speech recordings, impairments in gait, and other factors has also been shown in recent years (Gupta et al., 2023). Monzel et al. designed a Random Forest (RF) machine learning model to assess the neurotoxic potential of compounds on organoids by analyzing cellular traits while also establishing a human midbrain organoid system mimicking PD to serve as an in vitro platform for toxicity evaluation (Monzel et al., 2020). To establish an efficient drug testing pathway, Hughes et al. developed a zebrafish model of PD that employs an AI/ML-based approach to classify movement disorders in the model through high-resolution video Capture (Hughes et al., 2020).

14.10 Challenges and future directions

Diagnosing idiopathic PD is straightforward in typical cases but challenging in atypical ones, with misclassification rates of 15%–24% and an overall diagnostic accuracy of 80.6%. Even with strict criteria, 10% of PD diagnoses are incorrect. Early differentiation from essential tremor, secondary parkinsonism, and atypical parkinsonian disorders like MSA, progressive supranuclear palsy (PSP), and corticobasal degeneration (CBD) remains difficult, with diagnostic error rates ranging from 7% to 35%. Despite high sensitivity and specificity in diagnostic criteria, accuracy remains below 100%, but future biomarkers, AI-driven MRI analysis, and radiotracer imaging of α-syn hold promise for improvement (Tolosa et al., 2021). On the therapeutic front, nanomedicine has gained significant research attention over the past 2 decades, leading to numerous patents and clinical studies, yet its practical applications remain limited. Nano-drug delivery systems (NDDSs) offer a promising approach for neurological disorders like PD, enabling targeted drug delivery and enhanced protection. Future research should focus on improving drug absorption and stability while refining precise delivery mechanisms. While the benefits of nanomedicine are becoming more evident, its full impact on healthcare remains uncertain, and affordability is crucial for market adoption (Sharma et al., 2021). Nanotechnology could enhance symptom control and slow disease progression, offering personalized therapies. However, safety concerns, regulatory challenges, and potential neurotoxicity such as α-syn aggregation, oxidative stress, and neuroinflammation—necessitate further risk assessment before clinical application (Bougea, 2024; Yadav et al., 2025).

14.11 Conclusion

These findings suggest that advancements in diagnostic criteria, nanotechnology, and genetic insights collectively offer transformative potential for managing PD. The integration of these advances promotes earlier and more precise diagnoses, enabling personalized and targeted treatments that can significantly enhance patient outcomes and overall management of diseases. NDDS indicate a notably promising frontier in this context. NDDS offers a viable solution for the difficulties of neurological disorders such as PD by improving drug absorption and facilitating site-specific distribution. In conclusion, integrating nanotechnology into PD treatment, combined with advancements in diagnostic precision and genetic understanding, marks a significant step forward in addressing the challenges of PD. These developments not only enhance the effectiveness of existing therapies but also lay the foundation for a more precise, efficient, and patient-centered approach to managing PD.

References

Aires, I. D., Boia, R., Rodrigues-Neves, A. C., Madeira, M. H., Marques, C., Ambrósio, A. F., & Santiago, A. R. (2019). Blockade of microglial adenosine A 2A receptor suppresses elevated pressure-induced inflammation, oxidative stress, and cell death in retinal cells. *Glia, 67*(5), 896–914. https://doi.org/10.1002/glia.23579

Alabrahim, O. A. A., & Azzazy, H. M. E.-S. (2022). Polymeric nanoparticles for dopamine and levodopa replacement in Parkinson's disease. *Nanoscale Advances, 4*(24), 5233–5244. https://doi.org/10.1039/d2na00524g

Anekonda, T. S., & Quinn, J. F. (2011). Calcium channel blocking as a therapeutic strategy for Alzheimer's disease: The case for isradipine. *Biochimica et Biophysica Acta - Molecular Basis of Disease, 1812*(12), 1584–1590. https://doi.org/10.1016/j.bbadis.2011.08.013

Anekonda, T. S., Quinn, J. F., Harris, C., Frahler, K., Wadsworth, T. L., & Woltjer, R. L. (2011). L-type voltage-gated calcium channel blockade with isradipine as a therapeutic strategy for Alzheimer's disease. *Neurobiology of Disease, 41*(1), 62–70. https://doi.org/10.1016/j.nbd.2010.08.020

Ascierto, P. A., & Marincola, F. M. (2011). Combination therapy: The next opportunity and challenge of medicine. *Journal of Translational Medicine, 9*(1). https://doi.org/10.1186/1479-5876-9-115

Bahadur, S., Pardhi, D. M., Rautio, J., Rosenholm, J. M., & Pathak, K. (2020). Intranasal nanoemulsions for direct nose-to-brain delivery of actives for cns disorders. *Pharmaceutics, 12*(12), 1–27. https://doi.org/10.3390/pharmaceutics12121230

Banks, W. A., Rhea, E. M., Reed, M. J., & Erickson, M. A. (2024). The penetration of therapeutics across the blood-brain barrier: Classic case studies and clinical implications. *Cell Reports Medicine, 5*(11). https://doi.org/10.1016/j.xcrm.2024.101760

Barboza, J. N., da Silva Maia Bezerra Filho, C., Silva, R. O., Medeiros, J. V. R., & de Sousa, D. P. (2018). An overview on the anti-inflammatory potential and antioxidant profile of eugenol. *Oxidative Medicine and Cellular Longevity, 2018*. https://doi.org/10.1155/2018/3957262

Barker, R. A., Björklund, A., Gash, D. M., Whone, A., Van Laar, A., Kordower, J. H., Bankiewicz, K., Kieburtz, K., Saarma, M., Booms, S., Huttunen, H. J., Kells, A. P., Fiandaca, M. S., Stoessl, A. J., Eidelberg, D., Federoff, H., Voutilainen, M. H., Dexter, D. T., Eberling, J., … Lang, A. E. (2020). GDNF and Parkinson's Disease: Where Next? A Summary from a recent workshop. *Journal of Parkinson's Disease, 10*(3), 875–891. https://doi.org/10.3233/JPD-202004

Bezard, E., Pioli, E. Y., Li, Q., Girard, F., Mutel, V., Keywood, C., Tison, F., Rascol, O., & Poli, S. M. (2014). The mGluR5 negative allosteric modulator dipraglurant reduces dyskinesia in the MPTP macaque model. *Movement Disorders, 29*(8), 1074–1079. https://doi.org/10.1002/mds.25920

Björklund, T., Davidsson, M., Björklund, A., Bloem, B. R., Brundin, P., & Howard, F. (2021). Next-Generation gene therapy for parkinson's disease using engineered viral vectors. *Journal of Parkinson's Disease, 11*(s2), S209. https://doi.org/10.3233/jpd-212674

Blanchet, P. J., Konitsiotis, S., & Chase, T. N. (1998). Amantadine reduces levodopa-induced dyskinesias in parkinsonian monkeys. *Movement Disorders, 13*(5), 798–802. https://doi.org/10.1002/mds.870130507

Bloem, B. R., Okun, M. S., & Klein, C. (2021). Parkinson's disease. *The Lancet, 397*(10291), 2284–2303. https://doi.org/10.1016/S0140-6736(21)00218-X

Bougea, A. (2024). Some novel therapies in parkinson's disease: A promising path forward or not yet? A systematic review of the literature. *Biomedicines, 12*(3), 549. https://doi.org/10.3390/biomedicines12030549

Bratsos, S. P., Karponis, D., & Saleh, S. N. (2018). Efficacy and safety of deep brain stimulation in the treatment of parkinson's disease: A systematic review and meta-analysis of randomized controlled trials. *Cureus, 10*(10). https://doi.org/10.7759/cureus.3474

Butola, M., & Nainwal, N. (2024). Non-Invasive techniques of nose to brain delivery using nanoparticulate carriers: Hopes and hurdles. *AAPS PharmSciTech, 25*(8). https://doi.org/10.1208/s12249-024-02946-z

Calzoni, E., Cesaretti, A., Polchi, A., Di Michele, A., Tancini, B., & Emiliani, C. (2019). Biocompatible polymer nanoparticles for drug delivery applications in cancer and neurodegenerative disorder therapies. *Journal of Functional Biomaterials, 10*(1), 4. https://doi.org/10.3390/jfb10010004

Castonguay, A.-M., Gravel, C., & Lévesque, M. (2020). Treating parkinson's disease with antibodies: Previous studies and future directions. *Journal of Parkinson's Disease, 11*(1), 71–92. https://doi.org/10.3233/JPD-202221

Chen, J. J., Swope, D. M., Dashtipour, K., & Lyons, K. E. (2009). Transdermal rotigotine: A clinically innovative dopamine-receptor agonist for the management of parkinson's disease. *Pharmacotherapy: The Journal of Human Pharmacology and Drug Therapy, 29*(12), 1452–1467. https://doi.org/10.1592/phco.29.12.1452

Chen, Y., Xu, J., & Chen, Y. (2021). Regulation of neurotransmitters by the Gut Microbiota and effects on cognition in neurological disorders. *Nutrients, 13*(6), 2099. https://doi.org/10.3390/nu13062099

Chopade, P., Chopade, N., Zhao, Z., Mitragotri, S., Liao, R., & Chandran Suja, V. (2023). Alzheimer's and Parkinson's disease therapies in the clinic. *Bioengineering & Translational Medicine, 8*(1). https://doi.org/10.1002/btm2.10367

Cryan, J. F., O'riordan, K. J., Cowan, C. S. M., Sandhu, K. V., Bastiaanssen, T. F. S., Boehme, M., Codagnone, M. G., Cussotto, S., Fulling, C., Golubeva, A. V., Guzzetta, K. E., Jaggar, M., Long-Smith, C. M., Lyte, J. M., Martin, J. A., Molinero-Perez, A., Moloney, G., Morelli, E., Morillas, E., … Dinan, T. G. (2019). The microbiota-gut-brain axis. *Physiological Reviews, 99*(4), 1877–2013. https://doi.org/10.1152/physrev.00018.2018

Cubo, E., & Delgado-López, P. D. (2022). Telemedicine in the management of parkinson's disease: Achievements, challenges, and future perspectives. *Brain Sciences, 12*(12). https://doi.org/10.3390/brainsci12121735

Danysz, W., Parsons, C. G., Kornhuber, J., Schmidt, W. J., & Quack, G. (1997). Aminoadamantanes as NMDA receptor antagonists and antiparkinsonian agents — Preclinical studies. *Neuroscience & Biobehavioral Reviews, 21*(4), 455–468. https://doi.org/10.1016/s0149-7634(96)00037-1

Dinan, T. G., Stanton, C., & Cryan, J. F. (2013). Psychobiotics: A novel class of psychotropic. *Biological Psychiatry, 74*(10), 720–726. https://doi.org/10.1016/j.biopsych.2013.05.001

Dockendorf, M. F., Hansen, B. J., Bateman, K. P., Moyer, M., Shah, J. K., & Shipley, L. A. (2021). Digitally enabled, patient-centric clinical trials: Shifting the drug Development paradigm. *Clinical and Translational Science, 14*(2), 445–459. https://doi.org/10.1111/cts.12910

Doostmohammadi, A., Jooya, H., Ghorbanian, K., Gohari, S., & Dadashpour, M. (2024). Potentials and future perspectives of multi-target drugs in cancer treatment: The next generation anti-cancer agents. *Cell Communication and Signaling, 22*(1). https://doi.org/10.1186/s12964-024-01607-9

Duan, L., Xu, L., Xu, X., Qin, Z., Zhou, X., Xiao, Y., Liang, Y., & Xia, J. (2021). Exosome-mediated delivery of gene vectors for gene therapy. *Nanoscale, 13*(3), 1387–1397. https://doi.org/10.1039/d0nr07622h

Dunn, B., Stein, P., & Cavazzoni, P. (2021). Approval of aducanumab for alzheimer Disease—The FDA's perspective. *JAMA Internal Medicine, 181*(10), 1276. https://doi.org/10.1001/jamainternmed.2021.4607

Eisenreich, W., Sommer, B., Hartter, S., & Jost, W. H. (2010). Pramipexole extended release: A novel treatment option in Parkinson's Disease. *Parkinson's Disease, 2010*, 1–7. https://doi.org/10.4061/2010/612619

Elahi, B., Phielipp, N., & Chen, R. (2012). N-Methyl-D-Aspartate antagonists in levodopa induced dyskinesia: A meta-analysis. *Canadian Journal of Neurological Sciences/Journal Canadien des Sciences Neurologiques, 39*(4), 465–472. https://doi.org/10.1017/s0317167100013974

Erickson, M. A., & Banks, W. A. (2022). Transcellular routes of blood–brain barrier disruption. *Experimental Biology and Medicine, 247*(9), 788–796. https://doi.org/10.1177/15353702221080745

Fabbri, M., Rosa, M. M., & Ferreira, J. J. (2018). Adjunctive therapies in parkinson's disease: How to choose the best treatment strategy approach. *Drugs and Aging, 35*(12), 1041–1054. https://doi.org/10.1007/s40266-018-0599-2

Fong, Y. O., Huang, P., Hsu, C. Y., & Yang, Y. H. (2022). Effects of perampanel on seizure control, cognition, behavior, and psychological status in patients with epilepsy: A systematic review. *Journal of Clinical Neurology, 18*(6), 653–662. https://doi.org/10.3988/jcn.2022.18.6.653

Fox, S. H. (2013). Non-dopaminergic treatments for motor control in Parkinson's disease. *Drugs, 73*(13), 1405–1415. https://doi.org/10.1007/s40265-013-0105-4

Fricova, D., Harsanyiova, J., & Trancikova, A. K. (2020). Alpha-Synuclein in the gastrointestinal tract as a potential biomarker for early detection of parkinson's disease. *International Journal of Molecular Sciences, 21*(22), 8666. https://doi.org/10.3390/ijms21228666

Gaines, K. D., & Hinson, V. K. (2012). Adjunctive therapy in Parkinson'S disease: The role of rasagiline. *Neuropsychiatric Disease and Treatment, 8*, 285–294. https://doi.org/10.2147/NDT.S25142

Gao, S., Li, N., Wang, Y., Zhong, Y., & Shen, X. (2020). Blockade of adenosine A 2A receptor protects photoreceptors after retinal detachment by inhibiting inflammation and oxidative stress. *Oxidative Medicine and Cellular Longevity, 2020*, 1–12. https://doi.org/10.1155/2020/7649080

Garcia-Serna, R., & Mestres, J. (2010). Anticipating drug side effects by comparative pharmacology. *Expert Opinion on Drug Metabolism and Toxicology, 6*(10), 1253–1263. https://doi.org/10.1517/17425255.2010.509343

Gash, D. M., Gerhardt, G. A., Bradley, L. H., Wagner, R., & Slevin, J. T. (2020). GDNF clinical trials for Parkinson's disease: A critical human dimension. *Cell and Tissue Research, 382*(1), 65–70. https://doi.org/10.1007/s00441-020-03269-8

Gerritsen, J., Smidt, H., Rijkers, G. T., & De Vos, W. M. (2011). Intestinal microbiota in human health and disease: The impact of probiotics. *Genes & Nutrition, 6*(3), 209–240. https://doi.org/10.1007/s12263-011-0229-7

Getahun, M. J., Kassie, B. B., & Alemu, T. S. (2024). Recent advances in biopolymer synthesis, properties, & commercial applications: A review. *Process Biochemistry, 145*, 261–287. https://doi.org/10.1016/j.procbio.2024.06.034

Goñi, M., Eickhoff, S. B., Far, M. S., Patil, K. R., & Dukart, J. (2022). Smartphone-Based digital biomarkers for parkinson's disease in a remotely-administered setting. *IEEE Access, 10*, 28361–28384. https://doi.org/10.1109/ACCESS.2022.3156659. IEEE Access.

Gosselet, F., Azevedo Loiola, R., Roig, A., Rosell, A., & Culot, M. (2021). Central nervous system delivery of molecules across the blood-brain barrier. *Neurochemistry International, 144*, 104952. https://doi.org/10.1016/j.neuint.2020.104952

Güldenpfennig, W. M., Poole, K. H., Sommerville, K. W., & Boroojerdi, B. (2005). Safety, tolerability, and efficacy of continuous transdermal dopaminergic stimulation with rotigotine patch in early-stage idiopathic Parkinson disease. *Clinical Neuropharmacology, 28*(3), 106–110. https://doi.org/10.1097/01.wnf.0000162228.00154.ba

Gupta, R., Kumari, S., Senapati, A., Ambasta, R. K., & Kumar, P. (2023). New era of artificial intelligence and machine learning-based detection, diagnosis, and therapeutics in Parkinson's disease. *Ageing Research Reviews, 90*, 102013. https://doi.org/10.1016/j.arr.2023.102013

György, B., Lööv, C., Zaborowski, M. P., Takeda, S., Kleinstiver, B. P., Commins, C., Kastanenka, K., Mu, D., Volak, A., Giedraitis, V., Lannfelt, L., Maguire, C. A., Joung, J. K., Hyman, B. T., Breakefield, X. O., & Ingelsson, M. (2018). CRISPR/Cas9 mediated disruption of the Swedish APP allele as a therapeutic approach for early-onset Alzheimer's Disease. *Molecular Therapy Nucleic Acids, 11*, 429–440. https://doi.org/10.1016/j.omtn.2018.03.007

Hao, F., Feng, Y., & Guan, Y. (2019). A novel botulinum toxin TAT-EGFP-HCS fusion protein capable of specific delivery through the blood-brain barrier to the central nervous System. *CNS & Neurological Disorders - Drug Targets, 18*(1), 37–43. https://doi.org/10.2174/1871527317666181011113215

Hauser, R. A., Hattori, N., Fernandez, H., Isaacson, S. H., Mochizuki, H., Rascol, O., Stocchi, F., Li, J., Mori, A., Nakajima, Y., Ristuccia, R., & Lewitt, P. (2021). Efficacy of istradefylline, an adenosine A2A receptor antagonist, as adjunctive therapy to levodopa in Parkinson's Disease: A pooled analysis of 8 phase 2b/3 trials. *Journal of Parkinson's Disease, 11*(4), 1663–1675. https://doi.org/10.3233/jpd-212672

Henriksen, T., & Staines, H. (2021). Continuous subcutaneous apomorphine infusion in parkinson's disease: A Single-Center, long-term Follow-Up Study of the causes for discontinuation. *Journal of Personalized Medicine, 11*(6), 525. https://doi.org/10.3390/jpm11060525

Hersh, A. M., Alomari, S., & Tyler, B. M. (2022). Crossing the blood-brain barrier: Advances in nanoparticle technology for drug delivery in Neuro-Oncology. *International Journal of Molecular Sciences, 23*(8). https://doi.org/10.3390/ijms23084153

Hill, C., Guarner, F., Reid, G., Gibson, G. R., Merenstein, D. J., Pot, B., Morelli, L., Canani, R. B., Flint, H. J., Salminen, S., Calder, P. C., & Sanders, M. E. (2014). The International Scientific Association for Probiotics and Prebiotics consensus statement on the scope and appropriate use of the term probiotic. *Nature Reviews Gastroenterology & Hepatology, 11*(8), 506–514. https://doi.org/10.1038/nrgastro.2014.66

Hoang, D. M., Pham, P. T., Bach, T. Q., Ngo, A. T. L., Nguyen, Q. T., Phan, T. T. K., Nguyen, G. H., Le, P. T. T., Hoang, V. T., Forsyth, N. R., Heke, M., & Nguyen, L. T. (2022). Stem cell-based therapy for human diseases. *Signal Transduction and Targeted Therapy, 7*(1). https://doi.org/10.1038/s41392-022-01134-4

Holmqvist, S., Chutna, O., Bousset, L., Aldrin-Kirk, P., Li, W., Björklund, T., Wang, Z. Y., Roybon, L., Melki, R., & Li, J. Y. (2014). Direct evidence of Parkinson pathology spread from the gastrointestinal tract to the brain in rats. *Acta Neuropathologica, 128*(6), 805–820. https://doi.org/10.1007/s00401-014-1343-6

Houston, E., Kennedy, A. G., O'malley, D., Rabinowitz, T., Rose, G. L., & Boyd, J. (2022). Telemedicine in neurology: A scoping review of key outcomes in movement disorders. *Telemedicine and E-Health, 28*(3), 295–308. https://doi.org/10.1089/tmj.2021.0117

Hu, J., Zhang, D., Tian, K., Ren, C., Li, H., Lin, C., Huang, X., Liu, J., Mao, W., & Zhang, J. (2023). Small-molecule LRRK2 inhibitors for PD therapy: Current achievements and future perspectives. *European Journal of Medicinal Chemistry, 256*, 115475. https://doi.org/10.1016/j.ejmech.2023.115475

Hughes, G. L., Lones, M. A., Bedder, M., Currie, P. D., Smith, S. L., & Pownall, M. E. (2020). Machine learning discriminates a movement disorder in a zebrafish model of Parkinson's disease. *DMM Disease Models and Mechanisms, 13*(10). https://doi.org/10.1242/dmm.045815

Iovino, L., Tremblay, M. E., & Civiero, L. (2020). Glutamate-induced excitotoxicity in Parkinson's disease: The role of glial cells. *Journal of Pharmacological Sciences, 144*(3), 151–164. https://doi.org/10.1016/j.jphs.2020.07.011

Iqbal, S., Du, X., Wang, J., Li, H., Yuan, Y., & Wang, J. (2018). Surface charge tunable nanoparticles for TNF-α siRNA oral delivery for treating ulcerative colitis. *Nano Research, 11*(5), 2872–2884. https://doi.org/10.1007/s12274-017-1918-3

Islam, S. U., Shehzad, A., Ahmed, M. B., & Lee, Y. S. (2020). Intranasal delivery of nanoformulations: A potential way of treatment for neurological disorders. *Molecules, 25*(8), 1929. https://doi.org/10.3390/molecules25081929

Jenner, P. (2014). An overview of adenosine A2A receptor antagonists in Parkinson's disease. *International Review of Neurobiology, 119*, 71–86. https://doi.org/10.1016/B978-0-12-801022-8.00003-9

Jeong, S. H., Jang, J. H., & Lee, Y. B. (2023). Drug delivery to the brain via the nasal route of administration: Exploration of key targets and major consideration factors. *Journal of Pharmaceutical Investigation, 53*(1), 119–152. https://doi.org/10.1007/s40005-022-00589-5

Jones, L., Cerquera-Cleves, C., Schuh, A. F. S., Makarious, M. B., Iwaki, H., Nalls, M. A., Noyce, A. J., Blauwendraat, C., Singleton, A., Mata, I., & Bandres-Ciga, S. (2024). Multi-ancestry population attributable risk assessment of common genetic variation in Alzheimer's and Parkinson's diseases. *medRxiv*. https://doi.org/10.1101/2024.09.23.24314240

Kamei, N., Suwabe, S., Arime, K., Bando, H., Murata, K., Yamaguchi, M., Yokoyama, N., Tanaka, E., Hashimoto, A., Kanazawa, T., Ago, Y., & Takeda-Morishita, M. (2021). Investigation of the transport pathways associated with enhanced brain delivery of peptide drugs by intranasal coadministration with penetratin. *Pharmaceutics, 13*(11), 1745. https://doi.org/10.3390/pharmaceutics13111745

Kapoor, A., Hafeez, A., & Kushwaha, P. (2024). Nanocarrier mediated intranasal drug delivery systems for the management of parkinsonism: A review. *Current Drug Delivery, 21*(5), 709–725. https://doi.org/10.2174/1567201820666230523114259

Keller, L. A., Merkel, O., & Popp, A. (2022). Intranasal drug delivery: Opportunities and toxicologic challenges during drug development. *Drug Delivery and Translational Research, 12*(4), 735–757. https://doi.org/10.1007/s13346-020-00891-5

Khatri, D. K., Preeti, K., Tonape, S., Bhattacharjee, S., Patel, M., Shah, S., Singh, P. K., Srivastava, S., Gugulothu, D., Vora, L., & Singh, S. B. (2023). Nanotechnological advances for nose to brain delivery of therapeutics toImprove the parkinson therapy. *Current Neuropharmacology, 21*(3), 493–516. https://doi.org/10.2174/1570159X20666220507022701

Kiran, P., Kumar Debnath, S., Neekhra, S., Pawar, V., Khan, A., Dias, F., Pallod, S., & Srivastava, R. (2022). Designing nanoformulation for the nose-to-brain delivery in Parkinson's disease: Advancements and barrier. *WIREs Nanomedicine and Nanobiotechnology, 14*(1). https://doi.org/10.1002/wnan.1768

Kondo, T., Mizuno, Y., & Group, J. I. S. (2015). A long-term Study of istradefylline safety and efficacy in patients with parkinson disease. *Clinical Neuropharmacology, 38*(2), 41. https://doi.org/10.1097/WNF.0000000000000073

Kuwar, O. K., & Kalia, N. (2025). Anti-inflammatory and antioxidant effects of baicalein: Targeting Nrf2, and NFκB in neurodegenerative disease. *Inflammopharmacology, 33*(3), 1303–1310. https://doi.org/10.1007/s10787-025-01698-x

Laloux, C., Gouel, F., Lachaud, C., Timmerman, K., Do Van, B., Jonneaux, A., Petrault, M., Garcon, G., Rouaix, N., Moreau, C., Bordet, R., Duce, J. A., Devedjian, J. C., & Devos, D. (2017). Continuous cerebroventricular administration of dopamine: A new treatment for severe dyskinesia in Parkinson's disease? *Neurobiology of Disease, 103*, 24–31. https://doi.org/10.1016/j.nbd.2017.03.013

Lee, D., Amirthalingam, S., Lee, C., Rajendran, A. K., Ahn, Y.-H., & Hwang, N. S. (2023). Strategies for targeted gene delivery using lipid nanoparticles and cell-derived nanovesicles. *Nanoscale Advances, 5*(15), 3834–3856. https://doi.org/10.1039/D3NA00198A

Li, X., Hetjens, L., Wolter, N., Li, H., Shi, X., & Pich, A. (2023). Charge-reversible and biodegradable chitosan-based microgels for lysozyme-triggered release of vancomycin. *Journal of Advanced Research, 43*, 87–96. https://doi.org/10.1016/j.jare.2022.02.014

Li, T., & Le, W. (2020). Biomarkers for parkinson's disease: How good are they? *Neuroscience Bulletin, 36*(2), 183–194. https://doi.org/10.1007/s12264-019-00433-1

Liu, Q., Zhang, W., Chen, S., Zhuang, Z., Zhang, Y., Jiang, L., & Lin, J. S. (2020). SELEX tool: A novel and convenient gel-based diffusion method for monitoring of aptamer-target binding. *Journal of Biological Engineering, 14*(1). https://doi.org/10.1186/s13036-019-0223-y

Luqman, A., Nega, M., Nguyen, M. T., Ebner, P., & Götz, F. (2018). SadA-Expressing staphylococci in the human gut show increased cell adherence and internalization. *Cell Reports, 22*(2), 535–545. https://doi.org/10.1016/j.celrep.2017.12.058

Ma, Q., Xing, C., Long, W., Wang, H. Y., Liu, Q., & Wang, R. F. (2019). Impact of microbiota on central nervous system and neurological diseases: The gut-brain axis. *Journal of Neuroinflammation, 16*(1). https://doi.org/10.1186/s12974-019-1434-3

Marogianni, C., Sokratous, M., Dardiotis, E., Hadjigeorgiou, G. M., Bogdanos, D., & Xiromerisiou, G. (2020). Neurodegeneration and inflammation—an interesting interplay in parkinson's disease. *International Journal of Molecular Sciences, 21*(22), 1–15. https://doi.org/10.3390/ijms21228421

Marras, C., Canning, C. G., & Goldman, S. M. (2019). Environment, lifestyle, and Parkinson's disease: Implications for prevention in the next decade. *Movement Disorders, 34*(6), 801–811. https://doi.org/10.1002/mds.27720

Marucci, G., Dal Ben, D., Lambertucci, C., Navia, A. M., Spinaci, A., Volpini, R., & Buccioni, M. (2021). Combined therapy of A1AR agonists and A2AAR antagonists in neuroinflammation. *Molecules, 26*(4). https://doi.org/10.3390/molecules26041188

Metta, V., Dhamija, R. K., Batzu, L., Mrudula, R., Kumar, N. S. S., Arunan, S., Falup-Pecurariu, C., Rodriguez-Blazquez, C., Goyal, V., LK, P., Bhattacharya, K., Kumar, S., Chaudhuri, K. R., & Borgohain, R. (2023). Safety and tolerability of long-term apomorphine infusion in advanced Parkinson's disease: An Indian multicenter (APO-IND) experience. *Scientific Reports, 13*(1). https://doi.org/10.1038/s41598-023-46003-4

S.Mg, S.Ml, L.Vm, T.Jq, Alpha-synuclein in Lewy bodies. (1997).

Michel, A., Downey, P., Nicolas, J.-M., Scheller, D., & Lee, J. (2014). Unprecedented therapeutic potential with a combination of A2A/NR2B receptor antagonists as observed in the 6-OHDA lesioned rat model of Parkinson's Disease. *PLoS One, 9*(12), e114086. https://doi.org/10.1371/journal.pone.0114086

Mishima, T., Fujioka, S., Morishita, T., Inoue, T., & Tsuboi, Y. (2021). Personalized medicine in parkinson's disease: New options for advanced treatments. *Journal of Personalized Medicine, 11*(7), 650. https://doi.org/10.3390/jpm11070650

Montegiove, N., Calzoni, E., Emiliani, C., & Cesaretti, A. (2022). Biopolymer nanoparticles for nose-to-brain drug delivery: A new promising approach for the treatment of neurological diseases. *Journal of Functional Biomaterials, 13*(3), 125. https://doi.org/10.3390/jfb13030125

Monzel, A. S., Hemmer, K., Kaoma, T., Smits, L. M., Bolognin, S., Lucarelli, P., Rosety, I., Zagare, A., Antony, P., Nickels, S. L., Krueger, R., Azuaje, F., & Schwamborn, J. C. (2020). Machine learning-assisted neurotoxicity prediction in human midbrain organoids. *Parkinsonism & Related Disorders, 75*. https://doi.org/10.1016/j.parkreldis.2020.05.011

Morelli, M., Blandini, F., Simola, N., & Hauser, R. A. (2012). A 2A receptor antagonism and dyskinesia in Parkinson'S disease. *Parkinson's Disease*. https://doi.org/10.1155/2012/489853

Morris, H. R., Spillantini, M. G., Sue, C. M., & Williams-Gray, C. H. (2024). The pathogenesis of Parkinson's disease. *The Lancet, 403*(10423), 293–304. https://doi.org/10.1016/S0140-6736(23)01478-2

Neuron-Astrocyte Interactions in Parkinson's Disease. (2020).

Nimmons, D., Bhanu, C., Orlu, M., Schrag, A., & Walters, K. (2022). Orthostatic hypotension and antiparkinsonian drugs: A systematic review and meta-analysis. *Journal of Geriatric Psychiatry and Neurology, 35*(5). https://doi.org/10.1177/08919887211060017

Noack, C., Schroeder, C., Heusser, K., & Lipp, A. (2014). Cardiovascular effects of levodopa in Parkinson's disease. *Parkinsonism & Related Disorders, 20*(8), 815–818. https://doi.org/10.1016/j.parkreldis.2014.04.007

O'Mahony, S. M., Hyland, N. P., Dinan, T. G., & Cryan, J. F. (2011). Maternal separation as a model of brain-gut axis dysfunction. *Psychopharmacology, 214*(1), 71–88. https://doi.org/10.1007/s00213-010-2010-9

Olanow, C. W., Calabresi, P., & Obeso, J. A. (2020). Continuous dopaminergic stimulation as a treatment for parkinson's disease: Current status and future opportunities. *Movement Disorders: Official Journal of the Movement Disorder Society, 35*(10), 1731–1744. https://doi.org/10.1002/mds.28215

Papp, M. I., & Lantos, P. L. (1992). Accumulation of tubular structures in oligodendroglial and neuronal cells as the basic alteration in multiple system atrophy. *Journal of the Neurological Sciences, 107*(2), 172–182. https://doi.org/10.1016/0022-510X(92)90286-T

Pawar, A., & Patil, A. (2024). Nanotechnology-Based approaches for parkinson's disease: Progress in drug delivery and regenerative medicine. *Journal of Drug Delivery and Biotherapeutics, 1*(02). https://doi.org/10.61920/jddb.v1i02.148

Petrov, D., Pedros, I., De Lemos, M. L., Pallàs, M., Canudas, A. M., Lazarowski, A., Beas-Zarate, C., Auladell, C., Folch, J., & Camins, A. (2014). Mavoglurant as a treatment for Parkinson's disease. *Expert Opinion on Investigational Drugs, 23*(8), 1165–1179. https://doi.org/10.1517/13543784.2014.931370

Pfau, S. J., Langen, U. H., Fisher, T. M., Prakash, I., Nagpurwala, F., Lozoya, R. A., Lee, W. C. A., Wu, Z., & Gu, C. (2024). Characteristics of blood–brain barrier heterogeneity between brain regions revealed by profiling vascular and perivascular cells. *Nature Neuroscience, 27*(10), 1892–1903. https://doi.org/10.1038/s41593-024-01743-y

Pingale, T., & Gupta, G. L. (2021). Current and emerging therapeutic targets for Parkinson's disease. *Metabolic Brain Disease, 36*(1), 13–27. https://doi.org/10.1007/s11011-020-00636-w

Poewe, W. (1998). Adjuncts to levodopa therapy: Dopamine agonists. *Neurology, 50*(Issue 6, Suppl. 6), S23. https://doi.org/10.1212/WNL.50.6_Suppl_6.S23

Popoli, P., Minghetti, L., Tebano, M. T., Pintor, A., Domenici, M. R., & Massotti, M. (2004). Adenosine A2A receptor antagonism and neuroprotection: Mechanisms, lights, and shadows. *Critical Reviews in Neurobiology, 16*(1–2), 99–106. https://doi.org/10.1615/CritRevNeurobiol.v16.i12.110

Pouratian, N., Thakkar, S., Kim, W., & Bronstein, J. M. (2012). Deep brain stimulation for the treatment of Parkinson's disease: Efficacy and safety. *Degenerative Neurological and Neuromuscular Disease, 2012*(2), 107–117. https://doi.org/10.2147/DNND.S25750

Pourmirbabaei, S., Dolatshahi, M., & Rahmani, F. (2019). Pathophysiological clues to therapeutic applications of glutamate mGlu5 receptor antagonists in levodopa-induced dyskinesia. *European Journal of Pharmacology, 855*, 149–159. https://doi.org/10.1016/j.ejphar.2019.05.004

Quigley, E. M. M. (2017). Microbiota-Brain-Gut axis and neurodegenerative diseases. *Current Neurology and Neuroscience Reports, 17*(12). https://doi.org/10.1007/s11910-017-0802-6

Rabey, J. M., Nissipeanu, P., & Korczyn, A. D. (1992). Efficacy of memantine, an NMDA receptor antagonist, in the treatment of Parkinson's disease. *Journal of Neural Transmission - Parkinson's Disease and Dementia Section, 4*(4), 277–282. https://doi.org/10.1007/bf02260076

Reddy, M. S. B., Ponnamma, D., Choudhary, R., & Sadasivuni, K. K. (2021). A comparative review of natural and synthetic biopolymer composite scaffolds. *Polymers, 13*(7). https://doi.org/10.3390/polym13071105

Rhee, S. H., Pothoulakis, C., & Mayer, E. A. (2009). Principles and clinical implications of the brain-gut-enteric microbiota axis. *Nature Reviews Gastroenterology & Hepatology, 6*(5), 306–314. https://doi.org/10.1038/nrgastro.2009.35

Richardson, P. J. (2001). The adenosine A2A receptor of the basal ganglia. *Journal of Physiology, 532*(2), 284. https://doi.org/10.1111/j.1469-7793.2001.0284f.x

Ryszkiewicz, P., Malinowska, B., & Schlicker, E. (2023). Polypharmacology: Promises and new drugs in 2022. *Pharmacological Reports, 75*(4), 755–770. https://doi.org/10.1007/s43440-023-00501-4

Salas-Jara, M., Ilabaca, A., Vega, M., & García, A. (2016). Biofilm forming lactobacillus: New challenges for the development of probiotics. *Microorganisms, 4*(3), 35. https://doi.org/10.3390/microorganisms4030035

Sanches, E. S., Simões, D., Baptista, F. I., & Silva, A. P. (2025). Neurovascular dysfunction in psychiatric disorders: Underlying mechanisms and therapeutic approaches. *European Journal of Clinical Investigation, 55*(1). https://doi.org/10.1111/eci.14319

Sanders, M. E., Merenstein, D. J., Reid, G., Gibson, G. R., & Rastall, R. A. (2019). Probiotics and prebiotics in intestinal health and disease: From biology to the clinic. *Nature Reviews Gastroenterology & Hepatology, 16*(10), 605–616. https://doi.org/10.1038/s41575-019-0173-3

Sauter, A., & Rudin, M. (1990). Experimental studies with isradipine in stroke. *Drugs, 40*(Suppl. 2), 44–51. https://doi.org/10.2165/00003495-199000402-00012

Scheperjans, F., Aho, V., Pereira, P. A. B., Koskinen, K., Paulin, L., Pekkonen, E., Haapaniemi, E., Kaakkola, S., Eerola-Rautio, J., Pohja, M., Kinnunen, E., Murros, K., & Auvinen, P. (2015). Gut microbiota are related to Parkinson's disease and clinical phenotype. *Movement Disorders, 30*(3), 350–358. https://doi.org/10.1002/mds.26069

Shao, Y. M., Ma, X., Paira, P., Tan, A., Herr, D. R., Lim, K. L., Ng, C. H., Venkatesan, G., Klotz, K. N., Federico, S., Spalluto, G., Cheong, S. L., Chen, Y. Z., & Pastorin, G. (2018). Discovery of indolylpiperazinylpyrimidines with dual-target profiles at adenosine A2A and dopamine D2 receptors for Parkinson's disease treatment. *PLoS One, 13*(1). https://doi.org/10.1371/journal.pone.0188212

Sharma, S., Rabbani, S. A., Agarwal, T., Baboota, S., Pottoo, F. H., & Ka-Dian, R. (2021). Nanotechnology driven approaches for the management of parkinson's dis-ease: Current status and future perspectives. *Current Drug Metabolism, 22*(4), 287–298. https://doi.org/10.2174/1389200221666201124123405

Siegel, C. A., Rai, V., Outtier, A., Vermeire, S., Law, C. C. W., Sands, B. E., Abdulhamid, A., Gearry, R., McGuire, J., Lindsay, J. O., Panaccione, R., Schweistein, H., Dotan, I., Scarallo, L., Griffiths, A., & Dubinsky, M. C. (2024). Recommendations for broadening eligibility criteria in inflammatory bowel disease clinical trials. *Journal of Crohn's and Colitis, 18*(12), 1967–1975. https://doi.org/10.1093/ecco-jcc/jjae097

Simuni, T. (2020). Isradipine versus placebo in early Parkinson disease a randomized trial. *Annals of Internal Medicine, 172*(9), 591–598. https://doi.org/10.7326/M19-2534

Sisodia, V., Dubbeld, L., De Bie, R. M. A., Duarte, G. S., Costa, J., & Dijk, J. M. (2024). Efficacy and safety of adjunctive oral therapy in Parkinson's disease with motor complications: A systematic review and network meta-analysis. *BMJ Neurology Open, 6*(1). https://doi.org/10.1136/bmjno-2023-000573

Smith, L. J., Lee, C. Y., Menozzi, E., & Schapira, A. H. V. (2022). Genetic variations in GBA1 and LRRK2 genes: Biochemical and clinical consequences in Parkinson disease. *Frontiers in Neurology, 13*. https://doi.org/10.3389/fneur.2022.971252

Song, J., Lu, C., Leszek, J., & Zhang, J. (2021). Design and development of nanomaterial-based drug carriers to overcome the blood–brain barrier by using different transport mechanisms. *International Journal of Molecular Sciences, 22*(18), 10118. https://doi.org/10.3390/ijms221810118

Strandwitz, P. (2018). Neurotransmitter modulation by the gut microbiota. *Brain Research, 1693*(Pt B), 128–133. https://doi.org/10.1016/j.brainres.2018.03.015

Strandwitz, P., Kim, K. H., Terekhova, D., Liu, J. K., Sharma, A., Levering, J., McDonald, D., Dietrich, D., Ramadhar, T. R., Lekbua, A., Mroue, N., Liston, C., Stewart, E. J., Dubin, M. J., Zengler, K., Knight, R., Gilbert, J. A., Clardy, J., & Lewis, K. (2018). GABA-modulating bacteria of the human gut microbiota. *Nature Microbiology, 4*(3), 396–403. https://doi.org/10.1038/s41564-018-0307-3

Suez, J., Zmora, N., Segal, E., & Elinav, E. (2019). The pros, cons, and many unknowns of probiotics. *Nature Medicine, 25*(5), 716–729. https://doi.org/10.1038/s41591-019-0439-x

Sun, Y.-meng, Wang, Z.-yun, Liang, Y.-yuan, Chen-wei, H., & Shi, C.-he (2024). Digital biomarkers for precision diagnosis and monitoring in Parkinson's disease. *Npj Digital Medicine, 7*(1). https://doi.org/10.1038/s41746-024-01217-2

Takahashi, M., Fujita, M., Asai, N., Saki, M., & Mori, A. (2018). Safety and effectiveness of istradefylline in patients with Parkinson's disease: Interim analysis of a post-marketing surveillance study in Japan. *Expert Opinion on Pharmacotherapy, 19*(15), 1635–1642. https://doi.org/10.1080/14656566.2018.1518433

Tashima, T. (2020). Shortcut approaches to substance delivery into the brain based on intranasal administration using nanodelivery strategies for insulin. *Molecules, 25*(21), 5188. https://doi.org/10.3390/molecules25215188

Thakkar, S., Fung, V. S. C., Merola, A., Rollins, M., Soileau, M. J., & Kovács, N. (2021). 24-Hour levodopa-carbidopa intestinal gel: Clinical experience and practical recommendations. *CNS Drugs, 35*(2), 137–149. https://doi.org/10.1007/s40263-020-00782-w

Timpka, J., Mundt-Petersen, U., & Odin, P. (2016). Continuous dopaminergic stimulation therapy for Parkinson's disease – Recent advances. *Current Opinion in Neurology, 29*(4), 474–479. https://doi.org/10.1097/wco.0000000000000354

Tolosa, E., Garrido, A., Scholz, S. W., & Poewe, W. (2021). Challenges in the diagnosis of Parkinson's disease. *The Lancet Neurology, 20*(5), 385–397. https://doi.org/10.1016/S1474-4422(21)00030-2

Tyson, T., Steiner, J. A., & Brundin, P. (2016). Sorting out release, uptake and processing of alpha-synuclein during prion-like spread of pathology. *Journal of Neurochemistry, 139*(S1), 275–289. https://doi.org/10.1111/jnc.13449

Ullah, H., Arbab, S., Tian, Y., Liu, C. Q., Chen, Y., Qijie, L., Khan, M. I. U., Hassan, I. U., & Li, K. (2023). The gut microbiota–brain axis in neurological disorder. *Frontiers in Neuroscience, 17.* https://doi.org/10.3389/fnins.2023.1225875

Van Damme, P., Van den Bosch, L., Van Houtte, E., Callewaert, G., & Robberecht, W. (2002). GluR2-Dependent properties of AMPA receptors determine the selective vulnerability of motor neurons to excitotoxicity. *Journal of Neurophysiology, 88*(3), 1279–1287. https://doi.org/10.1152/jn.2002.88.3.1279

Van Wamelen, D. J., Grigoriou, S., Chaudhuri, K. R., & Odin, P. (2018). Continuous drug delivery aiming continuous dopaminergic stimulation in Parkinson's disease. *Journal of Parkinson's Disease, 8*(1), S65. https://doi.org/10.3233/JPD-181476

van Wamelen, D. J., Sringean, J., Trivedi, D., Carroll, C. B., Schrag, A. E., Odin, P., Antonini, A., Bloem, B. R., Bhidayasiri, R., & Chaudhuri, K. R. (2021). Digital health technology for non-motor symptoms in people with Parkinson's disease: Futile or future? *Parkinsonism & Related Disorders, 89,* 186–194. https://doi.org/10.1016/j.parkreldis.2021.07.032

Vargas, J. Y., Grudina, C., & Zurzolo, C. (2019). The prion-like spreading of α-synuclein: From in vitro to in vivo models of Parkinson's disease. *PubMed.* https://doi.org/10.1016/j.arr.2019.01.012. Epub 2019 Jan 25.

Vatansever, S., Schlessinger, A., Wacker, D., Kaniskan, H.Ü., Jin, J., Zhou, M. M., & Zhang, B. (2021). Artificial intelligence and machine learning-aided drug discovery in central nervous system diseases: State-of-the-arts and future directions. *Medicinal Research Reviews, 41*(3), 1427–1473. https://doi.org/10.1002/med.21764

Wang, X. L., Feng, S. T., Chen, B., Hu, D., Wang, Z. Z., & Zhang, Y. (2022). Efficacy and safety of istradefylline for Parkinson's disease: A systematic review and meta-analysis. *Neuroscience Letters*, 774. https://doi.org/10.1016/j.neulet.2022.136515

Wang, Y., Tong, Q., Ma, S. R., Zhao, Z. X., Pan, L. B., Cong, L., Han, P., Peng, R., Yu, H., Lin, Y., Gao, T. L., Shou, J. W., Li, X. Y., Zhang, X. F., Zhang, Z. W., Fu, J., Wen, B. Y., Yu, J. B., Cao, X., & Jiang, J. D. (2021). Oral berberine improves brain dopa/dopamine levels to ameliorate Parkinson's disease by regulating gut microbiota. *Signal Transduction and Targeted Therapy, 6*(1). https://doi.org/10.1038/s41392-020-00456-5

Wang, J., Wang, F., Mai, D., & Qu, S. (2020). Molecular mechanisms of glutamate toxicity in parkinson's disease. *Frontiers in Neuroscience, 14*, 585584. https://doi.org/10.3389/fnins.2020.585584

Wang, K., Zhang, C., Zhang, B., Li, G., Shi, G., Cai, Q., & Huang, M. (2022). Gut dysfunction may be the source of pathological aggregation of alpha-synuclein in the central nervous system through Paraquat exposure in mice. *Ecotoxicology and Environmental Safety, 246*, 114152. https://doi.org/10.1016/j.ecoenv.2022.114152

Wang, W. W., Zhang, X. R., Zhang, Z. R., Wang, X. S., Chen, J., Chen, S. Y., & Xie, C. L. (2018). Effects of mGluR5 antagonists on Parkinson's patients with L-Dopa-Induced dyskinesia: A systematic review and meta-analysis of randomized controlled trials. *Frontiers in Aging Neuroscience, 10.* https://doi.org/10.3389/fnagi.2018.00262

Wang, Q., Liu, Y., & Zhou, J. (2015). Neuroinflammation in Parkinson's disease and its potential as therapeutic target. *PubMed.* https://pubmed.ncbi.nlm.nih.gov/26464797/.

Witt, J. A., & Helmstaedter, C. (2022). The impact of perampanel on cognition: A systematic review of studies employing standardized tests in patients with epilepsy. *Seizure, 94,* 107–111. https://doi.org/10.1016/j.seizure.2021.12.001

Wright, B. A., & Waters, C. H. (2013). Continuous dopaminergic delivery to minimize motor complications in Parkinson's disease. *Expert Review of Neurotherapeutics, 13*(6), 719–729. https://doi.org/10.1586/ern.13.47

Xiao, B., & Tan, E. K. (2025). Prasinezumab slows motor progression in Parkinsons disease: Beyond the clinical data. *Npj Parkinson's Disease, 11*(1). https://doi.org/10.1038/s41531-025-00886-4

Xu, H., Li, Z., & Si, J. (2014). Nanocarriers in gene therapy: A review. *Journal of Biomedical Nanotechnology, 10* (12), 3483–3507. https://doi.org/10.1166/jbn.2014.2044

Yadav, V. K., Dhanasekaran, S., Choudhary, N., Nathiya, D., Thakur, V., Gupta, R., Pramanik, S., Kumar, P., Gupta, N., & Patel, A. (2025). Recent advances in nanotechnology for Parkinson's disease: Diagnosis, treatment, and future perspectives. *Frontiers of Medicine, 12*, 1535682. https://doi.org/10.3389/fmed.2025.1535682

Yang, Z.-xian, Zhang, Y., Wang, Q., Zhang, L., Liu, Y.-fei, Zhang, Y., Ren, Y., Zhou, C., Gao, H.-wen, Zhang, N.-xia, & Feng, L.-yin (2024). Addition of α-synuclein aggregates to the intestinal environment recapitulates Parkinsonian symptoms in model systems. *Acta Pharmacologica Sinica, 45*(1), 36–51. https://doi.org/10.1038/s41401-023-01150-2

Yoon, H. H., Ye, S., Lim, S., Jo, A., Lee, H., Hong, F., Lee, S. E., Oh, S. J., Kim, N. R., Kim, K., Kim, B. J., Kim, H., Lee, C. J., Nam, M. H., Hur, J. W., & Jeon, S. R. (2022). CRISPR-Cas9 gene editing protects from the A53T-SNCA overexpression-induced pathology of Parkinson's Disease in vivo. *CRISPR Journal, 5*(1), 95–108. https://doi.org/10.1089/crispr.2021.0025

Young, K. C., McGehee, D. S., & Brorson, J. R. (2007). Glutamate receptor expression and chronic glutamate toxicity in rat motor cortex. *Neurobiology of Disease, 26*(1), 78–85. https://doi.org/10.1016/j.nbd.2006.12.002

Zha, S., Liu, H., Li, H., Li, H., Wong, K. L., & All, A. H. (2024). Functionalized nanomaterials capable of crossing the blood-brain barrier. *ACS Nano, 18*(3), 1820–1845. https://doi.org/10.1021/acsnano.3c10674

Zheng, J., Zhang, X., & Zhen, X. (2019). Development of adenosine A 2A receptor antagonists for the treatment of parkinson's disease: A recent update and challenge. *ACS Chemical Neuroscience, 10*(2), 783–791. https://doi.org/10.1021/acschemneuro.8b00313

Zhu, M., Liu, X., Ye, Y., Yan, X., Cheng, Y., Zhao, L., Chen, F., Zongxin, L., & Microbiota, G. (2022). A novel therapeutic target for parkinson's disease. *Frontiers in Immunology, 13*. https://doi.org/10.3389/fimmu.2022.937555

CHAPTER

Future directions in Parkinson's disease pharmacotherapy 15

Dina Essam Abo-elnour[1], Mohamed Mohsen Helal[1], Basant Atef Ahmed[2], Moaz Elsayed Abouelmagd[3], Mahmoud Tarek Hefnawy[1], Hamza K. Alsalhi[4], Ahmed Abdelkader[5], Nada Mostafa Al-dardery[6] and Sakhr Alshwayyat[7, 8, 9]

[1]*Faculty of Medicine, Zagazig University, Zagazig, Egypt;* [2]*Faculty of Medicine, Tanta University, Tanta, Egypt;* [3]*Kasr-Alainy Faculty of Medicine, Cairo University, Cairo, Egypt;* [4]*The Hashemite University, Zarqa, Jordan;* [5]*Faculty of Medicine, New Vision University, Tbilisi, Georgia;* [6]*Faculty of Medicine, Fayoum University, Fayoum, Egypt;* [7]*Kern Medical (UCLA David Geffen School of Medicine Affiliate), Bakersfield, CA, United States;* [8]*Applied Science Research Center, Applied Science Private University, Amman, Jordan;* [9]*King Hussein Cancer Center, Amman, Jordan*

15.1 Introduction

15.1.1 Overview of Parkinson's disease

Parkinson's disease (PD) is a progressive neurological disorder that causes significant motor symptoms, including bradykinesia, postural instability, resting tremors, and muscle rigidity (Balestrino & Schapira, 2020). Along with motor symptoms, PD is associated with several non-motor symptoms (NMSs) such as anxiety, constipation, and dementia (Hayes, 2019), which often occur during a prodromal phase that can manifest years before motor dysfunction (Cabreira & Massano, 2019). Lewy bodies—abnormal aggregates of misfolded alpha-synuclein (α-syn) protein encoded by the SNCA gene—are a hallmark pathological feature of PD (Cerri et al., 2019). Their accumulation leads to the demise of dopaminergic neurons in the midbrain, particularly the substantia nigra (SN).

In spite of these pathological insights, diagnostic criteria for PD are established solely based on clinical aspects (Cabreira & Massano, 2019; Cerri et al., 2019). Genetic and environmental factors are believed to potentially contribute to the etiology of PD; however, the precise pathogenic mechanisms remain unclear (Homayoun, 2018). The loss of dopaminergic neurons in the SN is a defining characteristic of PD; however, the onset of the disease varies widely among individuals due to a combination of idiopathic, environmental, and genetic factors. Some individuals may develop the condition due to unidentified factors or environmental influences, while others may possess a strong genetic predisposition (Shah et al., 2024).

PD is believed to begin with a preclinical phase, during which anxiety, sleep disturbances, and autonomic dysfunctions may arise. These include impairments in digestion, respiration, salivation, thermoregulation (e.g., excessive sweating), bladder control, and sexual function. The clinical phase of PD begins with classical motor symptoms, such as resting tremors, bradykinesia, stiffness, and balance problems, which usually start on one side and progress slowly. Early manifestations may include a

Pharmacological Foundations of Parkinson's Disease. https://doi.org/10.1016/B978-0-443-27702-3.00025-X

softer voice, reduced arm swing while walking, and sporadic tremors. While current PD treatments provide symptomatic relief, their efficacy diminishes as the disease advances, and they often cause serious adverse effects.

15.1.2 The need for innovation in PD pharmacotherapy

The discovery of levodopa (L-DOPA), the metabolic precursor of dopamine, revolutionized the treatment of Parkinson's disease (PD). Despite decades of research into alternative therapies, levodopa remains the most effective and widely used treatment for motor symptoms. However, long-term use is associated with motor complications, including dyskinesia, dystonia, and motor fluctuations, particularly in patients with advanced disease (Pfeiffer, 2016; Salat & Tolosa, 2013). Furthermore, many axial symptoms, such as postural instability, freezing of gait, balance impairment, and falls, often become less responsive to dopaminergic therapy as the disease progresses. Adverse effects of levodopa may include nausea, dizziness, somnolence, and, particularly in older adults, neuropsychiatric manifestations such as hallucinations, delusions, agitation, and psychosis (Gandhi & Saadabadi, 2023).

Current pharmacological management primarily focuses on symptomatic relief. In addition to levodopa, therapies such as catechol-O-methyltransferase inhibitors, decarboxylase enzyme inhibitors, monoamine oxidase-B inhibitors, and dopamine agonists are used to enhance dopaminergic neurotransmission and improve motor symptoms (Tong et al., 2017; Maiti et al., 2017). A range of pharmacological agents, such as cholinesterase inhibitors, antidepressants, and sedatives, are employed in the management of non-motor symptoms. At present, no medication exists that can reverse disease progression. Early diagnosis remains a major challenge, as substantial dopaminergic neuronal loss and autonomic dysfunction often occur before the onset of characteristic motor symptoms. This highlights the need for reliable biomarkers and disease-modifying therapies capable of intervening during the prodromal stages of PD. Moreover, existing symptomatic treatments for are limited by poor drug reactions, short drug half-lives, and restricted passage across the blood-brain barrier (BBB) (Stoker et al., 2018; Pingale & Gupta, 2021).

In this context, the development of innovative therapeutic strategies has become a major research priority. This chapter explores emerging pharmacological targets, disease-modifying treatments, personalized medicine approaches, advanced drug delivery technologies, and ethical and legal issues surrounding novel interventions for PD. Collectively, these advances have the potential to improve disease management and patient outcomes.

15.2 Emerging therapeutic targets

15.2.1 Targeting α-synuclein

The loss of the SN pars compacta leads to dopamine depletion, the hallmark of PD. The defining pathological feature is the aggregation of Lewy bodies, primarily composed of aggregated α-syn, within affected neurons (Gautam et al., 2010). α-syn accumulation contributes to oxidative stress and mitochondrial dysfunction in dopaminergic neurons, leading to progressive neurodegeneration and worsening parkinsonian symptoms (Guo et al., 2018). Familial forms of PD have been linked to mutations and multiplications in SNCA gene, underscoring its critical role in disease pathology (Zhang et al., 2020; Ng et al., 2015).

Numerous emerging therapies are targeting α-syn to alleviate PD symptoms, with some existing drugs exhibiting anti-α-syn effects beyond their primary mechanisms. Most PD medications, except anticholinergics, have demonstrated disease-modifying properties by reducing α-syn aggregation or attenuating metabolic deficits and oxidative stress (Natalello et al., 2023; Nakamura et al., 2021; Braga et al., 2011; Müller, 2020; Di Giovanni et al., 2010; Ferreira et al., 2017; He et al., 2022; Pirchio et al., 2022; Li, Liu, et al., 2025). Given the systemic impact of PD, multi-mechanistic pharmacological approaches seem well-suited to addressing its neurodegenerative nature.

Recent therapeutic strategies have focused on α-syn immunotherapy, as well as interventions designed to inhibit its aggregation or promote its clearance.

15.2.1.1 Anti-α-syn immunotherapy

Immunotherapy against α-syn has emerged as a promising avenue for disease modification (Lee & Lee, 2016). Initially, the feasibility of immunization was uncertain due to the intracellular nature of α-syn. However, research suggests that α-syn is secreted through unconventional exocytosis, making it accessible to antibody-mediated clearance. Preclinical studies have demonstrated that immunization with *recombinant α-syn antigens* elicits an antibody response, reducing α-syn aggregation and behavioral deficits in PD models (Masliah et al., 2005). Similarly, passive immunization with monoclonal antibodies targeting the C-terminal region of α-syn has been shown to reduce α-syn accumulation and improve motor symptoms in transgenic mouse models (Masliah et al., 2011).

The underlying α-syn immunotherapy are not yet fully understood, but current research suggests their mechanisms may include.

1. Clearance of extracellular α-syn: antibodies facilitate microglia-mediated phagocytosis, enhancing α-syn clearance. (Bae et al., 2012)
2. Physical blockade of α-syn transmission: antibodies bind to extracellular α-syn, preventing its intercellular propagation and reducing its pathogenic effects. (Tran et al., 2014)

A meta-analysis of randomized controlled trials (RCTs) in 2022 evaluated the effects of anti-α-syn immunization in PD patients (Hu et al., 2022). While there was a trend toward improvement in motor symptoms (Unified Parkinson's Disease Rating Scale (UPDRS) III, MD: -0.72, $P = 0.099$), statistical significance was not achieved. The authors noted that the limited number and variable quality of included trials constrained interpretation. Since then, several new placebo-controlled RCTs have been conducted, further assessing α-syn immunotherapy (Nikolcheva et al., 2025; Pagano et al., 2024; Eijsvogel et al., 2024; Buur et al., 2024). Most of these trials support continued clinical development of anti-α-syn antibodies for PD.

15.2.1.2 Inhibition of α-syn aggregation

Among the promising candidates is UCB0599 (Minzasolmin), which has shown efficacy in preclinical models by reducing α-syn misfolding and preventing the formation of aggregates on lipid membranes, ultimately improving PD symptoms (Price et al., 2022, 2023). Phase 1 trials confirmed its safety, tolerability, and predictable pharmacokinetics, prompting further investigation in the Phase 2 ORCHESTRA study (NCT04658186) (Smit et al., 2022). This large, randomized, placebo-controlled trial enrolled 496 early-stage PD patients and was concluded on September 2024. However, the pharmaceutical company responsible for the trial announced that Minzasolmin failed to demonstrate superiority over placebo in primary and secondary clinical endpoints, and no published articles on the study data are currently available. Another trial (NCT05543252), sponsored by the same company, is currently active. This extension trial aims to assess the long-term effects of Minzasolmin and is anticipated to conclude in April 2025.

Another strategy involves targeting α-syn cell-to-cell transmission. Memantine, an NMDA (N-methyl-D-aspartate) receptor antagonist widely used in Alzheimer's disease, has gained interest in PD research due to its role in modulating α-syn propagation. Studies suggest that Memantine alters α-syn structure, reducing its internalization and attenuating α-syn-induced neurotoxicity (Lee et al., 2021; Jeong & Lee, 2025). Clinical trials have explored its potential in PD, with encouraging preliminary results, and a phase 3 trial is underway to assess its ability to slow disease progression (NCT03858270) (Emre et al., 2010; Wictorin & Widner, 2016; Stubendorff et al., 2014; Wesnes et al., 2015; Moreau et al., 2013; Kawashima et al., 2022).

Lithium has also been explored for its potential to enhance α-syn clearance (Sarkar et al., 2005). A Phase 1 trial reported modest effects on α-syn serum levels (Guttuso et al., 2023), and ongoing studies are investigating its repurposing for PD. These include trials NCT06339034, NCT06099886, and NCT06592014, all of which are expected to be completed by 2026.

Probiotics, live microorganisms with beneficial effects on health, have been proposed as a novel approach to reducing α-syn aggregates in PD. Preclinical studies indicate that probiotics lower α-syn accumulation in the SN, reduce neuroinflammation, and mitigate oxidative stress (Wang et al., 2022). Furthermore, they appear to modulate gut microbiota composition, potentially influencing α-syn pathology through the gut-brain axis. While several clinical trials have explored the use of probiotics in PD, ongoing research is now focusing on various probiotic formulations and synbiotics to assess their therapeutic potential in managing both motor and non-motor symptoms of PD (NCT05568498).

15.2.2 Mitochondrial dysfunction and oxidative stress

Oxidative stress is a well-established factor in the development and progression of neurodegenerative diseases, including PD. PD patients exhibit elevated levels of oxidized DNA, proteins, and lipids, alongside decreased levels of glutathione, a key endogenous antioxidant (Li, Liu, et al., 2025). Notably, oxidative stress has also been linked to the increased deposition of α-syn, which further exacerbates disease pathology (Huang et al., 2021). A hallmark of oxidative stress is the excessive release of reactive oxygen species (ROS) from mitochondria, underscoring the critical role of mitochondrial dysfunction in PD pathogenesis (Apostolova et al., 2020). Given the strong association between mitochondrial disruption and PD progression, various therapeutic agents are being developed to target these pathways.

One promising therapeutic approach is nicotinamide adenine dinucleotide (NAD) replenishment therapy using nicotinamide riboside (NR) (Gaare et al., 2023; Yulug et al., 2024; Brakedal et al., 2022; Berven et al., 2023). NAD is essential for cellular energy metabolism, functioning as a reversible electron donor (NADH) and acceptor (NAD+), thereby maintaining cellular homeostasis and counteracting oxidative stress-induced mitochondrial dysfunction and neuroinflammation (Brakedal et al., 2022). NR, a vitamin B3 derivative and a biosynthetic precursor of NAD, has gained attention as a potential therapeutic agent. The NADPARK study, a Phase 1 clinical trial published in 2022, demonstrated that NR administration increased cerebral NAD levels, improved motor function, and reduced inflammatory cytokines in both serum and cerebrospinal fluid (CSF) of PD patients (Brakedal et al., 2022). These findings were further supported by the NR-SAFE study in 2023 (Berven et al.,

2023). However, there is currently no consensus on the optimal dosing regimen. To address this, the N-DOSE trial, a Phase 2 dose-optimization study, is ongoing (NCT05589766). Additionally, a Phase 3 trial (NOPARK) has recently been launched to further investigate the long-term efficacy of NR in PD (NCT05546567) (NCT03568968).

Another potential therapeutic target is ursodeoxycholic acid (UDCA), a bile acid that has shown neuroprotective effects in PD models by enhancing brain adenosine triphosphate (ATP) levels (Abdelkader et al., 2016; Qi et al., 2021). Two clinical trials have evaluated UDCA in PD. The first, conducted in 2020, demonstrated its tolerability in a small cohort ($n = 5$) (Sathe et al., 2020). A subsequent double-blind, placebo-controlled Phase 2 trial assessed the safety and efficacy of long-term (48-week) UDCA administration. Motor improvements were observed in gait parameters, including cadence (steps per minute), in the UDCA group compared to placebo. However, no significant differences were noted in UPDRS-III scores between the groups (Payne et al., 2023). Another similar trial (NCT03840005) has been completed, but its results have not yet been published.

Given the oxidative nature of mitochondrial damage in PD, a wide range of antioxidant compounds and dietary interventions are being explored as potential therapeutic strategies. Antioxidants such as melatonin, vitamin E, and omega-3 fatty acids are currently under investigation for their role in mitigating oxidative stress in PD (NCT04491383) (Jiménez-Delgado et al., 2021; Hadi et al., 2022; Sugumaran et al., 2024; Tamtaji et al., 2019; Pantzaris et al., 2021). Additionally, exercise regimens and dietary interventions such as the ketogenic diet are being studied for their potential neuroprotective effects (NCT05854524) (NCT05469997).

Crocin, a bioactive compound derived from Crocus sativus (saffron), has also been evaluated in PD. An RCT investigating its effects on motor function and oxidative DNA damage found no significant impact on oxidative stress markers (Mohammad Soleymani et al., 2024). However, improvements were noted in UPDRS-II and III scores, suggesting potential benefits in daily functioning and motor symptom management as an adjunct to conventional PD therapies. Another ongoing clinical trial (NCT05696665) is investigating the combined effects of saffron and chamomile in PD, though its current status remains "unknown" on ClinicalTrials.gov. Given that crocin is one of the main active components of saffron, the outcomes of this study may provide further insights into its therapeutic potential.

Targeting mitochondrial dysfunction in PD, Yulug et al. conducted an RCT (NCT04044131) investigating a combination therapy comprising mitochondrial activators and protectors, including NR (1 g), N-acetyl-L-cysteine (2.55 g), L-serine (12.35 g), and L-carnitine tartrate (Yulug et al., 2024). While no significant differences were observed in motor function, cognitive performance improved markedly in the treatment group compared to placebo. Notably, patients in the placebo group did not show cognitive improvements over time. A comprehensive multi-omics analysis provided mechanistic insights into these cognitive benefits, leading the authors to conclude that this combination therapy acts as a metabolic enhancer with potential cognitive benefits in PD. Further investigations are warranted to explore therapeutic applications of such combinations.

15.2.3 Neuroinflammation as a therapeutic target

Neuroinflammation is the immune response within the central nervous system (CNS) aimed at protecting brain tissues. In its acute form, it is considered neuroprotective (Jankovic & Tan, 2020; Surmeier et al., 2017). However, in chronic states, such as PD, persistent inflammation contributes to dopaminergic neuronal death by disrupting neurochemical processes. Neuroinflammation in PD is closely linked to other pathological mechanisms, including α-syn accumulation and oxidative stress (Araújo et al., 2022). Moreover, neuroinflammatory processes extend beyond the well-known roles of glial cells (microglia and astrocytes) to include components like the inflammasome, particularly NLRP3 (Schroder & Tschopp, 2010). Inflammasome, a cytoplasmic multiprotein complex present in glial cells and other immune cells such as neutrophils and macrophages, triggers cytokine release upon activation, contributing to neuroinflammation and neurodegeneration (Araújo et al., 2022).

Several emerging therapies aim to mitigate neuroinflammation in PD, including those discussed in Sections 2.1 and 2.2, which target α-syn accumulation and mitochondrial dysfunction, respectively. Notably, these therapies have also demonstrated the ability to reduce neuroinflammation, highlighting the bidirectional relationship between inflammation, α-syn pathology, and mitochondrial dysfunction. Among the most promising approaches is targeting NLRP3 inhibition. Two NLRP3 inhibitors, VENT-02 and VTX3232, are currently being tested in phase 1 and phase 2 clinical trials, with expected completion dates in January 2026 and March 2025, respectively (NCT06822517) (NCT06556173). Another potential target is the P2X7 receptor, implicated in PD pathophysiology and progression. Preclinical studies have shown that P2X7 blockade provides neuroprotective effects; however, only one clinical trial (NCT03918616) has been completed in PD patients, with no reported results.

Targeting the β-glucocerebrosidase (GCase) pathway also holds promise. The most common genetic risk factor for PD is a mutation in the glucocerebrosidase 1 (GBA1) gene, which encodes GCase, a lysosomal enzyme that reduces α-syn accumulation and, consequently, neuroinflammation (Zhang, Wu, et al., 2024; Lin et al., 2024). Preliminary clinical trials of ambroxol, a GCase upregulator, demonstrated good safety and pharmacokinetic profiles (Mullin et al., 2020). Currently, six well-designed clinical trials of ambroxol in PD are registered or published as protocols, and many are still recruiting (NCT05778617) (NCT05830396) (NCT05287503) (NCT06193421) (NCT02914366) (NCT04388969).

Two therapeutic approaches targeting neuroinflammation in PD have gained attention in the past five years but currently lack active clinical trials. The first involves tyrosine kinase inhibitors, particularly Abl kinase inhibitors, which have been linked to both neurodegeneration and neuroinflammation in PD. Nilotinib, an Abl inhibitor, has undergone multiple small-scale trials with poor study designs, ultimately failing to provide sufficient evidence for further large-scale testing. The most recent trial on nilotinib was published in 2021. Another tyrosine kinase inhibitor, K0706, was evaluated in a phase 2 PD trial but was terminated in June 2024 due to unsatisfactory treatment outcomes (NCT03655236). The second approach involves sargramostim (Leukine), a granulocyte-macrophage colony-stimulating factor and immune modulator. Sargramostim was investigated in three clinical trials to assess its potential in inducing regulatory T-cell (Treg) immune responses, which has been shown to protect against nigrostriatal neurodegeneration in rodent PD models (NCT05677633). While these studies reported modest improvements in motor function in PD patients, all trials have now been completed, with no further ongoing investigations.

15.2.4 Glucagon-like peptide-1 receptor agonists

It has long been documented that glucose intolerance is prevalent in PD and that diabetes is a risk factor for its development (Bassil et al., 2022; Cullinane et al., 2023; Athauda et al., 2022). Previous cohort studies have shown that diabetics receiving glucagon-like peptide-1 receptor agonists (GLP-

1RAs) have a lower risk of PD compared to those using other antidiabetic medications, suggesting a potential neuroprotective effect (Svenningsson et al., 2016). Since then, GLP-1RAs have been extensively studied in PD models and well-designed clinical trials as potential disease-modifying agents.

To date, six published RCTs have evaluated GLP-1RAs in PD (Vijiaratnam et al., 2025; Meissner et al., 2024; McGarry et al., 2024; Athauda et al., 2017; Aviles-Olmos et al., 2013; Malatt et al., 2022). Findings related to improvements in the UPDRS-III scores are promising, particularly when assessed in the ON-medication state (Meissner et al., 2024; Aviles-Olmos et al., 2013; Malatt et al., 2022). However, these effects do not consistently translate to the OFF-medication state. Given that GLP-1RAs exhibit neuroprotective properties (Harkavyi et al., 2008; Zhang et al., 2015)—such as reducing neuroinflammation and oxidative stress, and promoting neurotrophic support in PD animal models—along with their promising results in other neurodegenerative diseases, further rigorous investigation is warranted to explore their disease-modifying potential.

What makes GLP-1RAs particularly appealing as candidates for PD therapy is their broad systemic effects (Goudra et al., 2024; Elahi et al., 2014). Since PD involves widespread systemic dysfunction, these agents hold considerable promise (Ezquerra et al., 2019). Additionally, unlike many other antidiabetic medications, GLP-1RAs are euglycemic rather than hypoglycemic, making them safer for long-term use (Keerie et al., 2021). Their favorable tolerability in non-diabetic patients further supports their potential role in PD treatment, regardless of diabetic status (Keerie et al., 2021; Hölscher, 2018).

Several clinical trials evaluating GLP-1RAs in PD, including (NCT03456687), (NCT04269642), (NCT03659682), and (NCT04305002), have either been completed or are still ongoing, but their results have not yet been published. Notably, one of these trials (NCT03659682) aims to follow PD patients for 4 years, which aims to provide valuable insights into the long-term therapeutic potential of GLP-1RAs in clinical practice.

15.2.5 Lysosomal and autophagy pathways

15.2.5.1 Lysosomal dysfunction in PD

Lysosomal dysfunction is a feature of PD that impairs cellular clearance and causes neurodegeneration. Genetic variants associated with PD are often exacerbated by pathogenic mutations affecting lysosomal pathways. For instance, Leucine-rich repeat kinase 2 (LRRK2) mutations lead to RAB8A phosphorylation, triggering lysosomal stress and a 35% increase in membrane permeabilization, ultimately causing neuronal death (Tengberg et al., 2024). Similarly, the PD-associated protein DJ-1 (PARK7) is secreted in response to autophagic activation following lysosomal damage and oxidative stress, which is accompanied by a 40% reduction in lysosomal proteolytic activity (Dash et al., 2024). Beyond lysosomal impairment, this dysfunction also disrupts mitochondrial homeostasis, with 70%–80% of damaged cells showing cristae loss, a 50% loss of the mitochondrial contact site and cristae organizing system (MICOS) integrity, and defective ATP production (Kraus et al., 2025).

15.2.5.2 Autophagy-targeted therapies for α-syn clearance

Autophagy plays a critical role in the clearance of misfolded proteins in PD. Through selective aggrephagy, toxic α-syn aggregates are targeted for degradation by autophagosomes and lysosomes. Autophagy receptors such as p62, NBR1, and TAX1BP1 receptors can promote the removal of these aggregates by up to 50% in PD models (Zhuang & Ma, 2025). Chaperone-mediated autophagy, a key pathway for the degradation of misfolded α-syn, is impaired in PD, resulting in reduced α-syn clearance and its subsequent accumulation (Koszła & Sołek, 2024). Pharmacological agents such as rapamycin, an mTOR inhibitor, and trehalose, a transcription factor EB (TFEB) activator, have been shown to enhance α-syn clearance by 45%–55%. In addition, activation of nuclear respiratory factor 1 (NRF1) increases proteasomal clearance by 60% and can replace disrupted autophagy (Hickey et al., 2024).

15.2.5.3 GBA gene mutations and GCase-targeted therapies

Mutations in the GBA1 gene are found in 5%–10% of PD patients worldwide and in 15% of Western populations, leading to impaired lysosomal function by reducing GCase activity (Koros et al., 2024). Efforts to target this pathway have yielded encouraging results. Pharmacological chaperones such as ambroxol can enhance GCase activity by 50% and decrease α-syn build-up (Montpeyo et al., 2024).

15.2.6 LRRK2-targeting therapies

LRRK2 is a key therapeutic target in PD and is associated with both familial and sporadic cases. Although LRRK2 mutations are responsible for 1%–2% of all PD cases, they account for up to 40% of certain familial forms. The G2019S mutation results in a 2- to 3-fold increase in kinase activity, which contributes to neuronal dysfunction. Increased LRRK2 activity is noted in both familial and idiopathic PD, with kinase levels increasing by 30%–60% (Tan et al., 2024). Current inhibitors can achieve 80%–90% inhibition of LRRK2 in preclinical models and selectively reduce Rab protein phosphorylation by up to 75% (Xiong & Yu, 2024; Bai et al., 2025). Moreover, DARPin E11, a non-kinase modulator that attaches to the WD40 domain, decreased Rab8A phosphorylation by 50%, presenting a novel approach beyond kinase inhibition (Dederer et al., 2024).

15.2.7 Adenosine A2A receptor antagonists

Adenosine A2A receptors (A2ARs) are predominantly found in the striatopallidal neurons of the indirect basal ganglia pathway, where they influence dopaminergic signaling and play a role in the motor impairments observed in PD. Excessive activation of these receptors suppresses dopamine D2 receptor function, exacerbating symptoms, such as bradykinesia and rigidity. A2AR antagonists help restore motor abilities by reestablishing the balance in dopaminergic transmission (Waggan et al., 2023; Nunes et al., 2024; Rivas-Santisteban et al., 2023). In rodent models of PD, the antagonist Scheme 5826 was shown to decrease early synaptic loss in the striatum by more than 50% and protect neurons in the SN by nearly 60%, although its effectiveness decreased with delayed treatment, indicating a time-dependent neuroprotective effect (Nunes et al., 2024).

Clinically, tradefylline, a selective A2AR antagonist, has been found to reduce daily "off" periods by 1–1.8 h when used alongside levodopa, with 45% of patients experiencing improved motor symptoms without an increase in dyskinesia (Offit et al., 2023). Recent advancements in drug development have produced potent quinazoline derivatives, such as compound 5m ($Ki = 5$ nM, $IC50 = 6$ μM), which offer enhanced solubility and pharmacokinetics (Laversin et al., 2024).

Additionally, dual A2A/A1 antagonists like compound 11o demonstrate strong affinities ($Ki = 13.3$ nM for A2A; 55 nM for A1) and have been shown to reverse catalepsy by 90% in animal models without causing cardiac or mutagenic side effects (Jung et al., 2022).

15.2.8 Calcium and iron targeting therapies

15.2.8.1 Dysregulation of calcium and iron in PD pathology

An imbalance between calcium (Ca^{2+}) and iron is a critical factor in PD, contributing to dopaminergic neurons death, oxidative stress, and mitochondrial dysfunction. Disruption of Ca^{2+} influx through voltage-gated calcium channels (VGCCs) and sodium-calcium exchangers (NCX) results in excitotoxicity and abnormal synaptic transmission. In PD, malfunctioning NCX leads to a 30%–50% increase in intracellular Ca^{2+} levels, causing mitochondrial overload and neuroinflammation (Maniscalchi et al., 2024). Iron accumulation in the SN initiates ferroptosis, with studies indicating a 40% increase in iron levels, 60% increase in lipid peroxidation, and heightened α-syn aggregation (Zhao et al., 2024).

15.2.8.2 Ca^{2+} channel blockers in PD

Ca^{2+} channel blockers have shown neuroprotective properties by lowering intracellular Ca^{2+} levels, alleviating mitochondrial stress, and enhancing neuronal survival. Isradipine reduces Ca^{2+} influx by 30%–50% and mitigates oxidative damage (Egunlusi et al., 2024). Modulators of small-conductance calcium-activated potassium channels decrease mitochondrial Ca^{2+} uptake, thereby reducing neurotoxicity marker levels by 40%–60% (Zhang, Shaabani, et al., 2024). Despite promising preclinical outcomes, isradipine did not show symptomatic benefits in large-scale clinical trials, indicating the need for optimized or combined therapeutic strategies.

15.2.8.3 Iron chelation therapies in PD

Iron build-up, especially in the SN, intensifies oxidative stress and ferroptosis in PD. Elevated iron levels are associated with a 50% increase in lipid peroxidation and the loss of dopaminergic neurons (Maniscalchi et al., 2024). Iron chelators decrease the iron load by 20%–30% and have shown neuroprotective effects in early trials. The ferroptosis inhibitor ferrostatin-1 also reduces neuronal loss by 35%–45% (Zhao et al., 2024). Mitochondrial iron imbalance disrupts electron transport and decreases ATP production by 40% (Xiao et al., 2024). Targeted chelation strategies that maintain essential enzymatic functions are currently under investigation.

15.2.9 Other emerging targets

New investigations have identified various novel therapeutic interventions directed against synaptic plasticity, epigenetic regulation, and the gut-brain axis in PD. Such interventions can modulate the onset of the disease, enhance neuroprotection, and promote motor and non-motor outcomes. An overview of these interventions and the mechanism underlying them is given in Table 15.1.

15.3 Advances in disease-modifying therapies (DMTs)

15.3.1 Gene therapy and gene editing

Managing PD becomes difficult because treatments like L-dopa stop working well and cause serious movement and mental health problems as the disease gets worse. This unmet need has driven research into alternative therapies, including gene therapy, which aims to address the disease's underlying mechanisms rather than merely alleviating symptoms (Saravanan et al., 2024). Genetic insights have

Table 15.1 Emerging therapies targeting epigenetic regulation, gut-brain axis, and synaptic plasticity in Parkinson's disease.

Therapeutic strategy	Target/ Mechanism	Therapy type	Reported benefits	Key studies
Epigenetic regulation				
Histone deacetylase (HDAC) inhibitors	Reverses hypoacetylation; promotes gene expression	Pharmacologic	Neuroprotection, restored gene regulation	Harrison and Dexter (2013)
DNA methyltransferase (DNMT) inhibitors	Prevent DNA hypermethylation	Pharmacologic	Gene reactivation, neuroprotection	Zhang et al. (2023)
microRNA (miRNA)-based therapies	Regulate protein expression (e.g., α-syn)	Molecular	Modulates disease-related pathways	Zhang et al. (2023)
Vitamin C–treated stem cells	Alters histone acetylation marks	Stem cell	Reduces α-syn expression	Mao et al. (2024)
Gut-brain axis				
Fecal microbiota transplantation (FMT)	Restores healthy microbiota	Microbiome	Reduces inflammation, improves symptoms	Ebedes and Borlongan (2024)
Vagus nerve stimulation (VNS)	Enhances gut–CNS signaling	Neuromodulation	Reduces α-syn spread	Bonaz (2024)
Gut barrier repair agents	Reduce intestinal permeability	Pharmacologic	Limits systemic inflammation	Jia et al. (2024)
Short-chain fatty acid (SCFA) modulation (e.g., butyrate)	Enhances anti-inflammatory gut metabolites	Metabolite therapy	Neuroprotection, immune modulation	Kollaparampil Kishanchand et al. (2025)
Synaptic plasticity				
L-dopa + NMDA modulation	Restores corticostriatal long-term potentiation; avoids maladaptive plasticity	Pharmacologic	Motor improvement, fewer dyskinesias	Bagetta et al. (2010)
Neural stem cells + ethyl stearate	Enhances brain-derived neurotrophic factor (BDNF) and synaptic protein	Cell therapy + small molecule	Increased synaptic density, behavioral recovery	Yi et al. (2024)

Table 15.1 Emerging therapies targeting epigenetic regulation, gut-brain axis, and synaptic plasticity in Parkinson's disease.—cont'd

Therapeutic strategy	Target/ Mechanism	Therapy type	Reported benefits	Key studies
	expression via Drd1/ERK/AP-1			
Environmental enrichment	Reduces α-syn-synaptic protein interaction	Behavioral/ Nutritional	Improves mood, motor function, synaptic protein expression	Kim et al. (2021)
Computationally guided STDP Modulation	Targets aberrant inhibitory spike-timing-dependent plasticity (iSTDP)	Neurostimulation modeling	Reverses maladaptive connectivity	Madadi et al. (2022)
PHF8 knockdown (epigenetic)	Alters histone demethylation and synaptic gene expression	Epigenetic	Decreases α-syn and synaptic proteins (e.g., SYNJ1)	Oey et al. (2023)

identified key targets, including mutations in *SNCA* (encoding α-synuclein, which aggregates into Lewy bodies), *GBA1* (linked to lysosomal dysfunction), and *LRRK2* (implicated in kinase overactivity) (Trevisan et al., 2024). Viral vector-based strategies, particularly adeno-associated viruses (AAVs), are being used to deliver genes such as aromatic L-amino acid decarboxylase (*AADC*) to enhance dopamine synthesis or neurotrophic factors like glial cell line-derived neurotrophic factor (*GDNF*) to support neuronal survival (Saravanan et al., 2024).

These approaches aim to provide sustained therapeutic effects, bypassing the fluctuating dopamine levels caused by oral medications. Several clinical trials highlight the promise and challenges of gene therapy in PD. In a recent systematic review, several trials—mostly utilizing AAV-delivery—demonstrated safety but variable putamen coverage and efficacy. Beyond dopamine restoration, strategies such as CRISPR/Cas9-mediated correction of *SNCA* duplications or *GBA1* loss-of-function mutations are being explored. Concurrently, small-molecule therapies like LTI-291 (a GCase activator) and ambroxol (which crosses the BBB) aim to modulate PD-linked pathways, with early trials showing target engagement in CSF.

GBA1 mutations, the most common genetic risk factor for PD, impair lysosomal GCase activity, contributing to α-syn aggregation and neurodegeneration (Granek et al., 2023). Ambroxol, a repurposed mucolytic agent, acts as a pH-dependent chaperone, rescuing misfolded GCase by facilitating its trafficking to lysosomes (Mullin et al., 2020). A pivotal 2020 open-label trial in PD patients, including GBA1 carriers, confirmed Ambroxol's CNS penetration, showing increased CSF GCase protein and α-syn levels—a potential biomarker of target engagement with well-tolerated side effects and no significant safety concerns, supporting its repurposing for disease modification (Mullin et al., 2020). Currently, a larger randomized, placebo-controlled trial evaluating high-dose Ambroxol (1.8 g/day) in GBA-PD patients over 48 weeks is ongoing (Siemeling et al., 2024). Other trials on other genetic therapies are also ongoing after initial promising results (NCT00643890, NCT02418598). The translation of gene therapy into clinical practice faces hurdles, including optimizing vector delivery to ensure adequate brain coverage, determining the ideal treatment window (early vs. late disease), and addressing the genetic heterogeneity of PD. Personalized approaches, informed by polygenic risk scores (PRS) and mutation-specific strategies, may enhance efficacy, particularly for high-risk genotypes like *GBA1* or *LRRK2* carriers. Nonviral methods, such as nanoparticle-delivered GDNF or Trojan horse liposomes, offer alternatives to invasive intracranial injections but require improved transfection efficiency (Pardridge, 2020). As trials evolve, combining gene therapy with other treatments can lead to significant advances in PD management.

15.3.2 RNA-based therapies

Nucleic acid therapies for PD are based on the initial hypothesis of their abilities to regulate α-syn expression and thereby block the progression of PD. As the case for genetic therapies, nucleic acid therapies are also first tested on genetically determined PD types, especially PARK 4, an autosomal dominantly inherited PD caused by SNCA gene multiplication, which leads to the accumulation of α-syn (Yasuda & Mochizuki, 2010). Researchers studied the possibility of decreasing this accumulation by reducing SNCA messenger RNA (mRNA) levels through various approaches. Approaches that included targeting SNCA mRNA through AAV or vectors expressing SNCA-targeting short hairpin RNA (shRNA) or short interfering RNA (siRNA) have led to promising results, achieving a 35%–50% decrease in α-syn levels in rat experiments (Lewis et al., 2008; Helmschrodt et al., 2017). Although these initial approaches were promising, challenges of stability and concerns about the toxicity of these compounds persisted. Recently, researchers designed Antisense oligonucleotides (ASOs) that target mRNA degradation through Gapmer configuration. This configuration consists of modified nucleic acids (linear single-stranded oligonucleotide) at both ends and a central DNA segment. When they bind to target mRNA, an enzyme called RNase H recognizes the DNA: RNA hybrid and degrades the mRNA. The modified nucleic acids at both ends enhance stability and affinity, and protect the central portion—responsible for starting the degradation process—from getting degraded by other enzymes before reaching its target. After that, the Gapmer ASOs can repeatedly target and destroy mRNA molecules for a long time before degrading. Although these strategies have been suggested for a while, their application in PD has not been available, especially after initial failure in Hungiton's disease trials and their termination and lessons from these experiments are used for further development (Aguti et al., 2024). MicroRNAs (miRNAs) are key regulators of gene expression and offer potential therapeutic strategies for PD. Two main approaches are being explored: miRNA mimics and anti-miRNAs. MiRNA mimics are small RNA molecules that reduce the expression of disease-related proteins. In contrast, anti-miRNAs bind to and deactivate overexpressed miRNAs. Among miRNAs, miRNA-7 is particularly promising, as it lowers α-syn, promotes its clearance, and reduces inflammation. MiRNA-124 protects neurons, while miRNA-155 drives neuroinflammation, making it a target for inhibition. Although no miRNA-based therapies for PD are currently in clinical trials, targeting miRNAs holds promise, particularly for regulating α-syn (Shaheen et al., 2024).

15.3.3 Stem cell therapies and regenerative medicine

Fetal ventral mesencephalon (VM) tissue contains dopaminergic neurons from the SN and other regions, which have been hypothesized to treat PD. Transplantation of fetal midbrain cells containing dopaminergic neurons began in the 1980s, with early clinical cases showing functional improvement in PD patients. Some concerns regarding their safety, especially after finding evidence for Lewy bodies in some of the transplanted cells, led to the fear of progressive neurodegeneration. However, later controlled trials did not support the efficacy of fetal VM. Early trials suffered from several limitations of inconsistent outcomes, populations, methods, and ethical concerns using fetal cells from abortions. While early trials used surgically obtained fetal tissue, recent approaches often employ medically derived sources. Preclinical data supported VM grafts in alleviating PD symptoms, and the TRANSEURO trial was initiated in 2012 to improve the variability of outcomes in previous trials using human fetal VM tissue for PD treatment by implementing stricter patient selection, cell handling, surgical technique, and immune suppression. However, logistical issues with tissue availability led to premature termination.

Striatal grafts of midbrain dopaminergic neurons can be obtained from various sources, such as fetal tissues, porcine fetal SN neurons, and immature retinal cells. Ethical concerns, inconsistent cell availability, and quality issues further limited fetal cell therapies, driving interest in pluripotent stem cell (PSC)-derived dopaminergic neurons as a scalable alternative. Human embryonic stem cells (hESCs) and adult stem cell sources such as mesenchymal stem cells (MSCs) are capable of generating dopaminergic neurons in cell culture models (Zeng & Couture, 2013).

Dopaminergic neurons generated from PSCs are hypothesized to replicate native midbrain neurons by producing dopamine, forming functional synapses, and integrating into host brain circuits. Whereas both adult and embryonic PSC sources have shown promise, hESC sources have made the most progress. To overcome these limitations, researchers developed STEM-PD, a standardized, scalable, and quality-controlled dopaminergic progenitor cell product derived from hESCs. Preclinical studies demonstrated that STEM-PD cells successfully reversed motor impairments in PD models, maintained genetic stability, and showed long-term safety (Kirkeby et al., 2023). The first-in-human clinical trial, STEM-PD, is currently underway in Europe to assess the safety, tolerability, and efficacy of these cells in patients with moderate PD. The first patient in the trial was transplanted at Skåne University Hospital, Lund, Sweden, in February 2023, and several patients have been administered the stem cells till now with no serious adverse effects reported.

MSCs that are sourced from bone marrow, adipose tissue, or umbilical cord can differentiate into dopaminergic neurons and also secrete neurotrophic factors (BDNF, GDNF) that reduce inflammation and protect dopaminergic neurons (Li et al., 2022). MSCs also possess unique characteristics such as genetic stability, absence of tumorigenicity, and minimal ethical concerns compared to embryonic stem cells. Their therapeutic effects stem from cellular differentiation and paracrine actions, with their secretome—rich in growth factors and cytokines—playing a key role in neuroprotection. Preclinical studies confirm MSC efficacy in PD models, demonstrating improved motor function and dopamine neuron restoration via various administration routes (intranasal, intravenous, intracerebral, intramuscular) (Tambe et al., 2024). Several case reports and open-label studies for the use of adipose-derived and bone marrow-derived MSCs revealed inconsistent results, with some studies showing significant improvements while others showed minimal efficacy. Schiess et al. found that a single intravenous infusion of bone marrow-derived MSCs at a dose of 10×10^6/kg was safe and well tolerated in PD, and led to a decrease of −14.4 ($P < .01$) in OFF-UPDRS motor score. However, there are concerns about patients liable to lymphocytic leukemia, dyskinesias, and embolization risk (Schiess et al., 2021).

Induced pluripotent stem cells (iPSCs) have emerged as a promising avenue for PD treatment, offering the potential to generate patient-specific dopaminergic neurons while minimizing immune rejection. Japan made history in 2018 with the first human trial using iPSC-derived cells for PD treatment (Cyranoski, 2017).

Ongoing clinical trials continue to evaluate the safety and efficacy of these approaches, with efforts focused on developing universal iPSC lines that bypass immunosuppression through major histocompatibility complex (MHC) gene editing or human leukocyte antigens (HLA) matching. Neural stem/progenitor cells (NSCs/NPCs) represent another promising therapeutic option for PD based on their ability to release neurotrophic factors and support neuroprotection. Animal studies on rats and monkeys suggest that NSC transplantation not only replaces lost neurons but also stimulates endogenous repair mechanisms, potentially offering synergistic benefits (Oz et al., 2023). However, they have restricted proliferation and differentiation potential compared to PSCs, and they often rely on fetal tissue, presenting ethical concerns. Despite these advancements, scalability, cost, the risk of contamination with undifferentiated cells, and concerns about tumorigenicity further complicate and hinder widespread application and clinical trials development (Yefroyev & Jin, 2022).

The current status of stem cell-based therapies for PD is advancing from its immature state 40 years ago. Several clinical trials are advancing stem cell-based therapies for PD. Kyoto University pioneered the first iPSC-derived dopaminergic neuron trial in 2018, transplanting 2.4 million Corin-sorted progenitor cells into seven patients. Chinese Academy of Sciences launched a Phase I/II trial in 2017 using hESC-derived neural precursors in 50 patients, showing safety in primates but awaiting human results. Cyto Therapeutics (Australia) conducted a Phase I trial with parthenogenetic stem cell-derived neurons (30–70 million cells), reporting dose-dependent motor improvement in PD monkeys and early human efficacy signals. More recent trials include the 2022 STEM-PD study, testing hESC-derived cells (3.5 to 7 million cells/putamen) in eight patients, with early safety data supporting dose escalation. Aspen Neuroscience (NCT06344026) is investigating autologous iPSC-derived dopaminergic neurons, showing preclinical efficacy without tumorigenicity. The University of California/SBMP (NCT06482268) follows Kyoto's protocol with bilateral putamen injections of 4.2–5.4 million iPSC progenitors. S.Biomedics (NCT05887466) is conducting a dose-escalation study of hESC-derived A9 progenitors (3.15–6.3 million cells), tracking safety and motor improvements over 2 years. These trials collectively aim to refine stem cell therapies for PD, addressing safety and efficacy, and may publish their results in the next few years. Madrazo et al. published the report of their study using stereotactic surgery to inject NPC suspensions into patients' dorsal putamina, demonstrating safety with no adverse effects. One year after cell grafting, all but one of the seven patients completing the study showed various degrees of motor improvement, and five of them showed better response to medication. However, the small sample sizes limit the generalizability and strength of the conclusions. A recent Phase 1 study found intranasal transplantation of human neural stem cells (ANGE-S003) to be generally safe and to have the ability to reduce impairment by significant 19 points (measured by MDS-UPDRS). Combined approaches of stem cells and gene editing represent the future for PD management and hold promise for conquering the "Parkinson's epidemic" (Hwang et al., 2018).

15.4 Personalized medicine in PD

15.4.1 Biomarkers for early diagnosis and monitoring treatment response

As the onset of clinical manifestations of PD occurs after the loss of a reasonable number of SN neurons, the need for biomarkers for early detection of the disease and monitoring of clinical condition is imminent (Miller & O'Callaghan, 2015; Simuni et al., 2024). Biomarkers are needed in detecting the susceptibility for the disease and monitoring its progression in each stage (Simuni et al., 2024; Mitchell et al., 2021). Biomarkers are broadly categorized as biochemical, imaging, and—more recently—digital biomarkers. Biochemical biomarkers are derived from blood, CSF, urine, saliva, or tissue biopsies, such as skin samples, and are analyzed using molecular and tissue-based techniques (Brumm et al., 2023).

Misfolded proteins, such as α-syn oligomers, α-syn aggregates, and phosphorylated α-syn, are elevated in the CSF of patients with PD compared to healthy controls (Parnetti et al., 2019). The α-syn species, neurofilaments, glial fibrillary acidic protein (GFAP), pTau181, and inflammatory cytokines are critical prospective biomarkers that could be detected in the plasma of PD patients (Youssef et al., 2023). Detection of phosphorylated α-syn through immunohistochemical examination of peripheral tissue samples is proven to be a reliable biomarker (Jiménez-Jiménez et al., 2023).

Imaging modalities form a milestone in diagnosing PD. As these modalities are noninvasive, can be used repeatedly, and reveal a wide range of neuroanatomical and pathophysiological processes in PD, their noteworthiness could overweigh biochemical markers (Gaurav et al., 2021). Many integral mechanisms contribute to diagnosing PD in all its stages, including structural magnetic resonance imaging (MRI) to assess regional tissue atrophy as in SN and locus coeruleus, functional MRI to detect reduced functional connectivity in basal ganglia of early-stage PD patients, single-photon emission computed tomography (SPECT) to measure the density of nigrostriatal nerve terminals, and positron emission tomography (PET) to assess neuroinflammations, pathogenic Aβ and tau protein buildup, cerebral glucose utilization, and dopamine system integrity (Gaurav et al., 2021; Saeed et al., 2017, 2020).

Research interest in digital biomarkers is growing. The use of incorporated sensors in portable devices of patients allows a longwise monitoring of those with neurodegenerative disease. Indeed, this gives a chance to predict motor symptoms prior to their onset, and even the course of the disease. Besides, it represents a systematic method of collecting valuable data on different disease parameters (Dorsey et al., 2017).

15.4.2 Pharmacogenomics

The complex of pharmacogenetics in PD involves pathogenic, mechanistic, metabolic, transporter, and pleiotropic genes (Cacabelos et al., 2016, 2022). These genes are controlled largely by epigenomic factors (e.g., DNA methylation, histone/chromatin remodeling, and mRNA regulation) (Cacabelos et al., 2016; Cacabelos & Torrellas, 2014). Evidence shows that the efficacy and safety of drugs in PD patients is affected largely by these pharmacogenetic factors. Genetic testing to detect these genes is either targeted testing looking for a particular gene, or a multigene panel screening for a set of genes (Cook et al., 2021). This method already has important relevance for families. For instance, the detection of a mutation by this test allows a deeper knowledge about the disease risks and potential family planning. Detection of one of the most commonly observed mutations in PD (LRRK-2 and GBA-1) should not be worrying for asymptomatic relatives, as they have low penetrance potential, thus a minimal risk of developing PD (Trevisan et al., 2024).

As drugs of PD have different mechanisms and wide targets, a mutation in any of the enzymes that are involved in their pharmaco-dynamics or -kinetics could affect the disease control and outcome (Politi et al., 2018). For instance, mutation (polymorphism) in catechol-O-methyltransferase (COMT) and monoamine oxidase B (MAO-B) genes, which encode enzymes involved in the metabolism of L-Dopa, thus control the bioavailability of dopamine, may significantly influence treatment response and disease risk (Bialecka et al., 2007). Polymorphisms of DRD-2 and DRD-3 genes that encode dopamine receptors, affect the response to a main drugs category which acts as dopaminergic agents on dopamine receptors, which are divided into either ergot-derived (e.g., bromocriptine) or non-ergot-derived (e.g., ropinirole) (Liu et al., 2009).

Accordingly, therapeutic advances aim to administer treatments according to the genetic mutation present, as patients with specific mutations have dominant clinical manifestations. For instance, LRRK2-PD patients typically develop clinical features and disease progression identical to idiopathic PD, and GBA1-PD commonly has early onset, poor motor function and high risk of cognitive impairment (Trevisan et al., 2024).

15.4.3 Precision medicine approaches

Precision medicine, also known as individualized medicine, aims to identify the acceptable treatment for a patient to ensure the best outcomes with the least harm. To apply this approach, PD patients are divided according to their genetic, clinical, and biomarker-based subtypes. PD according to genetics include GBA-, LRRK2-, and SNCA-associated parkinsonism (Schneider & Alcalay, 2020). Clinical subtyping is based on predominant motor features of the disease, age of onset, gender, or predominant nonmotor symptoms (Marras et al., 2020). One of the most crucial causes of this targeted patients' stratification is to simplify the guidance to clinical care and conduction of research. In clinical trials, patients' classification according to their disease subtypes enhances the similarity within the same group, so that more pathophysiological details related to a specific subtype could be identified, providing reliable evidence-based perspectives and increasing the quality of research.

The integration of various subtypes of PD into clinical care and personalizing treatments has been considered a breakthrough in managing PD patients. When age is taken into consideration, delaying motor symptoms in younger patients is a target, while in older patients' other comorbidities as Alzheimer's disease should never be deserted. Tremor-dominant disease, patients complaining of Akinetic-rigid subtype should be considered for early physical therapy to accommodate their motor limitations, and GPi-DBS (Brain Stimulation of the Globus Pallidus Internus) evaluation may be warranted if significant gait impairment develops (Seppi et al., 2019).

Every detail of subtypes has a therapeutic implication in PD, which should be considered to reach the best outcome. Although they have been intensively studied, only age and motor status have an actual influence on selecting appropriate treatment until now (Marras et al., 2020; Seppi et al., 2019). Multi-omics data enhance the understanding of PD by integrating multiple layers of biological and clinical data, including genomic, transcriptomic, proteomic, biomarker, and clinical information. This integrative strategy facilitates the identification of data-driven patient subtypes, enabling improved characterization of disease heterogeneity, differentiation of progression trajectories, and prediction of clinical outcomes (Fereshtehnejad et al., 2017). In simple words, it is a way so that we can apply the genetic background of the disease to clinical perspectives. Furthermore, machine learning was proven to be a reliable method of designing functional genomes, leading to precise predictability of the functional effect of a specific genome (Schilder et al., 2022).

15.4.4 Digital health and artificial intelligence in PD pharmacotherapy

Drug discovery has witnessed a significant transformation in the era of artificial intelligence (AI), by enhancing efficiency, reducing costs, and increasing success rates. Better outcomes are primarily achieved by the identification of feasible compounds, thus enhancing the development timeline. AI facilitates the analysis of a wide range of molecular compounds and stratify their binding affinities, designing the three-dimensional (3D) structure of a target protein, and projection of drug-protein interactions. Furthermore, it gives the chance to design new drug-alike molecules independently from any previous molecules (Blaschke et al., 2020; Hasselgren & Oprea, 2024). By integrating these features of AI with machine learning, we are able to produce platforms that could forecast the interactions of new drugs with already existing agents and anticipate alternative therapeutic applications with fewer adverse effects. Predictive capabilities could be extended to detect off-target interactions, enhancing our understanding of a drug's overall effects to for safer and more efficient treatments.

Body wearable sensors (BWS) are gaining traction in clinical trials and, recently, in practice. Inertial management units (IMU) are a typical type of these sensors, in which quantitative parameters are obtained to assess the motor condition of PD patients, including tremors, gait status, dyskinesia, and motor fluctuations (Artusi et al., 2018). Many devices have implicated these sensors and being clinically validated, such as PD monitor, Personal Kinetigraph, Stat-On, Kinesia technology, DynaPort, and Feet me monitor (Moreau et al., 2023). Other types of sensors have emerged to monitor the non-motor status of patients, as it is a crucial determinant of the quality of life and lead the therapeutic strategy, such as those designed to monitor the psycho-behavioral manifestations of PD (Evans et al., 2014).

The clinical application of BWS should never be underestimated, as it has a significant potential to be used as an independent method for monitoring the disease status and modify the therapeutics accordingly, in addition to the ability of some of these sensors to be used as a rehabilitation method, such as Feet me device (Moreau et al., 2023).

15.5 Novel drug delivery systems

A summary of the novel drug delivery methods in PD are presented in Table 15.2.

15.5.1 Overcoming the blood-brain barrier

One of the principal challenges in developing effective pharmacotherapies for PD is overcoming the restrictive nature of the BBB (Niazi, 2023). The BBB effectively shields the brain from potentially harmful agents, pathogens, and fluctuations in plasma composition (Dotiwala et al., 2025). Meanwhile, this protective function also restricts the entry of a wide range of therapeutic compounds, including most large molecule biologics and a significant proportion of small-molecule drugs (Wu et al., 2023).

Table 15.2 Comparison of novel drug delivery methods in Parkinson's disease.

Method	Mechanism	Application	Advantages	Challenges
Nanoparticles (Xie et al., 2019; Sadat et al., 2025)	Passive/active BBB crossing	CNS delivery of drugs	Targeted delivery, prolonged circulation	Clearance, toxicity, regulatory hurdles
Focused ultrasound (FUS) (Burgess et al., 2015)	Temporary BBB disruption via microbubbles	Localized brain delivery	Non-invasive, site-specific delivery	Equipment cost, safety, precise targeting
Receptor-mediated transcytosis (RMT) (Jones & Shusta, 2007; Haqqani et al., 2024)	Ligand-receptor interaction at BBB	Delivery of biologics	Exploits natural transport, applicable to large drugs	Receptor saturation, immune response
Levodopa-carbidopa intestinal gel (LCIG) (Batzu et al., 2023)	Continuous intestinal infusion	Advanced PD, motor fluctuation	Stable plasma levels, improved motor control	Invasive, requires device management
Subcutaneous infusions (Fung et al., 2024)	Continuous systemic delivery	Advanced PD	Non-oral, convenient, stable drug levels	Skin irritation, device limitations
Inhaled/Nasal delivery (Zhang et al., 2022)	Pulmonary or nasal mucosa absorption	Rapid relief of "off" episodes	Fast onset, non-invasive	Short duration, formulation challenges
Exosome-based delivery (Haney et al., 2015)	Natural vesicle-mediated BBB crossing	Gene therapy, neuroprotection	Biocompatibility, targeted delivery	Production scalability, clinical validation
3D printing/ Smart release (Gültekin et al., 2022; Peng et al., 2024)	Custom drug release profiles, responsive delivery	Personalized treatment	Tailored dosing, adaptive release	Technological and regulatory barriers

Overcoming the restrictive nature of the BBB remains a critical step in translating emerging therapies into clinical reality for PD (Hersh et al., 2022). As a result, the delivery of neuropharmacological agents intended to modify disease progression or manage symptoms in PD is severely limited. The challenge is further compounded by the fact that many of the most promising therapeutic candidates, such as neurotrophic factors, monoclonal antibodies, and gene-editing tools, are macromolecules that cannot traverse the BBB without specialized delivery systems (Hersh et al., 2022; Upadhyay, 2014). This has necessitated the exploration of innovative strategies to enhance CNS drug delivery, including nanotechnology-based carriers, receptor-mediated transport mechanisms, and physical methods for transient BBB disruption (Nguyen et al., 2021).

Recent innovations aim to modulate the BBB to enhance central drug delivery. Nanoparticle-based drug delivery systems have shown promise in preclinical models (Elumalai et al., 2024). These carriers, composed of biodegradable materials such as lipids or polymers, can encapsulate therapeutic agents and protect them from systemic degradation, prolonging circulation time and facilitating targeted delivery to the brain (Parveen et al., 2023; Yusuf et al., 2023). Surface modification of nanoparticles, such as PEGylation or ligand conjugation, can further optimize their transport across the BBB (Veronese & Mero, 2008; Teixeira et al., 2023). Focused ultrasound (FUS) in conjunction with microbubble administration represents a non-invasive strategy for temporarily disrupting the BBB (Burgess et al., 2015). This method enables localized, reversible permeability, allowing for site-specific drug delivery without systemic exposure (Chen et al., 2021). Early pre-clinical trials have demonstrated the safety and feasibility of this approach, suggesting its potential as a platform for delivering both conventional and novel PD therapeutics (Antoniou et al., 2024; Schregel et al., 2021). Another strategy is receptor-mediated transcytosis (RMT), where therapeutic agents are engineered to bind to endogenous BBB transporters such as transferrin or insulin receptors (Jones & Shusta, 2007). This technique exploits natural transport mechanisms to carry drugs across the BBB and into neuronal tissues. Although still in the early development, RMT offers a promising avenue for delivering biologics and other macromolecules in PD (Jones & Shusta, 2007; Lajoie & Shusta, 2015).

In addition to non-invasive and nanoparticle-mediated strategies, direct intracerebral gene delivery using viral vectors represents a powerful method to bypass the BBB entirely. This approach involves the stereotactic injection of modified viruses, such as adenoviruses or AAVs, into key brain regions such as the putamen (Liu, Li, et al., 2024). These vectors can carry genes encoding enzymes involved in dopamine synthesis or neuroprotective proteins, offering the potential for disease-modifying effects. A schematic of this gene delivery process is illustrated in Fig. 15.1.

15.5.2 Sustained-release and long-acting formulations

To address motor fluctuations and optimize dopaminergic stimulation, sustained-release and long-acting formulations have been developed. The levodopa-carbidopa intestinal gel (LCIG) represents a significant advancement over traditional oral levodopa therapy (Othman & Dutta, 2014). Administered via a percutaneous gastrojejunostomy, LCIG provides a continuous infusion of levodopa directly into the small intestine, reducing plasma fluctuations and enhancing motor control in patients with advanced PD (Fernandez et al., 2013; Abbruzzese et al., 2012). Clinical studies have reported improvements in "off" time, dyskinesias, and quality of life (Antonini et al., 2017, 2021; Fernandez et al., 2015).

Implantable infusion systems and subcutaneous delivery devices have also gained traction. These systems enable steady-state plasma levels of dopaminergic agents, minimizing peaks and troughs associated with oral dosing (Pons-Faudoa et al., 2019). Subcutaneous apomorphine infusions, for instance, have shown efficacy in managing motor complications and serve as a less invasive alternative to LCIG (Katzenschlager et al., 2018).

In addition, microsphere and nanosphere formulations offer the potential for depot drug delivery (van Vliet et al., 2023). These formulations, composed of biodegradable polymers such as PLGA (Poly Lactic-co-Glycolic Acid), can release active agents over days to weeks. Preclinical research supports their use for sustained delivery of dopamine agonists and neuroprotective agents, although clinical translation remains ongoing (Yang et al., 2024; Lagreca et al., 2020).

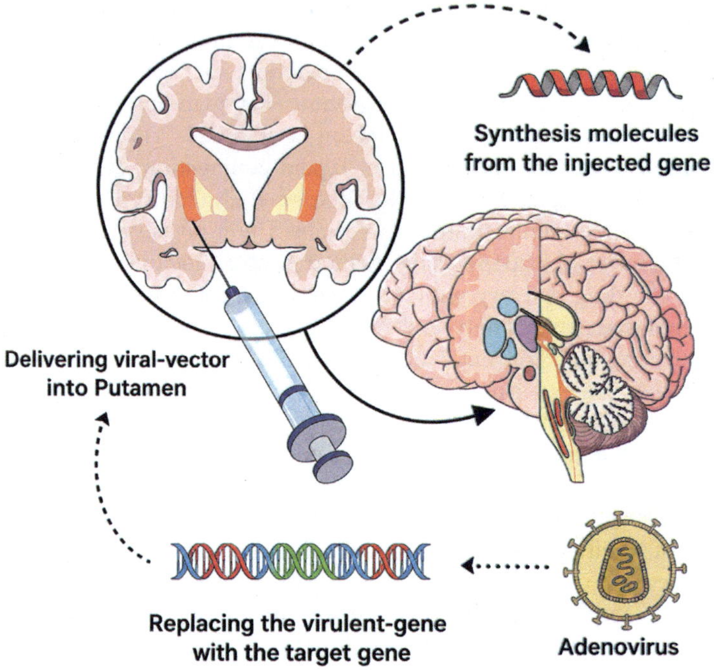

FIGURE 15.1 A schematic of targeted gene therapy using adenoviral vectors in PD.

Direct intracerebral gene delivery using viral vectors represents a powerful method to bypass the BBB entirely. This approach involves the stereotactic injection of modified viruses, such as adenoviruses or adeno-associated viruses (AAVs), into key brain regions such as the putamen. These vectors can carry genes encoding enzymes involved in dopamine synthesis or neuroprotective proteins, offering the potential for disease-modifying effects.

15.5.3 Non-invasive delivery methods

The pursuit of non-invasive drug delivery methods in PD is driven by the need to improve patient adherence, reduce treatment-related burdens, and optimize symptom control, especially in the context of long-term, chronic therapy. Traditional oral administration of anti-parkinsonian medications is often complicated by motor fluctuations, erratic gastrointestinal absorption, and delayed gastric emptying, which can substantially affect drug bioavailability and therapeutic consistency (Nyholm & Lennernäs, 2008). In this context, alternative routes of administration have gained increasing attention.

Transdermal delivery systems, such as the rotigotine patch, represent a clinically validated option that provides continuous dopaminergic stimulation over 24 hours (Wüllner et al., 2010). This approach avoids the peaks and troughs associated with oral dosing and circumvents first-pass hepatic metabolism, offering a more stable pharmacokinetic profile. It also serves as a practical alternative for patients with dysphagia or gastrointestinal complications and may reduce the overall pill burden (Rascol & Perez-Lloret, 2009).

Other non-invasive delivery modalities currently under investigation include inhalable, intranasal, and oral mucosal formulations. Inhaled levodopa (CVT-301) has been approved for the rapid relief of "off" episodes in PD patients already on a stable oral levodopa regimen (Glenardi et al., 2022; Hauser et al., 2019). Delivered via a dry-powder inhaler, it facilitates fast systemic absorption through the pulmonary epithelium, providing symptom relief within minutes. Similarly, intranasal sprays are being explored for their potential to bypass the BBB via the olfactory and trigeminal pathways, offering direct nose-to-brain delivery for a range of therapeutic agents (Al-Hajaj et al., 2025; Du et al., 2024).

Oral mucosal delivery systems, including sublingual and buccal formulations, are also under development (Lai et al., 2018). These approaches aim to provide a rapid onset of action while avoiding gastrointestinal degradation and hepatic first-pass metabolism.

Collectively, non-invasive drug delivery platforms not only enhance pharmacokinetic predictability but also align with patient-centric care models, especially for individuals experiencing advanced disease stages or treatment-related complications. As research continues, these strategies are expected to complement or even replace more invasive delivery options in specific patient populations.

15.5.4 Exosome-based drug delivery

Exosomes, nanoscale extracellular vesicles secreted by various cell types, have emerged as a novel vehicle for targeted drug delivery. These vesicles possess inherent biocompatibility, low immunogenicity, and the unique ability to cross the BBB, making them promising candidates for neurological drug delivery (Rana et al., 2025; Sen et al., 2023). In the context of PD, exosomes can be engineered to carry therapeutic cargo, such as small molecules, RNA-based drugs, or proteins (Li, Wang, et al., 2025). Their surface proteins can be modified for targeted delivery to dopaminergic neurons or other relevant cell types. Studies have demonstrated the potential of exosomes to deliver siRNA to downregulate α-syn expression (Pinnell et al., 2021; Liu, Cheng, et al., 2024). Although still in the early stages, exosome-based therapies represent a promising frontier in personalized and targeted PD treatment.

15.5.5 Other emerging technologies drug delivery

Several emerging technologies hold the potential to transform the landscape of PD pharmacotherapy. 3D printing has enabled the fabrication of customizable, patient-specific drug delivery systems, including multilayer tablets with programmed release kinetics (Gültekin et al., 2022; Peng et al., 2024). This technology allows precise dosing and release profiles tailored to individual pharmacokinetic needs.

Biodegradable implants are being investigated as long-term delivery devices for dopaminergic agents or neuroprotective compounds (Mogharbel et al., 2022). These implants can provide sustained drug release over months, reducing the burden of frequent dosing and enhancing adherence (Bellotti et al., 2021). Smart drug release systems, responsive to physiological triggers such as pH, temperature, or enzymatic activity, offer site or condition-specific drug delivery potentials (Boppana et al., 2024). These systems can adapt to disease fluctuations and deliver therapy in a controlled, dynamic manner, aligning with the complex pathophysiology of PD.

15.6 Targeting non-motor symptoms

15.6.1 Non-motor symptoms (NMSs) of PD

NMSs of PD include neuropsychiatric symptoms (such as depression, anxiety, and cognitive impairment), autonomic dysfunction (including orthostatic hypotension, constipation, and urinary impairment), sleep disorders, sensory disturbances, mood disorders, and psychosis. While these symptoms significantly impact the quality of life of PD patients—just as motor symptoms do—they are difficult to assess due to lack of standardized measures and variations in their definitions. As a result, the insufficient focus on NMSs, their costs, and quality of life implications reflects a significant unmet patient need. Research has shown that patients may experience NMSs several years before motor symptoms; furthermore, they can be more debilitating than motor symptoms in the later stages of PD. Consequently, patients often feel there is a lack of response from clinicians, the pharmaceutical industry, and academics regarding the burden posed by NMSs. The current lack of attention and underreporting of NMSs suggest that PD affects more people than is currently recorded (Jerčić et al., 2024; van der Meer et al., 2025; Radad et al., 2023).

15.6.2 Novel therapies for NMSs

- Atomoxetine, among the pharmacologic therapies, shows promise in terms of improving global cognition and attention-related symptoms, but has an insignificant effect on executive function. Rasagiline's cognitive benefits are inconsistent. Creatine and coenzyme Q10 may boost cognitive performance; however, the research is preliminary. Systematic cognitive training programs like NEUROvitalis seem to help people with dementia and other cognitive problems and improve their memory and overall thinking (Sun & Armstrong, 2021).
- According to previous research, type 2 diabetes mellitus drugs may have the potential to improve cognitive impairment in PD (Green et al., 2019).
- Cognitive Behavioral Therapy (CBT): CBT is effective in treating depression and anxiety in PD patients. A systematic review and meta-analysis showed significant improvements in mood disorders with CBT (Luo et al., 2021).
- Pimavanserin: this medicine is effective in treating PD Psychosis and is approved in the US (Phillips et al., 2023).
- New therapeutic targets, including Protein Abelson, Rabphilin-3 A, and Colony Stimulating Factor 1-Receptor (CSF1R), are being investigated. These targets are promising for regulating disease development and treating autonomic dysfunction in PD (Ntetsika et al., 2021).
- Deep Brain Stimulation (DBS): while predominantly used to treat motor symptoms, DBS has a promise in treating specific autonomic dysfunctions in PD patients (Ntetsika et al., 2021).

15.7 Challenges and ethical considerations

15.7.1 Regulatory hurdles in developing new therapies

The heterogeneity of PD symptoms, combined with limited understanding of its biology, poses significant challenges in clinical trial design and therapeutic development. The wide range of motor and non-motor symptoms, along with difficulties in selecting appropriate biomarkers, complicates the creation of standardized protocols and uniform assessment of treatment efficacy. Additionally, factors such as age, disease duration, and comorbid conditions contribute to clinical variability, complicating participant recruitment and outcome measurement. Given the slow progression of PD, trials require extended durations and increasing financial costs (Zhang, Liu, et al., 2024; Zeissler et al., 2023; McFarthing et al., 2024).

Balancing innovation with safety and efficacy in PD clinical trials remains a critical challenge. While innovative therapies hold promise for disease modification, they must undergo rigorous testing to ensure patient safety and therapeutic benefit. Many trials struggle in the transition from Phase 2 to Phase 3 due to difficulties in maintaining this balance, as early-stage results may not always apply to larger, more diverse populations. Adaptive trial designs incorporating interim analyses and real-world evidence could help address these challenges (Luo et al., 2021).

15.7.2 Ethical issues in emerging therapies

The International Society for Stem Cell Research (ISSCR) developed specific guidelines for the field of stem cell research to encourage appropriate and timely translation of stem cell research to clinical environments. The documents open with the statement: "The primary societal mission of basic biomedical research and its clinical translation is to alleviate and prevent human suffering caused by illness and injury." Such biomedical research is a collective effort. Some of the recommendations apply to basic research and clinical translation efforts, while others address challenges unique to stem cell-based research. These challenges include the vulnerability and pressing medical needs of patients with serious illnesses who currently lack effective treatments, as well as public expectations about medical advances and access. To ensure the validity of informed consent in early-phase stem cell trials, several measures have been recommended, including involving an independent individual in the consent process, clearly communicating the low likelihood of therapeutic benefit, assessing participants' comprehension before enrollment, implementing a cooling-off period between information disclosure and consent, avoiding language that may foster unrealistic therapeutic expectations, and providing supplementary educational materials to support informed decision-making. As appropriately specified, both legislation and guidelines of this type should be periodically revised to adapt to scientific progress and changes in social priorities.

Clinical trials for neurodegenerative diseases are now being conducted using stem cells. These trials may include the first human intracerebral transplantation of cells, including hESCs and iPSCs. Several publications have pointed out that when using PST-based therapy, especially when the target is the brain, the risks of early clinical trials are increased. This is because any adverse effects could potentially affect the cognitive functions of the patients. Getting proper informed consent from patients with cognitive impairments may be more challenging. Gene and cell therapies are approved under independent legal and regulatory systems in Europe and the US. However, the rapid evolution of these advanced therapies creates issues for both regulatory systems, which must constantly change through ongoing communication with all stakeholders involved. In the US, biological drug products, including cellular therapy products, human gene therapy products, and certain devices related to cell and gene therapy, are subject to pre-market approval by the US Food and Drug Administration (FDA). In 2015, the FDA's Center for Biologics Evaluation and Research (CBER), which specifically regulates cellular and human gene therapy products, provided guidance to assist sponsors and investigators in designing early-phase clinical trials for cellular therapy (CT) and gene therapy (GT) products, collectively referred to as CGT products. This guidance includes recommendations for clinical trials focused on initial assessments of safety, tolerability, or feasibility of administering the investigational products. It highlights aspects of early-phase clinical trial design that differ for CGT products compared to other types of products and stresses the need for a case-by-case approach in designing each trial. Furthermore, in 2018, the CBER released specific gene therapy guidelines tailored for certain classes of diseases, such as rare diseases and hemophilia (de Melo-Martín et al., 2015; Chapman, 2015; Collins

& Gottlieb, 2018; Complex Innovative Trial Design, 2025; Research CFBEA, 2025; Research CFBEA, 2020).

15.8 Conclusion

The future of PD management lies in a multidisciplinary approach, integrating innovative science with patient-centered care. Continued innovation in pharmacotherapy, combined with advances in precision medicine and drug delivery technologies, holds the promise of not just alleviating symptoms but ultimately slowing or halting disease progression. Collaborative efforts among researchers, clinicians, regulators, and patients will be essential to translate these scientific breakthroughs into real-world therapies, offering hope for a better quality of life for individuals living with PD.

References

Abbruzzese, G., Barone, P., Bonuccelli, U., Lopiano, L., & Antonini, A. (2012). Continuous intestinal infusion of levodopa/carbidopa in advanced Parkinson's disease: Efficacy, safety and patient selection. *Functional Neurology, 27*(3), 147–154.

Abdelkader, N. F., Safar, M. M., & Salem, H. A. (2016). Ursodeoxycholic acid ameliorates apoptotic Cascade in the rotenone model of parkinson's disease: Modulation of mitochondrial perturbations. *Molecular Neurobiology, 53*(2).

Aguti, S., Cheng, S., Ala, P., Briggs, S., Muntoni, F., & Zhou, H. (2024). Strategies to improve the design of gapmer antisense oligonucleotide on allele-specific silencing. *Mol Ther Nucleic Acids, 35*(3), Article 102237.

Al-Hajaj, N., Khalil, R., & Husseini, G. A. (2025). Intranasal drug delivery: Pathways, challenges, and advancements in CNS targeting. *Journal of Drug Delivery Science and Technology, 107*, Article 106825.

Antonini, A., Odin, P., Pahwa, R., Aldred, J., Alobaidi, A., Jalundhwala, Y. J., et al. (2021). The long-term impact of Levodopa/Carbidopa intestinal gel on 'Off'-time in patients with advanced parkinson's disease: A systematic review. *Advances in Therapy, 38*.

Antonini, A., Poewe, W., Chaudhuri, K. R., Jech, R., Pickut, B., Pirtošek, Z., et al. (2017). Levodopa-carbidopa intestinal gel in advanced Parkinson's: Final results of the GLORIA registry. *Parkinsonism Relat Disord, 45*.

Antoniou, A., Stavrou, M., Evripidou, N., Georgiou, E., Kousiappa, I., Koupparis, A., et al. (2024). FUS-mediated blood–brain barrier disruption for delivering anti-Aβ antibodies in 5XFAD Alzheimer's disease mice. *Journal of Ultrasound, 27*(2).

Apostolova, I., Lange, C., Frings, L., Klutmann, S., Meyer, P. T., & Buchert, R. (2020). Nigrostriatal degeneration in the cognitive part of the striatum in parkinson disease is associated with frontomedial hypometabolism. *Clinical Nuclear Medicine, 45*(2).

Araújo, B., Caridade-Silva, R., Soares-Guedes, C., Martins-Macedo, J., Gomes, E. D., Monteiro, S., et al. (2022). Neuroinflammation and parkinson's Disease—From neurodegeneration to therapeutic opportunities. *Cells, 11*.

Artusi, C. A., Mishra, M., Latimer, P., Vizcarra, J. A., Lopiano, L., Maetzler, W., et al. (2018). Integration of technology-based outcome measures in clinical trials of Parkinson and other neurodegenerative diseases. *Parkinsonism Relat Disord, 46*.

Athauda, D., Evans, J., Wernick, A., Virdi, G., Choi, M. L., Lawton, M., et al. (2022). The impact of type 2 diabetes in parkinson's disease. *Movement Disorders, 37*(8).

Athauda, D., Maclagan, K., Skene, S. S., Bajwa-Joseph, M., Letchford, D., Chowdhury, K., et al. (2017). Exenatide once weekly versus placebo in Parkinson's disease: A randomised, double-blind, placebo-controlled trial. *The Lancet, 390*(10103), 1664–1675.

Aviles-Olmos, I., Dickson, J., Kefalopoulou, Z., Djamshidian, A., Ell, P., Soderlund, T., et al. (2013). Exenatide and the treatment of patients with Parkinson's disease. *Journal of Clinical Investigation, 123*(6), 2730–2736.

Bae, E. J., Lee, H. J., Rockenstein, E., Ho, D. H., Park, E. B., Yang, N. Y., et al. (2012). Antibody-aided clearance of extracellular α-synuclein prevents cell-to-cell aggregate transmission. *Journal of Neuroscience, 32*(39).

Bagetta, V., Ghiglieri, V., Sgobio, C., Calabresi, P., & Picconi, B. (2010). Synaptic dysfunction in Parkinson's disease. *Biochemical Society Transactions, 38*(2), 493–497.

Bai, X., Zhu, J., Chen, Y., & Sun, H. (2025). The design and development of LRRK2 inhibitors as novel therapeutics for Parkinson's disease. *Future Medicinal Chemistry, 17*(2), 221–236.

Balestrino, R., & Schapira, A. H. V. (2020). Parkinson disease. *European Journal of Neurology, 27.*

Bassil, F., Delamarre, A., Canron, M. H., Dutheil, N., Vital, A., Négrier-Leibreich, M. L., et al. (2022). Impaired brain insulin signalling in Parkinson's disease. *Neuropathology and Applied Neurobiology, 48*(1).

Batzu L, Qamar MA, Leta V, Mhapankar K, Poplawska-Domaszewicz K, Chaudhuri KR. 2.4 Continuous dopaminergic stimulation and nonmotor symptoms of Parkinson's. 2023.

Bellotti, E., Schilling, A. L., Little, S. R., & Decuzzi, P. (2021). Injectable thermoresponsive hydrogels as drug delivery system for the treatment of central nervous system disorders: A review. *Journal of Controlled Release, 329.*

Berven, H., Kverneng, S., Sheard, E., Søgnen, M., Af Geijerstam, S. A., Haugarvoll, K., et al. (2023). NR-SAFE: A randomized, double-blind safety trial of high dose nicotinamide riboside in Parkinson's disease. *Nature Communications, 14*(1).

Bialecka, M., Klodowska-Duda, G., Honczarenko, K., Gawrońska-Szklarz, B., Opala, G., Safranow, K., et al. (2007). Polymorphisms of catechol-0-methyltransferase (COMT), monoamine oxidase B (MAOB), N-acetyltransferase 2 (NAT2) and cytochrome P450 2D6 (CYP2D6) gene in patients with early onset of Parkinson's disease. *Parkinsonism Relat Disord, 13*(4).

Blaschke, T., Arús-Pous, J., Chen, H., Margreitter, C., Tyrchan, C., Engkvist, O., et al. (2020). REINVENT 2.0: An AI Tool for de Novo Drug Design. *Journal of Chemical Information and Modeling, 60*(12).

Bonaz, B. (2024). The gut-brain axis in Parkinson's disease. *Revue Neurologique, 180*(1–2), 65–78.

Boppana, S. H., Kutikuppala, L. V. S., Sharma, S., Madhavrao, C., Rangari, G., Misra, A. K., et al. (2024). Current approaches in smart nano-inspired drug delivery: A narrative review. *Health Science Reports, 7*(4).

Braga, C. A., Follmer, C., Palhano, F. L., Khattar, E., Freitas, M. S., Romão, L., et al. (2011). The anti-parkinsonian drug selegiline delays the nucleation phase of α-synuclein aggregation leading to the formation of nontoxic species. *Journal of Molecular Biology, 405*(1).

Brakedal, B., Dölle, C., Riemer, F., Ma, Y., Nido, G. S., Skeie, G. O., et al. (2022). The NADPARK study: A randomized phase I trial of nicotinamide riboside supplementation in Parkinson's disease. *Cell Metabolism, 34*(3).

Brumm, M. C., Siderowf, A., Simuni, T., Burghardt, E., Choi, S. H., Caspell-Garcia, C., et al. (2023). Parkinson's progression markers initiative: A milestone-based strategy to monitor parkinson's disease progression. *Journal of Parkinson's Disease, 13*(6).

Burgess, A., Shah, K., Hough, O., & Hynynen, K. (2015). Focused ultrasound-mediated drug delivery through the blood-brain barrier. *Expert Review of Neurotherapeutics, 15.*

Buur, L., Wiedemann, J., Larsen, F., Ben Alaya-Fourati, F., Kallunki, P., Ditlevsen, D. K., et al. (2024). Randomized phase I trial of the α-Synuclein antibody Lu AF82422. *Movement Disorders, 39*(6), 936–944.

Cabreira, V., & Massano, J. (2019). Parkinson's disease: Clinical review and update. *Acta Med Port, 32*(10).

Cacabelos R, Naidoo V, Martínez-Iglesias O, Corzo L, Cacabelos N, Pego R, et al. Pharmacogenomics of Alzheimer's Disease: Novel Strategies for Drug Utilization and Development. In: Methods in Molecular Biology. 2022.

Cacabelos, R., & Torrellas, C. (2014). Epigenetic drug discovery for Alzheimer's disease. *Expert Opinion on Drug Discovery, 9.*

Cacabelos, R., Torrellas, C., Teijido, O., & Carril, J. C. (2016). Pharmacogenetic considerations in the treatment of Alzheimer's disease. *Pharmacogenomics, 17.*

Cerri, S., Mus, L., & Blandini, F. (2019). Parkinson's disease in women and men: What's the difference? *Journal of Parkinson's Disease, 9.*

Chapman, A. R. (2015). Refining Ethical Guidelines for early clinical trials of pluripotent stem-cell-derived therapeutics for parkinson's disease. *AJOB Neurosci, 6*(1), 65–66.

Chen, K. T., Wei, K. C., & Liu, H. L. (2021). Focused ultrasound combined with microbubbles in central nervous system applications. *Pharmaceutics, 13*(7).

Collins, F. S., & Gottlieb, S. (2018). The next phase of human gene-therapy oversight. *New England Journal of Medicine, 379*(15), 1393–1395.

Complex Innovative Trial Design - Emerging Approaches Internet. 2025. https://www.medidata.com/en/complex-trial-design-approaches/?qgad=710874935207&qgterm=clinical%20trial%20design%20and%20protocol&gad_source=1&gad_campaignid=21622932212&gclid=CjwKCAjw6ZTCBhBOEiwAqfwJd2CXT5APkqn5nPjSRgMfERegJxCNM6yyYnkH3Rc0PLh0ohxieVoZCRoCSBcQAvD_BwE.

Cook, L., Schulze, J., Naito, A., & Alcalay, R. N. (2021). The role of genetic testing for parkinson's disease. *Current Neurology and Neuroscience Reports, 21.*

Cullinane, P. W., de Pablo Fernandez, E., König, A., Outeiro, T. F., Jaunmuktane, Z., & Warner, T. T. (2023). Type 2 diabetes and parkinson's disease: A focused review of Current concepts. *Movement Disorders, 38.*

Cyranoski, D. (2017). Japanese man is first to receive "reprogrammed" stem cells from another person. *Nature.*

Dash, B. K., Urano, Y., & Noguchi, N. (2024). Lysosomal damage promotes autophagy-based unconventional secretion of the Parkinson's disease protein PARK7. *Redox Experimental Medicine., 2024*(1).

de Melo-Martín, I., Hellmers, N., & Henchcliffe, C. (2015). First-in-human cell transplant trials in Parkinson's disease: The need for an improved informed consent process. *Parkinsonism Relat Disord, 21*(8), 829–832.

Dederer, V., Sanz Murillo, M., Karasmanis, E. P., Hatch, K. S., Chatterjee, D., Preuss, F., et al. (2024). A designed ankyrin-repeat protein that targets Parkinson's disease-associated LRRK2. *Journal of Biological Chemistry, 300*(7), Article 107469.

Di Giovanni, S., Eleuteri, S., Paleologou, K. E., Yin, G., Zweckstetter, M., Carrupt, P. A., et al. (2010). Entacapone and tolcapone, two catechol O-methyltransferase inhibitors, block fibril formation of α-synuclein and β-amyloid and protect against amyloid-induced toxicity. *Journal of Biological Chemistry, 285*(20).

Dorsey, E. R., Papapetropoulos, S., Xiong, M., & Kieburtz, K. (2017). The first frontier: Digital biomarkers for neurodegenerative disorders. *Digital Biomarkers, 1.*

Dotiwala AK, McCausland C, Samra NS. Anatomy, head and neck: Blood brain barrier. 2025.

Du, S., Wen, Z., Yu, J., Meng, Y., Liu, Y., & Xia, X. (2024). Breath and beyond: Advances in nanomedicine for oral and intranasal aerosol drug delivery. *Pharmaceuticals, 17*(12), 1742.

Ebedes, D., & Borlongan, C. V. (2024). Going straight for the gut: Gut-brain axis pathology and treatment of Parkinson's disease. *Neural Regeneration Research, 19*(10), 2111–2112.

Egunlusi, A. O., Malan, S. F., Palchykov, V. A., & Joubert, J. (2024). Calcium modulating effect of polycyclic cages: A suitable therapeutic approach against excitotoxic-induced neurodegeneration. *Mini-Reviews in Medicinal Chemistry, 24*(13), 1277–1292.

Eijsvogel, P., Misra, P., Concha-Marambio, L., Boyd, J. D., Ding, S., Fedor, L., et al. (2024). Target engagement and immunogenicity of an active immunotherapeutic targeting pathological α-synuclein: A phase 1 placebo-controlled trial. *Nature Medicine, 30*(9), 2631–2640.

Elahi, D., Angeli, F. S., Vakilipour, A., Carlson, O. D., Tomas, E., Egan, J. M., et al. (2014). GLP-1(32–36)amide, a novel pentapeptide cleavage product of GLP-1, modulates whole body glucose metabolism in dogs. *Peptides (NY), 59*, 20–24.

Elumalai, K., Srinivasan, S., & Shanmugam, A. (2024). Review of the efficacy of nanoparticle-based drug delivery systems for cancer treatment. *Biomedical Technology, 5*.

Emre, M., Tsolaki, M., Bonuccelli, U., Destée, A., Tolosa, E., Kutzelnigg, A., et al. (2010). Memantine for patients with Parkinson's disease dementia or dementia with Lewy bodies: A randomised, double-blind, placebo-controlled trial. *Lancet Neurol, 9*(10), 969–977.

Evans, A. H., Kettlewell, J., McGregor, S., Kotschet, K., Griffiths, R. I., & Horne, M. (2014). A conditioned response as a measure of impulsive-compulsive behaviours in Parkinson's disease. *PLoS One, 9*(2).

Ezquerra, M., Martí, M. J., & Fernández-Santiago, R. (2019). Parkinson's disease as a systemic pathology. *Aging, 11*(4), 1081–1082.

Fereshtehnejad, S. M., Zeighami, Y., Dagher, A., & Postuma, R. B. (2017). Clinical criteria for subtyping Parkinson's disease: Biomarkers and longitudinal progression. *Brain, 140*(7).

Fernandez, H. H., Standaert, D. G., Hauser, R. A., Lang, A. E., Fung, V. S. C., Klostermann, F., et al. (2015). Levodopa-carbidopa intestinal gel in advanced Parkinson's disease: Final 12-month, open-label results. *Movement Disorders, 30*(4).

Fernandez, H. H., Vanagunas, A., Odin, P., Espay, A. J., Hauser, R. A., Standaert, D. G., et al. (2013). Levodopa-carbidopa intestinal gel in advanced Parkinson's disease open-label study: Interim results. *Parkinsonism Relat Disord, 19*(3).

Ferreira, D. G., Batalha, V. L., Miranda, H. V., Coelho, J. E., Gomes, R., Gonçalves, F. Q., et al. (2017). Adenosine A2A receptors modulate α-synuclein aggregation and toxicity. *Cerebral Cortex, 27*(1).

Fung, V. S. C., Aldred, J., Arroyo, M. P., Bergquist, F., Boon, A. J. W., Bouchard, M., et al. (2024). Continuous subcutaneous foslevodopa/foscarbidopa infusion for the treatment of motor fluctuations in Parkinson's disease: Considerations for initiation and maintenance. *Clinical Parkinsonism and Related Disorders, 10*.

Gültekin, H. E., Tort, S., & Acartürk, F. (2022). Fabrication of three dimensional printed tablets in flexible doses: A comprehensive study from design to evaluation. *Journal of Drug Delivery Science and Technology, 74*, Article 103538.

Gaare, J. J., Dölle, C., Brakedal, B., Brügger, K., Haugarvoll, K., Nido, G. S., et al. (2023). Nicotinamide riboside supplementation is not associated with altered methylation homeostasis in Parkinson's disease. *iScience, 26* (3).

Gandhi KR, Saadabadi A. Levodopa (L-Dopa) Internet. 2023.

Gaurav, R., Yahia-Cherif, L., Pyatigorskaya, N., Mangone, G., Biondetti, E., Valabrègue, R., et al. (2021). Longitudinal changes in neuromelanin MRI signal in parkinson's disease: A progression marker. *Movement Disorders, 36*(7).

Gautam, N., Das, S., Kar Mahapatra, S., Chakraborty, S. P., Kundu, P. K., & Roy, S. (2010). Age associated oxidative damage in lymphocytes. *Oxidative Medicine and Cellular Longevity, 3*(4).

Glenardi, G., Handayani, T., Barus, J., & Mangkuliguna, G. (2022). Inhaled levodopa (CVT-301) for the treatment of parkinson disease: A systematic review and meta-analysis of randomized controlled trials. *Neurology. Clinical Practice, 12*.

Goudra, B., Merli, G. J., & Green, M. (2024). Glucose-Lowering agents developed in the last two decades and their perioperative implications. *Pharmaceuticals, 18*(1), 4.

Granek, Z., Barczuk, J., Siwecka, N., Rozpędek-Kamińska, W., Kucharska, E., & Majsterek, I. (2023). GBA1 gene mutations in α-Synucleinopathies—Molecular mechanisms underlying pathology and their clinical significance. *International Journal of Molecular Sciences, 24*(3), 2044.

Green, H., Tsitsi, P., Markaki, I., Aarsland, D., & Svenningsson, P. (2019). Novel treatment opportunities against cognitive impairment in parkinson's disease with an emphasis on diabetes-related pathways. *CNS Drugs, 33* (2), 143–160.

Guo, J. D., Zhao, X., Li, Y., Li, G. R., & Liu, X. L. (2018). Damage to dopaminergic neurons by oxidative stress in Parkinson's disease (Review). *International Journal of Molecular Medicine, 41*.

Guttuso, T., Shepherd, R., Frick, L., Feltri, M. L., Frerichs, V., Ramanathan, M., et al. (2023). Lithium's effects on therapeutic targets and MRI biomarkers in Parkinson's disease: A pilot clinical trial. *IBRO Neurosci Rep, 14*.

Hölscher, C. (2018). Novel dual GLP-1/GIP receptor agonists show neuroprotective effects in Alzheimer's and Parkinson's disease models. *Neuropharmacology, 136*, 251–259.

Hadi, F., Agah, E., Tavanbakhsh, S., Mirsepassi, Z., Mousavi, S. V., Talachi, N., et al. (2022). Safety and efficacy of melatonin, clonazepam, and trazodone in patients with Parkinson's disease and sleep disorders: A randomized, double-blind trial. *Neurological Sciences, 43*(10).

Haney, M. J., Klyachko, N. L., Zhao, Y., Gupta, R., Plotnikova, E. G., He, Z., et al. (2015). Exosomes as drug delivery vehicles for Parkinson's disease therapy. *Journal of Controlled Release*, 207.

Haqqani, A. S., Bélanger, K., & Stanimirovic, D. B. (2024). Receptor-mediated transcytosis for brain delivery of therapeutics: Receptor classes and criteria. *Frontiers in Drug Delivery, 4*.

Harkavyi, A., Abuirmeileh, A., Lever, R., Kingsbury, A. E., Biggs, C. S., & Whitton, P. S. (2008). Glucagon-like peptide 1 receptor stimulation reverses key deficits in distinct rodent models of Parkinson's disease. *Journal of Neuroinflammation, 5*(1), 19.

Harrison, I. F., & Dexter, D. T. (2013). Epigenetic targeting of histone deacetylase: Therapeutic potential in Parkinson's disease? *Pharmacology & Therapeutics, 140*(1), 34–52.

Hasselgren, C., & Oprea, T. I. (2024). Artificial intelligence for drug discovery: Are we there yet? Vol. 64. *Annual Review of Pharmacology and Toxicology*, 527–550.

Hauser, R. A., Isaacson, S. H., Ellenbogen, A., Safirstein, B. E., Truong, D. D., Komjathy, S. F., et al. (2019). Orally inhaled levodopa (CVT-301) for early morning OFF periods in Parkinson's disease. *Parkinsonism Relat Disord, 64*.

Hayes, M. T. (2019). Parkinson's disease and parkinsonism. *The American Journal of Medicine, 132*.

He, Y., Huang, L., Wang, K., Pan, X., Cai, Q., Zhang, F., et al. (2022). α-Synuclein selectively Impairs Motor Sequence learning and value sensitivity: Reversal by the adenosine A2AReceptor antagonists. *Cerebral Cortex, 32*(4).

Helmschrodt, C., Höbel, S., Schöniger, S., Bauer, A., Bonicelli, J., Gringmuth, M., et al. (2017). Polyethylenimine nanoparticle-mediated siRNA delivery to reduce α-Synuclein expression in a model of parkinson's disease. *Mol Ther Nucleic Acids, 9*, 57–68.

Hersh, A. M., Alomari, S., & Tyler, B. M. (2022). Crossing the blood-brain barrier: Advances in nanoparticle technology for drug delivery in Neuro-Oncology. *International Journal of Molecular Sciences, 23*(8).

Hickey KL, Panov A, Whelan EM, Schäfer T, Mizrak A, Kopito RR, et al. Temporal control of acute protein aggregate turnover by UBE3C and NRF1-dependent proteasomal pathways. 2024.

Homayoun, H. (2018). Parkinson disease. *Annals of Internal Medicine, 169*(5).

Hu, F., Zhang, S., Wang, C., Zhou, H., & Shi, H. (2022). The safety and effectiveness of α-synuclein immunotherapy vs. placebo for the treatment of Parkinson's disease: A systematic review and meta-analysis. *Annals of Palliative Medicine, 11*(12).

Huang, M., Lou, D., Charli, A., Kong, D., Huajun, J., Zenitsky, G., et al. (2021). Mitochondrial dysfunction-induced H3K27 hyperacetylation perturbs enhancers in Parkinson's disease. *JCI Insight, 6*(17).

Hwang, J. Y., Won, J. S., Nam, H., Lee, H. W., & Joo, K. M. (2018). Current advances in combining stem cell and gene therapy for neurodegenerative diseases. *Precision and Future Medicine, 2*(2).

Jankovic, J., & Tan, E. K. (2020). Parkinson's disease: Etiopathogenesis and treatment. *Journal of Neurology Neurosurgery and Psychiatry, 91*(8).

Jeong, S. H., & Lee, P. H. (2025). Drug repositioning and repurposing for disease-modifying effects in parkinson's disease. *J Mov Disord, 18*(2), 113–126.

Jerčić, K. G., Blažeković, A., Borovečki, S., & Borovečki, F. (2024). Non-motor symptoms of parkinson's disease-insights from genetics. *Journal of Neural Transmission, 131*(11), 1277–1284.

Jia, X., Wang, Q., Liu, M., & Ding, J. Y. (2024). The interplay between gut microbiota and the brain-gut axis in Parkinson's disease treatment. *Frontiers in Neurology*, 15.

Jiménez-Delgado, A., Ortiz, G. G., Delgado-Lara, D. L., González-Usigli, H. A., González-Ortiz, L. J., Cid-Hernández, M., et al. (2021). Effect of Melatonin Administration on mitochondrial activity and oxidative stress markers in patients with parkinson's disease. *Oxidative Medicine and Cellular Longevity, 2021.*

Jiménez-Jiménez, F. J., Alonso-Navarro, H., García-Martín, E., Santos-García, D., Martínez-Valbuena, I., & Agúndez, J. A. G. (2023). Alpha-Synuclein in peripheral tissues as a possible marker for neurological diseases and other medical conditions. *Biomolecules, 13.*

Jones, A. R., & Shusta, E. V. (2007). Blood-brain barrier transport of therapeutics via receptor-mediation. *Pharmaceutical Research, 24.*

Jung, J., Lee, Y., Moon, A. N., Ann, J., Jeong, J. J., Do, N., et al. (2022). Discovery of novel dual adenosine A2A and A1 receptor antagonists with 1H-Pyrazolo[3,4-d]pyrimidin-6-amine core scaffold as anti-parkinson's disease agents. *Pharmaceuticals, 15*(8), 922.

Katzenschlager, R., Poewe, W., Rascol, O., Trenkwalder, C., Deuschl, G., Chaudhuri, K. R., et al. (2018). Apomorphine subcutaneous infusion in patients with Parkinson's disease with persistent motor fluctuations (TOLEDO): A multicentre, double-blind, randomised, placebo-controlled trial. *Lancet Neurol, 17*(9).

Kawashima, S., Shimizu, Y., Horiba, M., Ueki, Y., Akanabe, R., Kan, H., et al. (2022). Memantine for the patients with mild cognitive impairment in Parkinson's disease: A pharmacological fMRI study. *BMC Neurology, 22* (1).

Keerie, A., Brown-Wright, H., Kirkland, I., Grierson, A., Alix, J. J. P., Holscher, C., et al. (2021). The GLP-1 receptor agonist, liraglutide, fails to slow disease progression in SOD1G93A and TDP-43Q331K transgenic mouse models of ALS. *Scientific Reports, 11*(1), Article 17027.

Kim, K., Wi, S., Seo, J. H., Pyo, S., & Cho, S. R. (2021). Reduced interaction of aggregated α-Synuclein and VAMP2 by environmental enrichment alleviates hyperactivity and anxiety in a model of parkinson's disease. *Genes, 12*(3), 392.

Kirkeby, A., Nelander, J., Hoban, D. B., Rogelius, N., Bjartmarz, H., Storm, P., et al. (2023). Preclinical quality, safety, and efficacy of a human embryonic stem cell-derived product for the treatment of Parkinson's disease. *STEM-PD. Cell Stem Cell, 30*(10).

Kollaparampil Kishanchand, D., A. Ak, K., Chandrababu, K., Philips, C. A., Sivan, U., & Pulikaparambil Sasidharan, B. C. (2025). The intricate interplay: Microbial metabolites and the gut-liver-brain axis in parkinson's disease. *Journal of Neuroscience Research, 103*(1).

Koros, C., Bougea, A., Alefanti, I., Simitsi, A. M., Papagiannakis, N., Pachi, I., et al. (2024). A global perspective of GBA1-Related parkinson's disease: A narrative review. *Genes, 15*(12), 1605.

Koszła, O., & Sołek, P. (2024). Misfolding and aggregation in neurodegenerative diseases: Protein quality control machinery as potential therapeutic clearance pathways. *Cell Communication and Signaling, 22*(1), 421.

Kraus, F., He, Y., Swarup, S., Overmyer, K. A., Jiang, Y., Brenner, J., et al. (2025). Global cellular proteo-lipidomic profiling of diverse lysosomal storage disease mutants using nMOST. *Science Advances, 11*(4).

Lagreca, E., Onesto, V., Di Natale, C., La Manna, S., Netti, P. A., & Vecchione, R. (2020). Recent advances in the formulation of PLGA microparticles for controlled drug delivery. *Progress in Biomaterials, 9.*

Lai, K. L., Fang, Y., Han, H., Li, Q., Zhang, S., Li, H. Y., et al. (2018). Orally-dissolving film for sublingual and buccal delivery of ropinirole. *Colloids and Surfaces B: Biointerfaces, 163.*

Lajoie, J. M., & Shusta, E. V. (2015). Targeting receptor-mediated transport for delivery of biologics across the blood-brain barrier. *Annual Review of Pharmacology and Toxicology, 55.*

Laversin, A., Dufossez, R., Bolteau, R., Duroux, R., Ravez, S., Hernandez-Tapia, S., et al. (2024). Novel quinazoline derivatives as highly effective A2A adenosine receptor antagonists. *Molecules, 29*(16), 3847.

Lee, J. E., Kim, H. N., Kim, D. Y., Shin, Y. J., Shin, J. Y., & Lee, P. H. (2021). Memantine exerts neuroprotective effects by modulating α-synuclein transmission in a parkinsonian model. *Experimental Neurology, 344.*

Lee, J. S., & Lee, S. J. (2016). Mechanism of Anti-α-Synuclein immunotherapy. *J Mov Disord., 9*(1).

Lewis, J., Melrose, H., Bumcrot, D., Hope, A., Zehr, C., Lincoln, S., et al. (2008). In vivo silencing of alpha-synuclein using naked siRNA. *Molecular Neurodegeneration, 3*(1), 19.

Li, M., Chen, H., & Zhu, M. (2022). Mesenchymal stem cells for regenerative medicine in central nervous system. *Frontiers in Neuroscience, 16*.

Li, S., Liu, Y., Lu, S., Xu, J., Liu, X., Yang, D., et al. (2025). A crazy trio in Parkinson's disease: Metabolism alteration, α-synuclein aggregation, and oxidative stress. *Molecular and Cellular Biochemistry, 480*(1), 139–157.

Li, J., Wang, J., & Chen, Z. (2025). Emerging role of exosomes in cancer therapy: Progress and challenges. *Molecular Cancer, 24*(1), 13.

Lin, S. C., Chang, C. C., Tsou, S. H., Chiu, P. Y., Cheng, J. F., Hung, H. C., et al. (2024). Protective effects of ambroxol on Aβ and α-Synuclein-Induced neurotoxicity through glucocerebrosidase activation in HT-22 Hippocampal neuronal cells. *International Journal of Molecular Sciences, 25*(22), Article 12114.

Liu, Z., Cheng, L., Cao, W., Shen, C., Qiu, Y., Li, C., et al. (2024). Present and future use of exosomes containing proteins and RNAs in neurodegenerative diseases for synaptic function regulation: A comprehensive review. *International Journal of Biological Macromolecules, 280*, Article 135826.

Liu, D., Li, T., Liu, L., Che, X., Li, X., Liu, C., et al. (2024). Adeno-associated virus therapies: Pioneering solutions for human genetic diseases. *Cytokine & Growth Factor Reviews, 80*, 109–120.

Liu, Y. Z., Tang, B. S., Yan, X. X., Liu, J., Ouyang, D. S., Nie, L. N., et al. (2009). Association of the DRD2 and DRD3 polymorphisms with response to pramipexole in Parkinson's disease patients. *European Journal of Clinical Pharmacology, 65*(7).

Luo, F., Ye, M., Lv, T., Hu, B., Chen, J., Yan, J., et al. (2021). Efficacy of cognitive behavioral therapy on mood disorders, sleep, fatigue, and quality of life in parkinson's disease: A systematic review and meta-analysis. *Front Psychiatry, 12*.

Müller, T. (2020). Pharmacokinetics and pharmacodynamics of levodopa/carbidopa cotherapies for Parkinson's disease. *Expert Opinion on Drug Metabolism and Toxicology, 16*.

Madadi, A. M., Asadi, A., Enayati, J., & Valizadeh, A. (2022). Inhibitory spike-timing-dependent plasticity can account for pathological strengthening of Pallido-Subthalamic synapses in parkinson's disease. *Frontiers in Physiology, 19*, 13.

Maiti, P., Manna, J., Dunbar, G. L., Maiti, P., & Dunbar, G. L. (2017). Current understanding of the molecular mechanisms in Parkinson's disease: Targets for potential treatments. *Translational Neurodegeneration, 6*.

Malatt, C., Wu, T., Bresee, C., Hogg, E., Wertheimer, J., Tan, E., et al. (2022). Liraglutide improves non-motor function and activities of daily living in patients with parkinson's disease: A randomized, Double-Blind, placebo-controlled trial (P9-11.005). *Neurology, 98*(18_Suppl. ment).

Maniscalchi, A., Benzi Juncos, O. N., Conde, M. A., Funk, M. I., Fermento, M. E., Facchinetti, M. M., et al. (2024). New insights on neurodegeneration triggered by iron accumulation: Intersections with neutral lipid metabolism, ferroptosis, and motor impairment. *Redox Biology, 71*, Article 103074.

Mao, Q., Luo, Z., Wang, K., Chen, B., Wang, Z., Zhang, Y., et al. (2024). Modifications on histone tails in Parkinson's disease. *SciBase neurology, 2*(2).

Marras, C., Chaudhuri, K. R., Titova, N., & Mestre, T. A. (2020). Therapy of parkinson's disease subtypes. *Neurotherapeutics, 17*.

Masliah, E., Rockenstein, E., Adame, A., Alford, M., Crews, L., Hashimoto, M., et al. (2005). Effects of α-synuclein immunization in a mouse model of Parkinson's disease. *Neuron, 46*(6).

Masliah, E., Rockenstein, E., Mante, M., Crews, L., Spencer, B., Adame, A., et al. (2011). Passive immunization reduces behavioral and neuropathological deficits in an alpha-synuclein transgenic model of lewy body disease. *PLoS One, 6*(4).

McFarthing, K., Buff, S., Rafaloff, G., Pitzer, K., Fiske, B., Navangul, A., et al. (2024). Parkinson's disease drug therapies in the clinical trial pipeline: 2024 update. *Journal of Parkinson's Disease, 14*(5), 899–912.

McGarry, A., Rosanbalm, S., Leinonen, M., Olanow, C. W., To, D., Bell, A., et al. (2024). Safety, tolerability, and efficacy of NLY01 in early untreated Parkinson's disease: A randomised, double-blind, placebo-controlled trial. *Lancet Neurol, 23*(1), 37–45.

Meissner, W. G., Remy, P., Giordana, C., Maltête, D., Derkinderen, P., Houéto, J. L., et al. (2024). Trial of lixisenatide in early parkinson's disease. *New England Journal of Medicine, 390*(13), 1176–1185.

Miller, D. B., & O'Callaghan, J. P. (2015). Biomarkers of Parkinson's disease: Present and future. *Metabolism, 64* (3).

Mitchell, T., Lehéricy, S., Chiu, S. Y., Strafella, A. P., Stoessl, A. J., & Vaillancourt, D. E. (2021). Emerging neuroimaging biomarkers across disease stage in parkinson disease: A review. *JAMA Neurology, 78.*

Mogharbel, B. F., Cardoso, M. A., Irioda, A. C., Stricker, P. E. F., Slompo, R. C., Appel, J. M., et al. (2022). Biodegradable nanoparticles loaded with levodopa and curcumin for treatment of parkinson's disease. *Molecules, 27*(9).

Mohammad Soleymani, S., Assarzadegan, F., Habibi, S. A. H., Mahboubi, A., & Esmaily, H. (2024). The effect of crocin on movement disorders and oxidative DNA damage in Parkinson's disease: Insights from a randomized controlled trial. *Parkinsonism Relat Disord, 126*, Article 107051.

Montpeyo, M., Pérez-Carmona, N., Cubero, E., Delgado, A., Ruano, A., Carrillo, J., et al. (2024). Developing allosteric chaperones for GBA1-Associated Disorders—An integrated computational and experimental approach. *International Journal of Molecular Sciences, 26*(1), 9.

Moreau, C., Delval, A., Tiffreau, V., Defebvre, L., Dujardin, K., Duhamel, A., et al. (2013). Memantine for axial signs in Parkinson's disease: A randomised, double-blind, placebo-controlled pilot study. *Journal of Neurology Neurosurgery and Psychiatry, 84*(5).

Moreau, C., Rouaud, T., Grabli, D., Benatru, I., Remy, P., Marques, A. R., et al. (2023). Overview on wearable sensors for the management of Parkinson's disease. *Npj Parkinson's Disease, 9.*

Mullin, S., Smith, L., Lee, K., D'Souza, G., Woodgate, P., Elflein, J., et al. (2020). Ambroxol for the treatment of patients with parkinson disease with and without glucocerebrosidase gene mutations. *JAMA Neurology, 77*(4), 427.

Nakamura, Y., Arawaka, S., Sato, H., Sasaki, A., Shigekiyo, T., Takahata, K., et al. (2021). Monoamine oxidase-B inhibition facilitates α-synuclein secretion in vitro and delays its aggregation in rAAV-based rat models of Parkinson's disease. *Journal of Neuroscience, 41*(35).

Natalello, A., Brocca, S., Ponzini, E., Santambrogio, C., & Grandori, R. (2023). Modulation of Alpha-Synuclein conformational ensemble and aggregation pathways by dopamine and related molecules. *Frontiers in Bioscience - Landmark, 28.*

Ng, T. P., Feng, L., Nyunt, M. S. Z., Feng, L., Niti, M., Tan, B. Y., et al. (2015). Nutritional, physical, cognitive, and combination interventions and frailty reversal among older adults: A randomized controlled trial. *The American Journal of Medicine, 128*(11).

Nguyen, T. T., Dung Nguyen, T. T., Vo, T. K., Tran, N. M. A., Nguyen, M. K., Van Vo, T., et al. (2021). Nanotechnology-based drug delivery for central nervous system disorders. *Biomedicine & Pharmacotherapy, 143.*

Niazi, S. K. (2023). Non-Invasive drug delivery across the blood–brain barrier: A prospective analysis. *Pharmaceutics, 15.*

Nikolcheva, T., Pagano, G., Pross, N., Simuni, T., Marek, K., Postuma, R. B., et al. (2025). A Phase 2b, multicenter, randomized, double-blind, placebo-controlled study to evaluate the efficacy and safety of intravenous prasinezumab in early-stage Parkinson's disease (PADOVA): Rationale, design, and baseline data. *Parkinsonism Relat Disord, 132*, Article 107257.

Ntetsika, T., Papathoma, P. E., & Markaki, I. (2021). Novel targeted therapies for Parkinson's disease. *Molecular Medicine, 27*(1), 17.

Nunes, A. C. L., Carmo, M., Behrenswerth, A., Canas, P. M., Agostinho, P., & Cunha, R. A. (2024). Adenosine A2A receptor blockade provides more effective benefits at the onset rather than after overt neurodegeneration in a rat model of parkinson's disease. *International Journal of Molecular Sciences, 25*(9), 4903.

Nyholm, D., & Lennernäs, H. (2008). Irregular gastrointestinal drug absorption in Parkinson's disease. *Expert Opinion on Drug Metabolism and Toxicology, 4.*

Oey, N. E., Zhou, L., Chan, C. H. S., VanDongen, A. M. J., & Tan, E. K. (2023). A proteome-wide effect of PHF8 knockdown on cortical neurons shows downregulation of parkinson's disease-associated protein Alpha-Synuclein and its interactors. *Biomedicines, 11*(2), 486.

Offit M, Nagle B, Ozay G, Zhang I, Kerasidis A, Torres-Yaghi Y, et al. Adenosine A2A antagonists and Parkinson's disease. In 2023. p. 105–119.

Othman, A. A., & Dutta, S. (2014). Population pharmacokinetics of levodopa in subjects with advanced Parkinson's disease: Levodopa-carbidopa intestinal gel infusion vs. oral tablets. *British Journal of Clinical Pharmacology, 78*(1).

Oz, T., Kaushik, A., & Kujawska, M. (2023). Neural stem cells for Parkinson's disease management: Challenges, nanobased support, and prospects. *World Journal of Stem Cells, 15*(7).

Pagano, G., Monnet, A., Reyes, A., Ribba, B., Svoboda, H., Kustermann, T., et al. (2024). Sustained effect of prasinezumab on Parkinson's disease motor progression in the open-label extension of the PASADENA trial. *Nature Medicine, 30*(12), 3669–3675.

Pantzaris, M., Loukaides, G., Paraskevis, D., Kostaki, E. G., & Patrikios, I. (2021). Neuroaspis PLP10^{TM}, a nutritional formula rich in omega-3 and omega-6 fatty acids with antioxidant vitamins including gamma-tocopherol in early Parkinson's disease: A randomized, double-blind, placebo-controlled trial. *Clinical Neurology and Neurosurgery, 210.*

Pardridge, W. M. (2020). Brain delivery of nanomedicines: Trojan horse liposomes for plasmid DNA gene therapy of the brain. *Front Med Technol, 2.*

Parnetti, L., Gaetani, L., Eusebi, P., Paciotti, S., Hansson, O., El-Agnaf, O., et al. (2019). CSF and blood biomarkers for Parkinson's disease. *The Lancet Neurology, 18.*

Parveen, S., Gupta, P., Kumar, S., & Banerjee, M. (2023). Lipid polymer hybrid nanoparticles as potent vehicles for drug delivery in cancer therapeutics. *Medicine in Drug Discovery, 20.*

Payne, T., Appleby, M., Buckley, E., van Gelder, L. M. A., Mullish, B. H., Sassani, M., et al. (2023). A Double-Blind, randomized, placebo-controlled trial of ursodeoxycholic acid (UDCA) in parkinson's disease. *Movement Disorders, 38*(8).

Peng, H., Han, B., Tong, T., Jin, X., Peng, Y., Guo, M., et al. (2024). 3D printing processes in precise drug delivery for personalized medicine. *Biofabrication, 16*(3), Article 032001.

Pfeiffer, R. F. (2016). Non-motor symptoms in Parkinson's disease. *Parkinsonism Relat Disord, 22.*

Phillips, O., Ghosh, D., & Fernandez, H. H. (2023). Parkinson disease dementia management: An update of Current evidence and future directions. *Current Treatment Options in Neurology, 25*(5), 93–119.

Pingale, T., & Gupta, G. L. (2021). Current and emerging therapeutic targets for Parkinson's disease. *Metabolic Brain Disease, 36.*

Pinnell, J. R., Cui, M., & Tieu, K. (2021). Exosomes in Parkinson disease. *Journal of Neurochemistry, 157*(3), 413–428.

Pirchio, R., Graziadio, C., Colao, A., Pivonello, R., & Auriemma, R. S. (2022). Metabolic effects of prolactin. *Frontiers in Endocrinology, 13.*

Politi, C., Ciccacci, C., Novelli, G., & Borgiani, P. (2018). Genetics and treatment response in parkinson's disease: An update on pharmacogenetic studies. *Neuromolecular Medicine, 20.*

Pons-Faudoa, F. P., Ballerini, A., Sakamoto, J., & Grattoni, A. (2019). Advanced implantable drug delivery technologies: Transforming the clinical landscape of therapeutics for chronic diseases. *Biomedical Microdevices, 21*(2).

Price, D. L., Khan, A., Angers, R., Cardenas, A., Prato, M. K., Bani, M., et al. (2023). In vivo effects of the alpha-synuclein misfolding inhibitor minzasolmin supports clinical development in Parkinson's disease. *npj Parkinson's Disease, 9*(1).

Price, D., Khan, A., Angers, R., Cardenas, A., Prato, M. K., Citron, M., et al. (2022). Preclinical in vivo characterization of UCB0599, an orally available, small molecule inhibitor of α-Synuclein misfolding in development for parkinson's disease (S36.007). *Neurology, 98*(18_Suppl. ment).

Qi, H., Shen, D., Jiang, C., Wang, H., & Chang, M. (2021). Ursodeoxycholic acid protects dopaminergic neurons from oxidative stress via regulating mitochondrial function, autophagy, and apoptosis in MPTP/MPP+-induced Parkinson's disease. *Neuroscience Letters, 741*.

Radad, K., Moldzio, R., Krewenka, C., Kranner, B., & Rausch, W. D. (2023). Pathophysiology of non-motor signs in Parkinson's disease: Some recent updating with brief presentation. *Exploration of Neuroprotective Therapy, 27*, 24–46.

Rana, R., Devi, S. N., Bhardwaj, A. K., Yashavarddhan, M. H., Bohra, D., & Ganguly, N. K. (2025). Exosomes as nature's nano carriers: Promising drug delivery tools and targeted therapy for glioma. *Biomedicine & Pharmacotherapy, 182*, Article 117754.

Rascol, O., & Perez-Lloret, S. (2009). Rotigotine transdermal delivery for the treatment of Parkinson's disease. *Expert Opinion on Pharmacotherapy, 10*.

Research CFBEA. Human gene therapy for retinal disorders Internet. 2020. https://www.fda.gov/regulatory-information/search-fda-guidance-documents/human-gene-therapy-retinal-disorders.

Research CFBEA. Human gene therapy for hemophilia Internet. 2025. https://www.fda.gov/regulatory-information/search-fda-guidance-documents/human-gene-therapy-hemophilia.

Rivas-Santisteban, R., Rico, A. J., Muñoz, A., Rodríguez-Pérez, A. I., Reyes-Resina, I., Navarro, G., et al. (2023). Boolean analysis shows a high proportion of dopamine D2 receptors interacting with adenosine A2A receptors in striatal medium spiny neurons of mouse and non-human primate models of Parkinson's disease. *Neurobiology of Disease, 188*, Article 106341.

Sadat, R. Z., Sina, A. S., Sadat Razavi, F., Souri, M., & Soltani, M. (2025). Advancing neurological disorders therapies: Organic nanoparticles as a key to blood-brain barrier penetration. *International Journal of Pharmacy, 670*, Article 125186.

Saeed, U., Compagnone, J., Aviv, R. I., Strafella, A. P., Black, S. E., Lang, A. E., et al. (2017). Imaging biomarkers in Parkinson's disease and Parkinsonian syndromes: Current and emerging concepts. *Translational Neurodegeneration, 6*.

Saeed, U., Lang, A. E., & Masellis, M. (2020). Neuroimaging advances in parkinson's disease and atypical parkinsonian syndromes. *Frontiers in Neurology, 11*.

Salat, D., & Tolosa, E. (2013). Levodopa in the treatment of Parkinson's disease: Current status and new developments. *Journal of Parkinson's Disease, 3*.

Saravanan, C. R., Eisa, R. F. H., Gaviria, E., Algubari, A., Chandrasekar, K. K., Inban, P., et al. (2024). The efficacy and safety of gene therapy approaches in Parkinson's disease: A systematic review. *Disease-a-Month, 70*(7), Article 101754.

Sarkar, S., Floto, R. A., Berger, Z., Imarisio, S., Cordenier, A., Pasco, M., et al. (2005). Lithium induces autophagy by inhibiting inositol monophosphatase. *Journal of Cell Biology, 170*(7).

Sathe, A. G., Tuite, P., Chen, C., Ma, Y., Chen, W., Cloyd, J., et al. (2020). Pharmacokinetics, safety, and tolerability of orally administered ursodeoxycholic acid in patients with parkinson's Disease—A pilot Study. *Journal of Clinical Pharmacology, 60*(6).

Schiess, M., Suescun, J., Doursout, M. F., Adams, C., Green, C., Saltarrelli, J. G., et al. (2021). Allogeneic bone marrow–derived mesenchymal stem cell safety in idiopathic parkinson's disease. *Movement Disorders, 36*(8).

Schilder, B. M., Navarro, E., & Raj, T. (2022). Multi-omic insights into Parkinson's Disease: From genetic associations to functional mechanisms. *Neurobiology of Disease, 163*.

Schneider, S. A., & Alcalay, R. N. (2020). Precision medicine in Parkinson's disease: Emerging treatments for genetic Parkinson's disease. *Journal of Neurology, 267*.

Schregel, K., Baufeld, C., Palotai, M., Meroni, R., Fiorina, P., Wuerfel, J., et al. (2021). Targeted blood brain barrier opening with focused ultrasound induces focal Macrophage/Microglial activation in Experimental autoimmune encephalomyelitis. *Frontiers in Neuroscience, 15*.

Schroder, K., & Tschopp, J. (2010). The inflammasomes. *Cell, 140*.

Sen, S., Xavier, J., Kumar, N., Ahmad, M. Z., & Ranjan, O. P. (2023). Exosomes as natural nanocarrier-based drug delivery system: Recent insights and future perspectives. *3 Biotech, 13*(3), 101.

Seppi, K., Ray Chaudhuri, K., Coelho, M., Fox, S. H., Katzenschlager, R., Perez, L. S., et al. (2019). Update on treatments for nonmotor symptoms of Parkinson's disease—an evidence-based medicine review. *Movement Disorders, 34.*

Shah, S., Tereda, A., & Mansour, H. M. (2024). Molecular mechanisms of degeneration in parkinson's disease; deep brain stimulation, pluripotent stem cell therapy, and cutting edge technology in treatment of parkinson's disease. *Curr Genet Med Rep, 12*(1–4), 1–19.

Shaheen, N., Shaheen, A., Osama, M., Nashwan, A. J., Bharmauria, V., & Flouty, O. (2024). MicroRNAs regulation in Parkinson's disease, and their potential role as diagnostic and therapeutic targets. *npj Parkinson's Disease, 10*(1), 186.

Siemeling, O., Slingerland, S., van der Zee, S., & van Laar, T. (2024). Study protocol of the GRoningen early-PD Ambroxol treatment (GREAT) trial: A randomized, double-blind, placebo-controlled, single center trial with ambroxol in Parkinson patients with a GBA mutation. *BMC Neurology, 24*(1), 146.

Simuni, T., Chahine, L. M., Poston, K., Brumm, M., Buracchio, T., Campbell, M., et al. (2024). A biological definition of neuronal α-synuclein disease: Towards an integrated staging system for research. *The Lancet Neurology, 23.*

Smit, J. W., Basile, P., Prato, M. K., Detalle, L., Mathy, F. X., Schmidt, A., et al. (2022). Phase 1/1b studies of UCB0599, an oral inhibitor of α-Synuclein misfolding, including a randomized Study in parkinson's disease. *Movement Disorders, 37*(10).

Stoker, T. B., Torsney, K. M., & Barker, R. A. (2018). Emerging treatment approaches for Parkinson's disease. *Frontiers in Neuroscience, 12.*

Stubendorff, K., Larsson, V., Ballard, C., Minthon, L., Aarsland, D., & Londos, E. (2014). Treatment effect of memantine on survival in dementia with lewy bodies and Parkinson's disease with dementia: A prospective study. *BMJ Open, 4*(7).

Sugumaran, R., Sai Krishna, K. S., Saibaba, J., Narayan, S. K., Sandhiya, S., & Rajeswari, M. (2024). Melatonin on sleep in Parkinson's disease: A randomized double blind placebo controlled trial. *Sleep Medicine, 124*, 502–509.

Sun, C., & Armstrong, M. J. (2021). Treatment of parkinson's disease with cognitive impairment: Current approaches and future directions. *Behavioral Sciences, 11*(4), 54.

Surmeier, D. J., Obeso, J. A., & Halliday, G. M. (2017). Selective neuronal vulnerability in Parkinson disease. *Nature Reviews Neuroscience, 18.*

Svenningsson, P., Wirdefeldt, K., Yin, L., Fang, F., Markaki, I., Efendic, S., et al. (2016). Reduced incidence of Parkinson's disease after dipeptidyl peptidase-4 inhibitors—A nationwide case-control study. *Movement Disorders, 31.*

Tambe, P., Undale, V., Sanap, A., Bhonde, R., & Mante, N. (2024). The prospective role of mesenchymal stem cells in Parkinson's disease. *Parkinsonism Relat Disord, 127*, Article 107087.

Tamtaji, O. R., Taghizadeh, M., Aghadavod, E., Mafi, A., Dadgostar, E., Daneshvar Kakhaki, R., et al. (2019). The effects of omega-3 fatty acids and vitamin E co-supplementation on gene expression related to inflammation, insulin and lipid in patients with Parkinson's disease: A randomized, double-blind, placebo-controlled trial. *Clinical Neurology and Neurosurgery, 176.*

Tan, S., Liu, H., & Yao, X. (2024). LRRK2 inhibitors as promising treatment for parkinson's disease. *ACS Chemical Neuroscience, 15*(22), 4092–4094.

Teixeira, M. I., Lopes, C. M., Amaral, M. H., & Costa, P. C. (2023). Surface-modified lipid nanocarriers for crossing the blood-brain barrier (BBB): A current overview of active targeting in brain diseases. *Colloids and Surfaces B: Biointerfaces, 221.*

Tengberg, J. F., Russo, F., Benned-Jensen, T., & Nielsen, J. (2024). LRRK2 and RAB8A regulate cell death after lysosomal damage in macrophages through cholesterol-related pathways. *Neurobiology of Disease, 202*, Article 106728.

Tong, J., Rathitharan, G., Meyer, J. H., Furukawa, Y., Ang, L. C., Boileau, I., et al. (2017). Brain monoamine oxidase B and A in human parkinsonian dopamine deficiency disorders. *Brain, 140*(9).

Tran, H. T., Chung, C. H. Y., Iba, M., Zhang, B., Trojanowski, J. Q., Luk, K. C., et al. (2014). α-Synuclein immunotherapy blocks uptake and templated propagation of misfolded α-Synuclein and neurodegeneration. *Cell Reports, 7*(6).

Trevisan, L., Gaudio, A., Monfrini, E., Avanzino, L., Di Fonzo, A., & Mandich, P. (2024). Genetics in Parkinson's disease, state-of-the-art and future perspectives. *British Medical Bulletin, 149*(1), 60–71.

Upadhyay, R. K. (2014). Drug delivery systems, CNS protection, and the blood brain barrier. *BioMed Research International, 2014*.

van der Meer, F., Jorgensen, J., & Hiligsmann, M. (2025). Burden of non-motor symptoms of Parkinson's disease: Cost-of-illness and quality-of-life estimates through a scoping review. *Expert Review of Pharmacoeconomics & Outcomes Research, 25*(1), 17–27.

van Vliet, E. F., Knol, M. J., Schiffelers, R. M., Caiazzo, M., & Fens, M. H. A. M. (2023). Levodopa-loaded nanoparticles for the treatment of Parkinson's disease. *Journal of Controlled Release, 360*.

Veronese, F. M., & Mero, A. (2008). The impact of PEGylation on biological therapies. *BioDrugs, 22*.

Vijiaratnam, N., Girges, C., Auld, G., McComish, R., King, A., Skene, S. S., et al. (2025). Exenatide once a week versus placebo as a potential disease-modifying treatment for people with Parkinson's disease in the UK: A phase 3, multicentre, double-blind, parallel-group, randomised, placebo-controlled trial. *The Lancet, 405* (10479), 627–636.

Wüllner, U., Kassubek, J., Odin, P., Schwarz, M., Naumann, M., Häck, H. J., et al. (2010). Transdermal rotigotine for the perioperative management of Parkinson's disease. *Journal of Neural Transmission, 117*(7), 855–859.

Waggan, I., Rissanen, E., Tuisku, J., Joutsa, J., Helin, S., Parkkola, R., et al. (2023). Adenosine A2A receptor availability in patients with early- and moderate-stage Parkinson's disease. *Journal of Neurology, 270*(1), 300–310.

Wang, L., Zhao, Z., Zhao, L., Zhao, Y., Yang, G., Wang, C., et al. (2022). Lactobacillus plantarum DP189 reduces α-SYN aggravation in MPTP-Induced parkinson's disease mice via regulating oxidative damage, inflammation, and gut Microbiota disorder. *Journal of Agricultural and Food Chemistry, 70*(4).

Wesnes, K. A., Aarsland, D., Ballard, C., & Londos, E. (2015). Memantine improves attention and episodic memory in Parkinson's disease dementia and dementia with lewy bodies. *International Journal of Geriatric Psychiatry, 30*(1).

Wictorin, K., & Widner, H. (2016). Memantine and reduced time with dyskinesia in Parkinson's Disease. *Acta Neurologica Scandinavica, 133*(5).

Wu, D., Chen, Q., Chen, X., Han, F., Chen, Z., & Wang, Y. (2023). The blood–brain barrier: Structure, regulation, and drug delivery. *Signal Transduction and Targeted Therapy, 8*.

Xiao, Z., Wang, X., Pan, X., Xie, J., & Xu, H. (2024). Mitochondrial iron dyshomeostasis and its potential as a therapeutic target for Parkinson's disease. *Experimental Neurology, 372*, Article 114614.

Xie, J., Shen, Z., Anraku, Y., Kataoka, K., & Chen, X. (2019). Nanomaterial-based blood-brain-barrier (BBB) crossing strategies. *Biomaterials, 224*.

Xiong, Y., & Yu, J. (2024). LRRK2 in Parkinson's disease: Upstream regulation and therapeutic targeting. *Trends in Molecular Medicine, 30*(10), 982–996.

Yang, J., Zeng, H., Luo, Y., Chen, Y., Wang, M., Wu, C., et al. (2024). Recent applications of PLGA in drug delivery systems. *Polymers, 16*(18), 2606.

Yasuda, T., & Mochizuki, H. (2010). The regulatory role of α-synuclein and parkin in neuronal cell apoptosis; possible implications for the pathogenesis of Parkinson's disease. *Apoptosis, 15*(11), 1312–1321.

Yefroyev, D. A., & Jin, S. (2022). Induced pluripotent stem cells for treatment of alzheimer's and parkinson's diseases. *Biomedicines, 10*.

Yi, L., Ma, H., Yang, X., Zheng, Q., Zhong, J., Ye, S., et al. (2024). Cotransplantation of NSCs and ethyl stearate promotes synaptic plasticity in PD rats by Drd1/ERK/AP-1 signaling pathway. *Journal of Ethnopharmacology, 321*, Article 117292.

Youssef, P., Hughes, L., Kim, W. S., Halliday, G. M., Lewis, S. J. G., Cooper, A., et al. (2023). Evaluation of plasma levels of NFL, GFAP, UCHL1 and tau as Parkinson's disease biomarkers using multiplexed single molecule counting. *Scientific Reports, 13*(1).

Yulug, B., Altay, O., Li, X., Hanoglu, L., Cankaya, S., Velioglu, H. A., et al. (2024). Multi-omics characterization of improved cognitive functions in Parkinson's disease patients after the combined metabolic activator treatment: A randomized, double-blinded, placebo-controlled phase II trial. *Brain Commun, 7*(1).

Yusuf, A., Almotairy, A. R. Z., Henidi, H., Alshehri, O. Y., & Aldughaim, M. S. (2023). Nanoparticles as drug delivery systems: A review of the implication of nanoparticles' physicochemical properties on responses in biological systems. *Polymers, 15*.

Zeissler, M. L., Boey, T., Chapman, D., Rafaloff, G., Dominey, T., Raphael, K. G., et al. (2023). Investigating trial design variability in trials of disease-modifying therapies in Parkinson's disease: A scoping review protocol. *BMJ Open, 13*(12), Article e071641.

Zeng, X., & Couture, L. A. (2013). Pluripotent stem cells for Parkinson's disease: Progress and challenges. *Stem Cell Research & Therapy, 4*.

Zhang, Y., Chen, Y., Li, L., & Hölscher, C. (2015). Neuroprotective effects of (Val8)GLP-1-Glu-PAL in the MPTP Parkinson's disease mouse model. *Behavioural Brain Research, 293*, 107–113.

Zhang, Y., Liu, S., Xu, K., Zhou, Y., Shen, Y., Liu, Z., et al. (2024). Non-pharmacological therapies for treating non-motor symptoms in patients with Parkinson's disease: A systematic review and meta-analysis. *Frontiers in Aging Neuroscience, 16*.

Zhang, Y., Shaabani, S., Vowinkel, K., Trombetta-Lima, M., Sabogal-Guáqueta, A. M., Chen, T., et al. (2024). Novel SK channel positive modulators prevent ferroptosis and excitotoxicity in neuronal cells. *Biomedicine & Pharmacotherapy, 171*, Article 116163.

Zhang, X., Wu, H., Tang, B., & Guo, J. (2024). Clinical, mechanistic, biomarker, and therapeutic advances in GBA1-associated Parkinson's disease. *Translational Neurodegeneration, 13*(1), 48.

Zhang, Y. B., Xu, D., Bai, L., Zhou, Y. M., Zhang, H., & Cui, Y. L. (2022). A review of non-invasive drug delivery through respiratory routes. *Pharmaceutics, 14*.

Zhang, Y., Xu, X. J., Lian, T. Y., Huang, L. F., Zeng, J. M., Liang, D. M., et al. (2020). Development of frailty subtypes and their associated risk factors among the community-dwelling elderly population. *Aging, 12*(2).

Zhang, D., Zhang, J., Wang, Y., Wang, G., Tang, P., Liu, Y., et al. (2023). Targeting epigenetic modifications in Parkinson's disease therapy. *Medicinal Research Reviews, 43*(5), 1748–1777.

Zhao, X., Kang, Z., Han, R., Wang, M., Wang, Y., Sun, X., et al. (2024). JWA binding to NCOA4 alleviates degeneration in dopaminergic neurons through suppression of ferritinophagy in Parkinson's disease. *Redox Biology, 73*, Article 103190.

Zhuang, H., & Ma, X. (2025). Advances in aggrephagy: Mechanisms, disease implications, and therapeutic strategies. *Journal of Cellular Physiology, 240*(1).

Further reading

Guidelines—International Society for Stem Cell Research Internet. 2022.

CHAPTER 16

Pioneering the next generation therapies in Parkinson's disease

Hadeer N. Atalah[1], Mai Barakat[1] and Esraa M. Qansuwa[1,2]

[1]*Institute of Global Health and Human Ecology, School of Science and Engineering, The American University in Cairo, Cairo, Egypt;* [2]*Universal Health Insurance Authority (UHIA), Presidency of the Council of Ministers, Cairo, Egypt*

16.1 Introduction

Over 10 million individuals worldwide have Parkinson's disease, and this number is expected to double by 2040 due to aging populations and environmental changes (Dorsey et al., 2018). Clinically, Parkinson's disease is characterized by an increase in motor symptoms such as tremor, rigidity, and bradykinesia, along with non-motor symptoms that include cognitive decline and autonomic dysfunction. These symptoms significantly reduce individuals' quality of life (Chaudhuri et al., 2006; Wirdefeldt et al., 2011). The economic burden of Parkinson's disease includes significant direct healthcare expenditures and indirect costs related to reduced productivity and caregiving responsibilities, emphasizing a substantial societal impact (Koerts et al., 2016; Yang et al., 2020a; Yang, Hamilton, Kopil, Beck, Bandyopadhyay, et al., 2020).

Parkinson's Disease (PD) is defined as a progressive neurodegenerative disease, characterized mainly by motor deficiency and non-motor symptoms as a result of the loss of dopaminergic neurons in the substantia nigra (Rana et al., 2015). The etiology of PD extends beyond heredity or environmental factors; in addition, its characterization goes beyond its well-known motor symptoms and non-motor symptoms, which can significantly impact the quality of life for those affected (Wirdefeldt et al., 2011). The listed complexity of the disease makes it difficult to develop therapeutic agents or even an efficient experimental design for the clinical trials. In addition, PD diagnosis varies between patients; cognitive decline, mood disorders, and autonomic dysfunction are just a few examples of the multifaceted challenges faced by some patients. The interplay between motor and non-motor symptoms, along with the poorly understood origins of the disease and the lack of a This common characterization demonstrates the need for a more comprehensive approach to treatment. Current dopaminergic therapies mainly focus on motor symptoms, which means they don't always do a good job of treating non-motor problems. As a result, patients may experience a diminishing quality of life despite receiving what is considered standard care.

For many years, the main ways to treat PD have been dopaminergic drugs like levodopa and dopamine agonists. However, these medications primarily address motor symptoms like bradykinesia, tremor, and rigidity, and do little to manage the condition as a whole (Thanvi & Lo, 2004). Prolonged use of levodopa can lead to motor complications, including dyskinesias and motor fluctuations, which

Pharmacological Foundations of Parkinson's Disease. https://doi.org/10.1016/B978-0-443-27702-3.00020-0

may reduce treatment effectiveness and negatively impact patients' quality of life (Thanvi & Lo, 2004). More people are becoming aware that non-motor symptoms, such as cognitive decline, mood disorders, sleep problems, and autonomic dysfunction, can be just as debilitating as motor symptoms. However, current therapies often fail to adequately address these issues. Clinical practice frequently overlooks non-motor symptoms, despite their significant impact on patients' daily lives. The inability of dopaminergic medications to halt or slow the progression of the disease highlights their limitations (Lang & Obeso, 2004). Dopaminergic medications, including levodopa and dopamine agonists, have traditionally been the primary focus of treatment for PD. While these therapies effectively alleviate motor symptoms, they do not stop or reverse neurodegeneration (Bogetofte et al., 2020). Additionally, long-term use of these medications can result in motor complications, such as dyskinesias. Moreover, non-motor symptoms are still not adequately addressed, revealing significant gaps in available treatment options.

The research endeavors aimed at developing effective neuroprotective and neurodegenerative treatments for Parkinson's Disease (PD) have encountered numerous challenges, resulting in a frustrating stagnation in clinical outcomes (de la Fuente-Fernández et al., 2010). One major challenge is the heterogeneity of the disease itself and the lack of understanding of its etiology: PD manifests differently in each patient, complicating the development of universally applicable therapies. This variability means that clinical trials often struggle to reach a common ground among participants, making it difficult to draw meaningful conclusions about the efficacy of any given treatment (Clarke, 2004). These challenges are compounded by the current lack of validated methods to demonstrate genuine disease modification, particularly in the prediagnostic and early stages of PD (Salat et al., 2016; Lang, 2010). Furthermore, the diagnostic and prognostic biomarkers currently used to measure neurodevelopment after insult may not accurately reflect the underlying pathophysiological processes, leading to potential misinterpretations of trial results. Another major problem with the therapies that have been developed for PD is how clinical trials are set up and how long they last (de la Fuente-Fernández et al., 2010). Many studies are conducted over too short a time frame to capture the long-term effects of neuro-interventions. Because PD is a progressive neurodegenerative disorder, it may take years for changes in the disease to show up completely. Consequently, short-term trials may underestimate the potential benefits of a treatment, creating a misleading narrative about its effectiveness. Addressing these challenges requires a concerted effort in refining trial methodologies, improving patient selection, and establishing more reliable biomarkers that can truly reflect neuro-intervention outcomes in PD. According to (2010), two major limitations of the current PD therapies are related to research bench work and the treatment table for patients. Firstly, all of the presynaptic dopamine biomarkers that are currently utilized in functional neuroimaging studies, such as PET and SPECT, are naturally connected to the metabolic pathway of dopamine. Thus, dopamine may also control these presynaptic markers, making it difficult to tell if drugs or the condition caused the changes. Furthermore, it's vital to remember that functional neuroimaging shows "functional" rather than structural characteristics. Neuroimaging signals that diminish over time indicate structural alterations, including the depletion of dopamine nerve terminals. However, this process does not prove that dopamine nerve terminals have died. In other words, the present in vivo neuroimaging methods and markers cannot definitively show neuroprotection. The National Institutes of Health (NIH) put together a group of experts who agreed that "current evidence does not support the use of imaging as a diagnostic tool in clinical practice or as a surrogate endpoint in clinical trials." (Ravina et al., 2005). Second of all, clinical trial designs for PD therapies, such as the delayed-start approach, face challenges including unblinding, placebo effects, and rater bias, especially when the active treatment provides symptomatic relief. As a result, there are currently no objective tools that can reliably assess neurodegeneration in Parkinson's disease. Even in well-designed studies, existing methods fail to offer definitive evidence of neuro-intervention (de la Fuente-Fernández et al., 2010).

These limitations of current therapies and research in PD treatment have brought attention to the importance of innovative approaches in exploring PD therapy and treatment, whether through intervention or protection. In light of these challenges, researchers are actively exploring innovative therapeutic strategies that aim to alleviate symptoms and modify the disease course (Ali, 2024). Such work includes the investigation of neuroprotective agents, gene therapies, and novel compounds that target the underlying pathological processes of PD. Advancements in biomarker identification and imaging techniques also pave the way for better patient stratification and personalized treatment plans (Ali, 2024).

Current antiparkinsonian medications, including levodopa, dopamine agonists, monoamine oxidase-B inhibitors, and COMT inhibitors, primarily mitigate symptoms without modifying the fundamental disease process. These medications effectively ameliorate motor symptoms such as bradykinesia, rigidity, and tremor; however, they do not prevent or diminish the degeneration of dopaminergic neurons, which is a hallmark of PD. This fundamental limitation indicates that there are currently no treatments capable of curing PD, leaving many clinical needs unmet. Using these symptomatic therapies for an extended period can lead to significant complications. For example, long-term use of levodopa can result in motor fluctuations, characterized by periods when the medication is less effective ("off" times) and periods when it is overly effective, leading to dyskinesias. These motor issues tend to worsen as the disease progresses, complicating treatment efforts. Additionally, dopaminergic medications are often ineffective for addressing non-motor symptoms of PD, such as cognitive decline, mood disorders, autonomic dysfunction, and sleep disturbances, all of which can severely impact quality of life. Other issues include varying patient responses, the development of drug tolerance, and side effects such as hallucinations and impulse control problems. Since existing medications primarily address symptoms, they offer only short-term relief. This information indicates that over time, higher doses are required without altering the disease's progression. Additionally, this symptom-focused approach complicates the conduct of clinical trials, as demonstrating a change in the disease necessitates biomarkers and long-term outcomes that extend beyond mere symptom improvement. The lack of curative treatments capable of halting, delaying, or reversing neurodegeneration signifies a substantial deficiency in Parkinson's disease therapy. This deficiency drives ongoing research into next-generation approaches, including regenerative medicine, gene therapy, immunotherapies, and neuroprotective agents aimed at modifying the disease process rather than merely alleviating symptoms (Bogetofte et al., 2020; de la Fuente-Fernández et al., 2010; Lang & Obeso, 2004).

The limitations outlined emphasize the need to rush the development of next-generation medicines that go beyond merely alleviating symptoms to tackle the underlying causes of diseases. Emerging approaches include regenerative medicine, gene therapy, neuroengineering, and precision diagnostics. Collectively, these methods aim to restore neuronal function and alter the progression of diseases (Stocchi et al., 2024). This change in thinking aims to improve patient outcomes while lowering the costs and stress of medical care. By shifting the focus from merely managing symptoms to targeting the root causes of PD, the future holds promise for enhancing patient outcomes and redefining care standards in this debilitating condition (Stocchi et al., 2024). There is an urgent need for new treatments for PD. This chapter seeks to discuss and evaluate innovative approaches to treating dopamine-related disorders that extend beyond mere symptom relief. The emphasis will be on novel therapies that safeguard the brain and modify disease progression. Additionally, the chapter will explore novel methods of drug administration and strategies for addressing both motor and non-motor symptoms. This emerging class of medications could transform the treatment of Parkinson's disease by targeting the underlying causes of neurodegeneration and leveraging cutting-edge technologies.

16.2 Current therapeutic landscape: symptomatic treatments

Parkinson's disease (PD) is characterized by progressive loss of midbrain dopaminergic neurons, resulting in disabling motor and non-motor dysfunction. Current treatments focus on therapeutic interventions designed to alleviate the motor and non-motor symptoms without interfering with the underlying neurodegenerative process. The main target here is to improve the patients' quality of life by restoring dopaminergic neurotransmission or modulating neural circuits involved in motor control (Sprenger & Poewe, 2013). Pharmacological treatments or surgical procedures are employed to clinically address the manifestations of Parkinson's disease, including bradykinesia, rigidity, tremor, and postural instability, which generally arise at particular stages of the disease and adversely affect patients' quality of life. Symptomatic approaches do not alter disease progression like disease-modifying therapies, which slow or halt neuronal degeneration, but they provide significant functional relief that improves patients' DALYs. The current landscape of pharmacological medicine involves strategies such as mimicking depleted dopamine, stimulating dopamine agonists, or inhibiting dopamine metabolism. Surgical interventions, which enhance pathological neural activity in basal ganglia circuits, can help slow disease progression. However, neither of these approaches can completely halt the neurodegeneration process. Nonetheless, they provide disease management and symptom relief, positively impacting the patient's overall quality of life.

16.2.1 Pharmacological intervention for symptom relief

Pharmacological interventions for symptom relief are currently considered the primary approach in the clinical management of Parkinson's disease (PD) and other progressive neurodegenerative disorders. These interventions and medications have proven effective for addressing the main motor symptoms. However, they offer limited improvement for non-motor aspects. Levodopa and dopamine agonists are the standard treatments for motor symptoms. Those medicines are primarily targeting the dopaminergic pathways either by stimulating dopamine receptors or interfering with the breakdown of dopamine to address issues like bradykinesia, tremor, and rigidity (Church, 2021). Dopamine agonists can bind to dopamine receptors to activate them, thereby mimicking the influence of the dopamine neurotransmitter itself. These medicines include drugs like pramipexole, ropinirole, and rotigotine. These approved and commonly used medications have effective motor symptom management and a limited effect on non-motor symptoms. Although patients established on dopamine agonist therapies have experienced better motor abilities, researchers have concluded that some ergot-derived dopamine agonists can induce cardiovascular complications and fibrosis.

An indirect way to activate dopamine receptors was developed by levodopa, which can cross the blood-brain barrier and then be enzymatically converted into dopamine, increasing the dopamine level in the brain and replacing the depleted neurotransmitter dopamine (Church, 2021). Nausea, dizziness, headaches, and sleepiness are common side effects of levodopa. To help mitigate nausea, increasing the dose of carbidopa is recommended. If this adjustment does not alleviate the symptoms, considering domperidone may be beneficial. In elderly patients, levodopa can also lead to confusion, hallucinations, delusions, psychosis, and agitation (Huh et al., 2019). Furthermore, levodopa may cause a slight increase in homocysteine levels, potentially raising the risk of hip fractures. Patients with idiopathic Parkinsonian conditions undergoing levodopa treatment may experience decreased serum vitamin B12 levels, elevated methylmalonic acid concentrations, and an increased risk of sensorimotor peripheral neuropathy (Huh et al., 2019). Abruptly stopping or reducing the dose of levodopa heightens the risk of neuroleptic malignant syndrome (NMS), also known as Parkinsonism hyperpyrexia syndrome. In severe cases, symptoms can include hyperthermia, uncontrollable movements, and muscle stiffness (Huh et al., 2019). Management involves reinstating levodopa at previously prescribed dosages and providing intensive supportive care in an intensive care unit.

Interfering with the dopamine metabolism cascade is a crucial strategy to address progressive dopamine loss in treating various neurological and mental disorders, particularly Parkinson's disease. This approach aims to maintain or increase dopamine levels in the brain, compensating for the deficiencies observed in conditions like Parkinson's disease. Two primary enzymatic mechanisms inhibit dopamine metabolism: monoamine oxidase (MAO) inhibitors and catechol-O-methyltransferase (COMT) inhibitors (Sprenger & Poewe, 2013). MAO inhibitor medications prevent the MAO enzyme from breaking down dopamine in the brain, resulting in increased dopamine availability, which can enhance motor symptoms. Conversely, COMT inhibitors inhibit the COMT enzyme from breaking down dopamine outside of neuronal cells. By slowing this process, COMT inhibitors prolong the effects of dopamine and drugs like levodopa, leading to longer-lasting relief from symptoms. Both inhibitors enhance the positive effects of dopamine replacement therapies, such as levodopa. However, they do not cure These therapies do not cure the disease; instead, they focus on managing symptoms and addressing motor fluctuations, as well as the wearing-off phenomena that can occur with long-term dopamine therapy. Inhibiting dopamine metabolism effectively addresses motor symptoms; however, these targets do not encompass all facets of dopamine-related disorders (Sprenger & Poewe, 2013). Current therapies remain inadequate for addressing non-motor symptoms, which are significant contributors to disease progression and neurodegeneration. This gap indicates that there must be ongoing research into more comprehensive and restorative interventions.

16.2.2 Surgical intervention for symptom relief

Surgical interventions target the pathological neural activity within the basal ganglia circuits. For instance, deep-brain stimulation (DBS) involves implanting electrodes into specific brain areas, typically the subthalamic nucleus or the globus pallidus internus (Sprenger & Poewe, 2013). This procedure administers regulated electrical impulses aimed at normalizing neural activity and alleviating motor symptoms. DBS is suggested for alleviating tremors, rigidity, and motor fluctuations, as well as for treating symptoms unresponsive to medication (Williams & Okun, 2013). However, current research indicates that DBS does not slow the neurodegenerative process that leads to Parkinson's Disease (PD). Instead, it provides significant and lasting relief from symptoms, which can result in lower medication doses and an improved quality of life. Nonetheless, it does not appear to immediately halt or reverse neuronal loss or disease pathology. DBS, especially adaptive systems, can enhance abnormal brain activity by delivering real-time stimulation based on continuous neural signals (Williams & Okun, 2013). This approach increases the efficacy of the intervention while minimizing adverse effects (Sprenger & Poewe, 2013). As a method of neuroengineering, it is part of a broader strategy to restore functionality by reconnecting circuits and facilitating the integration of new technology into patient care. DBS and similar neuroengineering techniques are increasingly being integrated with regenerative and restorative approaches, such as stem cell transplantation and biomaterial scaffolds. This integration aims to provide not only symptomatic relief but also potential disease-modifying outcomes in the future (Williams & Okun, 2013). This combination illustrates the shift in how Parkinson's is treated—from merely controlling symptoms to employing strategies that may ultimately halt or modify the progression of the disease.

16.2.3 Limitations of current therapies and emerging strategies

Long-term use of dopamine replacement therapies can cause serious movement problems, like dyskinesias and motor fluctuations, which makes it harder to predict how well these drugs will work. Additionally, while these pharmacological therapies primarily focus on pain relief and improving motor symptoms, they have limited efficacy for non-motor symptoms, including cognitive decline, autonomic dysfunction, and overall disease progression. These treatments do not halt or slow the progression of the disease; rather, they function solely as therapies for symptom control (Sprenger & Poewe, 2013). Dopamine antagonists and levodopa are central to the management of Parkinson's disease (PD), but their limitations have prompted recent research into regenerative medicine, gene therapy, and other advanced approaches aimed at altering the disease's progression rather than merely alleviating symptoms. Researchers are also exploring new methods to administer levodopa and combination therapies to enhance efficacy and reduce adverse effects. While pharmacological therapies play a vital role in managing PD due to their effective symptom relief, challenges associated with long-term treatment necessitate additional therapeutic strategies for comprehensive care. The diversity in symptoms and disease progression among patients complicates standardized pharmaceutical therapy, rendering it generally inadequate. Researchers are developing emerging treatments, including regenerative medicine (such as stem cell therapy), gene therapies, and neuroengineering approaches, to go beyond merely alleviating symptoms and directly target the underlying disease processes. However, these therapies largely remain experimental and encounter significant challenges related to their translation into clinical practice and their associated costs. Current symptomatic therapies are relatively inexpensive for managing motor symptoms; however, the overall economic burden of the disease is significant, particularly when considering non-motor symptoms and the progression of impairment (Sprenger & Poewe, 2013). Emerging medications and delivery methods, such as exosome-based carriers and personalized gene therapies, may offer improvements in the future, but they also raise concerns regarding accessibility, costs, and regulatory complexities. Pharmacological intervention remains essential for symptomatic relief, particularly for motor symptoms, yet it constitutes merely one component of a comprehensive care plan. Improvements in customized medicine, combination therapy, and non-drug treatments (such as adaptive deep brain stimulation) are likely to have a big effect on the future plan. Nonetheless, deep-brain stimulation (DBS) has significant limitations (Williams & Okun, 2013). Before we can widely implement newer adaptive DBS methods and their combinations with regenerative treatments, we must address technical and regulatory challenges.

While DBS significantly enhances quality of life, it underscores the ongoing need to explore additional treatments for Parkinson's disease.

16.3 Emerging disease-modifying therapies

16.3.1 Gene therapy approaches: molecular fixing and neurotrophic support

Gene and cell therapies are at the forefront of advancements in treating Parkinson's disease (PD). Among these, AAV2-GAD represents a pioneering gene therapy, while stem cell-derived dopaminergic neurons offer the potential for a one-time intervention with long-lasting effects. Although the estimated cost of this therapy for PD ranges from $500,000 to $1 million per patient, maintaining its sustainability remains a significant challenge. Gene therapy presents revolutionary possibilities because it can act on the molecular origins of PD. There are various gene therapeutic strategies in development.

16.3.1.1 AAV-mediated gene delivery (e.g., GDNF, neurturin, AADC)

Adeno-associated virus (AAV)–mediated gene therapy has emerged as one of the most promising methods of changing the course of Parkinson's disease (PD). Recombinant AAV (rAAV) vectors are utilized because they are nonpathogenic, have low immunogenicity, and can transduce post-mitotic neurons with stable and long-term expression of therapeutic genes. Although packaging capacity in AAV is limited to approximately 4.7 kb, ongoing vector design enhancements like promoter optimization, codon optimization, and self-complementary genome configurations have significantly improved expression kinetics and transgene stability (Wang, 2024). Capsid engineering and directed evolution have also produced next-generation serotypes that exhibit enhanced neuronal specificity, improved penetration of the blood-brain barrier, and diminished peripheral off-target toxicity (Ghauri & Ou, 2023).

In PD, AAV vectors have been employed to provide genes for restoring enzymatic function or promoting neurotrophic support. Intrastriatal delivery of the aromatic L-amino acid decarboxylase (AADC) gene through AAV enhances local dopamine generation and has yielded enhanced motor function and reduced "off" periods in clinical trials (LeWitt, 2023). Parallel strategies with AAV vectors expressing glial cell line-derived neurotrophic factor (GDNF) or neurturin (NRTN) aim to rescue dying dopaminergic neurons by enhancing neuronal plasticity and survival (Bartus, 2022). Although earlier trials of AAV2-NRTN (CERE-120) were limited by defective vector diffusion and target coverage, developments in convection-enhanced delivery and gene promoter design have renewed interest in trophic gene delivery (Słyk et al., 2024).

Ongoing studies now assess combinatorial AAV approaches, such as dual-gene vectors that simultaneously express GBA1 and GDNF with synergistic neuroprotection in preclinical PD models (Zhang et al., 2024a). Additional efforts are being made to transcend lingering challenges—viz., immune response, vector durability, and control of expression—through the use of inducible promoter design, tissue-specific microRNA-based regulation, and sequential administration of orthogonal AAV serotypes (Marino, Callaerts & Holt, 2022). Clinically, AAV2-GAD gene therapy to the subthalamic nucleus remains one of the best-developed instances of successful gene delivery in PD, showing long-term functional benefit in randomized controlled trials (Kaplitt et al., 2022). The preclinical AAV-GDNF vector AB-1005, currently in Phase II trial, further testifies to the field's advancement

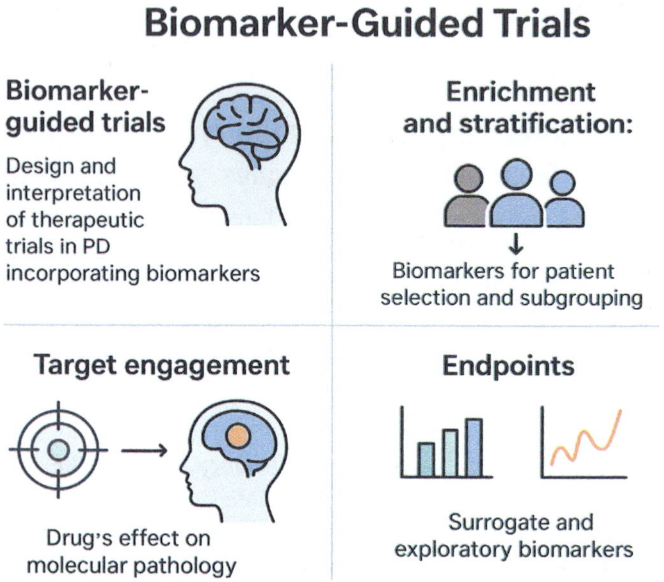

FIGURE 16.1

Integration of Biomarkers in Modern Parkinson's Disease trail.

toward safe and durable neurotrophic gene replacement therapy (Bankiewicz, 2024). In combination, these developments show how AAV vectors have evolved from single-gene delivery vehicles to broad-range molecular devices that have the ability to target multiple mechanisms in PD (Fig. 16.1). • Enzyme replacement: Vectors based on adeno-associated virus (AAV) that express aromatic L-amino acid decarboxylase (AADC) genes showed increased synthesis of dopamine and improved motor function (LeWitt, 2023). • Neurotrophic support: Administration of glial cell-derived neurotrophic factor (GDNF) and neurturin through viral vectors is an attempt to enhance neuronal survival and plasticity, but previous trials indicated restricted effectiveness. Recent advancements in targeting and vector construction are renewing enthusiasm for the strategy (Bartus, 2022).

16.3.1.2 Future of CRISPR and genome editing

While AAV-mediated gene therapy represents an important advance in the supply of neurotrophic and enzymatic support to dopaminergic neurons, the recent advances in CRISPR-based genome editing have unlocked the therapeutic window to irreversible genetic correction. Unlike viral gene replacement delivering surplus genes, CRISCR/Cas systems provide precise and long-lasting modification of the native genome, which offers a complementary strategy that addresses specifically the molecular roots of Parkinson's disease (PD) (Jin, 2023; Zhang et al., 2024b).

CRISPR/Cas9 system targets disease loci with single-guide RNAs (sgRNAs) to induce double-strand breaks, allowing the correction of hereditary PD mutations in genes such as LRRK2, PARK7, PINK1, and SNCA (Zhang, 2024c). Studies involving patient-derived induced pluripotent stem cells (iPSCs) and transgenic animal models have shown that such genome corrections restore mitochondrial function, correct autophagic flux, and lower α-synuclein aggregation, restoring dopaminergic neuron health (Qian, 2024). Importantly, these manipulations show the potential for a single-session, lifetime therapeutic benefit, positioning CRISPR as a disease-modifying therapy instead of a symptomatic management approach.

Besides traditional Cas9 nucleases, the development of base editors and prime editors now makes single-nucleotide exchange and small insertions or deletions possible without causing double-strand breaks—thereby reducing genotoxicity and off-targeting (Kim, 2024). Challenges in safe and efficient delivery to the central nervous system continue to hinder clinical translation. Viral vectors like AAVs can deliver CRISPR equipment but induce immune reactions or preserve unwanted long-term nuclease activity (Hsu, 2023). Therefore, research has focused on nonviral and hybrid delivery vehicles, namely extracellular vehicles (EVs) and exosomes, that pass naturally through the blood–brain barrier and have low immunogenicity (Dehghani et al., 2025a; Dehghani, Ocakcı et al., 2025).

Recent studies demonstrate that engineered exosomes derived from MSCs or iPSCs possess the capability to sequester Cas9 ribonucleoprotein complexes or therapeutic RNAs for the purpose of gene regulation. For instance, α-synuclein-targeted CRISPR/Cas9 or exosomes with siRNAs are able to effectively downregulate toxic α-synuclein levels and neuroinflammation in PD models (He et al., 2023a; He, Wang, et al., 2023; Singh, 2024). Moreover, MSC-derived exosomes carrying miR-133b or catalase enhance neuronal regeneration and antioxidative resistance, with synergistic neuroprotective effects when combined with CRISPR-guided gene repair (Zhao et al., 2023).

Together, these findings emphasize CRISPR's emergence as a second gene therapy platform to AAV-mediated approaches—offering unprecedented specificity, flexibility, and therapeutic cure potential. The integration of CRISPR with advanced delivery modes such as exosomes or second-generation AAVs is a direction toward non-invasive, personalized, and sustained treatments for Parkinson's disease.

16.3.2 Cell-based therapies

PD is not solely defined by dopaminergic cell loss but also involves a complex relationship between molecular and cellular dysfunction. The abnormal aggregation of α-synuclein into Lewy bodies is a key part of its pathogenesis. This condition affects synapses, mitochondria, oxidative stress, and the breakdown of proteins. Chronic neuroinflammation and, in many cases, peripheral alterations along the gut-brain axis accompany these degenerative changes. Early PD pathology often manifests in the enteric nervous system, which points to the importance of systemic biomarkers and peripheral targets. Such multifactorial pathology justifies a multi-pronged regenerative approach that goes beyond neuronal replacement to include immunomodulation, restoration of homeostasis, and reconstruction of neuronal circuitry.

16.3.2.1 Stem cell transplantation (iPSC-derived dopaminergic neurons)

Among the most promising reparative methods for PD is stem cell therapy. Pluripotent stem cells (PSCs), such as induced pluripotent stem cells (iPSCs) and embryonic stem cells (ESCs), can be differentiated into midbrain dopaminergic (mDA) neurons and possibly substitute for the dying neurons in the course of the disease. Clinical trials in humans have already adopted iPSC-derived dopaminergic progenitors transplanted in PD patients, showing promising safety and feasibility results (Schweitzer et al., 2020; Takahashi, 2024). Besides their therapeutic applications, stem cell cultures are essential for modeling PD pathogenesis and evaluating novel therapies in vitro. Patient-specific iPSC lines allow researchers to examine genetic heterogeneity and environmental susceptibility, paving the way for precision regenerative medicine (Qian, 2023).

16.3.2.2 Ethical and regulatory considerations

The ethical and regulatory challenges in cell-based therapy for degenerative diseases like PD encompass patient autonomy, informed consent, and the moral implications of using various types of stem cells (Jayaram et al., 2025). The use of embryonic stem cells (ESCs) is particularly controversial due to the destruction of human embryos, leading to calls for stringent governmental oversight and licensing (Jayaram et al., 2025). An example of such a regulatory framework is the UK's Human Fertilisation and Embryology Authority (HFEA). In contrast, induced pluripotent stem cells (iPSCs) mitigate some ethical concerns since they do not involve embryos. However, they introduce new issues related to genetic privacy, donor consent, and the potential for financial exploitation (Jayaram et al., 2025). The U.S. Food and Drug Administration (FDA) and other regulatory bodies have strict rules that are based on 21 CFR Part 1271. They mandate investigational new drug applications for significantly altered cells and require evidence of safety and efficacy through controlled clinical trials (Jayaram et al., 2025). Additionally, equitable access to these emerging therapies remains a significant concern, as high costs could exacerbate existing healthcare disparities. Therefore, it is crucial to implement measures that ensure treatments are both accessible and affordable.

16.3.3 Neuroprotective agents

16.3.3.1 Antioxidants, mitochondrial stabilizers

Oxidative stress and mitochondrial dysfunction are significant factors contributing to the loss of dopaminergic neurons during disease progression (Lang and Obeso, 2004). Oxidative stress typically occurs when there is an excess of reactive oxygen species (ROS) and insufficient antioxidant defenses. This imbalance leads to lipid peroxidation, DNA damage, and improper protein folding (Lang and Obeso, 2004). Antioxidants serve to neutralize ROS, thereby protecting nerve cells from oxidative stress-induced damage. In Parkinson's disease, mitochondrial activity is often disrupted, resulting in reduced ATP production and the activation of apoptotic pathways (Bogetofte et al., 2020). Mitochondrial stabilizers are designed to preserve this activity. Enhancing mitochondrial bioenergetics or repairing the electron transport chain may help sustain neuronal survival. These treatments work in concert to interrupt a critical pathogenic cascade, potentially slowing the progression of the disease (Bogetofte et al., 2020). These drugs enhance oxidative phosphorylation by reactivating the electron transport chain (ETC). This accelerates ATP production, which is vital for the survival and metabolism of neurons. Additionally, they reduce the production of reactive oxygen species (ROS), thereby protecting mitochondrial and cellular proteins, lipids, and DNA from oxidative damage. This two-part process helps keep the mitochondrial membrane potential stable and stops pro-apoptotic factors from being released. Together, these effects help maintain neuronal energy balance, inhibit cell death signaling, and disrupt the mitochondrial damage and oxidative stress cycles that lead to neurodegenerative diseases (Bogetofte et al., 2020). Examples of agents that enhance mitochondrial bioenergetics and act as antioxidants in PD include coenzyme Q10, creatine, and various compounds targeting mitochondrial complex I. Coenzyme Q10 acts as an electron carrier in the ETC and an antioxidant, which helps lower oxidative damage (Bogetofte et al., 2020). Creatine contributes to energy metabolism by buffering cellular ATP levels. Additionally, other mitochondrial stabilizers under investigation include agents that improve mitochondrial dynamics or biogenesis, such as PGC-1α activators (Bogetofte et al., 2020).

16.3.3.2 Alpha-synuclein aggregation inhibitors

The buildup and clumping of alpha-synuclein protein into Lewy bodies is a hallmark of PD, leading to the dysfunction and death of nerve cells. Therapeutic strategies aim to disrupt this aggregation process or enhance the clearance of toxic oligomers and fibrils (Schweitzer et al., 2020). Approaches include small compounds that prevent alpha-synuclein from misfolding, immunotherapies that target aggregated forms, and gene therapies that reduce the production of alpha-synuclein. Initial clinical trials of monoclonal antibodies, such as prasinezumab, have shown promise in targeting pathogenic alpha-synuclein; however, definitive evidence of disease modification is still awaited. These inhibitors aim to diminish neurotoxicity at its source, offering hope for treatments that may slow or halt disease progression (Stocchi et al., 2024). Anle138b is a small chemical that prevents the formation of fibrils, while prasinezumab and cinpanemab are monoclonal antibodies designed to target and help eliminate aggregated alpha-synuclein (Vallabh et al., 2023). These compounds serve as examples of alpha-synuclein aggregation inhibitors. Researchers are currently conducting human studies to evaluate whether these immunotherapies can alter the progression of the disease by dismantling harmful protein clumps (Vallabh et al., 2023). Additionally, there are emerging gene therapies aimed at reducing the production of alpha-synuclein or accelerating its breakdown (Stocchi et al., 2024). These treatments represent some of the most promising neuroprotective options for PD currently under investigation in clinical or preclinical settings.

16.3.3.3 Anti-inflammatory drugs

Chronic neuroinflammation plays a central role in the pathology of PD. Activation of microglia, astrocyte dysfunction, and influx of peripheral immune cells all contribute to a detrimental neural milieu. Stem cell-based immunomodulation, such as that derived from the bone marrow or Wharton's jelly, can exert anti-inflammatory properties through paracrine activity and exosomal secretion of cytokines such as IL-10 and TGF-β. Preclinical studies have shown that MSCs can reduce glial reactivity, protect dopaminergic neurons, and attenuate neuroinflammation in PD models. This suggests a synergistic role for immunomodulation alongside cell replacement in comprehensive regenerative strategies.

16.3.4 Circuitry restoration and neuroengineering advances

Not only is the replacement of dead cells critical, but so is the restoration of functional connectivity in PD-affected circuits. Techniques such as chemogenetics and optogenetics are being exploited to dissect and manipulate the basal ganglia circuitry. An exciting development with strong clinical promise is the advent of adaptive deep brain stimulation (DBS), in which implanted technologies are able to detect and respond to real-time neural activity and deliver personalized, dynamic stimulation with fewer off-target effects (Little, 2022). Alternatively, bioengineering advancements have currently made it possible to combine transplanted neurons with supportive biomaterials, including hydrogels or scaffolds. These materials provide cues for axonal growth and synaptic input, which enhance both the survival and integration of transplanted cells into the host brain (López-Tobón, 2023).

16.3.4.1 Organoids and 3D models

Human midbrain organoids derived from iPSCs mirror key aspects of human dopaminergic biology and provide valuable models for studying PD. These 3D models show dopaminergic neuron induction, synapse formation, and even α-synuclein aggregation resembling in vivo phenotypes. Production of patient-derived organoids has opened the possibility to evaluate genetic mutations, drug responses, and regenerative therapies and has brought a strong weapon into the hands of personalized medicine (Smits, 2023). Combined with single-cell omics and AI, organoid models enable the rapid screening of regenerative therapies with high predictive validity. Increasingly, organoid platforms are being paired with high-throughput, AI-assisted screening pipelines to accelerate drug discovery and disease modeling across neurodegenerative disorders (Chambers et al., 2023).

16.3.4.2 Advancements in delivery systems across the blood-brain barrier

The blood-brain barrier (BBB) represents a significant impediment to effective therapeutic delivery in Parkinson's disease treatment. To address this challenge, researchers have developed several innovative technologies designed to circumvent or temporarily compromise the BBB's protective mechanisms. Focused ultrasound (FUS) has emerged as a promising approach for safely disrupting the BBB, thereby facilitating enhanced localized delivery of therapeutic agents, including exosomes, nanoparticles, and viral vectors. This technique enables precise targeting while minimizing systemic exposure and potential adverse effects (Meng, 2024). Furthermore, advanced nanocarrier platforms, including lipid-based and polymeric nanoparticles, have been engineered to exploit receptor-mediated transcytosis mechanisms for BBB penetration. These sophisticated delivery systems demonstrate improved efficiency in therapeutic transport while enabling targeted drug delivery to specific brain regions. Biodegradable hydrogels and microspheres have also been created to deliver neuroprotective factors or therapeutic cells directly into the brain parenchyma in a controlled and long-lasting way. These platforms offer the advantage of localized treatment delivery, potentially reducing systemic side effects while maintaining therapeutic concentrations over extended periods (Rothenbücher et al., 2023). Complementary to these physical and pharmacological strategies, extracellular vesicles and exosome-based carriers exploit natural blood-brain-barrier-crossing mechanisms to shuttle genetic material, proteins, and neuroprotective cargo directly into the CNS (András and Toborek, 2016; Xie et al., 2022). These technological advances represent significant progress in overcoming the BBB challenge, offering new possibilities for more effective Parkinson's disease interventions.

16.4 Immunotherapy and targeted biologics

16.4.1 Alpha-synuclein monoclonal antibodies (e.g., prasinezumab)

Passive immunotherapy of Parkinson's disease (PD) is led by monoclonal antibodies targeting aggregated α-synuclein. Prasinezumab (RO7046015/PRX002), which binds C-terminal epitopes of aggregated α-synuclein, has been tested in early PD in the PASADENA and PADOVA studies. While PASADENA (52 weeks, double-blind placebo-controlled) did not show a statistically significant decrease in overall clinical progression as assessed by MDS-UPDRS total scores, it did show that motor signs—especially MDS-UPDRS Part III in the OFF state—worsened more slowly in patients treated with prasinezumab, with significant findings in subgroups and with early treatment initiation. It was also well-tolerated with satisfactory safety profiles (Pagano et al., 2024; Roche, 2025).

Subsequent findings from PADOVA, a Phase IIb study in over 500 early PD patients who were already taking symptomatic therapy, corroborated these findings. Prasinezumab did not achieve its primary endpoint (time to confirmed motor progression) with statistical significance (HR ≈ 0.84, $P \approx .0657$) but showed consistent, positive trends in motor progression—particularly in levodopa-treated patients (HR ≈ 0.79, $P \approx .043$ in prespecified analyses)—and in secondary or exploratory outcomes over ~104 weeks. Biomarker evidence from PADOVA indicates that prasinezumab has the potential to impact disease biology by reducing α-synuclein aggregation biomarkers (Roche, 2025).

Another monoclonal antibody, cinpanemab (BIIB054), binding the N-terminal region of α-synuclein with selectivity for aggregated forms, was also trialled in early PD (SPARK trial). It also failed to meet its primary clinical or imaging endpoints at 52 weeks (overall MDS-UPDRS change and DaT-SPECT), despite demonstrating target engagement (CSF α-synuclein binding) and dose-related pharmacokinetics. This outcome underscores that while monoclonals are mechanistically promising, it remains challenging to translate such effects into clinically meaningful disease modification (Lang et al., 2022).

Overall, the monoclonal antibody strategy is encouraging, especially in early or mild disease stages, with detectable biomarker effects and acceptable safety. The primary unresolved enquiries are whether trends can be replicated and amplified in Phase III, whether early intervention or stratification (e.g., by biomarkers or disease phenotype) enhances outcomes, and how to engineer antibodies for optimal epitope specificity, affinity, and cerebral penetration. Comparative analyses of binding, specificity for aggregated α-synuclein, and downstream effects of different epitope targets are ongoing (Kniazev, 2025).

16.4.2 Vaccine approaches

Active immunotherapy (vaccines) against pathological α-synuclein is intended to stimulate the patient's own immune system to produce antibodies that neutralize or eliminate aggregates or prevent them from spreading. One of the most advanced vaccine candidates is UB-312 (from Vaxxinity), in a Phase 1 trial of which target engagement was demonstrated: the immune responder formed antibodies that bound α-synuclein aggregates, and there was a measurable reduction in cerebrospinal fluid (CSF) levels of toxic aggregates compared with placebo, by seed amplification assays (SAA/PMCA) (Yu et al., 2022).

Vaccine approaches have some conceptual advantages over monoclonal antibodies: less costly, potentially longer in duration (if the memory response is maintained), and fewer injections. However, there are also disadvantages, such as autoimmunity, non-uniform titers of antibodies, and the potential for inferior responses in aged or immunosenescent hosts. Currently, phase 1 studies provide the majority of data, and many vaccine candidates are in the preclinical or Phase 1 development stages. Follow-up through years, dose discovery, adjuvanting effects, and safety will be required.

Recent news focuses on demonstrating target engagement—showing vaccine-induced antibodies bind to pathological α-synuclein forms in the CNS, reduce aggregate burden, or alter biomarkers—to validate vaccine approaches. Phase 1 results of UB-312 showed α-synuclein aggregate decreases in CSF and exhibited engagement with sensitive assays (SAA/PMCA) as a model for subsequent trials to add robust biomarker components (Yu et al., 2022).

16.4.3 Biomarker-guided trials

Biomarkers are also revolutionizing the design, execution, and analysis of disease-modifying trials in PD. Rather than being solely reliant on clinical scales that develop slowly and are susceptible to symptomatic therapies, modern trials are leveraging biomarkers for (1) cohort enrichment, (2) stratification, (3) target engagement, and (4) exploratory or surrogate endpoints (Fig. 16.2). Most potential therapies target molecular pathologies, including α-synuclein aggregation and lysosomal dysfunction; consequently, sensitive biomarkers can measure early biological effects years before clinical symptoms appear (Du et al., 2021).

Caption: Schematic overview illustrating how different biomarker types are incorporated into disease-modifying clinical trials for Parkinson's disease (PD).

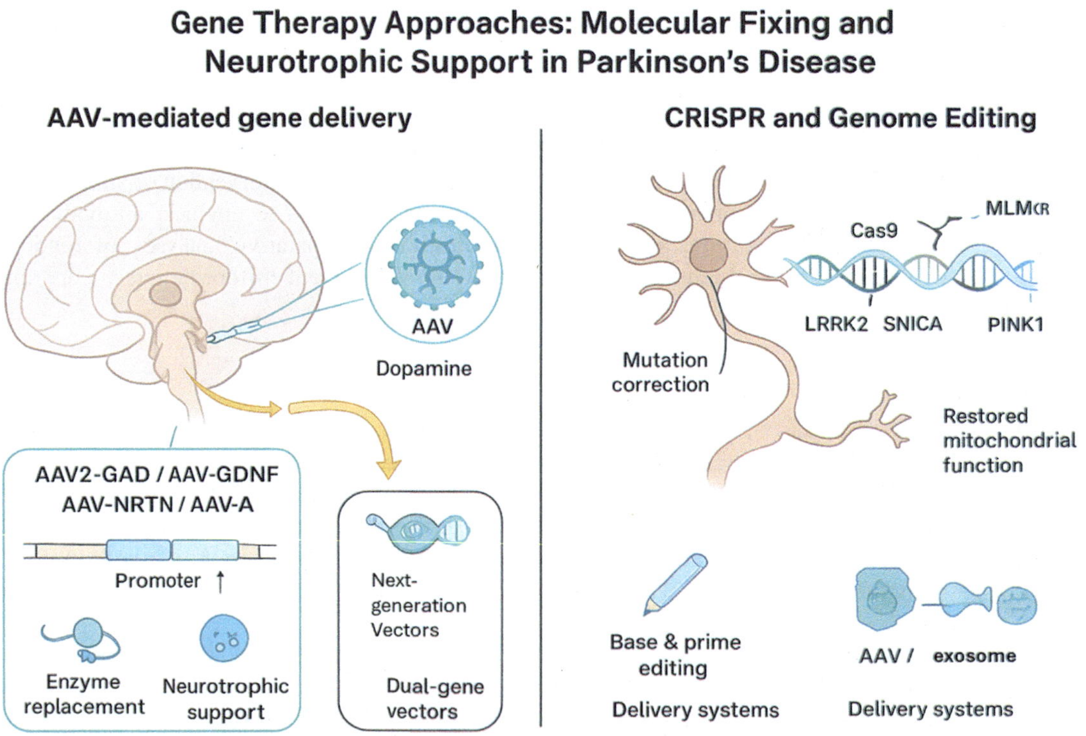

FIGURE 16.2 Gene Therapy Approaches in Parkinson's Disease: Molecular Fixing and Neurotrophic Support.

A schematic representation illustrating two principal gene therapy platforms for Parkinson's disease. Left: AAV-mediated gene delivery delivers genes encoding aromatic L-amino acid decarboxylase (AADC), glial cell line-derived neurotrophic factor (GDNF), or neurturin (NRTN) to enhance dopamine synthesis and neuronal survival. Right: CRISPR-based genome editing provides precise correction of PD-associated mutations (e.g., *LRRK2*, *SNCA*, *PINK1*) using Cas9, base editing, or prime editing systems. Engineered delivery tools such as exosomes and next-generation AAVs enable targeted, sustained molecular repair of dopaminergic neurons.

Dorsey, E. R., Sherer, T., Okun, M. S., & Bloem, B. R. (2018). The emerging evidence of the Parkinson pandemic. Journal of Parkinson's Disease, 8(s1), S3–S8.

Among fluid biomarkers, α-synuclein seed amplification assays (αSyn-SAA) have emerged as diagnostic and prognostic. CSF-based αSyn-SAA, and more recently blood-based versions, robustly discriminate PD from controls and predict conversion in prodromal cohorts. SAA kinetic parameters can be correlated with future clinical course and used as pharmacodynamic readouts for immunotherapy or anti-aggregation trials. Cross-laboratory and standardization studies are underway to harmonize SAA protocols (Giannakis et al., 2025).

Neurofilament light chain (NfL), measurable in plasma or serum, is a second valuable biomarker for prognostic enrichment and safety monitoring. Both elevated baseline NfL and more pronounced longitudinal increases have been associated with faster motor and cognitive decline (Brown et al., 2023). Neuroimaging biomarkers such as DAT-SPECT provide diagnostic confirmation and eligibility screening but are insensitive to short-term change because of their slow dynamic range. Novel PET tracers targeting α-synuclein and new MRI modalities such as neuromelanin imaging and quantitative susceptibility mapping promise more direct measures of pathology, but further validation is needed (He et al., 2023a; He, Wang, et al., 2023).

Passive monitoring, wearables, and smartphones—digital and remote-sensing biomarkers—are also maturing. These allow for continuous gait, activity, and sleep monitoring and motor fluctuation, correlating with clinical scales and with high temporal resolution for faster, smaller trials (Nguyen, 2025). Operationally, biomarker-guided trials increasingly utilize enrichment (e.g., αSyn-SAA-positive enrollment), stratified randomization, and adaptive designs with interim biomarker analyses to collapse doses or subgroups (Kluge & Iranzo, 2024). Multicenter harmonization, pre-established SOPs, and composite biomarker endpoints will be crucial as the field advances (Tanaka, 2025).

16.5 Precision and personalized medicine

By tailoring treatments to each patient's unique needs, precision and personalized medicine are revolutionizing the treatment of Parkinson's disease (PD). Pharmacogenomics plays a crucial role by demonstrating how genetic differences influence the effectiveness of medications (Titova & Chaudhuri, 2017). This enables doctors to develop better prescription plans that reduce side effects and enhance drug efficacy. Integrating genomics, proteomics, metabolomics, and other biological data with big data analytics enables a comprehensive understanding of the heterogeneity and progression of Parkinson's disease (PD). Artificial intelligence (AI) enhances this capability by forecasting patient responses to treatments and the progression of their diseases. This helps doctors create more accurate treatment plans. Stratification based on genetic alterations such as GBA1 and LRRK2 is crucial (Menozzi et al., 2023), as these mutations affect the risk of disease, symptoms, and treatment outcomes. This categorization supports the development of targeted therapies and personalized interventions that may impact disease progression. Progress in pharmacogenomics, multi-omics, AI, and genetic stratification is driving the transition to a precision medicine framework, which provides enhanced management strategies and novel therapeutic pathways for Parkinson's disease (Menozzi et al., 2023). Precision and personalized medicine represent a transformative approach by tailoring treatments according to each patient's unique genetic and molecular profile. Pharmacogenomics plays a vital role by examining how genetic variations affect drug metabolism and response, thus optimizing therapeutic strategies for greater efficacy and reduced side effects. The integration of multi-omics data—including genomic, transcriptomic, proteomic, and metabolomic information—with big data analytics provides a holistic view of the complex mechanisms underlying PD and enhances patient stratification. AI takes this field even further by using advanced computer models to predict how well drugs will work and how diseases will progress. This makes it easier to create personalized treatment options. Genetic stratification based on mutations such as GBA1 and LRRK2 is essential (Menozzi et al., 2023), as these variants affect disease susceptibility and prognosis, allowing for targeted therapies tailored to specific patient subgroups. Collectively, these advancements pave the way for precision medicine in PD, potentially leading to improved clinical outcomes and more effective, individualized treatments.

16.6 Non-dopaminergic and novel targets

16.6.1 Glutamatergic, serotonergic, and adenosinergic pathways

Targeting non-dopaminergic pathways presents opportunities to alleviate both motor and non-motor symptoms, enhance the effectiveness of existing medications, and reduce side effects, indicating a significant advancement in comprehensive Parkinson's disease (PD) management. The glutamatergic, serotonergic, and adenosinergic pathways are important non-dopaminergic neurotransmitter systems that play a role in the pathophysiology of PD and could be good targets for new treatments (Barone, 2010).

- **Glutamatergic Pathway: The primary neurotransmitter, glutamate, facilitates communication within the brain, especially in the compromised basal ganglia circuitry of Parkinson's disease (PD).** Abnormalities in glutamatergic signaling contribute to motor symptoms and excitotoxicity, which leads to neurological damage. Therapeutic approaches that focus on glutamate receptors, such as NMDA or AMPA antagonists, aim to reduce excitotoxicity and enhance motor control, including managing dyskinesias associated with levodopa treatment (Barone, 2010).
- **Serotonergic Pathway:** The serotonergic system plays a crucial role in regulating emotion, cognition, and movement. Disruptions in serotonin neurotransmission are linked to non-motor symptoms of Parkinson's disease (PD), including depression, anxiety, and cognitive decline. Research is ongoing into serotonin receptor modulators and selective serotonin reuptake inhibitors (SSRIs) to alleviate these symptoms and improve quality of life (Barone, 2010).
- **The Adenosinergic Pathway: Adenosine A2A receptors significantly influence dopaminergic signaling** in basal ganglia circuits. Istradefylline and other A2A receptor antagonists have been approved as supplementary therapies for levodopa, focusing on alleviating motor "off" periods and symptoms. This method makes dopaminergic drugs work better while reducing side effects (Barone, 2010).

By targeting these pathways, we can implement complementary strategies to manage the symptoms of Parkinson's disease. This approach addresses both motor and non-motor aspects beyond solely relying on dopamine replacement and also advances the development of comprehensive treatment options.

16.6.2 Gut-brain axis modulation

Modulating the gut-brain axis presents a promising approach to treating Parkinson's disease (PD) by pointing out the importance of gut microbiota and the enteric nervous system in the disease's pathogenesis and progression. The gut-brain axis involves bidirectional communication between the central nervous system and the gastrointestinal tract, which is facilitated by various pathways, including neuronal, immunological, endocrine, and metabolic mechanisms (Qansuwa et al., 2024). Initial pathological changes in Parkinson's disease (PD) often manifest in the enteric nervous system, characterized by atypical aggregation of alpha-synuclein. This data suggests that the gut may serve as a potential origin or early locus of the disease. Dysbiosis, which refers to an imbalance in gut microbiota, has been associated with inflammation. alters gut permeability, and systemic immune responses. These factors may contribute to neuroinflammation and neurodegeneration in individuals with Parkinson's disease (Qansuwa et al., 2024). Using probiotics, prebiotics, antibiotics, or fecal microbiota transplantation to modify the gut microbiota aims to restore microbial balance, reduce gut inflammation, and enhance the functionality of the intestinal barrier. These approaches may alleviate common gastrointestinal symptoms associated with Parkinson's disease (PD) and potentially influence both motor and non-motor symptoms. While gut-brain axis therapies show promise, clinical research is still in the early stages, and treatments tailored to each patient's specific microbiome composition may be necessary. In summary, targeting the gut-brain axis offers a novel approach to altering disease mechanisms that extends beyond conventional treatments focused solely on the brain.

16.6.3 Neurotrophic factors and neuromodulators

Neurotrophic factors and neuromodulators are critical components in the developing field of Parkinson's disease (PD) therapeutics, aimed at promoting neuronal survival, enhancing neural plasticity, and influencing disease progression beyond mere symptomatic relief. Key neurotrophic factors, such as glial cell line-derived neurotrophic factor (GDNF) and neurturin, play an essential role in the survival, proliferation, and maintenance of dopaminergic neurons that are affected by degeneration in Parkinson's disease. Experimental therapies entail either the direct administration of neuroprotective factors or the utilisation of gene therapy vectors, such as adeno-associated virus (AAV), to augment neuroprotection and promote neuronal repair, despite historical inconsistencies in clinical trial outcomes. Recent advancements in vector targeting, delivery techniques, and sustained-release formulations are making neurotrophic factor-based therapies increasingly promising as potential strategies to alter the disease's trajectory (Youssef et al., 2024).

Neuromodulators influence neurotransmitter systems and the dynamics of neural circuits, potentially improving non-motor symptoms. Examples of such drugs include adenosine A2A receptor antagonists, glutamate receptor modulators, and serotonergic substances, which target non-dopaminergic systems. These neuromodulators can complement dopaminergic therapy by addressing symptoms that are less responsive to dopamine replacement and by mitigating side effects like dyskinesias. Combining neurotrophic support with neuromodulation, gene therapy, and regenerative medicine may provide a promising approach to restore functionality and safeguard the brain. New technologies are being developed to enhance the efficacy of neurotrophic factors and neuromodulators, including modified extracellular vesicles (exosomes) for more effective transport and advanced biomaterials for sustained release (Youssef et al., 2024). Artificial intelligence and patient-derived organoid models are also making personalized medicine better by predicting how well treatments will work and customizing them to fit each person's disease profile. These approaches represent significant progress in addressing the underlying causes of Parkinson's disease while enhancing both motor and non-motor outcomes (Qansuwa et al., 2025). The ultimate objective is to restore neuronal function and improve the quality of life for patients.

16.7 Digital health and technological innovations

Digital health and technological innovation are fundamentally changing therapeutic approaches in Parkinson's disease, allowing for individualized, data-driven, and accessible care models. Wearables, closed-loop neuromodulation, and telemedicine are at the forefront of this movement; however, successful integration requires coordinated regulatory oversight and continuous ethical reflection.

16.7.1 Wearables and mobile applications for symptom tracking

Digital health tools, particularly wearables and mobile applications, are significantly reshaping the management of Parkinson's disease. These innovations facilitate real-time monitoring of both symptoms and patient behaviors in environments outside traditional clinical settings, providing a more comprehensive view of a patient's condition. Wearable devices, such as accelerometers and smartwatches, along with sensor-equipped clothing, are capable of capturing a range of vital motor metrics (Huang et al., 2025). Such information includes measurements of tremors, which can help diagnose the severity of motor symptoms, gait analysis to evaluate walking patterns, and assessments of bradykinesia, or the slowness of movement. Additionally, these devices track essential data related to sleep patterns, incidents of falls, and adherence to medication schedules, all of which are critical factors in managing Parkinson's disease effectively (Hoffman et al., 2024).

Evidence from recent studies has shown that the data collected by these technologies empowers clinicians and researchers with detailed longitudinal insights into patient health. This granular data allows for the early identification of changes in a patient's condition, which can lead to timely interventions and the development of personalized therapy plans tailored to individual needs. In parallel, mobile applications serve as an important complement to wearable technology (Negash & Hanum, 2025). They enable patients to self-report various non-motor symptoms, such as mood fluctuations and fatigue, along with their activities of daily living. This ability to self-report adds to the information that healthcare providers have and helps them work together more effectively (Marciano et al., 2023). By integrating both wearable data and self-reported information, healthcare teams can engage in shared decision-making and adapt care plans to accommodate the evolving needs of patients with Parkinson's disease. Such a holistic approach not only enhances patient engagement but also improves overall disease management outcomes (Marciano et al., 2023).

16.7.2 Closed-loop neuromodulation systems

Deep brain stimulation (DBS) has become an important treatment option for patients with motor symptoms that do not respond to standard therapies, such as medications. This technique involves surgically implanting electrodes in specific areas of the brain to deliver electrical impulses aimed at modulating neural activity and alleviating symptoms (Foote et al., 2025). Recently, the advent of closed-loop neuromodulation has introduced new possibilities for improving therapeutic precision and effectiveness. Closed-loop systems offer significant advantages over traditional DBS methods (Wang et al., 2023). Unlike conventional systems, which provide a constant level of stimulation regardless of the patient's condition, closed-loop systems continuously monitor neural and physiological signals, such as local field potentials or real-time movement patterns. This capability allows these systems to automatically adjust stimulation based on the patient's current state, optimizing the therapeutic effect while minimizing potential side effects (Foote et al., 2025).

Recent research suggests that adaptive deep brain stimulation (DBS) systems are safe and feasible for clinical use. Closed-loop DBS can provide personalized treatment strategies, allowing healthcare providers to tailor therapies to each patient's unique needs. This personalization can enhance treatment outcomes and improve quality of life (Wang et al., 2023). The integration of advanced machine learning algorithms further enhances these systems by analyzing data to refine stimulation parameters based on neural activity and symptom fluctuations. Future DBS therapy may not only respond to immediate changes but also predict long-term variations in symptoms, creating a more effective treatment approach (Foote et al., 2025). Overall, closed-loop neuromodulation has the potential to transform the management of treatment-resistant motor symptoms, fostering a more adaptive healthcare model (Wang et al., 2023).

16.7.3 Telemedicine and virtual clinical trials

Telemedicine is revolutionizing how patients with Parkinson's disease access and receive care in various regions. Remote consultations, digital follow-up appointments, and AI-powered screening tools enable timely clinical assessments and interventions while reducing travel burdens and exposure risks (Cubo & Delgado-López, 2022). Also, improvements in virtual clinical trials, like the use of wearable devices, electronic consent platforms, and cloud-based data aggregation, are speeding up research. These innovations allow for the enrollment of diverse participants, streamline data collection, and facilitate decentralized protocols. This approach not only promotes inclusivity but also enhances the ecological validity of research findings and expedites the regulatory approval process (Dou et al., 2025).

16.8 Regulatory and ethical considerations

The increasing integration of digital technologies in Parkinson's Disease (PD) care brings forth new regulatory and ethical demands, necessitating robust standards for data privacy, cybersecurity, and interoperability. Regulatory bodies are refining their frameworks to evaluate the effectiveness, safety, and usability of digital health solutions, which requires transparent validation and ongoing post-market monitoring. Ethical considerations encompass ensuring equitable access, obtaining informed consent in virtual settings, addressing algorithmic bias, and safeguarding patient autonomy. Stakeholders need to foster multidisciplinary collaborations to ensure that innovation remains patient-centered, ethically sound, and socially equitable (Esper et al., 2024).

Despite the considerable promise of regenerative therapies, several significant challenges persist in their development and implementation. Ethical considerations surrounding the use of embryonic stem cells continue to generate debate, while concerns regarding the long-term safety profile of iPSC-derived grafts and the associated risk of tumorigenesis require thorough investigation and resolution. Additionally, the development of combination therapies that integrate cellular, genetic, and device-based approaches presents substantial regulatory complexity, necessitating coordinated oversight across multiple therapeutic modalities. The successful translation of these therapies depends upon several critical factors, including the standardization of manufacturing protocols to ensure consistent quality and efficacy. Equally important is the establishment of equitable patient access mechanisms and the deliberate inclusion of genetically diverse populations in clinical trials to ensure broad applicability and safety across different demographic groups. The achievement of these goals will require regulatory harmonization and enhanced international collaboration to facilitate scalable implementation of regenerative therapies (Peterson & Haggerty, 2022).

According to Yang et al. (2020a, 2020b), the financial burden of Parkinson's disease (PD) encompasses a range of expenses that significantly surpass direct medical costs, including hospitalizations, prescription medications, and therapy. A significant portion of this burden arises from indirect costs, including lost productivity attributable to disabilities and time off work for both patients and their families. Furthermore, informal caregiving plays a significant role in the overall economic impact, often imposing substantial emotional and physical strain on friends and family members (Jerry et al., 2023). It is important to recognize the significant societal advantages that novel therapies designed to improve functional independence in Parkinson's disease patients can provide. By potentially improving the quality of life for these individuals, such therapies may enable them to remain in the workforce and ease some of the caregiving pressures on family members, thereby alleviating broader financial strains (Jerry et al., 2023; Yang et al., 2020a; 2020b).

The high upfront costs associated with novel therapies present a significant challenge, as they can worsen existing inequities in access to essential treatments. These advanced therapies are often prohibitively expensive for patients from lower socioeconomic backgrounds, leading to a situation where wealthier individuals receive superior care compared to those with fewer financial resources (Zaman et al., 2021). Policymakers are tasked with the vital responsibility of striking a balance between providing pharmaceutical companies with the necessary incentives to innovate and ensuring that these innovations remain accessible and affordable for all segments of society. Effective strategies to address these equity concerns include pooled procurement, where multiple organizations collaborate to purchase medications at discounted prices, and compulsory licensing, which permits governments to authorize the production of generic drugs without the consent of the patent holder (Zaman et al., 2021).

Cell-based therapies for PD require a complicated process for making and distributing them, which could make them harder to get and more expensive (Skidmore & Barker, 2023). The complexity of cell-based and gene therapies necessitates an established infrastructure with specific requirements, which contributes to their high production costs; without substantial support, these therapies are unaffordable, raising significant concerns. Therefore, the demand for these therapies may exceed supply, showing patient access and contributing to the high expenses of therapies (Skidmore & Barker, 2023).

16.9 Challenges and future perspectives

16.9.1 Current challenges in next-generation therapies

Despite remarkable advancements, significant challenges impede the development of therapies capable of halting or reversing PD. Chief among these is the difficulty in developing neuroprotective, disease-modifying interventions, as well as the persistent variability in treatment response and progression of non-motor symptoms. Moreover, cost, accessibility, and the necessity to reconcile innovation with regulatory, administrative, and ethical frameworks hinder therapeutic implementation (Filippi et al., 2022; Lucchetta et al., 2020). Integrating pharmacological, surgical, and technological modalities, identifying early biomarkers, and increasing diversity in clinical research are all priorities for future work (2023b).

16.9.2 Translational gaps and economic barriers

Translational obstacles remain between preclinical advances and widespread clinical application. Variations in trial outcomes, the lack of long-term safety and efficacy data, and inherent uncertainties associated with real-world implementation contribute to the high risk of health economic models (Filippi et al., 2022). Developing adaptive health technology assessment (HTA) frameworks and innovative financing models, such as outcomes-based agreements and annuity payments, is essential for the sustainable introduction of costly novel therapies (Sagoo et al., 2023; Zurynski et al., 2022).

16.9.3 Future perspectives in integrating digital health and advanced parkinson's therapies within universal health coverage

The integration of artificial intelligence (AI), machine learning (ML), and mobile/wearable platforms is rapidly transforming the management and research of Parkinson's disease (PD) (Qansuwa et al., 2025). Applications span predictive modeling of disease trajectories, optimization of interventions like deep brain stimulation, and analysis of large-scale omics data, thus advancing personalized and precision medicine approaches (Shokrpour et al., 2025; Twala, 2025). These innovations also enable adaptive, virtual clinical trial designs that may address inherent limitations of traditional trials. Universal Health Coverage (UHC) plays a pivotal role in promoting equitable access by embedding digital health innovations within national coverage policies to foster a supportive environment for cutting-edge research and therapy deployment. Leveraging telemedicine, AI-driven diagnostics, and interoperable health data systems through UHC can facilitate early detection and tailored management of PD's complex symptoms. Digital infrastructures support continuous remote monitoring of both motor and non-motor symptoms, enabling treatment adaptations aligned with individual disease progression. Furthermore, UHC-backed investment and dissemination of next-generation therapies—including gene therapy, targeted neuroprotective agents, and advanced neuromodulation—ensure equitable access beyond specialized centers (Ahmed et al., 2025; Hammad et al., 2025). By integrating such innovative therapies within UHC frameworks, the health system not only tackles PD's clinical challenges but also advances global health reform where sustainable financing and innovation converge to enhance long-term patient outcomes (Hammad et al., 2025).

16.9.4 Vision for a cure: realistic or futuristic?

The quest for a cure remains a central aspiration in PD research. Recent foundational advances in genetics, imaging, and cellular therapies lay essential groundwork for disease-modifying strategies. While transformative therapies may soon dramatically alter disease progression and quality of life, experts generally recognize that a definitive and universally effective cure is likely a long-term objective—contingent on deeper mechanistic understanding and persistent collaborative effort (Schweitzer et al., 2020; Takahashi, 2024). Implementing next-generation therapies in routine care will require not only continued scientific development but also robust, adaptive assessment of societal, ethical, and economic impacts (2023b). International partnerships and equitable access strategies are critical for ensuring these advances benefit diverse patient populations globally. Precision medicine, combinatorial approaches, and stakeholder-driven research will form the foundation of future progress.

16.10 Conclusion

Treatments for Parkinson's disease (PD) are undergoing significant change. New therapies are being created that aim to alter the illness, restore brain function, and enhance patient outcomes rather than merely treating its symptoms. Regenerative and restorative therapies, such as stem cell treatments, gene editing, and cutting-edge neuroengineering methods, can help combat the nerve damage caused by Parkinson's disease. Although there is enormous potential in these new developments, there are drawbacks as well, such as cost, availability, and complex regulations. Effective teamwork is essential, and the patient must come first in everything we do. To obtain the most out of new drugs, we also need to employ contemporary research, reliable clinical trial methods, and fair healthcare systems. To make these treatments accessible to as many people as possible, this entails resolving translation issues, ensuring that moral and legal requirements are fulfilled, and promoting international collaboration. Treatments for Parkinson's disease have the potential to significantly improve patient care and quality of life. However, we must address important policy, economic, and health issues early in the development process. Language barriers should be removed, new research areas should be explored, and the effects of these factors on the economy and society at large should be taken into account. To maximize the benefits of these innovative concepts for both patients and society, a comprehensive strategy is necessary. Investing in the collection of real-world data is also crucial because it can be used to develop flexible pricing and reimbursement plans that adapt to the needs of patients and the healthcare system. We can accelerate the development and application of these therapies by using tailored medicine, enhancing biomarker discoveries, and leveraging artificial intelligence. Millions of patients and their families around the world will have new hope if PD treatments shift from merely managing symptoms to significantly altering the course of the illness by emphasizing scalable, affordable solutions that promote global accessibility. This chapter makes it abundantly evident that to improve the future, we must continue to develop new concepts, collaborate, and invest in PD care. Innovative treatments for Parkinson's disease have enormous potential to improve patient care and enhance the quality of life. However, early in the development process, we must address the significant policy, economic, and health challenges that these innovations present. Overcoming translational barriers, embracing emerging research areas, and considering broader socioeconomic factors are critical. A comprehensive approach is necessary to fully leverage the benefits of these innovations for both patients and society. Additionally, investing in the generation of empirical evidence is essential, as this data will support flexible pricing and reimbursement strategies that can adapt to patient needs and the changing healthcare landscape.

AI disclosure

During the preparation of this work the author(s) used Grammarly in order to Grammar and spelling check/ language proficiency level. After using this tool/service, the author(s) reviewed and edited the content as needed and take(s) full responsibility for the content of the publication.

References

Ahmed, M. M., Okesanya, O. J., Olaleke, N. O., Adigun, O. A., Adebayo, U. O., Oso, T. A., Eshun, G., & Lucero-Prisno, D. E. (2025). Integrating digital health innovations to achieve universal health coverage: Promoting health outcomes and quality through global public health equity. *Healthcare (Switzerland), 13*(9). https://doi.org/10.3390/healthcare13091060

Ali, M. (2024). Neurodegenerative diseases: Insights into early diagnosis and therapeutic approaches. *Trends in Life Sciences and Biotechnology, 1*, 98–106.

Bankiewicz, K. (2024). Phase Ib trial of AB-1005 (AAV2-GDNF) in Parkinson's disease meets primary endpoint.

András, I. E., & Toborek, M. (2016). Extracellular vesicles of the blood-brain barrier. *Tissue Barriers, 4*(1), Article e1131804.

Barone, P. (2010). Neurotransmission in Parkinson's disease: Beyond dopamine. *European Journal of Neurology, 17*(3), 364–376. https://doi.org/10.1111/j.1468-1331.2009.02900.x

Bartus, R. T. (2022). Long-term effects of AAV2-neurturin gene therapy for parkinson's disease: A 5-year follow-up study. *Movement Disorders, 37*(3), 587–596.

Bogetofte, H., Alamyar, A., Blaabjerg, M., & Meyer, M. (2020). Levodopa therapy for parkinson's disease: History, current status and perspective. *CNS & Neurological Disorders-Drug Targets-CNS & Neurological Disorders), 19*(8), 572–583.

Brown, G., Hakun, J., Lewis, M. M., De Jesus, S., Du, G., Eslinger, P. J., … Huang, X. (2023). Frontostriatal and limbic contributions to cognitive decline in Parkinson's disease. *Journal of Neuroimaging, 33*(1), 121–133.

Chambers, B. E., Weaver, N. E., & Wingert, R. A. (2023). The "3Ds" of growing kidney organoids: advances in nephron development, disease modeling, and drug screening. *Cells, 12*(4), 549.

Chaudhuri, K. R., Healy, D. G., & Schapira, A. H. (2006). Non-motor symptoms of Parkinson's disease: Diagnosis and management. *The Lancet Neurology, 5*(3), 235–245.

Church, F. C. (2021). Treatment options for motor and non-motor symptoms of parkinson's disease. *Biomolecules, 11*(4), 612. https://doi.org/10.3390/biom11040612

Clarke, C. E. (2004). A "cure" for parkinson's disease: Can neuroprotection be proven with current trial designs? *Movement Disorders, 19*(5), 491–498. https://doi.org/10.1002/mds.20057

Cubo, E., & Delgado-López, P. D. (2022). Telemedicine in the management of parkinson's disease: Achievements, challenges, and future perspectives. *Brain Sciences, 12*(12), 1735. https://doi.org/10.3390/brainsci12121735

de la Fuente-Fernández, R., Schulzer, M., Mak, E., & Sossi, V. (2010). Trials of neuroprotective therapies for Parkinson's disease: Problems and limitations. *Parkinsonism & Related Disorders, 16*(6), 365–369. https://doi.org/10.1016/j.parkreldis.2010.04.008

Dehghani, S., et al. (2025). Exosome-based delivery systems for neurodegenerative disease therapy: Crossing the blood–brain barrier with precision. *Journal of Controlled Release, 375*, 210–225.

Dehghani, S., Ocakcı, O., Hatipoglu, P. T., Özalp, V. C., & Tevlek, A. (2025). Exosomes as biomarkers and therapeutic agents in neurodegenerative diseases: Current insights and future directions. *Molecular Neurobiology, 62*(7), 9190–9215. https://doi.org/10.1007/s12035-025-04825-5

Dorsey, E. R., Sherer, T., Okun, M. S., & Bloem, B. R. (2018). The emerging evidence of the Parkinson pandemic. *Journal of Parkinson's Disease, 8*(s1), S3–S8.

Dou, J., Wang, J., Gao, X., Wang, G., Bai, Y., Liang, Y., Yang, K., Yang, Y., & Zhang, L. (2025). Effectiveness of telemedicine interventions on motor and nonmotor outcomes in parkinson disease: Systematic review and network meta-analysis. *Journal of Medical Internet Research, 27*, Article e71169. https://doi.org/10.2196/71169

Du, T., Wang, L., Liu, W., Zhu, G., Chen, Y., & Zhang, J. (2021). Biomarkers and the role of α-Synuclein in Parkinson's disease. *Frontiers in Aging Neuroscience, 13*, 645996.

Esper, C. D., Valdovinos, B. Y., & Schneider, R. B. (2024). The importance of digital health literacy in an evolving Parkinson's Disease care System. *Journal of Parkinson's Disease, 14*(1), Article S181. https://doi.org/10.3233/JPD-230229

Filippi, M., Amato, M. P., Centonze, D., Gallo, P., Gasperini, C., Inglese, M., Patti, F., Pozzilli, C., Preziosa, P., & Trojano, M. (2022). Early use of high-efficacy disease-modifying therapies makes the difference in people with multiple sclerosis: An expert opinion. *Journal of Neurology, 269*(10), 5382–5394. https://doi.org/10.1007/s00415-022-11193-w

Foote, A., de Waal, E., Caiado, F., Samman, A., & Ukolov, A. (2025). A comprehensive review of deep brain stimulation for Parkinson's disease: The history, current state of the art and future possibilities. *Medicine in Novel Technology and Devices, 26*, Article 100362. https://doi.org/10.1016/j.medntd.2025.100362

Ghauri, M. S., & Ou, L. (2023). AAV engineering for improving tropism to the central nervous System. *Biology, 12*(2). https://doi.org/10.3390/biology12020186

Giannakis, A., Pechlivani, L., Sioka, C., Alexiou, G., Konitsiotis, S., & Kyritsis, A. P. (2025). Seed amplification assay for α-Synuclein: Diagnostic applications in synucleinopathies. *International Journal of Molecular Sciences, 26*(16), 7817.

Hammad, A. S., Khalifa, A. Y., ELKarim, G. G., Mataria, A., & Fouad, A. M. (2025). Effect of universal health insurance implementation on beneficiaries' evaluation of public health facilities in Egypt – a cross-sectional study. *International Journal for Equity in Health, 24*(1), 59. https://doi.org/10.1186/s12939-025-02402-9.

He, Q., et al. (2023). Engineered exosomes carrying CRISPR/Cas9 for α-synuclein gene editing ameliorate Parkinsonian pathology. *Advanced Science, 10*(12), Article 2300547.

He, S., Wang, Q., Chen, L., He, Y. J., Wang, X., & Qu, S. (2023). miR-100a-5p-enriched exosomes derived from mesenchymal stem cells enhance the anti-oxidant effect in a Parkinson's disease model via regulation of Nox4/ROS/Nrf2 signaling. *Journal of Translational Medicine, 21*(1). https://doi.org/10.1186/s12967-023-04638-x

Hoffman, S. L., Schmiedmayer, P., Gala, A. S., Wilkins, K. B., Parisi, L., Karjagi, S., Negi, A. S., Revlock, S., Coriz, C., Revlock, J., Ravi, V., & Bronte-Stewart, H. (2024). Comprehensive real time remote monitoring for Parkinson's disease using Quantitative DigitoGraphy. *Npj Parkinson's Disease, 10*(1). https://doi.org/10.1038/s41531-024-00751-w

Hsu, P. D. (2023). Delivery and safety considerations of CRISPR-based therapeutics in the central nervous system. *Nature Reviews Drug Discovery, 22*(11), 873–890.

Huang, G., Chen, X., & Liao, C. (2025). AI-Driven wearable bioelectronics in digital healthcare. *Biosensors, 15*(7), 410. https://doi.org/10.3390/bios15070410

Huh, Y., Kim, D. H., Choi, M., Park, J. H., Kwon, D. Y., Jung, J. H., Han, K., & Park, Y. G. (2019). Metoclopramide and levosulpiride use and subsequent levodopa prescription in the korean elderly: The prescribing cascade. *Journal of Clinical Medicine, 8*(9). https://doi.org/10.3390/jcm8091496

Jayaram, P., Danilkowicz, R. M., & Yuan, X. (2025). Ethical and regulatory considerations related to regenerative medicine. *HSS Journal*. https://doi.org/10.1177/15563316251361511

Jerry, M., Arcona, S., McMorrow, D., Schwartz, H., Princic, N., & Sasane, R. (2023). Work loss and direct and indirect costs associated with parkinson's disease. *ClinicoEconomics and Outcomes Research, 15*, 309–319. https://doi.org/10.2147/ceor.s398509

Jin, X. (2023). Correction of LRRK2-G2019S mutation by CRISPR/Cas9 rescues mitochondrial function in Parkinson's disease patient-derived neurons. *Stem Cell Reports, 18*(4), 765–779.

Kaplitt, M. G., Feigin, A., & Tang, C. (2022). Safety and tolerability of AAV2-GAD gene therapy in Parkinson's disease. *Lancet Neurology, 20*(X), xxx.

Kim, S. H. (2024). Expanding CRISPR precision: Base and prime editing applications in neurodegenerative disorders. *Trends in Biotechnology, 42*(3), 345–359.

López-Tobón, A. (2023). Bioengineered scaffolds for stem cell-based repair in neurodegenerative disorders. *Nature Biomedical Engineering, 7*(1), 48–60.

Kluge, A., & Iranzo, A. (2024). Biofluid detection of pathological α-synuclein in the prodromal phase of synucleinopathies. *Journal of Parkinson's Disease, 14*(S2), S323–S331.

Kniazev, R. (2025). Immunotherapy in early Parkinson's disease: A biomarker-driven trial framework for secondary prevention. *Cureus, 17*(11).

Koerts, J., König, M., Tucha, L., & Tucha, O. (2016). Working capacity of patients with Parkinson's disease–A systematic review. *Parkinsonism & Related Disorders, 27*, 9–24. https://pubmed.ncbi.nlm.nih.gov/27029582/.

Lang, A. E. (2010). Clinical trials of disease-modifying therapies for neurodegenerative diseases: the challenges and the future. *Nature Medicine, 16*(11), 1223–1226.

Lang, A. E., & Obeso, J. A. (2004). Challenges in Parkinson's disease: Restoration of the nigrostriatal dopamine system is not enough. *The Lancet Neurology, 3*(5), 309–316. https://doi.org/10.1016/S1474-4422(04)00740-9

Lang, A. E., Siderowf, A. D., Macklin, E. A., Poewe, W., Brooks, D. J., Fernandez, H. H., … Dam, T. (2022). Trial of cinpanemab in early Parkinson's disease. *New England Journal of Medicine, 387*(5), 408–420.

LeWitt, P. A. (2023). AAV2-hAADC gene therapy for advanced Parkinson's disease: Phase 1b trial results. *Lancet Neurology, 22*(1), 23–34.

Little, S. (2022). Adaptive deep brain stimulation in Parkinson's disease: Progress and challenges. *Nature Reviews Neurology, 18*(4), 239–252.

Lucchetta, R. C., Leonart, L. P., Gonçalves, M. V. M., Becker, J., Pontarolo, R., Fernandez-Llimós, F., & Wiens, A. (2020). Reliability in long-term clinical studies of disease-modifying therapies for relapsing-remitting multiple sclerosis: A systematic review. *PLoS ONE, 15*(6), Article e0231722. https://doi.org/10.1371/journal.pone.0231722.

Marciano, L., Vocaj, E., Bekalu, M. A., Tona, A. La, Rocchi, G., & Viswanath, K. (2023). The use of Mobile assessments for monitoring mental health in youth: Umbrella review. *Journal of Medical Internet Research, 25* (1), Article e45540. https://doi.org/10.2196/45540

Marino, M., Callaerts, P., Holt, M. (2022). Optimized AAV systems for the treatment of CNS-related diseases.

Meng, Y. (2024). Focused ultrasound-mediated blood-brain barrier disruption for targeted delivery of regenerative therapeutics in Parkinson's disease. *Nature Communications, 15*(1), 1250.

Menozzi, E., Schapira, A. H. V., Blandini, F., & Avenali, M. (2023). Who is at risk of parkinson disease? Refining the preclinical phase of GBA1 and LRRK2 variant carriers: A clinical, biochemical, and imaging approach. *Current Neurology and Neuroscience Reports, 23*(4), 121–130. https://doi.org/10.1007/s11910-023-01259-1

Negash, Y. T., & Hanum, F. (2025). An analytical framework for improving healthcare data management and organizational performance. *Healthcare Analytics, 8*, Article 100415. https://doi.org/10.1016/j.health.2025.100415

Nguyen, H. D. (2025). Elucidate biomarkers and the molecular pathways associated with genetic variants that contribute to the etiology of Parkinson's disease. *Acta Neurologica Belgica, 125*(6), 1621–1641.

Pagano, G., Taylor, K. I., Anzures Cabrera, J., Simuni, T., Marek, K., Postuma, R. B., … Prasinezumab Study Group. (2024). Prasinezumab slows motor progression in rapidly progressing early-stage Parkinson's disease. *Nature Medicine, 30*(4), 1096–1103.

Peterson, K., & Haggerty, K. (2022). Regulatory challenges in translational neuroregenerative therapies: Bridging innovation and oversight. *Journal of Neuroethics, 16*(2), 111–123.

Qansuwa, E. M., Atalah, H. N., Abdelkader, M. S., Russell, A. E., Dakhlallah, D., & Brown, C. M. (2024). *The contribution of the gut-brain-microbiota axis to brain health throughout the lifespan Handbook of Neurodegenerative Disorders* (pp. 17–41). Egypt: Springer Nature. https://doi.org/10.1007/978-981-99-7557-0_2

Qansuwa, E. M., Atalah, H. N., & Salama, M. M. (2025). Rehabilitation, neuroplasticity, and machine learning: Approaching artificial intelligence for equitable health systems. *Neuroscience, 587*, 38–46. https://doi.org/10.1016/j.neuroscience.2025.09.050

Qian, X. (2023). Modeling Parkinson's disease with patient-derived iPSCs: Toward personalized medicine. *Cell Stem Cell, 30*(5), 721–738.

Qian, L. (2024). Targeted correction of SNCA duplication using CRISPR prime editing restores dopaminergic homeostasis in Parkinson's models. *Molecular Therapy – Nucleic Acids, 38*, 1–14.

Rana, A. Q., Ahmed, U. S., Chaudry, Z. M., & Vasan, S. (2015). Parkinson's disease: A review of non-motor symptoms. *Expert Review of Neurotherapeutics, 15*(5), 549–562. https://doi.org/10.1586/14737175.2015.1038244

Ravina, B., Eidelberg, D., Ahlskog, J. E., Albin, R. L., Brooks, D. J., Carbon, M., Dhawan, V., Feigin, A., Fahn, S., Guttman, M., Gwinn-Hardy, K., McFarland, H., Innis, R., Katz, R. G., Kieburtz, K., Kish, S. J., Lange, N., Langston, J. W., Marek, K., … Holloway, R. (2005). The role of radiotracer imaging in Parkinson disease. *Neurology, 64*(2), 208–215. https://doi.org/10.1212/01.WNL.0000149403.14458.7F

Roche. (2025). *Roche advances novel investigational anti-alpha-synuclein antibody to Phase III for early-stage Parkinson disease*. PharmaExec. https://www.pharmexec.com/view/roche-advances-novel-investigational-anti-alpha-synuclein-antibody-phase-iii-early-stage-parkinsons-disease.

Rothenbücher, T., et al. (2023). Biodegradable hydrogel microspheres for local delivery of neurotrophic factors in Parkinson's disease. *Advanced Healthcare Materials, 12*(2), Article 2201302.

Słyk, Ż., Stachowiak, N., & Małecki, M. (2024). Recombinant adeno-associated virus vectors for gene therapy of the central nervous System: Delivery routes and clinical aspects. *Biomedicines, 12*(7), 1523. https://doi.org/10.3390/biomedicines12071523

Sagoo, G. S., Robinson, T., Coughlan, D., Meader, N., Rice, S., & Vale, L. (2023). Evaluating high-cost technologies–no need to throw the baby out with the bathwater. *Expert Review of Pharmacoeconomics & Outcomes Research, 23*(10), 1177–1183. https://doi.org/10.1080/14737167.2023.2263647

Salat, D., Noyce, A. J., Schrag, A., & Tolosa, E. (2016). Challenges of modifying disease progression in prediagnostic Parkinson's disease. *The Lancet Neurology, 15*(6), 637–648.

Schweitzer, J. S., Song, B., Herrington, T. M., Park, T. Y., Lee, N., Ko, S., Jeon, J., Cha, Y., Kim, K., Li, Q., Henchcliffe, C., Kaplitt, M., Neff, C., Rapalino, O., Seo, H., Lee, I. H., Kim, J., Kim, T., Petsko, G. A., … Kim, K. S. (2020). Personalized iPSC-derived dopamine progenitor cells for Parkinson's disease. *New England Journal of Medicine, 382*(20), 1926–1932. https://doi.org/10.1056/NEJMoa1915872

Shokrpour, S., MoghadamFarid, A. M., Bazzaz Abkenar, S., Haghi Kashani, M., Akbari, M., & Sarvizadeh, M. (2025). Machine learning for Parkinson's disease: A comprehensive review of datasets, algorithms, and challenges. *Npj Parkinson's Disease, 11*(1). https://doi.org/10.1038/s41531-025-01025-9

Singh, R. (2024). Therapeutic exosomes delivering CRISPR/Cas9 ribonucleoproteins for α-synuclein silencing in Parkinson's disease. *Frontiers in Molecular Neuroscience, 17*, Article 1465289.

Skidmore, S., & Barker, R. A. (2023). Challenges in the clinical advancement of cell therapies for Parkinson's disease. *Nature Biomedical Engineering, 7*(4), 370–386. https://doi.org/10.1038/s41551-022-00987-y

Smits, L. M. (2023). Patient-derived midbrain organoids for modeling genetic Parkinson's disease. *Nature Neuroscience, 26*(4), 592–604.

Sprenger, F., & Poewe, W. (2013). Management of Motor and Non-Motor symptoms in parkinson's disease. *CNS Drugs, 27*(4), 259–272. https://doi.org/10.1007/s40263-013-0053-2

Stocchi, F., Bravi, D., Emmi, A., & Antonini, A. (2024). Parkinson disease therapy: Current strategies and future research priorities. *Nature Reviews Neurology, 20*(12), 695–707. https://doi.org/10.1038/s41582-024-01034-x

Takahashi, J. (2024). Clinical applications of iPSC-derived dopaminergic progenitors for Parkinson's disease. *Nature Reviews Neurology, 20*(2), 76–88.

Tanaka, M. (2025). Parkinson's disease: Bridging gaps, building biomarkers, and reimagining clinical translation. *Cells, 14*(15), 1161.

Thanvi, B. R., & Lo, T. C. N. (2004). Long term motor complications of levodopa: Clinical features, mechanisms, and management strategies. *Postgraduate Medical Journal, 80*(946), 452–458. https://doi.org/10.1136/pgmj.2003.013912

Titova, N., & Chaudhuri, K. R. (2017). Personalized medicine in Parkinson's disease: Time to be precise. *Federation Movement Disorders, 32*(8), 1147–1154. https://doi.org/10.1002/mds.27027

Twala, B. (2025). AI-driven precision diagnosis and treatment in Parkinson's disease: A comprehensive review and experimental analysis. *Frontiers in Aging Neuroscience, 17*. https://doi.org/10.3389/fnagi.2025.1638340

Vallabh, S. M., Zou, D., Pitstick, R., O'Moore, J., Peters, J., Silvius, D., & Cabin, D. E. (2023). Therapeutic trial of anle138b in mouse models of genetic prion disease. *Journal of Virology, 97*(2), Article e01672-22.

Wang, Y., 2024. Optimization strategies for self-complementary AAV and promoter design in neuroscience gene therapy.

Wang, S., Zhu, G., Shi, L., Zhang, C., Wu, B., Yang, A., Meng, F., Jiang, Y., & Zhang, J. (2023). Closed-Loop Adaptive deep Brain stimulation in Parkinson's Disease: Procedures to achieve it and future perspectives. *Journal of Parkinson's Disease, 13*(4), 453–471. https://doi.org/10.3233/jpd-225053

Williams, N. R., & Okun, M. S. (2013). Deep brain stimulation (DBS) at the interface of neurology and psychiatry. *Journal of Clinical Investigation, 123*(11), 4546–4556. https://doi.org/10.1172/JCI68341

Wirdefeldt, K., Adami, H. O., Cole, P., Trichopoulos, D., & Mandel, J. (2011). Epidemiology and etiology of Parkinson's disease: A review of the evidence. *European Journal of Epidemiology, 26*(Suppl 1), 1.

Xie, Y. X., Lv, W. Q., Chen, Y. K., Hong, S., Yao, X. P., Chen, W. J., & Zhao, M. (2022). Advances in gene therapy for neurogenetic diseases: a brief review. *Journal of Molecular Medicine, 100*(3), 385–394.

Yang, W., Hamilton, J. D., Kopil, C., Beck, J. C., Bandyopadhyay, D., Altar, C. A., & Marras, C. (2020). Current and projected future economic burden of Parkinson's disease in the U.S. *npj Parkinson's Disease, 6*(1), 15.

Yang, W., Hamilton, J. L., Kopil, C., Beck, J. C., Tanner, C. M., Albin, R. L., Dorsey, E. R., Dahodwala, N., Cintina, I., Hogan, P., & Thompson, T. (2020a). Current and projected future economic burden of Parkinson's disease in the U.S. *npj Parkinson's Disease, 6*(1), 15. https://doi.org/10.1038/s41531-020-0117-1

Youssef, S. H., Atalah, H. N., Badawy, M. T., El-Fawal, H. N., & Salama, M. M. (2024). *Three neurodegenerative diseases: A single hope Handbook of Neurodegenerative Disorders* (pp. 43–66). Egypt: Springer Nature. https://doi.org/10.1007/978-981-99-7557-0_3

Yu, H. J., Thijssen, E., van Brummelen, E., van Der Plas, J. L., Radanovic, I., Moerland, M., … Dodart, J. C. (2022). A randomized first-in-human study with UB-312, a UBITh® α-synuclein peptide vaccine. *Movement Disorders, 37*(7), 1416–1424.

Zaman, M. S., Ghahari, S., & McColl, M. A. (2021). Barriers to accessing healthcare services for people with Parkinson's disease: A scoping review. *Journal of Parkinson's Disease, 11*(4), 1537–1553.

Zhang, L., et al. (2024a). Combinatorial AAV vector co-expressing GBA1 and GDNF for synergistic neuroprotection in Parkinsonian models. *[Journal name]* (Volume)(Issue).

Zhang, L., et al. (2024b). CRISPR/Cas9-mediated genome editing strategies for familial Parkinson's disease mutations. *Progress in Neurobiology, 236*, Article 102426.

Zhang, Y. (2024c). CRISPR-based gene therapy targeting LRRK2 in Parkinson's disease models. *Science Translational Medicine, 16*(730), eabc1234.

Zhao, Y., et al. (2023). Mesenchymal stem cell-derived exosomes enriched with miR-133b promote dopaminergic neuron survival in Parkinson's models. *Brain Research, 1817*, Article 148687.

Zurynski, Y., Herkes-Deane, J., Holt, J., McPherson, E., Lamprell, G., Dammery, G., Meulenbroeks, I., Halim, N., & Braithwaite, J. (2022). How can the healthcare system deliver sustainable performance? A scoping review. *BMJ Open, 12*(5), Article e059207. https://doi.org/10.1136/bmjopen-2021-059207

Index

'*Note:* Page numbers followed by "f" indicate figures and "t" indicate tables.'

E

Q

R

S

9780443277023